Cardiology
<u>1991</u>

Cardiology
1991

WILLIAM C. ROBERTS, MD, Editor

Chief, Pathology Branch
National Heart, Lung, and Blood Institute
National Institutes of Health, Bethesda, Maryland, and
Clinical Professor of Pathology and Medicine (Cardiology)
Georgetown University, Washington, D.C., and
Editor-in-Chief, The American Journal of Cardiology

JAMES T. WILLERSON, MD

Randall Professor of Medicine and Chairman
Department of Internal Medicine
University of Texas Medical School at Houston
And
Director of Cardiology Research
At The Texas Heart Institute, Houston, Texas

DEAN T. MASON, MD

Physician-in-Chief, Western Heart Institute
Chairman, Department of
Cardiovascular Medicine
St. Mary's Hospital and Medical Center
San Francisco, California
Editor-in-Chief, American Heart Journal

CHARLES E. RACKLEY, MD

Professor of Medicine
Division of Cardiology
Department of Medicine
Georgetown University Medical Center
Washington, D.C.

THOMAS P. GRAHAM, JR, MD

Professor of Pediatrics
Chief, Division of Pediatrics
Department of Pediatrics
Vanderbilt University
Nashville, Tennessee

Butterworth–Heinemann
Boston   London   Oxford   Singapore   Sydney   Toronto   Wellington

Recognizing the importance of preserving what has been written, it is the policy of Butterworth–Heinemann to have the books it publishes printed on acid-free paper, and we exert our best efforts to that end.

LC 84-644030

ISBN 0-7506-9082-8

ISSN 0275-0066

Butterworth–Heinemann
80 Montvale Avenue
Stoneham, MA 02180

10 9 8 7 6 5 4 3 2 1

Printed in the United States of America

Contents

7. Myocardial Heart Disease   350

Preface

Cardiology 1991 is the eleventh book to be published in this series. It contains summaries of 804 articles, all published in 1990. A total of 26 medical journals (Table I) were examined and at least 1 and usually many articles were summarized from each journal. The number of articles summarized by each of the 5 authors is summarized in Table II. All of Rackley's submissions were from *Circulation;* Mason's from *The American Heart Journal;* and Willerson's from *The Journal of American College of Cardiology.* The contributions of Graham and Roberts were from a variety of medical journals. The summaries from each contributor were submitted to me, organized into the various sections in each of the 10 chapters, and each summary was copyedited by me.

A book of this type is made possible because of unselfish contributions from several individuals, none of whom is rewarded by authorship. I am

TABLE I. *Journals containing articles summarized in* Cardiology 1991.

1. American Heart Journal
2. American Journal of Cardiology
3. American Journal of Hypertension
4. American Journal of Medicine
5. Annals of Internal Medicine
6. Annals of Thoracic Surgery
7. Archives of Internal Medicine
8. Archives of Pathology and Laboratory Medicine
9. Arteriosclerosis
10. British Heart Journal
11. British Medical Journal
12. Chest
13. Circulation
14. Cleveland Clinic Journal of Medicine
15. Clinical Cardiology
16. Current Problems in Cardiology
17. European Heart Journal
18. Human Pathology
19. Journal of American College of Cardiology
20. Journal of the American Medical Association
21. Journal of Thoracic and Cardiovascular Surgery
22. Lancet
23. Medicine
24. Morbidity and Mortality Weekly Report
25. Mayo Clinic Proceedings
26. New England Journal of Medicine

TABLE II. *Contributions of the 5 authors to* CARDIOLOGY 1991.

Author					CHAPTERS						Totals
	1	2	3	4	5	6	7	8	9	10	
1) WCR	88	82	93	47	46	28	12	4	23	26	449 (55.85%)
2) JTW	1	29	23	12	0	9	12	0	2	10	98 (12.19%)
3) DTM	4	20	17	10	6	12	4	7	5	11	96 (11.94%)
4) CER	6	32	15	8	5	4	7	0	8	8	93 (11.57%)
5) TPG, Jr	0	0	0	3	0	0	3	59	0	3	68 (8.46%)
TOTALS	99	163	148	80	57	53	38	70	38	58	804 (100%)
Figures	19	29	22	5	4	5	5	9	3	19	120 ⎫
Tables	28	5	6	4	5	5	3	0	1	4	61 ⎬ 181 ⎭

enormously grateful to Marjorie Hadsell for typing perfectly the 449 summaries contributed by me; to Angie Ruiz, Leslie Silvernail-Flatt, Azora L. Irby, and Joy Phillips also for typing many summaries; to Coleen Traynor for all her work obtaining permissions and to Barbara Murphy for efficiently coordinating the publishing of the book in Boston.

William C. Roberts, M.D.
Editor

Conversion of Units

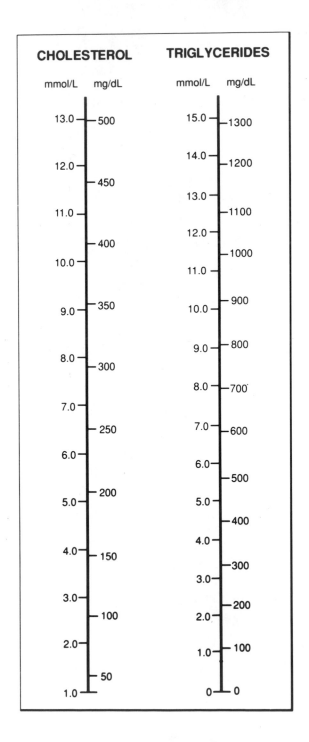

Cholesterol mg/dL = mmol/L x 38.6
Triglyceride mg/dL = mmol/L x 88.5

1

Factors Causing, Accelerating, or Preventing Coronary Arterial Atherosclerosis

Blood pressure and fatness in 5- and 6-year-olds

Gutin and associates[1] from New York, New York, studied cross-sectional relations among BP, aerobic fitness, body fatness, and fat patterning in 216 primarily Hispanic inner-city 5- and 6-year-olds. Fitness was measured with a submaximal treadmill test, and fatness was measured with 5 skin folds. Diastolic BP was inversely related to fitness in the boys and girls, and positively related to fatness for the boys. Systolic BP was positively related to fatness for the boys and girls. Using multiple regression and including parental BPs, fatness explained significant proportions of the variance in systolic BP for both the boys and girls and in diastolic BP for the boys. There were tendencies for central skin folds to explain more of the variation in BP than peripheral skin folds only for the boys. Fitness and fatness were inversely related for the boys and girls. Thus, at 5 and 6 years of age children have some of the same risk factors for cardiovascular disease seen in adults.

Among Chinese Americans ≥60 years of age

Choi and associates[2] from Boston, Massachusetts, surveyed in 1981 to 1983 the nutrition and health status of 346 Chinese immigrants to Boston, Massachusetts, aged 60 to 96 years. These Chinese were physically active and seldom obese and consumed a high-carbohydrate (57% of total energy intake), low-fat (24% of total energy intake), low-ascorbic acid (0.62 mmol/d) diet. Current cigarette smoking was common (39%) only in men, while alcoholism was rare in both sexes. Compared with similarly aged whites, they had lower mean BP and blood levels of total LDL and HDL cholesterol, apolipoproteins A-1 and B, and ascorbic acid (Table 1-1). These characteristics resemble those of the urban population in mainland China, where hemorrhagic stroke is the major cause of cardiovascular mortality.

Multiple risk factor intervention trial

The Multiple Risk Factor Intervention Trial was a primary prevention trial to test the effect of multifactor intervention on CAD mortality in high-risk men who were randomly assigned to special intervention (n = 6428) or to their usual sources of health care (n = 6438). As previously reported, after 6 to 8 years of intervention, mortality from CAD and from all causes did not differ significantly between men assigned to special intervention and men assigned to their usual sources of health care. The Multiple Risk Factor Intervention Trial Research Group now described a mortality finding after 10.5 years (an average of 3.8 years after the end of intervention).[3] Mortality rates were lower for men who received special intervention than for men who received their usual care by 10.6% for CAD and by 7.7% for all causes (Table 1-2). Differences in mortality rates were

TABLE 1-1. *Plasma lipid, lipoprotein, and apolipoprotein levels of elderly (aged ≥60 y) Chinese and white Americans.* Reproduced with permission from Choi, et al.[2]*

		Men		Women	
	Group	N	Mean ± 1 SD	N	Mean ± 1 SD
TC, mmol/L	Chinese	112	5.51 ± 1.32	175	5.64 ± 1.24
	White	355	5.59 ± 0.98	339	6.03 ± 1.11
LDL-C, mmol/L	Chinese	110	3.70 ± 1.27	175	3.59 ± 1.19
	White	355	3.78 ± 0.88	339	4.01 ± 1.09
HDL-C, mmol/L	Chinese	112	1.25 ± 0.37	175	1.42 ± 0.42
	White	355	1.32 ± 0.42	339	1.57 ± 0.45
TG, mmol/L	Chinese	113	1.25 ± 0.90	175	1.38 ± 0.89
	White	355	1.51 ± 1.11	339	1.51 ± 1.07
Apo A-I, μmol/L	Chinese	53	41.3 ± 11.0	88	49.1 ± 10.6
	White	60	48.0 ± 12.4	34	57.5 ± 13.1
Apo B, μmol/L	Chinese	53	1.40 ± 0.51	88	1.42 ± 0.47
	White	78	2.02 ± 0.60	88	1.93 ± 0.56

*Data on lipid and lipoprotein levels in white Americans were derived from the Lipid Research Prevalence Study Population in the United States and Canada. Apolipoprotein assays of both Chinese and white subjects were performed at the Lipid Metabolism Laboratory of the US Department of Agriculture Human Nutrition Research Center, Boston, Mass; the white Americans were part of the Framingham Cohort Study.

TABLE 1-2. *Cause of death for MRFIT SI and UC men through December 31, 1985.* Reproduced with permission from Mult. Risk Factor Intervention Trial Research Group.*[3]

Cause of Death	ICD-9 Code†	No. (%) of Deaths SI (n = 6428)	No. (%) of Deaths UC (n = 6438)	Relative Difference, %‡
All cardiovascular	390-459	266 (4.14)	290 (4.50)	−7.9
Acute myocardial infarction	410	106 (1.65)	140 (2.17)	−24.3§
Other ischemic heart disease	411-414, 429.2‖	96 (1.49)	86 (1.34)	+11.7
Cardiac dysrhythmias	427	10 (0.16)	10 (0.16)	−1.0
Hypertensive heart disease	402	5 (0.08)	5 (0.08)	...
Other hypertensive	401, 403-405	2 (0.03)	0 (0.0)	...
Cerebrovascular	430-438	20 (0.31)	23 (0.36)	−13.0
Other cardiovascular disease	...	27 (0.42)	26 (0.40)	+4.0
All noncardiovascular		229 (3.56)	245 (3.82)	−7.1
Neoplastic	140-239	140 (2.2)	149 (2.3)	−6.2
Lip, oral cavity, and pharynx	140-149	4 (0.06)	6 (0.09)	...
Digestive organs and peritoneum	150-159	34 (0.53)	42 (0.65)	−19.3
Colorectal	153-154	10 (0.16)	13 (0.20)	−22.8
Other gastrointestinal	150-152, 155-159	24 (0.37)	29 (0.45)	−17.7
Respiratory and intrathoracic organs	160-165	66 (1.03)	55 (0.85)	+20.1
Lung	162	65 (1.01)	54 (0.84)	+20.5
Other neoplasms	...	36 (0.56)	46 (0.71)	−22.0
Respiratory	460-519	13 (0.20)	16 (0.25)	−19.0
Digestive system	520-579	22 (0.34)	16 (0.25)	+36.8
Accidents, suicides, and homicides	800-999	38 (0.59)	43 (0.67)	−11.7
Other noncardiovascular disease	...	16 (0.25)	22 (0.34)	−26.2
Cause unknown (death certificate not found)	...	1 (0.02)	1 (0.02)	...
Total	...	**496 (7.72)**	**537 (8.34)**	**−7.7**

*MRFIT indicates Multiple Risk Factor Intervention Trial; SI, special intervention; and UC, usual care.
†ICD-9 indicates *International Classification of Diseases, Ninth Revision, Clinical Modification.*
‡(1 − RR) × 100%, where the RR (relative risk) is estimated from the proportional hazards regression model. The relative difference is not given if there were fewer than 10 deaths in either the SI or UC group.
§$P = .02; P > .05$ for all the other relative differences.
‖In *ICD-9*, 429.2 is cardiovascular disease, unspecified; in *ICD-8* this is coded as 412.4.

substantially larger after the end of intervention than observed to that point. Differences in mortality rates after 10.5 years were primarily due to a 24% reduction in the death rate from AMI in men receiving special intervention compared with men receiving their usual care. As before, mortality differences between special intervention and usual care varied according to the presence of resting electrocardiographic abnormalities. These data suggest that multiple risk factor intervention confers a mortality benefit in middle-aged men over a period of about 10 years.

Changes with education and effect on mortality

A decline in mortality from cardiovascular disease over the past 30 years has been well documented, but the reasons for the decline have remained unclear. Stykowski and associates[4] from Watertown and Boston, Massachusetts, analyzed the 10-year incidence of cardiovascular disease and death from cardiovascular disease in 3 groups of men aged 50 to 59 years at baseline in 1950, 1960, and 1970 (the 1950, 1960, and 1970 cohorts) to determine the contribution of secular trends in the incidence of cardiovascular disease, risk factors, and medical care to the decline in mortality (Figure 1-1). The 10-year cumulative mortality from cardiovascular disease in the 1970 cohort was 43% less than that in the 1950 cohort and 37% less than that in the 1960 cohort. Among the men who were free

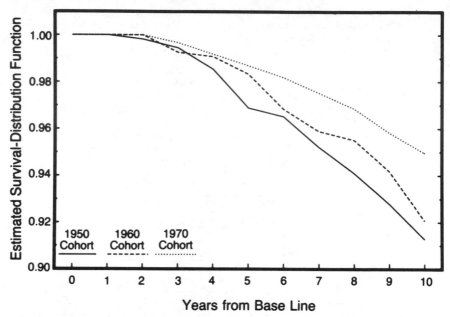

Fig. 1-1. Ten-year cardiovascular disease survival-distribution functions for men who were 50–59 years old at base line. Reproduced with permission from Sytkowski, et al.[4]

of cardiovascular disease at base line, the 10-year cumulative incidence of cardiovascular disease declined approximately 19%, from 190 per 1000 in the 1950 cohort to 154 per 1000 in the 1970 cohort, whereas the 10-year rate of death from cardiovascular disease declined 60% (relative risk for the 1950 cohort as compared with the 1970 cohort, 2.53; 95% confidence interval, 1.22 to 5.97). Significant improvements were found in risk factors for cardiovascular disease among the men initially free of cardiovascular disease in the 1970 cohort as compared with those in the 1950 cohort, including a lower serum cholesterol level (mean ± SD, 5.72 ± 0.98 mmol/L [221 ± 38 mg per deciliter], as compared with 5.90 ± 1.03 mmol/L [228 ± 40 mg/dl]) and a lower systolic BP (mean ± SD, 135 ± 19 mm Hg, as compared with 139 ± 25 mm Hg), better management of hypertension (22% vs. 0% were receiving antihypertensive medication), and reduced cigarette smoking (34% vs. 56%) (Table 1-3). The authors propose that these improvements may have had more pronounced effects on mortality from cardiovascular disease than on the incidence of cardiovascular disease in this population. The data suggest that the improvement in cardiovascular risk factors in the 1970 cohort may have been an important contributor to the 60% decline in mortality in that group as compared with the 1950 cohort, although a decline in the incidence of cardiovascular disease and improved medical interventions may also have contributed to the decline in mortality.

To test whether communitywide health education can reduce stroke and CAD, Farquhar and associates[5] from Palo Alto, California, compared 2 treatment cities (n = 122,800) and 2 control cities (n = 197,500) for changes in knowledge of risk factors, BP, plasma cholesterol level, cigarette smoking rate, body weight, and resting heart rate. Treatment cities received a 5-year, low-cost, comprehensive program using social learning theory, a communication-behavior change model, community organization principles, and social marketing methods that resulted in about

TABLE 1-3. *Selected risk factors at base-line examinations of men who were 50 to 59 years old at base line.* Reproduced with permission from Sytkowski, et al.[4]*

Risk Factor	Free of CVD at Base Line			Incident CVD within 10 Years of Base Line		
	1950	1960	1970	1950	1960	1970
Serum cholesterol (mg/dl)†	228±40	243±37	221±38‡	239±44	246±35	227±40§
Smokers (%)	56	52	34¶	64	60	57
Definite hypertension (%)‖	21	23	15¶	36	41	20¶
Use of antihypertensive medication (%)**	0	11	22¶	0	11	15
Systolic blood pressure (mm Hg)	139±25	137±21	135±19††	152±30	148±22	140±19§
Diastolic blood pressure (mm Hg)	85±13	86±12	84±10‡	91±15	91±12	85±11§
Metropolitan relative weight (%)‡‡	120±15	120±15	123±17‡	121±17	123±15	121±18

*The data are from the Framingham Heart Study, 1950 through 1979. Plus–minus values are means ±SD. CVD denotes cardiovascular disease.

†To convert values for serum cholesterol to millimoles per liter, multiply by 0.02586.

‡P<0.001 for the comparison of the three cohorts, by the general-linear-models procedure.

§P<0.01 for the comparison of the three cohorts, by the general-linear-models procedure.

¶P<0.05 for the comparison of the three cohorts, by the Mantel–Haenszel test.

‖Defined as systolic blood pressure >160 mm Hg, diastolic blood pressure >95 mm Hg, or both. See Gordon and Shurtleff.

**Percentages refer to all subjects with hypertension (systolic blood pressure >140 mm Hg and diastolic blood pressure >90 mm Hg).

††P<0.05 for the comparison of the three cohorts, by the general-linear-models procedure.

‡‡The measured body weight divided by the average U.S. age-specific and sex-specific weight for height, based on data from the Metropolitan Life Insurance Company.

26 hours of exposure to multichannel and multifactor education. Risk factors were assessed in representative cohort and cross-sectional surveys at baseline and in 3 later surveys. After 30 to 64 months of education, significant net reductions in community averages favoring treatment occurred in plasma cholesterol level (2%), BP (4%), resting pulse rate (3%), and smoking rate (13%) of the cohort sample. These risk factor changes resulted in important decreases in composite total mortality risk scores (15%) and CAD risk scores (16%). Thus, such low-cost programs can have an impact on risk factors in broad population groups.

BLOOD LIPIDS

Accuracy of measurements

Kaufman and associates[6] from Boston and Framingham, Massachusetts, evaluated 5 compact chemistry analyzers for the measurement of lipids. Fresh plasma or serum specimens from a standardized research laboratory were assayed for total cholesterol on all five analyzers. Triglycerides and HDL cholesterol were assayed on the 3 analyzers that could measure both of these analytes. Study results were interpreted by assessing accuracy and precision and by defining the percentage of patient specimens classified in the same categories as the reference laboratory, according to National Cholesterol Education Program guidelines. Two analyzers met standards for accuracy of cholesterol measurement. Three analyzers met performance standards for precision of cholesterol measurement. Agreement with National Cholesterol Education Program classification of specimens compared with the reference laboratory for total cholesterol ranged from 73% to 96% and was less for indirect LDL cholesterol. The authors concluded that under controlled conditions, compact chemistry analyzers vary in the reliability of lipid determination and classification of patients.

To determine the accuracy of portable cholesterol analyzers in public settings, Naughton and associates[7] from Minneapolis, Minnesota, accompanied 4 screening organizations to cholesterol screenings where consenting participants completed the finger-stick procedure and provided a blood sample by venipuncture. The finger-stick values were compared later with the participants' blood cholesterol values obtained in a reference laboratory. The results indicated that only 1 of the organizations produced cholesterol measurements entirely within the acceptable range (± 14.2%), while the accuracy of the other 3 organizations ranged from 76% to 96%. Those finger-stick values that did not fall within the acceptable range tended to underestimate the laboratory cholesterol values. Additionally, classification of the persons screened based on the National Cholesterol Education Program risk categories indicated that the finger-stick values primarily tended to produce false-negative results. The variability of the results across organizations was caused partially by insufficient operator training. Inadequate quality-control procedures for field settings and dilution of capillary blood by tissue fluid also may have contributed to the inaccurate finger-stick results.

Screening program

Bradford and associates[8] for the Lipid Research Clinics Cholesterol Screening Study Group performed a multicenter study of blood cholesterol screening in several typical environments, such as community sites (such as shopping malls and a supermarket), health care sites, work sites, a blood bank, and a school. Cholesterol was measured with a portable, dry-chemistry analyzer using capillary blood obtained by finger-stick. Data are reported from a total of 13,824 participants, spanning the entire age spectrum. Overall, 25% of screened subjects had blood cholesterol levels above the age-specific cutpoints used in the current study. Although in the aggregate this screening experience very closely approximates the expected level of referrals, the proportion of referred screened subjects differed significantly among the 5 types of screening environments and by gender. Follow-up telephone interviews indicated that 53% of referrals had initiated a physician contact. More than 75% of those who had seen a physician reported that the diagnosis of hypercholesterolemia had been confirmed, and almost 72% had been prescribed a diet. A large proportion of referred screened subjects reported having modified their diet, particularly when recommended to do so by a physician. This study has yielded encouraging evidence that physicians gave referred screened subjects appropriate initial advice for managing hypercholesterolemia. The new technology for blood cholesterol measurement evaluated in the current study has proven to be a feasible and reliable means for measuring blood cholesterol in typical screening settings.

Health departments participating in the Behavioral Risk Factor Survey System (BRFSS) conduct monthly random-digit-dialed telephone surveys of persons ≥18 years of age using a standardized questionnaire. In 1987 and 1988, respondents were asked whether they ever had their cholesterol "checked" and, if so, how long had it been since their cholesterol level was last checked and whether they had been told their cholesterol level.[9] Persons who reported they had been told their cholesterol level were asked to state their level; those who reported a number from 100–450 mg/dl were considered to know their cholesterol level. Survey results were adjusted according to the age, sex, and race distribution of adults in each state. In 1988, the percentage of adults who reported ever having their cholesterol checked ranged from 40% in New Mexico to 50% in Maine (median = 50%). From 1987 to 1988, statistically significant increases in cholesterol screening occurred in 17 (52%) of 33 states (median difference = 4%). Of the remaining 16 (48%) states, 4 had negligible decreases, 1 had no change, and 11 had small increases in cholesterol screening. In 1988, the percentage of adults who reported ever being told their cholesterol level ranged from 18% in South Carolina, and Tennessee to 40% in Wisconsin (median = 28%). All states had increases in the percentage of adults who were ever told their cholesterol level; these increases were statistically significant for 32 (97%) states. In 1988, the percentage of adults who reported knowing their cholesterol level ranged from 6% in the District of Columbia to 21% in Maine, Washington, and Wisconsin (median = 13%). In all states, the percentage of adults who reported knowing their cholesterol level increased (median difference = 7%); for 32 (97%) states, this increase was statistically significant. When the data for all states were combined, 54% of persons surveyed in 1988 who reported having their cholesterol level checked during the previous year were told their cholesterol level; in contrast, 40% of those surveyed in 1987 had been told their cholesterol level during the previous year. Similarly, 54% of those surveyed in 1988 who were told their level reported knowing their level, compared with 36% of those surveyed in 1987. As a result, the proportion of persons who knew their cholesterol level among those who reported having their cholesterol checked during the previous year increased from 15% in 1987 to 29% in 1988. The proposed health objectives for the USA state that by the year 2000 at least 90% of persons aged ≥18 years should have had their cholesterol checked within the previous 5 years and at least 75% should be able to report their cholesterol level. These data from the BRFSS indicate that substantial progress was made in most states toward meeting these objectives from 1987 to 1988. National surveys conducted by the National Heart, Lung, and Blood Institute and the Food and Drug Administration have also demonstrated substantial increases in cholesterol screening and awareness. In these surveys, the proportion of persons who reported ever having their blood cholesterol checked rose from 35% in 1983 to 58% in 1988, and the proportion who reported knowing their cholesterol level rose from 3% in 1983 to 17% in 1988.

Since November 1985, when the National Cholesterol Education Program (NCEP) was initiated by the National Heart, Lung, and Blood Institute, cholesterol screening and awareness of cholesterol levels have increased substantially in the USA. Cholesterol screening and awareness patterns, however, vary by state. To assess whether these variations may be related to demographic differences between states, data from the Behavioral Risk Factor Surveillance System (BRFSS) for 1989 were analyzed.[10] Health departments in the 39 participating states and the District of Columbia use a standardized questionnaire when conducting monthly random-digit-dialed telephone surveys of persons ≥18 years of age. In 1989, respondents were asked whether they had ever had their cholesterol checked. If so, they were asked to provide the duration since their last test and whether they had been told their cholesterol level. Persons who reported being told their cholesterol level were asked to state their level: those who reported a number from 100 mg/dl–450 mg/dl were considered to know their cholesterol level. The overall percentage of adults who reported ever having had their cholesterol level checked ranged from 48% in Alabama and New Mexico to 64% in Connecticut, Florida, and Washington. The percentage of adults who reported knowing their cholesterol level ranged from 12% in the District of Columbia to 33% in Washington. Cholesterol screening and awareness were slightly higher among women than among men (Table 1-4). Younger persons (18–34 years of age), blacks, and persons with lower education attainment (≤ 12 years of education) were less likely to have had their cholesterol level checked and were less likely to report knowing their cholesterol level. Persons with diabetes mellitus, systemic hypertension, or obesity were more likely to have had their cholesterol level checked and were more likely to know their cholesterol level than were persons who did not report having these risk factors (Table 1-5). Cholesterol screening and awareness were lower among persons who reported having a sedentary lifestyle and among persons who reported smoking than among persons who did not report having these risk factors.

The National Cholesterol Education Program (NCEP) has endorsed physician case findings as the primary method to detect individuals with elevated serum or plasma cholesterol levels. Despite this recommendation, promotional and for-profit public screening programs have flourished. Fischer and associates[11] from Augusta, Georgia, surveyed participants of a mall-based cholesterol screening program 1 year after their screening. Sixty-four percent of those screened had not previously

TABLE 1-4. *Cholesterol screening and awareness of cholesterol levels, by demographic category—Behavioral Risk Factor Surveillance System (BRFSS), 1989.* Reproduced with permission from Massachusetts Medical Society, et al.[10]*

| Category | Sample size | Respondents having had their cholesterol level checked | | | | Respondents knowing their cholesterol level | | | |
| | | Overall | | Standardized[†] | | Overall | | Standardized[†] | |
		(%)	95% CI[§]	(%)	95% CI	(%)	95% CI	(%)	95% CI
Sex									
Male[¶]	26,519	(56)	±1	(52)	±1	(23)	±1	(19)	±1
Female	37,394	(59)**	±1	(55)**	±1	(24)	±1	(21)	±1
Age (yrs)									
18–34[¶]	22,091	(37)	±1	(33)	±1	(12)	±1	(9)	±1
35–49	17,736	(61)**	±1	(55)**	±1	(27)**	±1	(23)**	±1
50–64	11,519	(75)**	±1	(73)**	±1	(35)**	±1	(33)**	±1
⩾65	12,567	(77)**	±1	(78)**	±1	(31)**	±1	(31)**	±1
Race									
White[¶]	57,998	(58)	±1	(54)	±1	(25)	±1	(21)	±1
Black	5,915	(50)**	±2	(50)**	±2	(9)**	±1	(8)**	±1
Education (yrs)[††]									
<12	10,921	(53)**	±1	(44)**	±2	(14)**	±1	(12)**	±1
12	21,736	(53)**	±1	(53)**	±1	(21)**	±1	(21)**	±1
>12[¶]	31,099	(62)	±1	(64)	±1	(29)	±1	(29)	±1

*Based on data from 39 states and the District of Columbia.
[†]Standardized for other demographic variables using 1980 U.S. census data. For example, age is adjusted for sex, race, and educational attainment.
[§]Confidence interval.
[¶]Referent group.
**Differs significantly from the referent group (p<0.05, z-test).
[††]Level unknown for 157 BRFSS respondents.

TABLE 1-5. *Awareness of cholesterol levels in relation to other cardio-vascular disease risk factors—Behavioral Risk Factor Surveillance System (BRFSS), 1989.* Reproduced with permission from Massachusetts Medical Society, et al.*[10]

| Risk factor | Sample size[§] | Respondents having had their cholesterol level checked | | | | Respondents knowing their cholesterol level | | | |
| | | Overall | | Standardized[†] | | Overall | | Standardized[†] | |
		(%)	95% CI[¶]	(%)	95% CI	(%)	95% CI	(%)	95% CI
Diabetes	3,223	(77)**	±2	(64)**	±3	(28)**	±2	(22)	±2
No diabetes	58,960	(56)	±1	(53)	±1	(23)	±1	(20)	±1
Hypertension[††]	11,923	(78)**	±1	(66)**	±2	(33)**	±1	(27)**	±2
No hypertension	51,773	(53)	±1	(51)	±1	(21)	±1	(19)	±1
Overweight[§§]	13,471	(64)**	±1	(58)**	±1	(26)**	±1	(23)**	±1
Not overweight	47,637	(56)	±1	(53)	±1	(23)	±1	(20)	±1
Sedentary[¶¶]	37,832	(54)**	±1	(51)**	±1	(20)**	±1	(18)**	±1
Not sedentary	26,004	(62)	±1	(59)	±1	(28)	±1	(24)	±1
Smoking***	15,510	(49)**	±1	(49)**	±1	(16)**	±1	(16)**	±1
Not smoking	48,267	(60)	±1	(55)	±1	(26)	±1	(22)	±1

*Based on data from 39 states and the District of Columbia.
[†]Standardized for age, sex, race, and educational attainment using 1980 U.S. census data.
[§]Risk factor information unknown for some BRFSS respondents.
[¶]Confidence interval.
**Differs significantly from persons who did not report having the risk factor (p<0.05, z-test).
[††]Persons who reported one or more of the following: 1) being told they had hypertension on two or more occasions, 2) having an antihypertensive medication currently prescribed, or 3) having high blood pressure at the time of the survey.
[§§]Body mass index (weight [kg] ÷ height [m^2]) ⩾27.8 for men and ⩾27.3 for women.
[¶¶]Persons who reported leisure-time physical activity fewer than three times per week and/or <20 minutes per session.
***Current cigarette smoker.

known their cholesterol levels. Those who were newly screened were less likely to benefit from this testing than the general public, since they were older (mean age, 55 years), more likely to be female (67%), and nonsmokers (88%). Screenees had excellent recall of their cholesterol level (mean absolute reporting error, 0.24 mmol/l [9 mg/dl]) and a good understanding of cholesterol as a CAD risk. Those with elevated cholesterol levels reported high distress from screening but no reduction in overall psychosocial well-being and an actual decrease in absenteeism. Only 54% of all who were advised to seek follow-up because of an elevated screening value had done so within the year following the screening program. However, of those with values greater than 6.2 mmol/L (240 mg/dL), 68% had sought follow-up. Many of those who participate in public screening programs have been previously tested, fall into low-benefit groups, or fail to comply with recommended follow-up. The authors therefore concluded that cholesterol screening programs of the type now commonly offered are unlikely to contribute greatly to the national efforts to further reduce CAD.

Within-person fluctuations

The National Cholesterol Education Program has begun a National Campaign to screen millions of adult Americans for serum total cholesterol level. To determine whether such random samples represent an individual's true lipoprotein status, Mogadam and associates[12] from Washington, D.C., and Alexandria and Fairfax, Virginia, measured fasting total serum cholesterol and lipoproteins on a weekly basis for 4 weeks in 20 subjects aged 22–63 years. Duplicate samples were tested by 2 standardized laboratories, each on 5 consecutive days. Variations of more than ± 20% in the serum levels of total, LDL, and HDL cholesterol were seen in 75%, 95%, and 65% of the subjects, respectively (Table 1-6). On retesting, 40% of the subjects moved in or out of 1 "risk category"; and in 10%, 2 categories, from "desirable" to "high risk," or vice versa. These data demonstrate that random testing may fail to detect wide fluctuations in the levels of serum lipoproteins, and therefore result in erroneous risk assignment or therapeutic intervention.

To test the impact of biologic and analytical variability on the ability of a single lipid measurement to assess risk accuracy, Bookstein and associates[13] from Chicago, Illinois, measured lipids on 3 occasions in 51 volunteers. Notable day-to-day variability of total cholesterol (5%) (Figure 1-2), triglyceride (20%), HDL cholesterol (10%), and calculated LDL cholesterol (8%) levels (Figure 1-3) was found. Analytic variability contributed significantly to total variability of HDL cholesterol levels and calculated LDL cholesterol levels. Confidence intervals constructed around National Cholesterol Education Program cutoff points suggested that classification was reliable from a single measurement if total cholesterol value was below 4.78 (<185 mg/dl), between 5.56 and 5.81 (215 and 225 mg/dl), or above 6.59 mmol/l (>225 mg/dl). LDL cholesterol value classification from a single measurement was only accurate at below 3.00 (<116 mg/dl) or above 4.50 mmol/l (>174 mg/dl). This study documents significant day-to-day variability of serum lipids and suggests that patients near the National Cholesterol Education Program cutoff points may require repeated measurements to assign risk accurately.

The article by Mogadam and associates[12] and by Bookstein and associates[13] was accompanied by an editorial by Carlos A. Dujovne and William S. Harris[14] from Kansas City, Kansas. These authors simply emphasized that the fact that there is some uncertainty in these lipid determinations should not be an excuse for physician to fail to test and to diagnose and treat dyslipidemic patients.

Familial dyslipidemic syndromes

Williams and associates[15] from Salt Lake City, Utah, determined the frequency of familial dyslipidemia syndromes from blood tests in 33 objectively ascertained families with early CAD (≥2 siblings with CAD by

TABLE 1-6. *The magnitude of overall percentage differences in serum lipid levels (due to within-person, interlaboratory, and intralaboratory fluctuations). Reproduced with permission from Mogadam, et al.*[12]

Lipid	No. (%) of Subjects	% Difference
Total cholesterol	15 (75)	>20
	9 (45)	>25
Low-density lipoprotein cholesterol	19 (95)	>20
	9 (45)	>40
High-density lipoprotein cholesterol	13 (65)	>20
	3 (15)	>30
Very-low-density lipoprotein cholesterol	18 (90)	>30
	14 (70)	>50
Triglycerides	19 (95)	>30
	14 (70)	>50

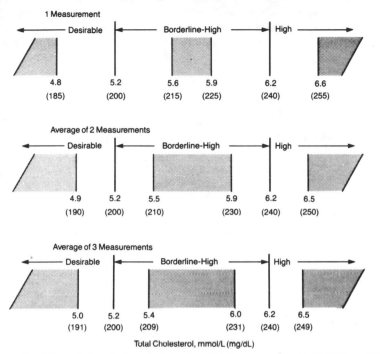

Fig. 1-2. Confidence intervals for accurate classification according to the National Cholesterol Education Program criteria for 1, 2 and 3 measurements are shown. Solid areas depict regions where the classification is reliable based on the number of measurements performed. In the unshaded areas, the classification could change if more measurements were obtained. Reproduced with permission from Bookstein, et al.[13]

the age of 55 years). Three-fourths of persons with early CAD in these families had 90th percentile lipid abnormalities (cholesterol level ≥90th percentile, triglyceride level ≥90th percentile, and/or HDL cholesterol level ≤10th percentile). The HDL cholesterol and triglyceride abnormalities were twice as common as LDL cholesterol abnormalities. The most common syndromes found were familial combined hyperlipidemia (36% to 48% of families with CHD), familial dyslipidemic systemic hypertension (21% to 54% of families with CHD), and isolated low levels of HDL cholesterol (15%), with overlapping familial dyslipidemic hypertension with familial combined hyperlipidemia and low-level HDL cholesterol. Well-defined monogenic syndromes were uncommon: familial hypercholesterolemia being 3% and familial type III hyperlipidemia, 3%. Another 15% of families with CHD had no lipid abnormalities at the 90th percentile. Physicians should learn to recognize and treat these common familial syndromes before the onset of CAD by evaluating family history and all 3 standard blood lipid determinations. Failure to recognize and treat them leaves affected family members at high risk of premature CAD.

In persons ≥65 years of age

Benfante and Reed[16] from Honolulu, Hawaii, evaluated reported findings of a diminished association between serum total cholesterol level and CAD in older persons. In the Honolulu (Hawaii) Heart Program, 1480 men aged ≥65 years and free of CAD were followed for an average of 12 years. Incidence rates of CAD increased progressively from the lowest to

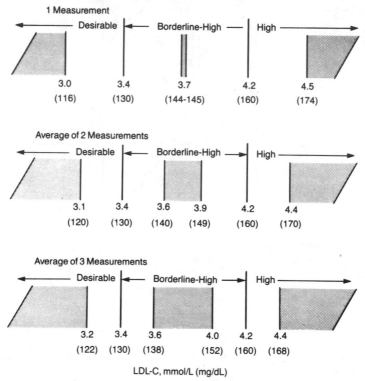

Fig. 1-3. As in Fig 1-2, solid areas show where low-density lipoprotein cholesterol (LDL-C) can be reliably classified according to National Cholesterol Education Program criteria for 1, 2 and 3 measurements. For the borderline-high group, multiple measurements are needed to ensure accurate classification. Reproduced with permission from Bookstein, et al.[13]

the highest quartile of serum cholesterol level. The independent role of serum cholesterol level as a predictor of CAD risk was evaluated with other major risk factors using a Cox multivariate regression model. The upper-lower quartile relative risk for serum cholesterol level was 1.64. The relative risk for middle-aged men was also 1.64. The results suggest that serum cholesterol level is an independent predictor of CAD, even among men older than 65 years. Thus, an elevated serum cholesterol level in older persons should be regarded, as in middle-aged men, to be an indicator for further evaluation of lipoprotein levels and possible intervention.

Various fats in diet

Trevisan and associates and a research group of the Italian National Research Council[17] analyzed the cross-sectional association between consumption of various fats (e.g., butter, olive oil, and vegetable oil) and the risk for CAD in a sample of 4,903 Italian men and women aged 20 to 59 years (Table 1-7). The intake of fats was ascertained by an interviewer-administered questionnaire. Increased consumption of butter was associated with significantly higher BP and serum cholesterol and glucose levels for men; in women only the association with glucose reached statistical significance. In both sexes consumption of olive oil and vegetable oil was inversely associated with serum cholesterol and glucose

TABLE 1-7. *Reported frequency of consumption of various fats in the Italian Nine Communities Study. Reproduced with permission from Trevisan, et al.*[17]

	In Cooking			Not In Cooking		
	6: Large Amount	3: Small Amount	0: No Use	2: Large Amount	1: Small Amount	0: No Use
Butter and margarine	11.4*	43.0	45.6	9.8	41.9	48.3
Olive oil	28.2	28.5	43.3	43.4	40.9	15.7
Peanut oil	6.5	16.2	77.3	2.0	5.1	92.9
Oils rich in polyunsaturated fat	22.5	39.3	38.2	12.2	19.8	68.0

*The percentage of subjects reporting that frequency category for each item; the percentage is calculated separately for use in cooking and not in cooking.

TABLE 1-8. *Typical fatty acid composition of the principal vegetable oils and animal fats.* Reproduced with permission from Bohigian, et al.*[18]

	% of Total Fatty Acids†		
Oil or Fat	Saturated	Monounsaturated	Polyunsaturated
Coconut oil	92	6	2
Palm kernel oil	82	15	2
Butterfat	63	31	3
Cocoa butter	61	34	3
Palm oil	50	40	10
Beef tallow	46	47	4
Lard	42	48	10
Cottonseed oil	26	20	55
Olive oil	17	72	11
Soybean oil	15	24	61
Peanut oil	14	50	32
Corn oil	13	28	59
Sunflower oil	12	19	69
Safflower oil	9	13	78
Low–erucic acid rapeseed oil (canola oil)	6	62	32

*Adapted from *Food Fats and Oils.*
†Component fatty acids may not add to 100% because of rounding.

levels and systolic BP. These findings were adjusted for confounding effects of other risk factors for cardiovascular disease. These cross-sectional findings from a large population sample suggest that consumption of butter may detrimentally affect coronary risk factors, while polyunsaturated and monounsaturated fats may be associated with a lower coronary risk profile.

The Council on Scientific Affairs of the American Medical Association[18] presented a Council report entitled, "Saturated Fatty Acids in Vegetable Oils." The Food and Drug Administration's proposed rule on food labeling requires that quantitative information be provided on both fatty acid and cholesterol content if either one is declared on the label. The American Medical Association is on record as supporting such an action and continues to support efforts to increase public awareness of the composition and nutritional values of foods. Tables 1-8, 1-9, and 1-10 show the percent of fatty acids in the various oils.

Oat bran

Studies in the past have shown that supplementation of the diet with oat bran may lower serum cholesterol levels. It has not been known,

TABLE 1-9. *Saturated fatty acid composition of some vegetable oils and animal fats.* Reproduced with permission from Bohigian, et al.[18]

Oil or Fat	% of Total Fatty Acids						
	Caproic (6)†	Caprylic (8)	Capric (10)	Lauric (12)	Myristic (14)	Palmitic (16)	Stearic (18)
Beef tallow	...	...	...	...	3	24	19
Coconut oil	1	8	6	47	18	9	3
Corn oil	...	...	...	...	...	11	2
Cottonseed oil	...	...	...	...	1	22	3
Lard	...	...	...	...	2	26	14
Palm oil	...	...	...	...	1	45	4
Palm kernel oil	...	3	4	48	16	8	3

*Adapted from Food Fats and Oils.
†Numbers in parentheses indicate the number of carbon atoms.

TABLE 1-10. *Fats and oils used in foods.* Reproduced with permission from Bohigian, et al.[18]

Source Oils	Fiscal Year Totals			
	1970/1971	1975/1976	1980/1981	1985/1986
Vegetable oils				
Soybean	5780	7431	8610	10004
Corn	403	520	624	837
Cottonseed	805	578	555	627
Palm	160	737	291	364
Coconut	220	506	338	333
Peanut	181	229	119	137
Sunflower	...	...	79	86
Meat fats				
Edible tallow	508	595	740	1021
Lard	1612	155	415	355

*Source: Economic Research Service of the US Department of Agriculture. Values are expressed as millions of pounds.

however, whether oat bran diets lower serum cholesterol levels by replacing fatty foods in the diet or by direct effect of the dietary fiber contained in the oat bran. To determine which is the case, Swain and associates[19] from Boston, Massachusetts, compared the effect of isocaloric supplements of high-fiber oat bran (87 g per day) and a low-fiber refined-wheat product on the serum lipoprotein cholesterol of 20 healthy subjects, 23 to 49 years old. After a 1-week base-line period during which they consumed their usual diets, the subjects were given each type of supplement for 6-week periods in a double-blind, crossover trial. Mean serum cholesterol levels (± SD) were not significantly different during the high-fiber and low-fiber periods: total cholesterol, 4.44 ± 0.73 and 4.46 ± 0.64 mmol/L (172 ± 28 and 172 ± 25 mg/dl); LDL, 2.69 ± 0.63 and 2.77 ± 0.59 mmol/L (104 ± 24 and 107 ± 23 mg/dl); and HDL 1.40 ± 0.39 and 1.32 ± 0.39 mmol/L (54 ± 15 and 51 ± 15 mg/dl), respectively. Both types of supplements lowered the mean base-line serum cholesterol level, 4.80 ± 0.80 mmol/L (186 ± 31 mg/dl), by 7 to 8%. The subjects ate less saturated fat and cholesterol and more polyunsaturated fat during both periods of supplementation than at base line. Those changes in dietary fats were sufficient to explain all of the reduction in serum cholesterol levels caused by the high-fiber and low-fiber diets. The average BP was 112/68 mm Hg at base line and did not change during either dietary period. The authors concluded that oat bran has little cholesterol-lowering effect and that high-fiber and low-fiber dietary grain supplements reduce serum cholesterol levels about equally, probably because they replace dietary fats.

This article was followed by an editorial entitled "Dietary Fiber—Nostrum or Critical Nutrient?" by William E. Connor[20] from Portland,

Oregon. Connor agreed with the aforementioned authors saying, "Its cholesterol lowering effect in normal people, however, is probably indirect, acting through replacement of dietary saturated fat and cholesterol."

Oral contraceptive agents

Oral contraceptives can induce changes in lipid and carbohydrate metabolism similar to those associated with an increased risk of CAD, including increased serum triglyceride, LDL cholesterol, and insulin levels and decreased HDL cholesterol levels. Godsland and associates[21] from London, UK, examined whether modification of the type or dose of progestin in oral-contraceptive preparation diminished these changes. The authors measured plasma lipoprotein levels and performed oral glucose-tolerance tests in a cross section of 1,060 women who took 1 of 9 types of oral contraceptives for at least 3 months and 418 women who took none. Seven of the contraceptive formulations contained various doses and types of progestin: levonorgestrel in low (150 µg), high (250 µg), and triphasic (50 to 125 µg) doses; norethindrone in low (500 µg), high (1000 µg), and triphasic (500 to 1000 µg) doses; and a new progestin, desogestrel, in 1 dose (150 µg). All 7 contained 30 to 40 µg of ethinyl estradiol. Two additional formulations contained progestin alone. As compared with controls, women taking combination drugs did not have increased serum total cholesterol levels but did have increases of 13 to 75% in fasting triglyceride levels. Levels of LDL cholesterol were reduced by 14% in women taking the combination containing desogestrel and by 12% in those taking low-dose norethindrone. Levels of HDL cholesterol were lowered by 5% and 16% by the combinations containing low-dose and high-dose levonorgestrel, respectively; these decreases were due to reductions of 29% and 43%, respectively, in the levels of HDL subclass 2. The combination pill containing high-dose norethindrone did not affect HDL cholesterol levels, whereas that containing low-dose norethindrone increased HDL cholesterol levels by 10%. The desogestrel combination increased HDL cholesterol levels by 12%. Levels of apolipoproteins A-1, A-II, and B were generally increased by combination drugs. Depending on the dose and type of progestin, combination drugs were associated with plasma glucose levels on the glucose-tolerance test that were 43 to 61% higher than in controls, insulin responses 12 to 40% higher, and C-peptide responses 18 to 45% higher. Progestin-only formulations had only minor metabolic effects. The appropriate dose and type of progestin may reduce the adverse effects of oral contraceptives on many metabolic markers of risk for CHF. Progestin-only formulations or combinations containing desogestrel or low-dose norethindrone were associated with the most favorable profiles.

In predicting future coronary death

Goldbourt and Yaari[22] from Tel Aviv and Tel-Hashamer, Israel, in a 23-year follow-up study of 10,059 40- to 60-year old participants in the Israeli Ischemic Heart Disease Study found that of 3,473 deaths (35%) in 1,098 (11%) CAD was the underlying cause. Total serum cholesterol was measured in 9,902 individuals. During the study, CAD mortality was elevated primarily in individuals in quintiles 4 and 5 (total cholesterol levels ≥217 mg/dl) (Table 1-11, Figure 1-4). Although CAD mortality increased marginally with increasing total cholesterol at levels below 217 mg/dl, this was entirely explained by age and other correlated risk factors in a

TABLE 1-11. *23-year all-cause mortality in deciles of lipid levels. Reproduced with permission from Goldbourt, et al.*[22]

Total serum cholesterol		Percentage of HDL cholesterol	
Decile (mg/dl)	Rate/10 000	Decile (%)	Rate/10 000
<161	149 (271)	<11.7	228 (266)
161–176	150 (316)	11.7–13.5	199 (266)
177–187	149 (282)	13.5–14.9	177 (235)
188–197	166 (317)	14.9–16.1	168 (215)
198–206	142 (278)	16.1–17.3	166 (231)
207–216	156 (339)	17.3–18.7	145 (212)
217–227	173 (374)	18.7–20.2	155 (203)
228–241	178 (380)	20.2–22.3	156 (215)
242–260	204 (376)	22.3–25.5	141 (201)
>260	233 (472)	>25.5	142 (189)
Total	170 (3405)		167 (2233)*

The values are age-adjusted rates per 10 000 person years. The number of deaths are given in parentheses. *Only 2233 subjects who subsequently died had both total cholesterol and high density lipoprotein (HDL) cholesterol levels assessed.

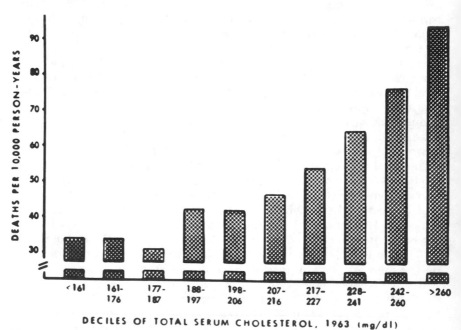

Fig. 1-4. Age-adjusted coronary heart disease mortality in deciles of cholesterol during 1963 to 1986 (rates per 10,000 person-years). Reproduced with permission from Goldbourt, et al.[22]

multi-variant adjustment of the survival curves. The net 23- year survival in terms of CAD was 87% in quintile 5 (total cholesterol >241) versus 93% in quintile 1 (total cholesterol <176 mg/dl). CAD mortality also was inversely related to the percent of cholesterol in HDL.

To determine whether high blood cholesterol is an important risk factor for mortality from CAD in elderly men, Rubin and associates[23] from San Francisco and Oakland, California, studied 2,746 white men and followed them a mean of 10.1 years. A total of 260 deaths occurred during 27,842 person years of follow-up. The relative risk for mortality from CAD in men 60 to 79 years of age in the highest serum cholesterol quartile was 1.5 compared to those in the 3 lower quartiles combined. The relative risk did not change greatly with age, ranging from 1.4 in men 60 to 64 years of age to 1.7 in men 75 to 79 years of age. However, because mortality from CAD increased with age, the excess risk for such mortality attributable to elevated serum cholesterol levels increased fivefold over these 20 years, from 2.2 deaths per 1000 person-years to 11.3 deaths per 1000 person-years. The authors' results support those of other observational studies in elderly men. If treatment of high blood cholesterol is as effective in reducing cholesterol-related risk for CAD after 65 years of age as it is in middle-aged men, in might actually produce greater reductions in mortality due to CAD.

Changes from weight loss

Williams and colleagues[24] in Berkeley, California, studied separately the effects of weight loss by calorie restriction (dieting) and by calorie expenditure (running) on lipoprotein subfraction concentrations in sedentary, moderately overweight men assigned at random into three groups as follows: exercise without calorie restriction, calorie restriction without exercise, and control. Plasma lipoprotein mass concentrations were measured by analytic ultracentrifugation for flotation rates within HDL, LDL, IDL, and VLDL particle distributions. Total body weight was reduced significantly more in dieters and exercisers than controls. As compared with mean changes in control, the exercisers and dieters significantly increased HDL^2, decreased VLDL mass, and increased LDL peak particle diameter. When adjusted to an equivalent change in body mass index by analysis of covariance, 1) exercise-induced and diet-induced weight loss produced comparable mean changes in the mass of small LDL and VLDL, and in LDL peak particle diameter; 2) the exercisers versus control group difference in HDL^2 was attributed to the exercisers' reduced body mass index; and 3) HDL^2 increased significantly less in dieters than in exercisers. In dieters, low calorie intake might mitigate the effects of weight loss on HDL^2.

Effects of exercise training

Exercise training has been associated with decreases in total cholesterol and increases in HDL cholesterol. The effect of the intensity of the exercise on alterations in cholesterol and lipoprotein fractions has not been defined and is the subject of this study. Stein and associates[25] from Brooklyn, New York, divided 49 healthy men (aged 44 ± 8 years) into 4 groups and evaluated them before and after 12 weeks of cycle ergometer exercise training at 1) an intensity of 65% of maximal achieved heart rate, 2) 75% maximal heart rate, 3) 85% maximal heart rate, and 4) a 12-week nonexercise control period. Pre- and post-training evaluations included maximal ergometer exercise electrocardiographic examinations with measurement of maximal minute oxygen consumption and serum total cholesterol, HDL cholesterol, and triglyceride levels. LDL and VLDL cholesterol levels were calculated. Dietary histories were obtained before and after the training period, and body weight and percentage of body fat were measured. Post-training oxygen uptake was significantly increased (training effect) in the groups exercising to 65%, 75%, and 85% maximal heart rate. Results of within-group analysis showed significant increases in the HDL cholesterol fractions in the 75% and 85% groups but not in the 65% group or the control group. Significant decreases in calculated LDL fractions occurred only in the 75% exercise-trained group with maximal heart rate. Aerobic exercise training favorably alters plasma lipoprotein profiles. A minimum training intensity equal to 75% maximal heart rate is required to increase HDL cholesterol level.

Effects of body fat distribution

Freedman and co-workers[26] in Milwaukee, Wisconsin, studied the role of body fat distribution, as assessed by the ratio of waist-to-hip circumferences in statistically explaining differences in levels of lipoproteins between men and women using data collected in 1985-86 from employed adults. As compared with 415 women, the 709 men had higher mean levels of triglycerides and apolipoprotein B as well as lower mean levels of HDL cholesterol and apolipoprotein A-1. Additionally, men were more overweight, consumed more alcohol, and exercised more frequently than women but were less likely to smoke cigarettes. Controlling for these characteristics, however, did not alter the differences in lipoprotein levels between men and women. In contrast, adjustment for waist-to-hip ratios (which was greater among men) reduced the sex differences in levels of apolipoprotein B, triglycerides, HDL cholesterol, and apolipoprotein A-1. Whereas generalized obesity and body fat distribution are associated with lipid levels, fat distribution (or a characteristic influencing fat patterning) can be an important determinant of sex differences in levels of triglycerides, HDL cholesterol, and apolipoproteins B and A-1.

Familial hypercholesterolemia

Rubba and co-workers[27] in Naples, Italy, performed repeat LDL apheresis and blood flow determinations in the forearm and leg in 10 patients (ages ranged from 13 to 49 years; 4 male, 6 female) with familial hypercholesterolemia. To perform LDL apheresis, plasma was first separated by a polysulphone hollow fiber filter; then, LDL was selectively removed from plasmal by dextran sulphate cellulose beads packed in columns. Blood flows in the forearm and leg were determined at rest and during a reactive hyperemia test. This test was performed noninvasively by a strain-gauge plethysmograph with semicontinuous registration of arterial blood flow variables before the first apheresis and three weeks after the last of 6 procedures for apheresis. Resting arterial blood flows in the forearm and leg were slightly increased after repeat LDL apheresis. Peak blood flow in the leg significantly increased by 34%. No change in peak blood flow in the forearm was observed. Systolic blood pressures were slightly but significantly reduced; forearm peripheral resistances were also reduced. Flow response was not related to LDL receptor status. Blood and plasma viscosities were determined before and seven days after the last apheresis. Blood viscosity was significantly reduced after LDL apheresis at shear rates of 11.25–450 sec^{-1}. Plasma viscosity did not change.

Effects of lowering on coronary artery mortality and total mortality

Holme[28] in Oslo, Norway, analyzed randomized trials of cholesterol reduction. The primary aim of this study was to estimate the relation between cholesterol reduction and total mortality and CAD incidence. Secondarily, the clinical issues of whether the efficacy of cholesterol lowering is dependent on the treatment modality, presence of CAD at baseline, or the simultaneous introduction of other interventions was explored. All randomized clinical intervention trials of cholesterol reduction were used in an overview analysis of total mortality rate and CAD incidence; analysis was performed with weighted linear regression. The trials included those that used primary and secondary intervention, diet and drugs, and single or multifactor design. Nineteen trials were analyzed for total mortality and of the 19, 16 were analyzed for CAD incidence rate. Net difference in cholesterol change between study groups was used as the independent variable, and the 3 previously mentioned dichotomous design characteristics were used as additional independent variables. For every 1% reduction in cholesterol, estimated 2.5% reduction in CHD incidence is indicated. With regard to CAD drug trials tended toward better efficiency in cholesterol lowering than the dietary trials. With regard total mortality, this efficiency was higher in secondary than in primary prevention trials. The efficiency was also somewhat dependent on the baseline cholesterol level. This study shows that cholesterol reduction is effective in lowering CAD incidence, but cholesterol reduction must be at least 8–9% to be effective in lowering total mortality.

Lowering effect of hydroxychloroquine

Wallace and associates[29] from Los Angeles, California, and New York, New York, studied the effects of hydroxychloroquine on serum levels of total cholesterol, total triglycerides, HDL and LDL cholesterol in patients with rheumatoid arthritis or systemic lupus erythematosus. A total of 155 women were divided into the following treatment groups: Group A: patients taking hydroxychloroquine and no steroids (n = 58); Group B: patients taking steroids and no hydroxychloroquine (n = 35); Group C: patients receiving both hydroxychloroquine and steroids (n = 18); and Group D: patients receiving neither HCQ nor steroids (n = 44). Hydroxychloroquine therapy had a high statistical association with low serum levels of cholesterol (181 mg/dl), triglycerides (106 mg/dl), and LDL (101 mg/dl), irrespective of concomitant steroid administration. The hydroxychloroquine-treated group (A) had lower cholesterol (181 mg/dl) and LDL (101 mg/dl) levels than those receiving neither hydroxychloroquine nor steroids (205 mg/dl) and (128 mg/dl) (Group D). No HDL differences were observed. The effects of hydroxychloroquine do not appear to be due to changes in diet or weight, and the drug was well tolerated. Although the mechanism of cholesterol lowering by hydroxychloroquine is not known, this drug deserves further investigation for its lipid-lowering properties.

In the nephrotic syndrome

Patients with the nephrotic syndrome characteristically have multiple abnormalities of lipoprotein metabolism, but the cause and exact nature of these abnormalities are uncertain. Joven and associates[30] from Barcelona, Spain, measured serum lipids and apoproteins in 57 patients with the nephrotic syndrome. They also determined the kinetic indexes of LDL metabolism in 6 patients and again in 3 of the 6 after recovery. The patients with the nephrotic syndrome had elevated serum concentrations of cholesterol, triglycerides, and phospholipids, which were confined to the lipoproteins containing apoprotein B (Figure 1-5). The serum concentrations of HDL and the associated A-I and A-II apoproteins were similar in the patients with the nephrotic syndrome and normal subjects. The relative proportions of lipids and their positive association with the increased serum concentrations of apoproteins B, C-II, C-III, and E sug-

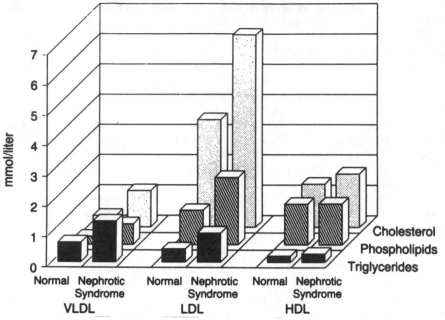

Fig. 1-5. Mean cholesterol, triglyceride, and phospholipid distribution in the lipoprotein fractions of serum of normal subjects and patients with the nephrotic syndrome. Reproduced with permission from Joven, et al.[30]

gest quantitative rather than qualitative differences in the lipoproteins. All the patients had lipiduria, which probably reflected the excretion of HDL, although no intact immunoreactive apoprotein A-I was found in urine. Serum albumin concentrations were inversely related to serum lipid concentrations in the patients, the severity of the hypoalbuminemia corresponding to the degree of change in serum lipoprotein concentrations. The kinetic studies of lipoprotein metabolism revealed an overproduction of LDL apoprotein B that returned to normal after recovery. The elevated serum concentrations of LDL cholesterol, other lipids, and apoprotein B in patients with uncomplicated nephrotic syndrome are due to reversible increases in lipoprotein production.

This article was followed by an editorial by Keane and Kasiske[31] entitled: "Hyperlipidemia in the Nephrotic Syndrome". These authors concluded the following: "The reasons for using pharmacologic agents to treat hyperlipidemia in selected patients with the nephrotic syndrome are growing in number and persuasiveness. Dietary measures to reduce serum lipid concentrations are often unsuccessful in patients with the nephrotic syndrome, whereas newer antilipemic agents may be effective. At present, it seems reasonable to extend the treatment guidelines adopted by the National Cholesterol Education Program to patients with unremitting nephrotic syndrome. A better understanding of the adverse effects of hyperlipidemia in such patients may ultimately justify even more aggressive treatment.

Effect of knowing level on behavior

To investigate the effect of screening for an elevated cholesterol level and compliance with follow-up recommendations, Gordon and associates[32] from Baltimore, Maryland, surveyed 375 participants in a free-screening program at a shopping mall walk-in clinic. One hundred thirty-nine participants (37%) had desirable (<5.17 mmol/L [<200 mg/dL]), 135 (36%) had borderline (5.17 to 6.18 mmol/L [200 to 239 mg/dL]), and 101 (27%) had high (>6.18 mmol/L [>239 mg/dL]) cholesterol levels. Persons in the borderline and high categories were instructed to see their physicians within 2 months for confirmation of their levels. Of the 338 (90%) who responded to a follow-up questionnaire at 3 months, 8 (7%) in the desirable, 23 (22%) in the borderline, and 44 (50%) in the high group had been to see physicians concerning their cholesterol levels since the screening (Table 1-12). In multiple logistic regression analyses only cholesterol category at time of screening, current use of antihypertensive drugs, history of CAD, and history of a high cholesterol level were associated with physician follow-up. Our results suggest that labeling persons as being at high rather than borderline risk results in greater physician follow-up.

Knowledge of lipoprotein levels in mmol/L is difficult for physicians in the USA. Most USA physicians use the units mg/ml. Two important numbers are necessary to remember when the units are mmol/L and they are 5.18, which is equivalent to 200 mg/dL and 6.18 which is equivalent to 240 mg/dL.

Effect of threat of unemployment

To assess whether the threat of unemployment effects risk factors for cardiovascular disease, Mattiasson and associates[33] from Malmo, Sweden, performed a longitudinal study of a cohort of middle-aged shipyard workers followed for a mean of 6.2 ± 1.9 years and a group of controls observed for the same period. The first investigation took place during a period of relative economic stability for the shipyard and the second during the phase of its closure. A total of 715 male shipyard workers and 261 age-matched male controls were studied. Serum cholesterol concentrations increased more (mean 0.25 ± 0.68 mmol/l vs. 0.08 ± 0.66 mmol/l) and serum calcium concentrations decreased less in the shipyard workers than in the controls. A correlation was found between scores for sleep disturbances and changes in serum total cholesterol concentration. In the whole series there was a greater increase in serum total cholesterol concentrations among men threatened with unemployment (437/976 = 45%) than among those who were not. A positive correlation was found between change between total cholesterol concentration and change in BP, indicating that the overall risk profile had worsened among men with increased serum total cholesterol concentrations. The authors concluded

TABLE 1-12. *Percent respondents seeing a physician about their cholesterol level within 3 months after screening.* Reproduced with permission from Gordon, et al.*[32]

Cholesterol Category	n	Percent Having Seen a Physician
Overall	338	24
Desirable, <5.17 mmol/L (<200 mg/dL)	126	7
Borderline, 5.17 to 6.18 mmol/L (200 to 239 mg/dL)	121	22
High, >6.18 mmol/L (>239 mg/dL)	91	50

*Difference between borderline and high categories, 28% (P<.001).

that risk of unemployment increases the serum total cholesterol concentration in middle-aged men, the increase being more pronounced in those with sleep disturbance.

Relation of sex hormones and HDL cholesterol

Duell and Bierman[34] from Seattle, Washington, sought to clarify the complex and uncertain relation between endogenous sex hormones and HDL cholesterol levels in healthy men. Fifty-five healthy adult men were consecutively recruited from an ongoing cross-sectional study of cardiovascular disease risk factors from a lipid research clinic at the University of Washington, Seattle. Subjects receiving medication were excluded. Multiple linear regression analysis identified several factors that correlated highly significantly with HDL cholesterol levels, including alcohol intake; frequency of strenuous exercise; age; levels of total cholesterol, LDL cholesterol, and triglyceride; and carbohydrate intake. Nearly 80% of the heterogeneity in HDL cholesterol levels could be accounted for by these factors. Despite finding significant correlations with factors known to influence HDL cholesterol levels, no correlation with estradiol level, testosterone level, or the ratio of estradiol to testosterone levels was apparent. In conclusion, endogenous sex hormones do not appear to influence HDL cholesterol levels in healthy adult men. Alternatively, a large proportion of the heterogeneity in HDL levels in this group of men can be accounted for by environmental factors. The disparity between this conclusion and others may be partially due to differences in accounting for these confounding variables.

Lipoprotein(a)

Familial hypercholesterolemia carries a marked increase in the risk of CAD, but there is considerable variation between individuals in susceptibility to CAD. To investigate the possible role of lipoprotein(a) as a risk factor for CAD, Seed and associates[35] from London, UK, studied the association between serum lipoprotein(a) levels, genetic types of apolipoprotein(a) (which influence lipoprotein(a) levels), and CAD in 115 patients with heterozygous familial hypercholesterolemia. The median lipoprotein(a) level in the 54 patients with CAD was 57 mg/dl, which is significantly higher than the corresponding value of 18 mg/dl in the 61 patients without CAD (Figure 1-6, Table 1-13). According to discriminant-function analysis, the lipoprotein(a) level was the best discriminator between the 2 groups (as compared with all other lipid and lipoprotein levels, age, sex, and smoking status). Phenotyping for apolipoprotein(a) was performed in 109 patients. The frequencies of the apolipoprotein(a) pheno-types and alleles differed significantly between the patients with and those without CAD. The allele Lp^{s2}, which is associated with high lipoprotein(a) levels, was found more frequently among the patients with CAD (0.33 vs. 0.12). In contrast, the Lp^{s4} allele, which is associated with low lipoprotein(a) levels, was more frequent among those without CAD (0.27 vs. 0.15). The authors concluded that an elevated level of lipoprotein(a) is a strong risk factor for CAD in patients with familial hypercholesterolemia, and the increase in risk is independent of age, sex, smoking status, and serum levels of total cholesterol, triglyceride, or HDL cholesterol. The higher level of lipoprotein(a) observed in the patients with CAD is the result of genetic influence.

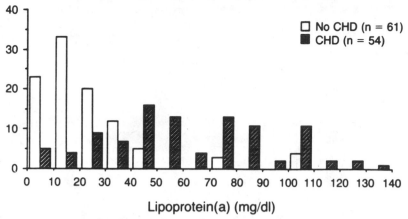

Fig. 1-6. Frequency distribution of serum lipoprotein(a) concentrations among patients with familial hypercholesterolemia who did not have CHD. Reproduced with permission from Seed, et al.[35]

TABLE 1-13. *Fasting serum lipid and lipoprotein levels, according to study group.** *Reproduced with permission from Seed, et al.[35]*

VARIABLE	No CHD (N = 61)	CHD (N = 54)	P VALUE
Total cholesterol (mmol/liter)†	9.9±1.5	10.1±2.08	NS‡
LDL cholesterol (mmol/liter)†	8.2±1.5	8.1±2.2	NS‡
HDL cholesterol (mmol/liter)†	1.18±0.28	1.19±0.37	NS‡
Triglyceride (mmol/liter)§	1.39±0.68	1.85±1.11	0.0041¶
Log triglyceride (mmol/liter)	0.09	0.21	<0.01‖
Lipoprotein(a) (mg/dl)	18	57	0.0001¶
Log lipoprotein(a) (mg/dl)	1.21	1.68	<0.0001‖

*Plus–minus values are means ±SD. Lipoprotein(a) concentrations are median values.

†To convert to milligrams per deciliter, multiply by 38.7.

‡No significant difference.   §To convert to milligrams per deciliter, multiply by 88.5.

¶By Mann–Whitney test.   ‖By Student's t-test.

Wiklund and associates[36] from Gothenburg, Sweden, measured serum concentrations of apolipoprotein(a) in patients with heterozygous familial hypercholesterolemia (Figure 1-7, Table 1-14). The levels in 47 patients were a median of 2.5 times higher than those in controls matched for age and sex (240 [range 25–1245] vs. 97 [7–1040] mg/l). Among patients with familial hypercholesterolemia apo(a) levels were higher in those with (n = 48) than in those without (n = 72) CAD (283 [18–1245] vs. 144 [7–741] mg/l); both in inivariate and multivariate analysis serum apo(a) was the most significant variable distinguishing between the groups. Despite reducing LDL cholesterol by 30%, treatment with cholestyramine or pravastatin did not reduce apo(a) levels in these patients. These findings support the concept that apo(a) concentration is a genetic trait predisposing to CAD and imply that it may be useful in the identification of familial hypercholesterolemia patients at high risk of CAD.

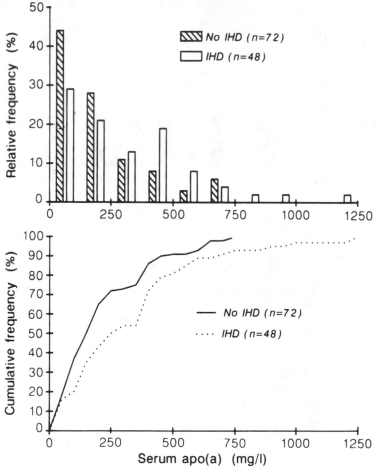

Fig. 1-7. Relative distribution of serum apo(a) levels in patients with familial hypercho-lesterolaemia with or without ischaemic heart disease (IHD). Reproduced with permission from Wiklund, et al.[36]

To determine the relation among serum lipids in predicting CAD, Hearn and associates[37] from Atlanta, Georgia, studied 213 patients undergoing diagnostic angiography for suspected CAD. Twenty-one pa-tients had normal coronary arteries and 192 had CAD in 1 to 3 arteries at angiography with measurements obtained with digital calipers. Li-poproteins were measured and lipoprotein(a) [Lp(a)] was also assayed in a subset of 98 patients with CAD. Statistical analysis was performed using uni- and multivariate techniques to test the association among age, gender, systemic hypertension, diabetes mellitus, cigarette smoking, fam-ily history, total cholesterol, triglycerides, HDL cholesterol, LDL choles-terol, very low density lipoprotein cholesterol, apolipoproteins (apo) A-1 and apo B, ratio of apo A-1 to apo B, and ratio of HDL cholesterol to total cholesterol, to Lp(a) and to CAD. All factors except gender, systemic hypertension, diabetes mellitus and cigarette smoking were univariate predictors of CAD. Multivariate predictors were, in decreasing order of significance, family history, age, HDL/total cholesterol ratio and apo B. When Lp(a) was included, multivariate predictors were age, family history, apo B and Lp(a), in that order. Lipid parameters alone showed that the HDL/total cholesterol ratio and that Lp(a) provide the best predictive tests

TABLE 1-14. *Characteristics of familial hypercholesterolaemia patients with and without ischaemic heart disease (IHD). Reproduced with permission from Wiklund, et al.*[36]

—	No IHD (n = 72)	IHD (n = 48)	p
Mean (SD) age (yr)	48 (14)	54 (10)	0·03
Male/female	36/36	26/22	NS
No of patients with			
Xanthomatosis	22	11	NS
Heredity for IHD	52	35	NS
No with smoking score			
1/2/3/4/5/6	31/23/1/9/3/1	11/25/0/3/8/1	0·03
Mean (SD) serum level (mmol/l)			
Total cholesterol	10·0 (2·0)	9·6 (2·0)	NS
Triglycerides	1·5 (0·6)	1·8 (0·8)	0·02
HDL-cholesterol	1·3 (0·6)	1·2 (0·3)	NS
LDL-cholesterol	8·2 (1·9)	7·8 (2·0)	NS
Mean (SD) serum level (g/l)			
Apo AI	1·40 (0·30)	1·32 (0·29)	NS
Apo B	1·97 (0·43)	1·97 (0·35)	NS
Apo (a)*	144 (7-741)	283 (18-1245)	0·006

NS = not significant.
*Median (range).

for the detection of CAD in this referral population and may ultimately become important screening tests for CAD.

To examine the association between the serum lipoprotein (a) concentration and subsequent CAD, Rosengren and associates[38] from Gothenburg, Sweden, performed a 6-year follow-up of a general population sample of men aged 50 at baseline in 1983–1984. Serum samples were frozen at the time of the baseline examination and kept at −7°C for 6 years, after which the lipoprotein (a) concentrations in the samples were measured in cases and controls. Twenty-six men, from a general population sample of 776 men, had had an AMI or died of CAD during the 6 years and 109 randomly selected controls from the same sample had remained free of AMI. In neither cases nor controls was there a history of AMI at baseline. The men who had CAD had significantly higher serum lipoprotein (a) concentrations than controls (mean difference 105 mg/l). Men with the highest fifth of serum lipoprotein (a) concentrations (cutoff point 365 mg/l) had a CAD rate which was more than twice that of men with the lowest four-fifths of concentrations. Logistic regression analysis showed the serum lipoprotein (a) concentration to be significantly associated with CAD independently of other risk factors.

LDL-uptake by tendon xanthomas

Technetium-labeled LDL appear to be useful for describing LDL biodistribution in normal and dyslipidemic subjects. Ginsberg and associates[39] from New York, New York, injected [99m]technetium-labeled LDL into subjects with large tendon xanthomas secondary to homozygous familial hypercholesterolemia or sitosterolemia. Rapid (4 hours) accumulation of

Tc-99m activity in xanthomas was observed, and this accumulation increased over a 24-hour period. No comparable accumulations of Tc-99m activity were noted in normal subjects or in a subject with heterozygous familial hypercholesterolemia who had very small tendon xanthomas. These findings support previous biopsy data indicating active uptake of LDL by macrophages within xanthoma and suggest that ^{99m}Tc-LDL imaging of xanthomas may be useful in studies of the effects of diet and drugs on the accumulation of lipoproteins by atherosclerotic plaques.

Apolipoproteins A-I and B

Reinhart and associates[40] from Marshfield, Wisconsin measured apolipoprotein A-I and B concentrations in 502 patients undergoing diagnostic cardiac catheterization to assess the predictive power of apolipoproteins B and A-I to discriminate between patients with CAD and those with normal coronary arteries as defined by coronary angiography (Table 1-15). The strength of the associations was compared with that of the associations between traditional risk factors (eg, smoking status, cholesterol levels) and CAD. The study population consisted of 154 women (mean age, 63 years) and 348 men (mean age, 60 years). The apolipoprotein A-I concentration averaged (± SD) 124 ± 25 mg/dl and the apolipoprotein measures showed a larger univariate difference between the "normal" (no CAD) group (66 patients) and the group with CAD (436 patients) than did the corresponding standard lipoprotein measures. The variable with the strongest association with CAD was the ratio of apolipoprotein A-I to apolipoprotein B, followed by apolipoprotein B level. These findings were confirmed using logistic regression, adjusting for other CAD risk factors. Fasting status did not affect apolipoprotein A-I or B concentrations. The authors concluded that the use of apolipoprotein A-I and B concentrations gives additional information to that supplied by lipoprotein measures to help predict the presence of CAD. Since traditional lipid measures may be changed by a meal, apolipoproteins A-I and B might be more useful measures when the fasting status of a patient is in question.

HDL lipoprotein comprises 2 major types of lipoprotein particles: (1) those that contain apolipoproteins A-I and A-II, designated LpA-I:A-II, and (2) those that contain apolipoprotein A-I but not apolipoprotein A-II, designated LpA-I. Both have been extensively studied and are believed to represent distinct metabolic entities that may confer differing protection against CAD risk. Puchois and associates[41] from Lille and Sophia Antipolis, France, previously suggested that LpA-I might represent the antiatherogenic effect, which has been ascribed mainly to its effect on HDL cholesterol. These authors now investigated in 344 men the relation

TABLE 1-15. *Relationship of laboratory variables to sex and presence of CAD.** *Reproduced with permission from Rheinhart, et al.*[40]

	Men			Women		
	No CAD	CAD	P	No CAD	CAD	P
Apo A-I	121 ± 17.0	119 ± 23.8	NS	140 ± 25.9	131 ± 26.9	NS
Apo B	82 ± 16.7	98 ± 22.5	.001	89 ± 26.9	104 ± 27.8	.01
Apo A-I/apo B ratio	1.49	1.23	.001	1.66	1.31	.001
TC	5.09 ± 0.97	5.69 ± 1.14	.003	5.72 ± 1.22	6.10 ± 1.30	NS
HDL-C	0.98 ± 0.22	0.98 ± 0.28	NS	1.22 ± 0.36	1.09 ± 0.30	NS
LDL-C	3.13 ± 0.82	3.78 ± 1.01	.001	3.85 ± 1.08	4.03 ± 1.13	NS
HDL-C/TC ratio	0.20 ± 0.5	0.18 ± 0.05	.017	0.22 ± 0.07	0.19 ± 0.06	.030
TC	2.25 ± 1.24	2.38 ± 1.84	NS	1.58 ± 0.87	2.37 ± 1.36	.004
Non–HDL-C	3.96 ± 0.82	4.63 ± 1.11	.001	4.42 ± 1.16	4.86 ± 1.22	NS

*CAD indicates coronary artery disease; apo, apolipoprotein; NS, not significant (P<.05); TC, total cholesterol; HDL-C, high-density lipoprotein cholesterol; LDL-C, low-density lipoprotein cholesterol; and TG, triglyceride. Values are mean ± SD, in milligrams per deciliter for apolipoproteins and in millimoles per liter for remaining measures. P values are two-tailed.

between LpA-I:A-II and LpA-I levels in cholesterol consumption. They found as the alcohol intake rose that LpA-I:A-II levels increased, while LpA-I levels fell. On the assumption that LpA-I is the antiatherogenic fraction of HDL, the putative protective action of alcohol consumption against CAD should be reconsidered. This article was followed by an editorial entitled "Role of apolipoprotein Levels in Clinical Practice" by Scott M. Grundy and Gloria Lena Vega[42] from Dallas, Texas. These authors concluded that considerably more research must be carried out before tests for levels of apolipoproteins can be employed clinically. They stated, "In general, clinicians should avoid the temptation of using currently available measurements of apolipoproteins for making decisions about patient care, especially when these decisions relate to drug therapy."

Dietary trans fatty acids

Fatty acids that contain a trans double bond are consumed in large amounts as hydrogenated oils, but their effect on serum lipoprotein levels is unknown. Mensink and Katan[43] from Wageningen, The Netherlands, placed 34 women (mean age 26 years) and 25 men (mean age 25 years) on 3 mixed natural diets of identical nutrient composition, except that 10% of the daily energy intake was provided as oleic acid (which contains 1 cis double bond), trans isomers of oleic acid, or saturated fatty acids. The 3 diets were consumed for 3 weeks each, in random order. On the oleic acid diet, the mean ($\pm$ SD) serum values for the entire group for total, LDL and HDL cholesterol were 4.46 $\pm$ 0.66, 2.67 $\pm$ 0.54, and 1.42 $\pm$ 0.32 mmol/l (172 $\pm$ 26, 103 $\pm$ 21, and 55 $\pm$ 12 mg/dl, respectively. On the trans-fatty-acid diet, the subjects' mean HDL cholesterol level was 0.17 mmol/l (7 mg/dl) lower than the mean value on the diet high in oleic acid; 95% confidence interval, 0.13 to 0.20 mmol/l). The HDL cholesterol level on the saturated-fat diet was the same as on the oleic acid diet. The LDL cholesterol level was 0.37 mmol/l (14 mg/dl) higher on the trans-fatty-acid diet than on the oleic acid diet (95% confidence interval, 0.28 to 0.45 mmol/l) and 0.47 mmol/l (18 mg/dl) higher on the saturated-fat diet (95% confidence interval, 0.39 to 0.55 mmol/l) than on the oleic acid diet. The effects on lipoprotein levels did not differ between women and men. The effect of trans fatty acids on the serum lipoprotein profile is at least as unfavorable as that of the cholesterol-raising saturated fatty acids, because they not only raise LDL cholesterol levels but also lower HDL cholesterol levels.

Lipid levels with angiographic coronary artery disease

The National Cholesterol Education Program treatment guidelines defined a plasma total cholesterol of <200 as "desirable" and recommended no further evaluation of plasma lipid or lipoprotein levels in patients with CAD. To determine the prevalence if dyslipidemias in the presence of coexistent CAD and total cholesterol ≤200 mg/dl, Miller and associates[44] from Baltimore, Maryland, performed a retrospective case control study of 100 patients who underwent diagnostic coronary angiography (Table 1-16). Of 351 patients with total cholesterol ≤200 mg/dl, 76% of the men (244) and 44% of the women (107) had angiographically demonstrated CAD. In men with CAD and total cholesterol ≤200 mg/dl, there was a significantly greater prevalence of low levels of HDL cholesterol (≤35 mg/dl), age >50 years, systemic hypertension and diabetes mellitus compared to non-CAD control subjects. In women with CAD

TABLE 1-16. *Mean levels of plasma lipids and lipoproteins with or without CAD and total cholesterol ≤200 mg/dl by sex. Reproduced with permission from Miller, et al.[44]*

	Men				Women			
	CAD		No CAD		CAD		No CAD	
	No.	Mean ± SD	No.	Mean ± SD	No.	Mean ± SD	No.	Mean ± SD
Age (yrs)	139	56 ± 9†	55	49 ± 11	37	56 ± 10	57	52 ± 9
TC (mg/dl)	139	175 ± 20*	55	167 ± 25	37	176 ± 23	57	169 ± 26
TG (mg/dl)	139	123 ± 62*	55	97 ± 73	37	126 ± 61†	57	85 ± 37
HDL (mg/dl)	138	34 ± 9*	55	40 ± 15	37	39 ± 10*	56	45 ± 12
LDL (mg/dl)	126	119 ± 22*	53	110 ± 21	35	113 ± 25	51	112 ± 26
VLDL (mg/dl)	120	23 ± 14*	50	18 ± 15	34	22 ± 13†	49	12 ± 6
TC:HDL	138	6 ± 2†	55	5 ± 2	37	5 ± 1*	56	4 ± 1
LDL:HDL	126	4 ± 2*	53	3 ± 1	35	3 ± 1	51	3 ± 1

* p <0.05; † p <0.001.
CAD = coronary artery disease; HDL = high density lipoprotein; LDL = low density lipoprotein; SD = standard deviation; TC = total cholesterol; TG = triglycerides; VLDL = very low density lipoprotein.

TABLE 1-17. *Age, serum total cholesterol, HDL cholesterol, triglycerides, and the ratio of HDL cholesterol to total cholesterol in patients without coronary artery disease and in those with single, double, or triple vessel disease. Reproduced with permission from Nikkila, et al.[45]*

Variable	No lesion (n = 63)	Single vessel (n = 124)	Double vessel (n = 192)	Triple vessel (n = 319)	Statistical significance in ANOVA
Age	52·2 (0·91)	49·4 (0·74)	53·5 (0·67)	54·9 (0·33)	
Total cholesterol (mmol/l)	5·93 (0·15)	6·34 (0·12)	6·53 (0·09)	6·52 (0·06)	p < 0·01
HDL cholesterol (mmol/l)	1·29 (0·05)	1·13 (0·03)	1·10 (0·03)	1·07 (0·01)	p < 0·001
Triglycerides (mmol/l)	1·77 (0·11)	2·39 (0·13)	2·50 (0·13)	2·59 (0·11)	p < 0·01
HDL:Total cholesterol	0·22 (0·01)	0·18 (0·01)	0·17 (0·01)	0·17 (0·01)	p < 0·001

Values are given as mean (SEM). ANOVA, analysis of variance. In Student-Newman-Keuls test the statistical difference was significant between the group without coronary artery disease and all other groups with coronary artery disease, but not between groups with single, double, and triple vessel disease.

and total cholesterol ≤200 mg/dl, HDL cholesterol ≤45 mg/dl and diabetes mellitus were also significantly prevalent. Multiple logistic regression analyses revealed that HDL cholesterol, hypertension and age in men and very LDL-cholesterol in women were significantly associated with CAD after adjustment for other risk factors. These results suggest that a complete lipid and lipoprotein analysis be obtained in all patients with CAD, irrespective of the plasma (or serum) total cholesterol level.

Nikkila and associates[45] from Tampere, Finland, measured serum triglycerides, HDL cholesterol, and total cholesterol in the serum in 698 patients examined by coronary angiography. The ratio of HDL cholesterol to total cholesterol was significantly lower in patients with 1, 2, and 3 vessel CAD than in patients without CAD (Table 1-17). The serum concentration of triglyceride was significantly higher in patients with 1, 2, and 3 vessel CAD than in those without CAD. Similar proportion of patients with CAD and without had serum total cholesterol concentrations of ≥6.5 mmol/l, but total cholesterol was significantly higher in patients with 1, 2, and 3 vessel CAD than in those without. HDL cholesterol (<1.0 mmol/l), triglycerides (>2.0 mmol/l), and the ratio of HDL cholesterol to total cholesterol (<0.20) were significantly better than total cholesterol as indicators of CAD risk.

Effects of coffee

Rossmarin and associates[46] from Memphis, Tennessee, in a prospective, randomized, cross-over clinical trial, studied 21 healthy white men who consumed an average of 3.6 cups of coffee a day. No effect of coffee consumption was found on serum total cholesterol, HDL cholesterol, LDL cholesterol, or apolipoprotein B.

Zock and associates[47] from Wageningen, the Netherlands, found that Scandinavian-style boiled coffee raised serum total cholesterol and that it contained more lipid material than drip filter coffee which does not raise serum total cholesterol. They studied 10 volunteers who consumed a lipid-enriched fraction from boiled coffee for 6 weeks: the supplement provided 77 g of water, 1.3 g of lipid, and 1.6 g of other solids per day. Serum cholesterol rose in every subject; the mean rise was 0.74 mmol/l after 3 weeks (range -0.09 to 1.48 mmol/l) and 1.06 SD 0.37 mmol/l or 23% after 6 weeks (range 0.48 to 1.52 mmol/l). The increase was mainly due to LDL cholesterol, which rose by 29%, but VLDL cholesterol was also raised, as evidenced by a 55% rise in triglycerides. HDL cholesterol was unchanged. After supplementation had ended, lipid levels returned to baseline. Boiled coffee thus contains a lipid that powerfully raises serum cholesterol.

Waist-to-hip circumference

High plasma levels of HDL_2, a subfraction of HDL cholesterol, are associated with a reduced risk of CAD. To investigate the characteristics related to HDL_2 cholesterol levels, Ostlund and associates[48] from St. Louis, Missouri, measured lipoprotein levels and several metabolic and anthropometric variables in 146 healthy subjects (77 men and 69 women) in the 7th decade of life. The level of HDL_2 cholesterol was inversely correlated with the ratio of the waist-to-hip circumference and the plasma insulin level. In a multiple regression model including both sexes, 41% of the variance in the HDL_2 level was explained by the combined effect of the waist-to-hip ratio, the plasma insulin level, and the degree of glucose tolerance indicated by the integrated area under the plasma glucose curve after an oral glucose-tolerance test. The body-mass index, total percentage of body fat, maximal oxygen uptake, diet, and sex were not significant predictors of the HDL_2 level when added to this model, whereas the original variables remained significant predictors. The HDL_2 cholesterol level in subjects at the 25th percentile for waist-to-hip ratio was 153% of that in subjects at the 75th percentile. The authors concluded that HDL_2 levels are inversely correlated with truncal fat, plasma insulin levels, and the presence of glucose intolerance and are not independently associated with sex or total body fat.

High plasma levels of HDL_2, a subfraction of HDL cholesterol, are associated with a reduced risk of CAD. To investigate the characteristics related to HDL_2 cholesterol levels, Ostlund and associates[49] measured lipoprotein levels and several metabolic and anthropometric variables in 146 healthy subjects (77 men and 69 women) in the 7th decade of life. The level of HDL_2 cholesterol was inversely correlated with the ratio of the waist-to-hip circumference and the plasma insulin level (Figure 1-8). In a multiple regression model including both sexes, 41% of the variance in the HDL_2 level was explained by the combined effect of the waist-to-hip ratio, the plasma insulin level, and the degree of glucose tolerance indicated by the integrated area under the plasma glucose curve after an oral glucose-tolerance test. The body-mass index, total percentage of body fat, maximal oxygen uptake, diet, and sex were not significant predictors of the HDL_2 level when added to this model, whereas the original variables remained significant predictors. The HDL_2 cholesterol level in subjects at the 25th percentile for waist-to-hip ratio was 153% of that in

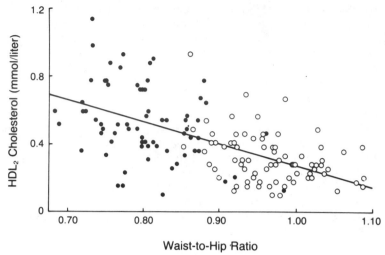

Fig. 1-8. HDL2 cholesterol level and waist-to-hip ratio in men (open circles) and women (solid circles). Reproduced with permission from Ostlund, Jr., et al.[48]

subjects at the 75th percentile. The authors concluded that HDL_2 levels are inversely correlated with truncal fat, plasma insulin levels, and the presence of glucose intolerance and are not independently associated with sex or total body fat.

Before diagnosis of colonic cancer

Winawer and associates[50] from New York and Yorktown Heights, New York, reported the results of a 10-year, time-trend, case-control study in which serum total cholesterol level was determined at several points in time preceding the diagnosis of colon cancer in a population of individuals who sought general checkups at an ambulatory care screening facility. Each of the 69 patients with colon cancer (32 men and 37 women) was matched with a control patient who was randomly selected. At the time of diagnosis, the patients with colon cancer had significantly lower serum cholesterol values than control patients (5.56 ± 0.31 mmol/L (SEM) vs 6.47 ± 0.34 mmol/L). This difference did not vary with sex or Dukes' stage of the cancer. The percent of matched pairs in which the cancer patient had a lower serum cholesterol level increased from 42% at 10 years prior to cancer diagnosis to 77% at diagnosis. The ratio of serum cholesterol at each period to the level at time of diagnosis demonstrated an average decline of 13% during the 10 years prior to diagnosis for case patients vs an average rise of 2% in the same period for control patients. The authors concluded that individuals in whom colorectal cancer develops share the same level of serum cholesterol as the general population initially, but during the 10 years preceding the cancer demonstrate a decline in serum cholesterol level that is opposite to the rising level seen with age in the general population.

Effects of alcohol

Handa and associates[51] from Fukuoka, Japan, examined the relation of alcohol consumption to serum lipids and the severity of CAD in 212 men undergoing coronary angiography. The severity of CAD was assessed in terms of the presence of ≥75% diameter stenosis and the Gensini severity score. Alcohol consumption was divided into 4 categories: none (0 ml alcohol/week), light (1–100 ml alcohol/week), moderate (101–300 ml alcohol/week) and heavy (≥301 ml alcohol/week). Alcohol consumption was positively related to HDL cholesterol and inversely related to total cholesterol, but was not associated with triglyceride. After adjustment for these serum lipids as well as for cigarette smoking and systemic hypertension, the risk of coronary stenosis was significantly decreased in the moderate drinkers. A decreased risk among moderate drinkers also was noted in terms of Gensini's severity score. These findings suggest that moderate alcohol consumption may protect against severe coronary atherosclerosis.

THERAPY OF HYPERLIPIDEMIA

Diet

The design of diets to achieve optimal changes in plasma lipid levels is controversial. In a randomized, double-blind trial involving 36 healthy young men, Ginsberg and associates[52] from New York, New York, evaluated the effects on plasma lipid levels of both an American Heart Association Step 1 diet (in which 30% of the total calories were consumed as fat: 10% saturated, 10% monounsaturated, and 10% polyunsaturated fats, with 250 mg of cholesterol per day) and a monounsaturated fat-enriched Step 1 diet (with 38% of the calories consumed as fat: 10% saturated, 18% monounsaturated, and 10% polyunsaturated fats, with 250 mg of cholesterol per day). The effects of these diets were then compared with those of an average American diet, in which 38% of the total calories were consumed as fat: 18% saturated, 10% monounsaturated, and 10% polyunsaturated fats, with 500 mg of cholesterol per day (Figure 1-9). The men consumed the average American diet for 10 weeks before random assignment to 1 of the 2 Step 1 diets or to continuation of the average diet for an additional 10 weeks. Caloric intake was adjusted to maintain a constant body weight. As compared with the mean (± SD) change in the plasma total cholesterol level in the group that followed the average American diet throughout the study (−0.05 ± 0.36 mmol/L), there were statistically significant reductions in the plasma total cholesterol level in the group on the Step 1 diet (−0.37 ± 0.27 mmol per liter) and in the group on the monounsaturated fat-enriched Step 1 diet (−0.46 ± 0.36 mmol/L). There were parallel reductions in the plasma low-density lipoprotein cholesterol levels in these 2 groups. Neither the plasma triglyceride levels nor the high-density lipoprotein cholesterol concentrations changed significantly with any diet. The authors concluded that enrichment of the Step 1 diet with monounsaturated fat does not alter the beneficial effects of the Step 1 diet on plasma lipid concentrations.

Insull and associates[53] from several USA medical centers conducted a 2-year randomized clinical trial to test whether free-living women aged 45 to 69 years can reduce the fat content of their diet from the typical US level of approximately 39% to 20% of energy from fat, using readily available foods, when given nutritional and behavioral counseling and social support. Three clinical units randomized 303 selected volunteers

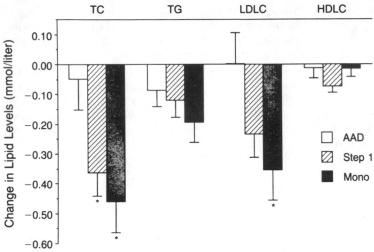

Fig. 1-9. Mean changes in plasma lipid concentrations in the three study groups. Each bar represents the mean (±SE) difference between the mean of the values obtained at weeks 4, 7, and 10 of the diet period and the mean of the values obtained at weeks 4, 6, and 9 of the control period. Asterisks indicate significant differences (P<0.025) between the changes in the average-American-diet (AAD) and Step 1 groups, and between those in the AAD and Mono groups. TC denotes total cholesterol, TG triglycerides, LDLC low-density lipoprotein cholesterol, and HDLC high-density lipoprotein cholesterol. Reproduced with permission from Ginsberg, et al.[52]

into intervention (low-fat eating plan) or control (customary diet) groups. The 2 groups were comparable at baseline. The intervention group received nutrition instruction and behavioral counseling largely in permanent groups of 12 to 15 participants meeting weekly, then biweekly, and finally monthly. At 6 months, they had substantially reduced the mean proportion of total energy from fat from 39.1% to 20.9%, compared with the control group's nonsignificant reduction from 39.0% to 38.1%. At 12 and 24 months, they sustained the reduction of energy from fat. Weight loss and plasma cholesterol level changes in the intervention group supported the self-recorded dietary intake changes. Attendance at intervention sessions averaged 75% during the first 6 months and, subsequently, 60% to 70%. Four-day food records for the randomized women were obtained at 6 and 12 months from approximately 95% and at 24 months from 87%. A clinical trial of a low-fat diet is feasible in women.

Dreon and associates[54] from Stanford and Berkeley, California, studied the effect on plasma lipoprotein of exchanging fat type within currently recommended reduced-fat diets in a free-living group of 19 men and 20 women who consumed both a polyunsaturated fat-enriched diet and a monounsaturated fat-enriched diet, each for a 12-week period, with saturated fat and cholesterol held constant. Mean plasma concentrations of LDL cholesterol and LDL total mass and HDL cholesterol and HDL total mass did not change significantly on exchanging fat type. HDL_2 cholesterol concentration, however, was 50% higher and HDL_3 cholesterol concentration was 7% lower for polyunsaturated compared with monounsaturated fat. Mean total mass of HDL_2 was also 24% higher in concentration of apolipoprotein B was 5.4% lower on transfer to the polyunsaturated fat diet. Contrary to frequent assertions, these authors found no advantage with respect to plasma HDL concentrations in using predominantly monounsaturated rather than polyunsaturated fats in subjects who consumed reduced-fat, solid-food diets.

To examine the contentious relation between diet and plasma lipids within a population, Thorogood and associates[55] from Oxford, UK, and Dunedin, New Zealand, studied a cross-sectional sample from a large prospective cohort of people eating different diets in Britain. Blood samples and diet records were collected from all subjects. The subjects were volunteers eating 1 of 4 distinct diets: vegans, vegetarians, fish eaters who did not eat meat, and meat eaters. Fifty-two subjects were selected from each group (Table 1-18). After controlling for age, sex, and body mass index, the correlation between plasma total cholesterol and the key score (which includes dietary cholesterol and saturated and polyunsaturated fat) was .37. The mean saturated fat intake in all groups was low (6–14% of energy), but polyunsaturated fat intake was high, so mean total fat intake was generally above the recommended. A high dietary fiber intake was not associated with high carbohydrate intake. Plasma HDL values were not associated with any measure of fat intake, but there was a significant correlation between HDL cholesterol values and alcohol intake. The authors concluded that the nature rather than quantity of dietary fat was an important determinant of cholesterol concentrations. Health conscious individuals, therefore, should select a fat modified, rather than a low fat-high carbohydrate diet.

The Cholesterol Lowering Atherosclerosis Study (CLAS), a randomized, placebo-controlled trial of blood lipid lowering, demonstrated significant benefit in 2-year coronary angiograms. Using angiograms of subjects in the CLAS who received a placebo and 24-hour dietary recall data, Blankenhorn and associates[56] performed an epidemiologic study of risk factors for formation of new atherosclerotic narrowings. Age and baseline plus on-trial lipid levels, BP levels, and diet variables were included. Significant dietary energy sources were protein, carbohydrate, alcohol, total fat, and polyunsaturated fat. Each quartile of increased consumption of total fat and polyunsaturated fat was associated with a significant increase in risk of new lesions. Increased intake of lauric, oleic, and linoleic acids significantly increased risk. Subjects in the Cholesterol Lowering Atherosclerosis Study in whom new lesions did not develop increased dietary protein to compensate for reduced intake of fat by substituting low-fat meats and dairy products for high-fat meats and dairy products. These results indicate that when total and saturated fat intakes

TABLE 1-18. *Mean (SE) of plasma lipid values in four diet groups by gender. Reproduced with permission from Thorogood, et al.[55]*

Diet group	Total cholesterol (mmol/l)	Low density lipoprotein cholesterol (mmol/l)	High density lipoprotein cholesterol (mmol/l)
	Men		
Vegan (Vg)	5·00 (0·15)	2·89 (0·11)	1·56 (0·05)
Vegetarian (Vt)	5·30 (0·15)	3·14 (0·15)	1·57 (0·05)
Fish eater (F)	5·59 (0·20)	3·36 (0·19)	1·64 (0·09)
Meat eater (M)	5·90 (0·18)	3·52 (0·21)	1·56 (0·07)
	Women		
Vegan (Vg)	4·84 (0·16)	2·72 (0·13)	1·62 (0·06)
Vegetarian (Vt)	5·38 (0·16)	3·19 (0·15)	1·68 (0·06)
Fish eater (F)	5·71 (0·19)	3·56 (0·21)	1·85 (0·13)
Meat eater (M)	5·95 (0·20)	3·79 (0·18)	1·73 (0·08)
	Analysis of variance		
Among men (p)	0·003	0·047	NS
Significant difference	Vg<M	None	None
Among women (p)	<0·001	p<0·001	NS
Significant difference	Vg<F, M	Vg<F, M	None

are reduced to levels recommended by the National Cholesterol Education Program, protein and carbohydrate are preferred substitutes for fat calories, rather than monounsaturated or polyunsaturated fat.

Barnard[57] from Los Angeles, California, reported the changes in serum lipid levels achieved by 2,685 men and 1,902 women who attended a residential program at the Pritikin Longevity Center between 1977 and 1988. This lifestyle modification program consisted of a diet high in complex carbohydrates, high in fiber, low in fat and low in cholesterol, combined with daily aerobic exercise, primarily walking. The diet provided 35 to 40 g of dietary fiber per 1,000 kcal with less than 4 g of sodium chloride per day. Less than 10% of total calories were derived from fat (ratio of polyunsaturated to saturated fat = 2.4), 15% from protein, and the remainder from carbohydrate (90% unrefined). Cholesterol intake was before 25 mg per day. During the 3-week program, 99% of the participants reduced their serum total cholesterol levels (Figure 1-10). Reductions ranged from a high of 51% in 1 person to no change in a few who entered the program with cholesterol levels less than 3.9 mmol/l (150 mg/dl). As shown in the figure, total and LDL cholesterol levels decreased an average of 23% and triglyceride levels by an average of 33%. The HDL cholesterol level was reduced by 16%, but the ratio of total cholesterol to HDL cholesterol was reduced 11%, from 5.7 ± .04 to 5.1 ± .03. By the end of the program, 74% of the participants had a cholesterol level below that rec-

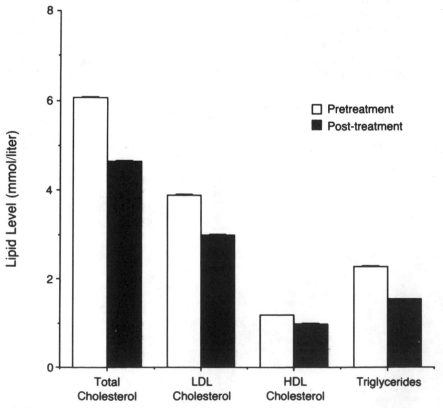

Fig. 1-10. Changes in serum lipid levels in 4587 adults during a three-week lifestyle-intervention program. Values and means ± SE for all post-treatment values were significantly reduced from pretreatment values (P<0.001). Reproduced with permission from Barnard, et al.[57]

ommended by the National Cholesterol Education Program. These results indicate that most persons can substantially lower their serum lipid levels through lifestyle modification.

In a prospective, randomized, controlled trial to determine whether comprehensive lifestyle changes affect coronary atherosclerosis after 1 year, Ornish and associates[58] from San Francisco, California, and Houston, Texas, and Richmond, Virginia, assigned 28 patients to an experimental group (low-fat vegetarian diet, stopping cigarette smoking, stress management training, and moderate exercise) and 20 to a usual-care control group (Figure 1-11; Tables 1-19 and 1-20). One-hundred ninety-five coronary artery lesions were analyzed by quantitative coronary angiography. The average percentage diameter stenosis regressed from 40 (SD 17)% to 38 (17)% in the experimental group yet progressed from 43 (16)% to 46

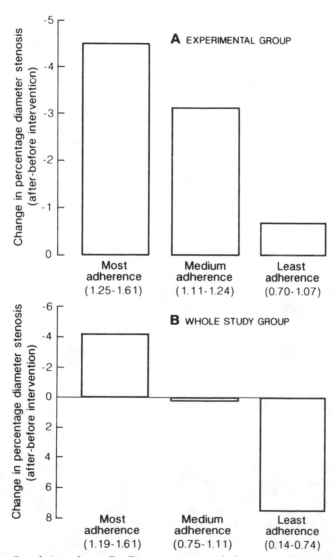

Fig. 1-11. Correlation of overall adherence score and changes in percentage diameter stenosis in experimental group only (A) and in whole study group (B). A = 7 subjects in each tertile; B = 13, 14, 13. Reproduced with permission from Ornish, et al.[58]

TABLE 1-19. *Compliance with exercise, stress management, and dietary changes. Reproduced with permission from Ornish, et al.*[58]

—	Mean (SD) at baseline		Mean (SD) at 12 mo		p (two-sided)
	Experimental (n = 20–22)	Control (n = 17–19)	Experimental (n = 20–22)	Control (n = 17–19)	
Exercise					
Times/day	0·26 (0·37)	0·35 (0·39)	0·69 (0·20)	0·39 (0·37)	0·0008
Min/day	11·0 (17·7)	18·4 (27·7)	38·1 (17·4)	20·6 (27·7)	0·0004
Stress reduction					
Times/day	0·50 (1·21)	0·16 (0·34)	5·94 (2·62)	0·42 (0·74)	<0·0001
Min/day	5·09 (12·7)	1·76 (4·34)	82·1 (36·6)	4·50 (10·2)	<0·0001
Fat intake					
g/day	67·4 (18·6)	58·2 (25·9)	14·0 (8·6)	55·2 (21·1)	<0·0001
% of energy intake	31·5 (7·6)	30·1 (10·7)	6·8 (3·5)	29·5 (8·6)	<0·0001
Dietary cholesterol (mg/day)	213 (111)	205 (127)	12·4 (45·8)	190 (99)	<0·0001
Energy intake (MJ/day)	8·2 (1·8)	7·2 (2·2)	7·6 (2·1)	7·1 (1·9)	0·5082
Total adherence score*	0·55 (0·22)	0·56 (0·30)	1·22 (0·22)	0·62 (0·30)	<0·0001

*Percentage of minimum recommended level of combined lifestyle change; includes all the above plus smoking cessation.

TABLE 1-20. *Changes in risk factors. Reproduced with permission from Ornish, et al.*[58]

—	Mean (SD) at baseline		Mean (SD) at 12 mo		p p (two-sided)
	Experimental group (n = 20–22)	Control group (n = 17–19)	Experimental group (n = 20–22)	Control group (n = 17–19)	
Serum lipids (mmol/l)					
Total cholesterol	5·88 (1·29)	6·34 (1·02)	4·45 (1·15)	6·00 (1·55)	0·0192
LDL cholesterol	3·92 (1·25)	4·32 (0·77)	2·46 (1·55)	4·07 (1·17)	0·0072
HDL cholesterol	1·00 (0·26)	1·35 (0·52)	0·97 (0·40)	1·31 (0·38)	0·8316
Triglycerides	2·38 (1·26)	2·45 (2·47)	2·91 (1·47)	2·24 (1·79)	0·2472
Apolipoproteins (mg/dl)					
A-I	133 (21)	156 (36)	135 (26)	166 (47)	0·4612
B	104 (33)	104 (21)	79 (23)	105 (28)	0·0104
Lipid ratios					
Total/HDL cholesterol	6·33 (2·14)	5·32 (1·89)	5·15 (2·23)	4·93 (1·59)	0·1734
LDL/HDL cholesterol	4·18 (1·53)	3·59 (1·37)	2·89 (1·92)	3·33 (1·42)	0·0348
Blood pressure (mm Hg)					
Systolic	134 (13)	140 (26)	127 (13)	131 (20)	0·7550
Diastolic	83 (8)	82 (13)	79 (7)	77 (11)	0·8987
Weight (kg)	91·1 (15·5)	80·4 (22·8)	81·0 (11·4)	81·8 (25·0)	<0·0001

(19)% in the control group. When only lesions greater than 50% stenosed were analyzed, the average percentage diameter stenosis regressed from 61 (9)% to 56 (11)% in the experimental group and progressed from 62 (10%) to 64 (16)% in the control group. Overall, 82% of experimental-group patients had an average change towards regression. Comprehensive lifestyle changes may be able to bring about regression of even severe coronary atherosclerosis after only 1 year, without use of lipid-lowering drugs.

Psyllium hydrophilic mucilloid vs cellulose

Levin and associates[59] from Washington, D.C., and Cincinnati, Ohio, compared the effects of the administration of 5.1 g of psyllium or placebo (cellulose) twice daily for 16 weeks as adjuncts to a prudent diet in the management of moderate hypercholesterolemia in 96 male and female subjects aged 21 to 70 years with plasma total cholesterol levels >200 mg/dl (>5.17 mmol/l) and lower than the 90th percentile for subject age and sex; plasma triglyceride levels <3.39 mmol/l; and body weight <30% above ideal after an 8-week diet stabilization period. The study was a parallel double-blind one. Psyllium decreased the total cholesterol level by 6% and the LDL cholesterol level by 9%, whereas the levels were unchanged in the placebo group (Figure 1-12). The HDL cholesterol level decreased during the diet stabilization period in both groups and returned to near baseline levels by week 16. Plasma triglyceride levels did not change substantially in either group. Subject compliance to treatment

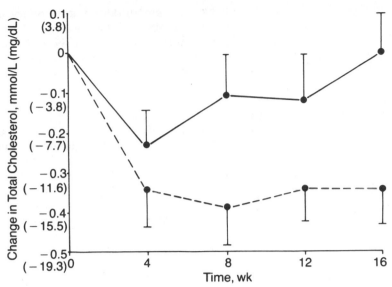

Fig. 1-12. Effects of psyllium and placebo (cellulose) on total plasma cholesterol levels. The change in total cholesterol levels after the diet stabilization period is shown for psyllium (broken line) and cellulose (solid line) for the 16-week treatment period. Each value represents the mean ± SD change in total cholesterol level. Reproduced with permission from Levin, et al.[59]

was greater than 95%. These data suggest that psyllium hydrophilic mucilloid in a twice daily regimen may be a useful and safe adjunct to a prudent diet in the treatment of moderate hypercholesterolemia.

Fish-oil supplements

Fish oil has consistently been shown to lower triglyceride levels, but its effects on LDL cholesterol remain controversial. Reis and associates[60] from Boston, Massachusetts, compared the long-term effects of 2 different fish oil preparations (ethyl ester and triglyceride) versus olive oil in patients with CAD. Eighty-nine subjects were randomly assigned to receive capsules containing 6 g/day (triglyceride group) or 7 g/day (ethyl ester group) of n–3 fatty acids, or capsules containing 12 g/day of olive oil for 6 months. Mean triglyceride levels decreased by 28% in the ester and 32% in the triglyceride fish oil groups. LDL cholesterol levels increased by 3% (difference not significant) in the ester and 12% in the triglyceride fish oil groups; in hypertriglyceridemic subjects the increase was 23% and 14% (difference not significant), respectively. Plasma phospholipid fatty acid analysis showed a fivefold increase in eicosapentaenoic acid levels in both fish oil groups, and a long-term decrease in arachidonic acid levels. Achieved eicoarachidonic acid level correlated with the degree of increase in LDL cholesterol (r = 0.38). These data suggest that fish oil administration is associated with an increase in LDL cholesterol levels in a diverse group of patients with CAD; this change appears to be correlated with n–3 fatty acid absorption. The impact of this increase in LDL is unknown, but should be considered as potentially adverse.

Estrogen replacement

Sullivan and associates[61] from Memphis, Tennessee, examined the relation among postmenopausal estrogen use, coronary artery stenosis, and survival retrospectively in 2,268 women undergoing coronary angiography. The patients were selected for study if their age was 55 years or older at the time of angiography or if they had previously undergone bilateral oophorectomy. Postmenopausal estrogen use in 1,178 patients with CAD (70% stenosis) and 644 patients with mild to moderate CAD (5% to 69% stenosis) was compared with 446 control subjects (9% stenosis) using life-table analysis. Over 10 years of follow-up, there was no significant difference in survival among patients initially free of coronary lesions on arteriography who had either never used (n = 377) or ever used (n = 69) estrogens. Among patients with mild to moderate coronary stenosis, 10-year survival of those who had never used estrogens was 85% and it was 96% among 99 "ever users." Survival was 60% among those with more than 70% coronary stenosis who had never used estrogen and it was 97% among 70 ever users. The "never users" group were older (65 vs 59 years), had a lower proportion of cigarette smokers (40% vs 57%), a higher proportion of subjects with diabetes (22% vs 13%) and hyperlipidemia (58% vs 44%), and approximately equal numbers of hypertensives (56% vs 54%). Cox's proportional hazards model was used to estimate survival as a function of multiple covariables. Estrogen use was found to have a significant, independent effect on survival in women. The authors concluded that estrogen replacement after menopause prolongs survival when CAD is present, but it has less effect in the absence of CAD.

Prescriptions of lipid-lowering drugs in the USA

Wysowski and associates[62] from Rockville, Maryland, used data from 2 pharmaceutical marketing research databases, the National Prescription Audit and the National Disease and Therapeutic Index, to study trends and outpatient use of cholesterol-lowering drugs in the USA from 1978 through 1988. Retail pharmacies dispensed an estimated 4.4 million prescriptions for cholesterol-lowering drugs in 1978 (Figure 1-13; Table 1-21). This declined to 2.6 million in 1983 and increased dramatically to nearly 13 million in 1988 (Table 1-22). This 5-fold increase between 1983 and 1988 was accounted for primarily by the introduction and use of 2 new drugs, gemfibrozil and lovastatin, and, to a lesser extent, by the increasing use of some older drugs. In 1988, after 1 full year of marketing, lovastatin was the leading cholesterol-lowering drug, followed closely by gemfibrozil; both drugs are currently considered second-line agents. Clofibrate and dextrothyroxine, drugs that ranked first and second in 1978, declined to ranks of 6th and 8th out of 8 in 1988. Cholestyramine, gemfibrozil, and lovastatin accounted for about 75% of all lipid-lowering prescriptions in 1988. From 1978 through 1988, an average 54% of individuals using cholesterol-lowering drugs were 60 years of age or older. The 13 million prescriptions for cholesterol-lowering drugs in 1988 represent a maximum estimate of 13 million treated individuals. This number compares with the 60 million Americans with high cholesterol levels who are candidates for dietary advice, and, if cholesterol levels do not improve, for combined diet and drug intervention.

Nicotinic acid

Nicotinic acid has been recommended as a first-line hypolipidemic drug. To determine the effectiveness of nicotinic acid in dyslipidemic patients with non-insulin-dependent diabetes mellitus, Garg and Grundy[63]

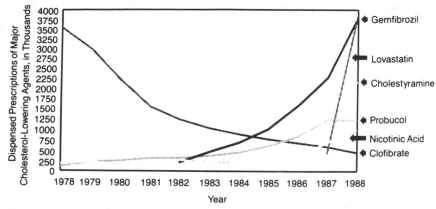

Fig. 1-13. Estimated number of dispensed prescriptions of major cholesterol-lowering medications from 1978 through 1988 in the United States. These data are from the National Prescription Audit and do not include over-the-counter use of nicotinic acid. The following major clinical trial results and guidelines influenced trends in use: reports from the Coronary Drug Project in 1972, 1975, and 1986; reports from the World Health Organization Cooperative Trial in 1978 and 1984; a report from the Lipid Research Clinics-Coronary Primary Prevention Trial in 1984, the 1985 guidelines from the National Institutes of Health Consensus Development Conference on Lowering Blood Cholesterol; a report from the Helsinki Heart Study in 1987; and the 1988 guidelines of the National Cholesterol Education Program Expert Panel on Detection, Evaluation, and Treatment. Reproduced with permission from Wysowski, et al.[62]

TABLE 1-21. *Dispensed prescriptions for cholesterol-lowering medications in the United States.* Reproduced with permission from Wysowski, et al.[62]

Generic Name	Trade Name(s)	Date Marketed	Dispensed Prescriptions for Cholesterol-Lowering Medications					
			1978		1983		1988	
			No. (%)†	Rank	No. (%)†	Rank	No. (%)†	Rank
Bile acid sequestrants								
Cholestyramine	Questran	1967‡	177 (4.0)	3	261 (10.2)	4	2206 (17.1)	3
Colestipol	Colestid	1977	12 (0.3)	6	52 (2.0)	7	290 (2.2)	7
Fibric acid derivatives								
Clofibrate	Atromid-S	1967	3555 (80.9)	1	1049 (41.2)	1	452 (3.5)	6
Gemfibrozil	Lopid	1982	. . .		462 (18.1)	2	3788 (29.4)	2
HMG CoA reductase inhibitor§								
Lovastatin	Mevacor	1987	. . .		. . .		3835 (29.7)	1
Others								
Nicotinic acid‖	Nicobid, Nicolar, Niacin	1974	168 (3.8)	4	204 (8.0)	5	1019 (7.9)	5
Probucol	Lorelco	1977	94 (2.1)	5	366 (14.4)	3	1261 (9.8)	4
Dextrothyroxine	Choloxin	1967	390 (8.9)	2	155 (6.1)	6	49 (0.4)	8
Total	. . .	. . .	4396 (100.0)		2549 (100.0)		12 900 (100.0)	

*These data are from the National Prescription Audit.
†These values are given in thousands.
‡Approved for use as a cholesterol-lowering agent in 1973.
§HMG CoA indicates 3-hydroxy-3-methylglutaryl coenzyme A.
‖These values do not include over-the-counter use.

from Dallas, Texas, treated 13 patients in a randomized cross-over trial. Patients received either nicotinic acid (1.5 g 3 times daily) or no therapy (control period) for 8 weeks each. Compared with the control period, nicotinic acid therapy reduced the plasma total cholesterol level by 24%, plasma triglyceride level by 45%, VLDL cholesterol level by 58%, and LDL cholesterol level by 15%, and it increased the HDL cholesterol level by 34%. However, nicotinic acid therapy resulted in the deterioration of glycemic control, as evidenced by a 16% increase in mean plasma glucose concentrations, a 21% increase in glycosylated hemoglobin levels, and the induction of marked glycosuria in some patients. Furthermore, a consistent increase in plasma uric acid levels was observed. Therefore,

TABLE 1-22. *Characteristics of individuals using and physicians prescribing cholesterol-lowering drugs.* Reproduced with permission from Wysowski, et al.*[62]

Characteristic	1978	1988	1978 Through 1988 Average
	Patients		
Age (y), %			
<20	2	1	3
20-39	3	7	6
40-59	36	34	37
≥60	60	59	54
Sex, %			
M	50	39	48
F	48	55	48
Unspecified	2	7	4
Therapy, %			
New	16	24	20
Continued	84	76	80
Concomitant drug use, %			
Used alone†	59	77	66
Coronary vasodilator and nitrites/nitrates	8	0	5
Diuretics	6	1	4
Other antihypertensives	6	8	7
Cholesterol reducers	0	10	6
	Physicians		
Physician specialty, %			
Internal medicine	39	40	40
General/family practice	37	26	28
Cardiology	9	16	13
Osteopathy	6	8	7
Gastroenterology	2	3	4
General surgery	4	3	3
Pediatrics	2	1	2
All others	1	3	3

*These data are from the National Disease and Therapeutic Index.
†For the primary indication mentioned.

despite improvement in lipid and lipoprotein concentrations, because of worsening hyperglycemia and the development of hyperuricemia, nicotinic acid must be used with caution in patients with non-insulin-dependent diabetes mellitus with dyslipidemia. The authors suggest that the drug not be used as a first-line hypolipidemic drug in patients with non-insulin-dependent diabetes mellitus.

Niacin (nicotinic acid) is available in several forms, including crystalline preparations and various types of sustained-release preparations. Evidence exists that sustained-release niacin, with respect to both the dosage and severity, is more hepatotoxic than crystalline niacin. Henkin and associates[64] from Birmingham, Alabama, and Baltimore, Maryland, described 3 patients who developed hepatitis during treatment with sustained-release niacin and were rechallenged with equivalent or higher doses of crystalline niacin and developed no evidence of recurring hepatocellular damage. Although the mechanism for niacin-induced hepatitis is unknown, these cases support previous observations that crystalline niacin may be less hepatotoxic than sustained-release preparations in certain patients.

Lovastatin

Many patients with high levels of serum total cholesterol have a concomitant elevation of serum triglyceride levels and thus have mixed hyperlipidemia. Vega and Grundy[65] from Dallas, Texas, treated 13 patients with mixed hyperlipidemia with the cholesterol lowering drug lovastatin to determine its effectiveness. In 9 of these patients, lovastatin therapy used alone was compared with the drug combination of lovastatin and gemfibrozil. In the 13 patients, lovastatin therapy produced a 31% reduction in total cholesterol level and a 32% decrease in triglyceride levels compared with placebo (Table 1-23). It lowered very-low-density plus intermediate-density lipoprotein cholesterol levels by 40%, LDL cholesterol levels by 36%, and total apolipoprotein B levels by 28%. Concentrations of HDL cholesterol and apolipoprotein A-1 were unchanged, but total cholesterol (and LDL cholesterol)/HDL cholesterol ratios were markedly reduced. Compared with lovastatin alone, lovastatin plus gemfibrozil produced greater decreases in very-low-density plus intermediate-density lipoprotein cholesterol levels and an increase in HDL cholesterol levels, but, in view of the higher risk for severe myopathy with this combination, lovastatin used alone may be adequate therapy for many patients with mixed hyperlipidemia.

Bates and associates[66] from Lexington, Kentucky, reviewed the progress of 56 consecutive patients with types 2A and 2B hyperlipoproteinemia following treatment with a 20 mg a day dose of lovastatin in 56 patients with known CAD studied prospectively and with fasting lipid values being measured at baseline and after 6, 12, 18, and 24 weeks of a 20 mg per day lovastatin therapy given as a single evening dose. The total serum cholesterol fell 26% from a mean baseline of 8.12 mmol/l (314 mg/dL) and triglyceride levels fell by 12% from a mean baseline of 2.46 mmol/L (Figure 1-14). The HDL levels increased 7.6%. One patient with known preexisting liver disease was withdrawn from the study owing to an asymptomatic significant rise in liver function test results; one subject

TABLE 1-23. *Effect of combined therapy on plasma lipids, lipoprotein cholesterol, and plasma apolipoproteins B and A-I (n = 9).* Reproduced with permission from Vega, et al.[65]

| Variable | Concentration, mmol/L (mg/dL) (±SEM) | | |
	Placebo	Lovastatin	Lovastatin and Gemfibrozil
Total cholesterol	· 7.55 ± 0.28 (292 ± 11)	5.22 ± 0.26† (202 ± 10)	4.94 ± 0.31 (191 ± 12)
Triglyceride	5.48 ± 0.54 (485 ± 48)	3.79 ± 0.42† (336 ± 37)	2.08 ± 0.26†‡ (184 ± 23)
VLDL cholesterol	2.95 ± 0.2 (114 ± 9)	1.8 ± 0.2† (70 ± 8)	0.88 ± 0.2†‡ (34 ± 7)
LDL cholesterol	3.83 ± 0.31 (148 ± 12)	2.5 ± 0.2† (97 ± 9)	2.97 ± 0.26† (115 ± 10)
HDL cholesterol	0.72 ± 0.05 (28 ± 2)	0.80 ± 0.08 (31 ± 3)	0.98 ± 0.2§ (38 ± 6)
Apolipoprotein B‖	(149 ± 10)	(108 ± 8†)	(98 ± 9†)
Apolipoprotein A-I‖	(83 ± 9)	(85 ± 6)	(111 ± 7§)

*VLDL indicates very-low-density lipoprotein; LDL, low-density lipoprotein; and HDL, high-density lipoprotein.
†Significantly lower than placebo (*P*<.05).
‡Significantly lower than lovastatin (*P*<.05).
§Significantly higher than placebo and lovastatin (*P*<.05).
‖These values are in mg/dL only.

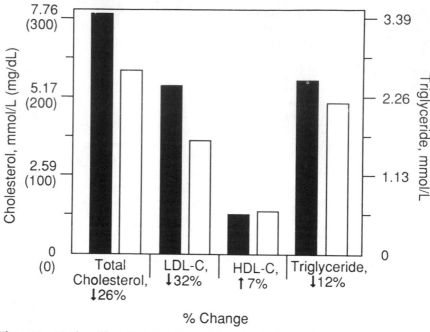

Fig. 1-14. Lipid profiles of total cholesterol, low-density lipoprotein cholesterol (LDL-C), high-density lipoprotein cholesterol (HDL-C), and triglyceride before (solid bars) and after (open bars) treatment with lovastatin. Only HDL-C value did not change significantly. Reproduced with permission from Levin, et al.[59]

complaining of proximal muscle weakness was also withdrawn. The maximal decrease in total cholesterol level occurred within 6 weeks of initiation of therapy (Figure 1-15). The authors concluded that low-dose (20 mg per day) lovastatin was effective in lowering serum cholesterol levels in patients with primary type 11a or 11b hyperlipoproteinemia with minimal short-term side effects. Further studies are needed to establish the long-term safety and effectiveness of this drug.

Laties and associates[67] from Philadelphia, Pennsylvania, and Baltimore, Maryland, and West Point, Pennsylvania, and Research Triangle Park, North Carolina, analyzed frequency of lens opacity and visual acuity after 48 weeks of lovastatin or placebo in 8,245 patients treated with lovastatin for 48 weeks plus a cholesterol lowering diet when participating in a 362-center, randomized, double-blind, placebo-controlled, parallel study lasting 48 weeks. The study design and base-line characteristics of the patients were described in an article in the American Journal of Cardiology in 1990. In brief, 5 groups, each composed of approximately 1,650 patients, received placebo or 20 mg of lovastatin once daily, 20 mg twice daily, 40 mg once daily, or 40 mg twice daily. The average age of the patients was 56 years (range 21–75), 59% were men, and 57% had cardiovascular disease. At baseline and after 24 and 48 weeks, the lens of each eye was assessed by slit-lamp examination (after dilation of the pupil to >6 mm); best-corrected visual acuity was also determined. Lens opacities were recorded with a standardized and reliable grading system of severity in 6 categories. From 79 to 82% of the patients in each group completed the study and provided sufficient data for analysis. The lens characteristics and changes in patients not included in the analysis were similar among treatment groups. Analyses of the distribution of cortical,

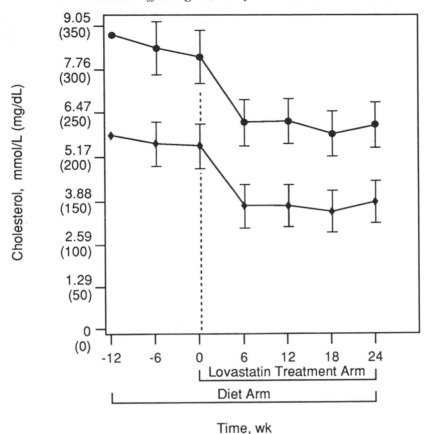

Fig. 1-15. The maximal fall in total cholesterol (circles) and low-density lipoprotein cholesterol (diamonds) values occurred by 6 weeks of treatment and then reached a plateau. Reproduced with permission from Bates, et al.[56]

nuclear, and subcapsular grades at 48 weeks showed no significant difference between the placebo and lovastatin groups. In patients without posterior subcapsular opacities at base line (92% of the sample), 97% of those in the placebo group and 96 to 98% of those in the lovastatin groups had no opacities after 48 weeks. In patients with a posterior subcapsular opacity at base line, the distribution of grades after 48 weeks also was similar in the placebo and lovastatin groups. Thus, these authors found no evidence of an effect of lovastatin on the human lens after 48 weeks of treatment.

Earnest Schaefer reported in 1988 (New England Journal of Medicine 319:1222) 9 (18%) of 51 patients taking lovastatin by prescription had decreased sleep of 1 to 3 hours compared to none of 33 patients receiving another 3-hydroxy-3-methylglutaryl coenzyme A (HMG CoA) reductase inhibitor, pravastatin, in a clinical trial. Black and associates[68] from Cincinnati, Ohio, assessed the prevalence of sleep disorders more systematically using a standard questionnaire in 409 hyperlipidemic patients (67% male) being treated by diet alone (n = 102), receiving 3 different types of HMG CoA reductase inhibitors (lovastatin [n = 161], simvastatin [n = 47], and pravastatin [n = 45]), or receiving non-HMG CoA reductase-inhibiting lipid-lowering agents (n = 54), gemfibrozil, niacin, and bile acid sequestrants. A standard questionnaire assessed the days during the past 30 on which subjects experienced trouble falling asleep, woke up several times per night, had trouble staying asleep, and woke up after their usual amount of sleep feeling tired and worn out. Analysis compared subjects experiencing no problems with those experiencing any problems. The results were as follows. (1) Falling asleep: analysis of subjects receiving lovastatin, simvastatin, pravastatin, or treatment by diet alone showed women had more problems than men, irrespective of whether they were treated with diet only or with medication. Analysis of the subjects taking lovastatin compared with those treated with diet alone revealed no significant differences. Among those subjects treated with diet, HMG CoA reductase inhibitor, or non-HMG CoA reductase inhibitor, the non-HMG CoA reductase inhibitor group had more problems falling asleep. (2) For the other 3 sleep categories, no significant differences were seen between the diet group and any of the HMB CoA reductase inhibitor groups individually or combined, or for those receiving non-HMG CoA reductase inhibitor. Similarly, comparison of diet only and lovastatin failed to reveal any differences. No sex differences were detected, except for awaking tired and worn out, where women, again, experienced more problems. In conclusion, this study, like others, indicates that insomnia is an extremely common problem in adults with greater prevalence in women. Therefore, studies assessing sleep disorders should be controlled for sex and age and include nontreated controls as well as prospective, double-blind design. To date, no report that indicates sleep alterations with lovastatin or simvastatin fulfill these requirements. The present study suggests that the prevalence of significant sleep disturbances in subjects taking lovastatin is not different from that in subjects treated with diet alone, other types of HMG CoA reductase inhibitors, or non-HMG CoA reductase inhibitors.

Lovastatin + colestipol vs Niacin + colestipol

The effect of intensive lipid-lowering therapy on coronary atherosclerosis among men at high risk of cardiovascular events was assessed by quantitative arteriography by Brown and associates[69] from Seattle, Washington. Of 146 men no more than 62 years of age who had apolipoprotein B levels >125 mg/dl documented CAD, and a family history of vascular disease, 120 completed the 2.5-year double-blind study, which included arteriography at base line and after treatment (Table 1-24). Patients were given dietary counseling and were randomly assigned to 1 of 3 treatments: lovastatin (20 mg twice a day) and colestipol (10 g 3 times a day); niacin (1 g 4 times a day) and colestipol (10 g 3 times a day); or conventional therapy with placebo (or colestipol if the LDL cholesterol level was elevated). The levels of LDL and HDL cholesterol changed only slightly in the conventional-therapy group (mean changes, −7 and +5%, respectively), but more substantially among patients treated with lovastatin and colestipol (−46 and +15%) or niacin and colestipol (−32 and +43%) (Table 1-25). In the conventional-therapy group, 46% of the patients had definite lesion progression (and no regression) in at least 1 of 9 proximal coronary segments; regression was the only change in 11%. By comparison, progression (as the only change) was less frequent among patients who received lovastatin and colestipol (21%) and those who received niacin and colestipol (15%) and those who received niacin and colestipol (15%), and regression was more frequent (lovastatin and colestipol, 32%; niacin and colestipol, 39%). Multivariate analysis indicated that a reduction in the level of apolipoprotein B (or LDL cholesterol) and in systolic BP, and an increase in HDL cholesterol correlated indepen-

TABLE 1-24. *Base-line risk factors among patients who did and did not complete the study. Reproduced with permission from Brown, et al.*[69]

VARIABLE	COMPLETED STUDY			DID NOT COMPLETE STUDY (N = 26)
	CONVENTIONAL THERAPY (N = 46)	LOVASTATIN– COLESTIPOL (N = 38)	NIACIN– COLESTIPOL (N = 36)	
Mean age (yr)	47	48	47	44
History of high blood pressure (%)	28	34	44	38
History of smoking (%)	72	74	92	85
Current smoking (%)	26	23	22	38
Cigarettes/day*	26	17	15	19
Pack-years*	41	25	28	46
Type A score (percentile)†	49	47	55	—
Body-mass index‡	26	27	27	27
Premature-disease index (father/mother)§	0.40/0.36	0.36/0.34	0.40/0.38	0.46/0.37
Previous myocardial infarction (%)	40	42	50	54
Angina at entry (%)	67	63	72	88
Positive exercise-tolerance test (≥2 mm) (%)	45	54	58	67
Mean % proximal stenosis¶	30	36	36	34
Mean no. of proximal lesions causing ≥50% stenosis	1.4	1.6	1.7	1.7

*Smokers only.

†From Jenkins Activity Survey, Harcourt Brace Jovanovich.

‡The weight in kilograms divided by the square of the height in meters.

§Proportion of first-degree relatives of the patient's father and mother who had premature cardiovascular disease.

¶Average of the most severe stenosis in each of nine proximal segments.

dently with regression of coronary lesions. Clinical events (death, myocardial infarction, or revascularization for worsening symptoms) occurred in 10 of 52 patients assigned to conventional therapy, as compared with 3 of 46 assigned to receive lovastatin and colestipol and 2 of 48 assigned to receive niacin and colestipol. In men with CAD who were at high risk for cardiovascular events, intensive lipid-lowering therapy reduced the frequency of progression of coronary lesions, increased the frequency of regression, and reduced the incidence of cardiovascular events.

Lovastatin + gemfibrozil

The Food and Drug Administration documents the receipt of 12 case reports of severe myopathy or rhabdomyolysis associated with concomitant use of lovastatin and gemfibrozil, including 10 voluntary postmarketing, and 2 required reports, and these cases were summarized by

TABLE 1-25. *Lipid and lipoprotein levels before, during, and after therapy, according to treatment group. Reproduced with permission from Brown, et al.*[69]

Index	Conventional Therapy (N = 46)			Lovastatin–Colestipol (N = 38)			Niacin–Colestipol (N = 36)		
	At Base Line	During Therapy	After Therapy	At Base Line	During Therapy	After Therapy	At Base Line	During Therapy	After Therapy
Cholesterol (mmol/liter)*									
Total	6.79	6.55	7.15	7.12	4.71†	7.59	6.99	5.41†	7.56
VLDL	1.24	1.30	1.37	1.19	0.93†	1.14	1.09	0.60†	1.06
LDL	4.53	4.20‡	4.66	5.08	2.77†	5.39	4.92	3.34†	5.31
HDL	0.98	1.04‡	1.09	0.91	1.06§	1.04	1.01	1.42†	5.31
HDL$_2$	0.11	0.11	0.18	0.08	0.13§	0.11	0.11	0.34†	0.16
Triglyceride (mmol/liter)¶									
Total	2.59	2.98	3.02	2.27	2.07	2.37	2.19	1.55†	2.35
VLDL	2.09	2.05	2.21	1.85	1.62	1.80	1.63	1.14†	1.77
Other lipoproteins (mg/dl)									
Lp(a) lipoprotein	41.1	36.4‡	38.6	33.4	30.1	31.3	32.6	24.2§	29.4
Apolipoproteins (mg/dl)									
B	149	142†	144	159	103†	162	155	111†	160
A-I	132	131	126	129	138§	127	132	151§	138
A-II	30.0	29.8	29.4	28.5	28.1	28.8	29.8	28.0‡	31.3

*To convert cholesterol values to milligrams per deciliter, multiply by 38.6.   †P<0.001 for the comparison with the base-line value, by paired t-test.

‡P<0.05 for the comparison with the base-line value, by paired t-test.

§P<0.01 for the comparison with the base-line value, by paired t-test.   ¶To convert triglyceride values to milligrams per deciliter, multiply by 88.5.

Pierce and associates[70] in Rockville, Maryland. All patients had serum creatine kinase levels of more than 10,000 U/L, 4 tested showed myoglobinuria, and 5 had acute renal failure. The patients' symptoms resolved when both drugs were discontinued. For the first year of marketing of lovastatin, spontaneous reports of myopathy with documentation of creatine kinase level were reviewed for the use of lovastatin, gemfibrozil, and combination therapy. The median creatine kinase level in reports involving concomitant lovastatin and gemfibrozil use was 15,250 U/L, 20 times that in reports with gemfibrozil use alone and 30 times that in reports with lovastatin use alone. Because of the potential for severe myopathy and life-threatening rhabdomyolysis, and given alternative drug combinations for treating hyperlipoproteinemia, the use of lovastatin in combination with gemfibrozil is to be discouraged.

Lovastatin vs gemfibrozil

A common pattern of dyslipidemia is elevated levels of plasma triglyceride, borderline high total cholesterol, reduced HDL cholesterol, and increased apolipoprotein B. This pattern of dyslipidemia frequently is associated with premature CAD. Nicotinic acid is the drug of first choice for this pattern. Vega and Grundy[71] from Dallas, Texas, compared gemfibrozil and lovastatin for their effects on the overall lipoprotein profile in 13 men with this type of dyslipidemia. Both drugs significantly reduced VLDL and intermediate density lipoprotein cholesterol levels, and both modestly raised HDL cholesterol levels. Gemfibrozil therapy, however, failed to reduce total cholesterol or total apolipoprotein B levels, whereas lovastatin therapy lowered levels of total cholesterol by 28%, LDL cholesterol by 33%, and total apolipoprotein B by 32%. Moreover, lovastatin therapy caused greater declines in lipoprotein cholesterol ratios than did gemfibrozil therapy. Lovastatin thus seems to have certain advantages over gemfibrozil for treatment of elevated plasma triglyceride levels accompanied by borderline high total cholesterol and raised apolipoprotein B levels. Therefore, lovastatin therapy should be considered as a primary approach for management of this condition.

Simvastatin ± cholestyramine

Stein and associates[72] from several USA medical centers compared simvastatin, a potent inhibitor of 3-hydroxy-3-methylglutaryl coenzyme

A reductase, with cholestyramine resin in a randomized open-label 12-week multicenter study of 251 high-risk patients with familial or nonfamilial hypercholesterolemia. Simvastatin, 20 mg and 40 mg daily, produced mean reductions in total cholesterol of 26% and 33%, respectively, and reductions in LDL cholesterol level of 32% and 40%. Cholestyramine resin, 4 to 12 g twice daily, reduced total cholesterol and LDL cholesterol levels 15% and 21%, respectively. HDL cholesterol levels were increased 8% to 10% by all treatments. Plasma triglyceride levels were moderately decreased by simvastatin treatment, while triglyceride levels increased with cholestyramine treatment (Table 1-26). Simvastatin was better tolerated than cholestyramine, which had numerous gastrointestinal tract side effects. No patient had a serious drug-related adverse event.

Emmerich and associates[73] from St. Mande, France, investigated the effects and safety of simvastatin, an inhibitor of 3-hydroxy-3-methylglutaryl coenzyme A reductase, alone and combined with cholestyramine in 66 patients with type IIa (43 patients) or type IIb (23 patients) hypercholesterolemia in a 1-year study. In 30 patients the LDL cholesterol ranged from 190 to 300 mg/dl (4.9–7.7 mmol/l) and in 36 patients the LDL cholesterol was ≥300 mg/dl. In the type IIb subjects the plasma triglyceride levels were >150 mg/dl (>1.71 mmol/l), but they were below 400 mg/dl (<4.56 mmol/l). The subjects ranged in age from 22 to 72 years.[44] The dose of simvastatin was 40 mg once a day before dinner and cholestyramine was added to simvastatin if the LDL cholesterol level remained above 190 mg/dl. A total of 39 patients were treated with simvastatin alone and 37 patients received simvastatin plus cholestyramine (8 g twice daily before breakfast and lunch). In the type IIa patients (41 patients)

TABLE 1-26. *Mean percentage change at 12 weeks.* Reproduced with permission from Stein, et al.*[72]

| | | % Change | | |
| | | Simvastatin | | |
	Baseline (n = 250)	20 mg Every Night (n = 84)	40 mg Every Night (n = 81)	Cholestyramine Resin (n = 85)
Total cholesterol, mmol/L	8.33	−26.5†‡	−32.7†‡	−14.8†
LDL cholesterol, mmol/L	6.34	−32.3†‡	−40.5†‡	−21.1†
HDL cholesterol, mmol/L	1.16	9.5†	10.0†	7.9†
LDL-C/HDL-C ratio	5.8	−36.3†‡	−45.3†‡	−24.7†
Median VLDL, mmol/L	0.65	−7.6	−27.9‡§	7.0
APO B, g/L	1.894	−28.1†	−35.8†‡	−23.6†
APO A-I, g/L	1.37	2.7	2.0	6.0§
Triglycerides, mmol/L	1.87	−13.0†‡	−21.0†‡	15.3†

*LDL indicates low-density lipoprotein; HDL, high-density lipoprotein; VLDL, very low density lipoprotein; and APO, apolipoprotein. Numbers of patients are maximum numbers in the efficacy analyses.
†$P ≤ .01$ vs. baseline.
‡$P ≤ .01$ vs cholestyramine.
§$P ≤ .05$ vs baseline.

the combination of simvastatin plus cholestyramine was more effective than simvastatin alone in lowering the total cholesterol level (37% vs 29%) and LDL cholesterol (45% vs 37%). In type IIb hypercholesterolemia (23 patients) combined simvastatin-cholestyramine was not more effective than simvastatin alone. The only side effect was myolysis which occurred in 2 patients and was diagnosed by a marked increase in creatine phosphokinase.

Pravastatin

Inhibitors of the rate-limiting enzyme of cholesterol biosynthesis, 3-hydroxy-3-methylglutaryl coenzyme A (HMG-CoA) reductase, are now used frequently to treat patients with hypercholesterolemia. Reihner and associates[74] from Stockholm, Sweden, studied the effects of specific inhibition of cholesterol synthesis by pravastatin on the hepatic metabolism of cholesterol in patients with gallstone disease who were scheduled to undergo cholecystectomy. Ten patients were treated with pravastatin (20 mg twice a day) for 3 weeks before cholecystectomy; 20 patients not treated served as controls. A liver specimen was obtained from each patient at operation, and the activities of rate-determining enzymes in cholesterol metabolism as well as LDL receptor binding activity were determined. Pravastatin therapy reduced plasma total cholesterol by 26% and LDL cholesterol by 39%. Serum levels of free lathosterol, a precursor of cholesterol whose concentration reflects the rate of cholesterol synthesis in vivo, decreased by 63%, indicating reduced de novo biosynthesis of cholesterol. Microsomal HMG-CoA reductase activity, when analyzed in vitro in the absence of the inhibitor, was increased 12 fold (1344 ± 311 vs 105 ± 14 pmol per minute per milligram of protein in the controls. The expression of LDL receptors was increased by 180%, whereas the activities of cholesterol 7 a-hydroxylase (which governs bile acid synthesis) and of acyl-coenzyme A:cholesterol O-acyltransferase (which regulates cholesterol esterification) were unaffected by treatment. Inhibition of hepatic HMG-CoA reductase by pravastatin results in an increased expression of hepatic LDL receptors, which explains the lowered plasma levels of LDL cholesterol.

Gemfibrozil

The Helsinki Heart Study demonstrated a 34% reduction in the incidence of cardiac end points (AMI and sudden coronary death) with the use of gemfibrozil compared with the use of a placebo in dyslipidemic middle-aged men. The major effect was confined to nonfatal myocardial infarctions. In this study, Mänttäri and associates[75] from Helsinki, Finland, analyzed the effect of gemfibrozil therapy on the incidences of Q wave and non-Q wave infarctions, since the long-term prognoses of these 2 types of myocardial infarction may be different. The analyses indicated a 45% reduction in the cumulative incidence of Q wave AMI in the gemfibrozil group without a statistically significant effect on either the rate of non-Q wave AMI or of CAD death. The reduction in the incidence of Q wave AMI became evident during the second half of the 5-year study period.

EXERCISE

Morris and associates[76] from London, UK, followed 9,376 male civil servants, aged 45–64 years at entry, with no history of CAD for a mean of 9 years and 4 months during which time 474 had a coronary attack. The 9% of men who reported that they often participated in vigorous sports or did considerable amounts of cycling or rated the pace of their regular walking as fast (>4 mph, 6.4 km/h) experienced less than half the non-fatal and fatal CAD of the other men. In addition, entrants aged 55–64 who reported the next lower degree of this vigorous aerobic exercise had rates less than two-thirds of the remainder; entrants of 45–54 did not show such an effect. When these forms of exercise were not vigorous they were no protection against the disease, nor were other forms of exercise or high totals of physical activity per se. A history of vigorous sports in the past was not protective. Indications in these men are of protection by specific exercise: vigorous, aerobic, with a threshold of intensity for benefit and "dose response" above this threshold, exercise that has to be habitual, and continuing, which suggests that protection is against the acute phases of the disease. Those men who took vigorous aerobic exercise were demonstrably a favorably "selected" group; they suffered less of the disease, however, whether at low risk or high by the several risk factors that were studied. Men with exercise-related reduction in CAD also had lower death rates from the total of other causes, and so lower total death rates than the rest of the men.

OBESITY

Williamson and associates[77] from Atlanta, Georgia, and Madison, Wisconsin, estimated the 10 year incidence of major weight gain (a gain in body mass index of ≥5 kg/m^2 and overweight (a body mass index of ≥27.8 for men and ≥27.3 for women) in US adults using data from the First National Health and Nutrition Examination Survey Epidemiologic Follow-up Study. Persons aged 25 to 74 years at baseline were reweighed a decade after their initial examination (men, 3,727; women, 6,135). The incidence of major weight gain was twice as high in women and was highest in persons aged 25 to 34 years (men, 4%; women, 8%). Initially overweight women aged 25 to 44 years had the highest incidence of major weight gain of any subgroup (14%). For persons not overweight at baseline (men, 2,760; women, 4,925), the incidence of becoming overweight was similar in both sexes and was highest in those aged 35 to 44 years (men, 16%; women, 14%). The authors concluded that obesity prevention should begin among adults in their early twenties and that special emphasis is needed for young women who are already overweight.

Manson and associates[78] from Boston, Massachusetts, examined the incidence of nonfatal and fatal CAD in relation to obesity in a prospective cohort study of 115,886 U.S. women aged 30 to 55 years in 1976 and free of diagnosed CAD, stroke, and cancer. During 8 years of follow-up (775,430 person-years), the authors identified 605 first coronary events, including 306 nonfatal AMIs, 83 deaths due to CAD, and 216 cases of confirmed angina pectoris (Figure 1-16). A higher quetelet index (weight in kilograms divided by the square of the height in meters) was positively associated with the occurrence of each category of CAD. For increasing levels of current Quetelet index (<21, 21 to <23, 23 to <25, 25 to <29, and ≥29), the relative risks of nonfatal AMI and fatal CAD combined, as adjusted for age and cigarette smoking, were 1.0, 1.3, 1.3, 1.8, and 3.3. As expected, control for a history of hypertension, diabetes mellitus, and hypercho-lesterolemia—conditions known to be biologic effects of obesity—atten-

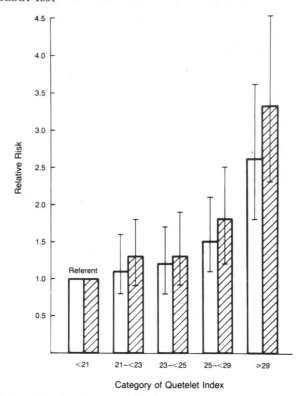

Fig. 1-16. Relative risks of nonfatal myocardial infarction and fatal coronary heart disease (combined). According to category Quetelet index in a cohort of U.S. women 30 to 55 years of age in 1976. The reference category was that with an index under 21. For the other categories, open bars show the relative risks as adjusted for age, and hatched bars show the relative risks as adjusted for both age and smoking. The vertical lines represent 95 percent confidence intervals. Reproduced with permission from Manson, et al.[78]

uated the strength of the association (Figure 1-17). The current Quetelet index was a more important determinant of coronary risk than that at the age of 18; an intervening weight gain increased risk substantially. These prospective data emphasize the importance of obesity as a determinant of CAD in women. After control for cigarette smoking, which is essential to assess the true effect of obesity, even mild-to-moderate overweight increased the risk of CAD in middle-aged women.

CIGARETTE SMOKING

A splendid group of articles[79-88] on cigarette smoking appeared in the September 26, 1990, issue of the Journal of the American Medical Association. These articles concerned the following topics: (1) depression and the dynamics of cigarette smoking; (2) relation of smoking and smoking sensation to major depression; (3) socio-demographic characteristics of cigarette smoking initiation in the USA and implications for a smoking-prevention policy; (4) the effect of cigarette smoking on hemoglobin levels and anemia screening; (5) effects of drinking coffee and carbonated beverages on absorption of nicotine from nicotine polacrilex gum; (6) evaluation of smoking prevalence and in-door air pollution after ending

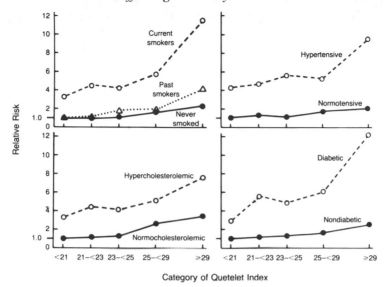

Fig. 1-17. Relative risks of nonfatal myocardial infarction and fatal coronary heart disease (combined). According to Quetelet index and coronary risk-factor status, after adjustment for age and smoking. The reference group in each panel comprised the women in the leanest Quetelet-index category who did not have the specified coronary risk factor. The diabetic group included women who received their diagnosis at ≥30 years of age. In all strata, the relative risk in the heaviest Quetelet category was at least twice that in the leanest. Reproduced with permission from Manson, et al.[78]

smoking at the Johns Hopkins Medical Institutions; (7) development of a state-wide antitobacco use campaign in California; (8) comparison of smoking patterns in the People's Republic of China to those in the USA. These articles were followed by 3 excellent editorials about smoking.

DIABETES MELLITUS

Although type II diabetes mellitus is associated with both microvascular and macrovascular complications, duration of the diabetes and severity of glycemia are strongly associated only with the former. Since prediabetic individuals are hyperinsulinemic, and since hyperinsulinemia may be a cardiovascular risk factor, Haffner and associates[89] from San Antonio, Texas, hypothesized that prediabetic individuals might have an atherogenic pattern of risk factors even before the onset of clinical diabetes, thereby explaining the relative lack of an association of macrovascular complications with either glycemic severity or disease duration. The authors documented the cardiovascular risk factor status of 614 initially nondiabetic Mexican Americans who later participated in an 8-year follow-up of the San Antonio Heart Study, a population-based study of diabetes and cardiovascular disease. Individuals who were nondiabetic at the time of baseline examination, but who subsequently developed type II diabetes (i.e., confirmed prediabetic subjects, n = 43), had higher levels of total and low-density lipoprotein cholesterol, triglyceride, fasting glucose and insulin, 2-hour glucose, body mass index, and BP, and lower levels of HDL cholesterol than subjects who remained nondiabetic (n = 571). Most of these differences persisted after adjustment for obesity and/

or level of glycemia, but were abolished after adjustment for fasting insulin concentration. When subjects with impaired glucose tolerance at baseline (n = 106) were eliminated, the more atherogenic pattern of cardiovascular risk factors was still evident (and statistically significant) among initially normoglycemic prediabetic subjects. These results indicate that prediabetic subjects have an atherogenic pattern of risk factors (possibly caused by obesity, hyperglycemia, and especially hyperinsulinemia), which may be present for many years and may contribute to the risk of macrovascular disease as much as the duration of clinical diabetes itself.

Moy and co-workers[90] in Pittsburgh, Pennsylvania, examined the relation between cigarette smoking and mortality prospectively in a population of adult insulin-dependent diabetes mellitus patients. In 1981, information on smoking history and other health lifestyle factors was obtained by questionnaire from 93% of the 723 patients included in the Children's Hospital of Pittsburgh insulin-dependent diabetes mellitus registry who were diagnosed between 1950 and 1964. Vital status as of January 1, 1988, was ascertained for 98% of 548 patients who participated in the baseline survey and were alive as of January 1, 1982. Fifty-four cases died during the 6-year follow-up (32 male, 22 female). Proportional hazards analysis revealed that heavy smoking was a significant independent predictor of all-cause mortality among females but not males. The excess mortality in female diabetics was explained primarily by a marked excess risk of coronary heart disease mortality in smokers. These data strongly suggest that cigarette smoking, especially among diabetic females, should be avoided to improve longevity.

Uusitupa and co-investigators[91] in Kuopino, Finland, examined the 5-year incidence of AMI and claudication in a group of middle-aged patients (70 men and 63 women) with newly diagnosed non-insulin-dependent diabetes and nondiabetic control subjects (62 men and 82 women). The effects of general risk factors, plasma insulin level, and lipoprotein abnormalities on the incidence of AMI and claudication were also evaluated by univariate analyses in both diabetic patients and nondiabetic subjects and by multivariate analyses combining both groups. The age-adjusted incidence of AMI was higher both in diabetic men (20%) and diabetic women (11%) than in nondiabetic men (3%) and nondiabetic women (3%). None of the general risk factors (LDL cholesterol, blood pressure, smoking, and HDL cholesterol) showed an association with the risk of AMI either in the diabetic or nondiabetic groups of subjects, but an ischemic electrocardiographic abnormality at the baseline examination predicted AMI in diabetic men. In multivariate analyses including both diabetic and control subjects, only diabetes had an independent association with AMI, whereas smoking, high LDL triglycerides or very low density lipoprotein cholesterol and high fasting plasma insulin showed independent relations to claudication. The present results indicate that changes in lipoprotein composition characteristic of non-insulin-dependent diabetes are atherogenic and increase the risk of atherosclerotic vascular disease. Furthermore, high plasma insulin might also be involved in atherogenesis, independent of lipoprotein abnormalities.

To determine the prevalence of cardiac disorders, Phillips and associates[92] from Rochester, Minnesota, conducted a survey in 1986 in a stratified random sample of the population of Rochester, Minnesota, 35 years of age or older (Table 1-27). The medical records of the 2,122 subjects in the sample were retrieved with use of the Rochester Epidemiology Project medical records linkage system. The data were used to estimate (1) the reliability of self-reported information about cardiac and cerebro-

TABLE 1-27. *Age- and sex-specific prevalence of diabetes mellitus and cardiac conditions among 2,122 randomly selected residents of Rochester, Minnesota, 35 years of age or older.* Reproduced with permission from Phillips, et al.[92]

	Men (by age group)					Women (by age group)					
	35-44	45-54	55-64	65-74	≥75	35-44	45-54	55-64	65-74	≥75	
Condition	No. (%)	No. (%)	No. (%)	No. (%)	No. (%)	No. (%)	No. (%)	No. (%)	No. (%)	No. (%)	Total no.
CHF	0	0	1 (0.5)	5 (2.3)	12 (6.9)	0	1 (0.5)	1 (0.5)	0	21 (8.0)	41
MI	1 (0.5)	4 (2.0)	17 (8.1)	23 (10.7)	29 (16.7)	2 (0.9)	1 (0.5)	3 (1.5)	6 (3.0)	15 (5.7)	101
Angina without MI	1 (0.5)	7 (3.4)	11 (5.3)	20 (9.3)	23 (13.2)	0	3 (1.4)	5 (2.4)	12 (5.9)	35 (13.3)	117
Hypokinetic segment†	2 (0.9)	4 (2.0)	16 (7.7)	23 (10.7)	22 (12.6)	2 (0.9)	4 (1.9)	3 (1.5)	6 (3.0)	13 (4.9)	95
LV aneurysm†	0	1 (0.5)	2 (1.0)	1 (0.5)	1 (0.6)	0	1 (0.5)	0	0	2 (0.8)	8
Intracardiac thrombus†	0	0	2 (1.0)	2 (0.9)	1 (0.6)	0	0	0	0	0	5
MV disease	0	1 (0.5)	0	5 (2.3)	5 (2.9)	0	5 (2.4)	3 (1.5)	0	13 (4.9)	32
MV prolapse	2 (0.9)	1 (0.5)	2 (1.0)	6 (2.8)	3 (1.7)	9 (4.2)	12 (5.7)	9 (4.4)	12 (5.9)	9 (3.4)	65
MAC†	0	0	0	4 (1.9)	15 (8.6)	1 (0.5)	0	0	3 (1.5)	21 (8.0)	44
Aortic valve disease	3 (1.4)	0	1 (0.5)	4 (1.9)	10 (5.7)	0	1 (0.5)	1 (0.5)	1 (0.5)	1 (3.0)	29
LVH	5 (2.3)	5 (2.5)	10 (4.8)	19 (8.8)	27 (15.5)	2 (0.9)	1 (0.5)	8 (3.9)	13 (6.4)	29 (11.0)	119
Dilated CM	0	0	0	1 (0.5)	1 (0.6)	0	0	0	0	0	2
Hypertrophic CM	0	0	0	0	0	0	0	0	0	1 (0.4)	1
CHD	2 (0.9)	0	0	1 (0.5)	0	1 (0.5)	0	3 (1.5)	0	0	7
Atrial fibrillation	0	1 (0.5)	2 (1.0)	13 (6.0)	28 (16.1)	0	1 (0.5)	3 (1.5)	6 (3.0)	32 (12.2)	86
Atrial flutter‡	0	0	1 (0.5)	1 (0.5)	5 (2.9)	0	0	2 (1.0)	1 (0.5)	8 (3.0)	18
PSVT	0	0	4 (1.9)	6 (2.8)	9 (5.2)	1 (0.5)	1 (0.5)	0	3 (1.5)	11 (4.2)	35
Sinus node dysfunction§	0	0	0	0	5 (2.9)	0	0	0	1 (0.5)	4 (1.6)	10

*CHD = congenital heart disease; CHF = congestive heart failure; CM = cardiomyopathy; LV = left ventricular; LVH = left ventricular hypertrophy; MAC = mitral annulus calcification; MI = myocardial infarction; MV = mitral valve; PSVT = paroxysmal supraventricular tachycardia.
†Of the sample, 12% had echocardiography, on which this diagnosis is dependent; 4% of the sample had radionuclide ventriculography, which contributes to this diagnosis.
‡Of the 18 subjects with atrial flutter, 14 also had atrial fibrillation.
§Sick sinus syndrome.

vascular disorders and (2) the age- and sex-specific prevalence of diabetes mellitus and various cardiac and cerebrovascular conditions. The estimated prevalence for selected risk factors in the population 35 years of age or older was 5.8% for diabetes mellitus, 3.3% for myocardial infarction, 1.2% for mitral valve disease, 4.2% for LV hypertrophy, and 2.8% for AF or flutter.

PARENTAL HISTORY

Family history of CAD, defined as parental death by CAD, was found to be a significant independent predictor of CAD in a logistic regression model controlling for standard risk factors and length of follow-up among the 5209 participants in the Framingham Study.[93] Persons with a positive parental history have a 29% increased risk of CAD, and the strength of the association between parental history and CAD was similar to that found for other standard risk factors such as systolic BP, cholesterol level, and cigarette smoking. No evidence was found that persons with a family history of CAD have a decreased capacity to cope with the deleterious effects of known risk factors; that is, no significant interaction was found between any of the risk factors and parental history of CAD. Among men with low risk for CAD by risk-factor profile (nonsmoking, thin, nonhypertensive persons), >⅔ of those who experienced CAD had a positive parental history. This study suggests that CAD among persons who are predicted to be a low risk by standard risk factors may have a substantial genetic component and that the risk associated with parental history may not be reduced by modification of these factors. Nevertheless, among persons with a positive family history, those with a favorable risk profile are at substantially less risk for CAD than those with an unfavorable risk profile.

SEDENTARY LIFESTYLE

During 1987, CAD accounted for 27.5% of the 2.1 million deaths in the U.S.A. Well-documented risk factors for CAD include sedentary lifestyle, elevated serum cholesterol, cigarette smoking, hypertension, diabetes, and obesity. A report using data from the 1988 Behavioral Risk Factor Surveillance System (BRFSS) and the 1976–1980 Second National Health and Nutrition Examination Survey (NHANES II)[94] estimated the number of persons at risk for CAD due to sedentary lifestyle and compared the prevalence of this risk factor with other risk factors for CAD. The 37 state health departments participating in the BRFSS used standard questionnaires and methods to conduct monthly random-digit-dialed telephone interviews of adults ≥18 years of age. For the BRFSS, sedentary lifestyle was defined as no physical activity reported or irregular physical activity reported (i.e., fewer than 3 times per week and/or <20 minutes per session). NHANES II, a nationwide probability sample of 28,000 persons aged 6 months to 74 years, described the relation between age and cholesterol levels for men and women aged 20–57 years; because this sample used direct serum measurement instead of self-report to record cholesterol levels, it provides the best national estimate for this CAD risk factor. In the BRFSS survey, sedentary lifestyle was the most prevalent (58%) modifiable risk factor for CAD reported, followed by cigarette smoking, 25%; obesity, 22%, systemic hypertension, 17%; and diabetes, 5% (Figure 1-18). Based on NHANES II, the estimate for serum cholesterol levels ≥200 mg/dL among persons 20–74 years of age was 31%. To reduce the burden of CAD attributable to sedentary lifestyle, 13 states are promoting physical activity as part of comprehensive cardiovascular disease prevention programs. Based on a median adjusted relative risk of 1.9 (2) (i.e., sedentary persons are approximately twice as likely as physically active persons to die from CAD) and the reported prevalence of sedentary lifestyle ranging from 45% (Washington) to 74% (New York), the percentage of CAD deaths attributable to sedentary lifestyle for these 13 states is 29%–40%. Based on population-attributable risk, the estimated number of preventable CAD deaths (i.e., deaths that might have been prevented if this risk factor had not been present in each of the 13 states) ranged from 1130 (Rhode Island) to 22,225 (New York).

FIBRINOGEN

In a study by Kannel and associates[95] from Boston, Massachusetts, the influence of fibrinogen on the risk of cardiovascular disease was examined over 16 years of follow-up in 1314 individuals who were initially

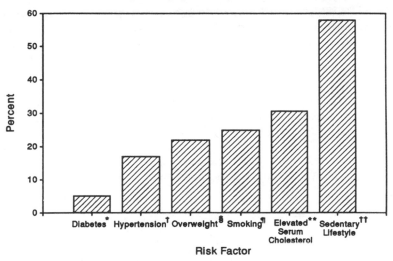

*Respondent self-reported having been told by physician that respondent has diabetes.
†Respondent self-reported having been told by a physician that blood pressure is high on multiple checks, or respondent is on medication for high blood pressure.
§Based on body mass index ≥27.8 for men and ≥27.3 for women from self-reported height and weight of respondent.
¶Respondent self-reported currently smoking.
**Measured ≥200 mg/dL by NHANES II.
††Respondent self-reported no physical activity or irregular physical activity (i.e., fewer than three times per week and/or <20 minutes per session).

Fig. 1-18. Prevalences of modifiable risk factors for coronary heart disease—Behavioral Risk Factor Surveillance System, 1988, and Second National Health and Nutrition Evaluation Survey (NHANES II), 1976–1980. Reproduced with permission from the Massachusetts Medical Society.[10]

free of cardiovascular disease in the Framingham Study. Of these individuals, 46 men and 43 women developed diabetes mellitus, and 56 men and 53 women had blood sugar levels >120 mg/dl. Diabetes predisposed individuals to all of the 408 major cardiovascular disease outcomes. Diabetics had higher levels of fibrinogen, hypertension, hypertriglyceridemia, and obesity, but lower HDL cholesterol values. The influence of diabetes on cardiovascular disease was greatly dependent on these coexistent risk factors, but there was a substantial independent effect of glucose intolerance when all the standard risk factors had been taken into account. There was a rise in fibrinogen values through the range of blood sugar levels, which suggests a thrombogenic explanation for the unique diabetic effect. However, multivariate analysis indicates no further reduction in diabetic cardiovascular risk ratios after adjustment for fibrinogen; thus, there is a residual effect for glucose intolerance after all of the standard risk factors and fibrinogen have been taken into account.

HOMOCYSTEINE

Genest and colleagues[96] in Boston and Framingham, Massachusetts and Beaverton, Oregon measured plasma homocyst(e)ine levels and its oxidized forms, homocystine and homocysteine-cysteine mixed disulfide, levels in 170 men with a mean age of 50 ± 7 years with premature CAD diagnosed at coronary arteriography and in 255 control subjects clinically free of CAD with a mean age of 49 ± 6 years. Patients with CAD had higher homocyst(e)ine levels than control subjects. HDL-cholesterol levels were lower and triglyceride levels were higher in the CAD group. Plasma total cholesterol and LDL-cholesterol levels were not significantly different between patients with CAD and control subjects. Systemic hypertension, smoking or diabetes mellitus did not alter homocyst(e)ine levels in the patients or the control group. Patients who were not taking a beta-blocking agent had slightly higher homocyst(e)ine levels than did patients taking this drug. No significant correlations were observed between homocyst(e)ine levels and age, serum cholesterol, LDL-cholesterol, HDL cholesterol, or triglyceride levels. Thus, an elevated plasma homocyst(e)ine level occurs in at least some patients with premature CAD.

COFFEE AND CAFFEINE

Tverdal and associates[97] from Oslo, Norway, studied the association between number of cups of coffee consumed per day and CAD death in all middle-aged people in 3 counties of Norway: 19,398 men and 19,168 women aged 33 to 54 years who reported neither cardiovascular disease nor diabetes mellitus nor symptoms of angina pectoris or claudication. At initial screening total serum cholesterol concentration, HDL cholesterol, BP, height, and weight were measured and self-reported information about cigarette smoking history, physical activity, and coffee drinking habits were recorded. Altogether 168 men and 16 women died of CAD during follow up. Mean cholesterol concentrations for men and women were almost identical and increased from the lowest to highest coffee consumption group (13.1% and 10.9% respectively). With the proportional hazards model and adjustment for age, total serum and HDL cholesterol concentrations, systolic BP, and number of cigarettes per day the coefficient for coffee corresponded to a relative risk between 9 or more cups of coffee and <1 cup of 2.2 for men and 5.1 for women (Table 1-28). For men the relative risk varied among the 3 counties. The authors concluded that coffee may affect mortality from CAD over and above its effect in raising cholesterol concentrations.

For many years, an association between coffee consumption and the risk of CAD has been suspected. Although based on small numbers of

TABLE 1-28. *Coffee consumption, cholesterol concentration, and deaths from coronary heart disease in Norwegians aged 35–54. Reproduced with permission from Tverdal, et al.*[97]

	No of cups of coffee						Linear trend coefficient (95% confidence interval)
	<1	1-2	3-4	5-6	7-8	≥9	
Men							
No at risk	870	1651	4995	5845	3481	2556	
Mean cholesterol (adjusted for age) (mmol/l)	5·80	5·96	6·15	6·25	6·37	6·56	
No of deaths	3	6	29	45	42	43	
Deaths per 100 000 observed years adjusted for:							
Age	62	61	92	119	186	244	0·33 (0·21 to 0·45)
Age and No of cigarettes per day	100	83	111	121	158	179	0·17 (0·05 to 0·29)
Age and serum cholesterol	81	73	96	121	177	203	0·25 (0·13 to 0·37)
Women							
No at risk	593	1771	6656	6164	2629	1353	
Mean cholesterol (adjusted for age) (mmol/l)	5·80	6·01	6·14	6·25	6·34	6·43	
No of deaths	0	2	1	3	4	6	
Deaths per 100 000 observed years, adjusted for:							
Age		18	2	8	24	69	0·79 (0·34 to 1·24)
Age and No of cigarettes per day		24	3	7	21	50	0·45 (0·01 to 0·89)
Age and serum cholesterol		24	3	7	21	50	0·49 (0·05 to 0·93)

endpoints, a prospective study has suggested a particular strong association between recent coffee drinking and the incidence of cardiovascular disease. Grobbee and associates[98] from Boston, Massachusetts, and Rotterdam, The Netherlands, examined prospectively the relation of coffee consumption with the risk of AMI, need for CABG and PTCA, and risk of stroke in a cohort of 45,589 U.S. men who were 40 to 75 years of age in 1986 and who had no history of cardiovascular disease. During 2 years of follow-up observation, 221 participants had a nonfatal AMI or died of CAD, 136 underwent CABG or angioplasty, and 54 had a stroke. Total coffee consumption was not associated with an increased risk of CAD or stroke. The age-adjusted relative risk for all cardiovascular disease among participants who drank 4 or more cups of coffee per day was 1.04. Increasing levels of consumption of caffeinated coffee were not associated with higher risks of cardiovascular disease. Higher consumption of decaffeinated coffee, however, was associated with a marginally significant increase in the risk of CAD. Finally, the authors observed no pattern of increased risk across the subgroups of participants with increasing intakes of caffeine from all sources. Adjustment for major cardiovascular-risk indicators, dietary intake of fats, and cholesterol intake did not materially alter these associations. These findings do not support the hypothesis that coffee or caffeine consumption increases the risk of CAD or stroke.

LEFT VENTRICULAR MASS

A pattern of LV hypertrophy evident on the electrocardiogram is a harbinger of morbidity and mortality from cardiovascular disease. Echocardiography permits the noninvasive determination of LV mass and the examination of its role as a precursor of morbidity and mortality. Levy and associates[99] from Framingham and Boston, Massachusetts, examined the relation of LV mass to the incidence of cardiovascular disease, mortality from cardiovascular disease, and mortality from all causes in 3,220 subjects enrolled in the Framingham Heart Study who were 40 years of age or older and free of clinically apparent cardiovascular disease, in whom LV mass was determined echocardiographically. During a 4-year follow-up period, there were 208 incident cardiovascular events, 37 deaths from cardiovascular disease, and 124 deaths from all causes. LV mass, determined echocardiographically, was associated with all outcome events (Figures 1-19 and 1-20). This relation persisted after adjustment for age, diastolic BP, pulse pressure, treatment for hypertension, cigarette smoking, diabetes, obesity, the ratio of total cholesterol to HDL cholesterol, and electrocardiographic evidence of LV hypertrophy. In men, the risk factor-adjusted relative risk of cardiovascular disease was 1.49 for each increment of 50 g/m in LV mass corrected for the subject's height; in women, it was 1.57. LV mass (corrected for height) was also associated with the incidence of death from cardiovascular disease (relative risk, 1.73 in men and 2.12 in women). LV mass (corrected for height) was associated with death from all causes (relative risk, 1.49 in men and 2.01 in women). The authors concluded that the estimation of LV mass by echocardiography offers prognostic information beyond that provided by the evaluation of traditional cardiovascular risk factors. An increase in LV mass predicts a higher incidence of clinical events, including death, attributable to cardiovascular disease.

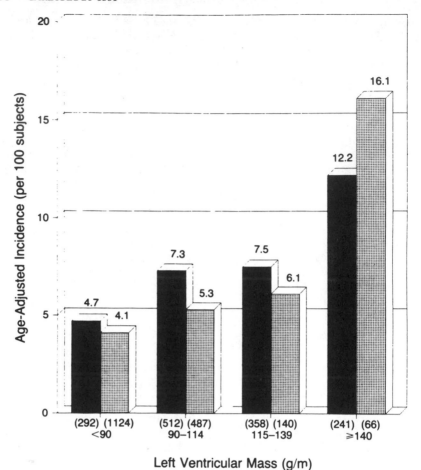

Fig. 1-19. Four-year age-adjusted incidence of cardiovascular disease, according to left-ventricular mass (corrected for height). The numbers in parentheses indicate the numbers of subjects at risk. The rates for men are represented by solid black bars, and those for women by stippled bars. The four corresponding categories based on left ventricular mass corrected for body-surface area are less than 75, 75 to 94, 95 to 116, and more than 116 g per square meter. Reproduced with permission by Levy, et al.[99]

References

1. Gutin B, Basch C, Shea S, Contento I, Delozier M, Rips J, Irigoyen M, Zybert P: Blood pressure, fitness, and fatness in 5- and 6-year-old children. JAMA 1990 (Sept 5);264:1123–1127.

2. Choi ESK, McGandy RB, Dallal GE, Russell RM, Jacob RA, Schaefer EJ, Sadowski JA: The prevalence of cardiovascular risk factors among elderly chinese americans. Arch Intern Med 1990 (Feb);150:413–418.

3. Multiple Risk Factor Intervention Trial Research Group: Mortality rates after 10.5 years for participants in the multiple risk factor intervention trial: Findings related to a priori hypotheses of the trial. JAMA 1990 (Apr 4);263:1795–1801.

4. Sytkowski PA, Kannel WB, D'Agostino RB: Changes in risk factors and the decline in mortality from cardiovascular disease: The Framingham Heart Study. N Engl J Med 1990 (June 7);322:1635–1641.

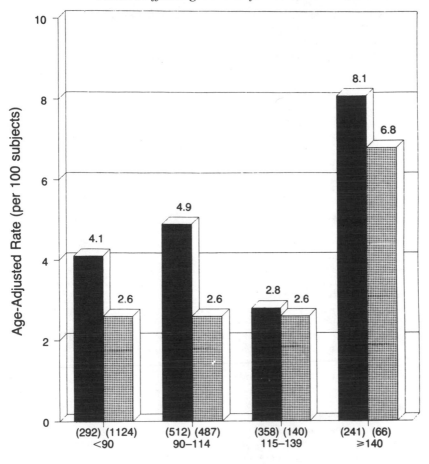

Left Ventricular Mass (g/m)

Fig. 1-20. Four-year age-adjusted rate of death from all causes, according to left ventricular mass (corrected for height). The numbers in parentheses indicate the numbers of subjects at risk. The rates for men are represented by solid black bars, and those for women by stippled bars. For the corresponding categories based on left ventricular mass corrected for body-surface area, see the legend to Figure 1-19. Reproduced with permission from Levy, et al.[99]

5. Farquhar JW, Fortmann SP, Flora JA, Taylor CB, Haskell WL, Williams PT, MacCoby N, Wood PD: Effects of communitywide education on cardiovascular disease risk factors: The Stanford five-city project. JAMA 1990 (July 18);264:359–365.
6. Kaufman HW, McNamara JR, Anderson KM, Wilson PWF, Schaefer EJ: How reliably can compact chemistry analyzers measure lipids? JAMA 1990 (Mar 2);263:1245–1249.
7. Naughton MJ, Luepker RV, Strickland D: The accuracy of portable cholesterol analyzers in public screening programs. JAMA 1990 (Mar 2);263:1213–1217.
8. Bradford RH, Bachorik PS, Roberts K, Williams OD, Gotto AM Jr, Lipid Research Clinics Cholesterol Screening Study Group: Blood cholesterol screening in several environments using a portable, dry-chemistry analyzer and fingerstick blood samples. Am J Cardiol 1990 (Jan. 1);65:6–13.
9. State-specific changes in cholesterol screening and awareness—United States, 1987–1988. MMWR 1990 (May 11);39:304–314.
10. Factors related to cholesterol screening and cholesterol level awareness—United States, 1989. MMWR 1990 (Sept 21) ;39/37:633–637.
11. Fischer PM, Guinan KH, Burke JJ, Karp WB, Richards JW Jr: Impact of a public cholesterol screening program. Arch Intern Med 1990 (Dec);150:2567–2572.

12. Mogadam M, Ahmed SW, Mensch AH, Godwin ID: Within-person fluctuations of serum cholesterol and lipoproteins. Arch Intern Med 1990 (Aug);150:1645–1648.

13. Bookstein L, Gidding SS, Donovan M, Smith FA: Day-to-day variability of serum cholesterol, triglyceride, and high-density lipoprotein cholesterol levels: Impact on the assessment of risk according to the National Cholesterol Education Program Guidelines. Arch Intern Med 1990 (Aug);150:1653–1657.

14. Dujovne CA, Harris WS: Variabilities in serum lipid measurements: Do they impede proper diagnosis and treatment of dyslipidemia. Arch Intern Med 1990 (Aug);1583–1585.

15. Williams RR, Hopkins PN, Hunt SC, Wu LL, Hasstedt SJ, Lalouel JM, Ash KO, Stults BM, Kuida H: Population-based frequency of dyslipidemia syndromes in coronary-prone families in Utah. Arch Intern Med 1990 (Mar);150:582–588.

16. Benfante R, Reed D: Is elevated serum cholesterol level a risk factor for coronary heart disease in the elderly? JAMA 1990 (Jan 19);263:393–396.

17. Trevisan M, Krogh V, Freudenheim J, Blake A, Muti P, Panico S, Farinaro E, Mancini M, Menotti A, Ricci G, Research Group ATS-RF2 of The Italian National Research Council. JAMA 1990 (Feb 2);263:688–692.

18. Council on Scientific Affairs: Saturated fatty acids in vegetable oils. JAMA 1990 (Feb 2);263:693–695.

19. Swain JF, Rouse IL, Curley CB, Sacks FM: Comparison of the effects of oat bran and low-fiber wheat on serum lipoprotein levels and blood pressure. N Engl J Med 1990 (Jan. 18);322:147–152.

20. Connor, WE: Dietary fiber—nostrum or critical nutrient: N Engl J Med 1990 (Jan. 18);322:193–195.

21. Godsland IF, Crrok D, Simpson R, Proudler T, Felton C, Lees B, Anyaoku V, Devenport M, Wynn V: The effects of different formulations of oral contraceptive agents on lipid and carbohydrate metabolism. N Engl J Med 1990 (Nov 15);323:1375–1381.

22. Goldbourt U, Yaari S: Cholesterol and coronary heart disease mortality: A 23-year follow-up study of 9902 men in Israel. Arteriosclerosis 1990 (July/Aug);10:512–519.

23. Rubin SM, Sidney S, Black DM, Browner WS, Hulley SB, Cummings SR: High blood cholesterol in elderly men and the excess risk for coronary heart disease. An Intern Med 1990 (Dec 15);113:916–920.

24. Williams P, Krauss R, Vranizan K, Wood P: Changes in Lipoprotein Subfractions During Diet-Induced and Exercise-Induced Weight Loss in Moderately Overweight Men. Circulation 1990 (April);81:1293–1304.

25. Stein RA, Michielli DW, Glantz MD, Sardy H, Cohen A, Goldberg N, Brown CD: Effects of different exercise training intensities on lipoprotein cholesterol fractions in healthy middle-aged men. Am Heart J 1990 (February);119:277–283.

26. Freedman D, Jacobsen S, Barboriak J, Sobocinski K, Anderson A, Kissebah A, Sasse E, Gruchow H: Body Fat Distribution and Male/Female Differences in Lipids and Lipoproteins. Circulation (May);81:1498–1506.

27. Rubba P, Iannuzzi A, Postiglione A, Scarpato N, Montefusco S, Gnasso A, Nappi G, Cortese C, Mancini M: Hemodynamic changes in the peripheral circulation after repeat low density lipoprotein apheresis in familial hypercholesterolemia: Circulation 1990 (February);81:610–616.

28. Holme I: An analysis of Randomized Trials Evaluating the Effect of Cholesterol Reduction on Total Mortality and Coronary Heart Disease Incidence. Circulation 1990 (December);82:1916–1924.

29. Wallace DJ, Metzger AL, Stecher VJ, Turnbull BA, Kern PA: Cholesterol-lowering effect of hydroxychloroquine in patients with rheumatic disease: Reversal of deleterious effects of steroids on lipids. Am J Med 1990 (Sept);89:322–326.

30. Joven J, Villabona C, Vilella E, Masana L, Alberti R, Valles M: Abnormalities of lipoprotein metabolism in patients with the nephrotic syndrome. N Engl J Med 1990 (Aug 30);323:579–584.

31. Keane WF, Kasiske BL: Hyperlipidemia in the nephrotic syndrome. N Engl J Med 1990 (Aug 30) 323:603–604.

32. Gordon RL, Klag MJ, Whelton PK: Community cholesterol screening: Impact of labeling on participant behavior. Arch Intern Med 1990 (Sept);150:1957–1960.

33. Mattiasson IN, Lindgarde F, Nilsson JA, Theorell T: Threat of unemployment and cardiovascular risk factors: Longitudinal study of quality of sleep and serum cholesterol

concentrations in men threatened with redundancy. Br Med J 1990 (Sept 8);301:461–466.

34. Duell PB, Bierman EL: The relationship between sex hormones and high-density lipoprotein cholesterol levels in healthy adult men. Arch Intern Med 1990 (Nov);150:2317–2320.

35. Seed M, Hoppichler F, Reaveley D, McCarthy S, Thompson GR, Boerwinkle E, Utermann G: Relation of serum lipoprotein(a) concentration and apolipoprotein(a) phenotype to coronary heart disease in patients with familial hypercholesterolemia. N Engl J Med 1990 (May 24);322:1494–1499.

36. Wiklund O, Angelin B, Olofsson SO, Eriksson M, Fager G, Berglund L, Bondjers G: Apolipoprotein(a) and ischemic heart disease in familial hypercholesterolemia. Lancet 1990 (June 9);335:1360–1363.

37. Hearn JA, Demaio SJ Jr, Roubin GS, Hammarstrom M, Sgoutas D: Predictive value of lipoprotein (a) and other serum lipoproteins in the angiographic diagnosis of coronary artery disease. Am J Cardiol 1990 (Nov 15);66:1176–1180.

38. Rosengren A, Wilhelmsen L, Eriksson E, Risberg B, Wedel H: Lipoprotein (a) and coronary heart disease: A prospective case-control study in a general population sample of middle aged men. Br Med J 1990 (Dec 1);301:1248–1251.

39. Ginsberg HN, Goldsmit SJ, Vallabhajosula S: Noninvasive imaging of [99m]technetium-labeled low density lipoprotein uptake by tendon xanthomas in hypercholesterolemic patients. Arteriosclerosis 1990 (March/April);10:256–262.

40. Reinhart RA, Gani K, Arndt MR, Broste SK: Apolipoproteins A-I and B as predictors of angiographically defined coronary artery disease. Arch Intern Med 1990 (Aug);150:1629–1633.

41. Puchois P, Ghalim N, Zylberberg G, Flevet P, Demarquilly C, Fruchart JC: Effect of alcohol intake on human apolipoprotein A-I-containing lipoprotein subfractions. Arch Intern Med 1990 (Aug);150:1638–1641.

42. Grundy SM, Vega GL: Role of apolipoprotein levels in clinical practice. Arch Intern Med 1990 (Aug);150:1579–1582.

43. Mennsink RP, Katan MB: Effect of dietary trans fatty acids on high-density and low-density lipoprotein cholesterol levels in healthy subjects. N Engl J Med 1990 (Aug 16);323:439–445.

44. Miller M, Mead LA, Kwiterovich PO Jr, Pearson TA: Dyslipidemias with desirable plasma total cholesterol levels and angiographically demonstrated coronary artery disease. Am J Cardiol 1990 (Jan 1);65:1–5.

45. Nikkila M, Koivula T, Niemela K, Sisto T: HIgh density lipoprotein cholesterol and triglycerides as markers of angiographically assessed coronary artery disease. Br Heart J 1990 (Feb);63:78–81.

46. Rosmarin PC, Applegate WB, Somes GW: Coffee consumption and serum lipids: A randomized, crossover clinical trial. Am J Med 1990 (Apr);88:349–356.

47. Zock PL, Katan MB, Merkus MP, Van Dusseldorp M, Harryvan JL: Effect of a lipid-rich fraction from boiled coffee on serum cholesterol. Lancet 1990 (May 26);335:1235–1237.

48. Ostlund RE Jr, Staten M, Kohrt WM, Schultz J, Malley M: The ratio of waist-to-hip circumference, plasma insulin level, and glucose intolerance as independent predictors of the HDL_2 cholesterol level in older adults. N Engl J Med 1990 (Jan 25);322:229–234.

49. Ostlund RE Jr, Staten M, Kohrt WM, Schultz J, Malley M: The ratio of waist-to-hip circumference, plasma insulin level, and glucose intolerance as independent predictors of the HDL_2 cholesterol level in older adults. N Engl J Med 1990 (Jan 25);322:229–234.

50. Winawer SJ, Flehinger BJ, Buchalter J, Herbert E, Shike M: Declining serum cholesterol levels prior to diagnosis of colon cancer: A time-trend, case-control study. JAMA 1990 (Apr 18);263:2083–2085.

51. Handa K, Sasaki J, Saku K, Kono S, Arakawa K: Alcohol consumption, serum lipids and severity of angiographically determined coronary artery disease. Am J Cardiol 1990 (Feb 1);65:287–289.

52. Ginsberg HN, Barr SL, Gilbert A, Karmally W, Deckelbaum R, Kaplan K, Ramakrishnan R, Holleran S, Dell RB: Reduction of plasma cholesterol levels in normal men on an

American Heart Association Step 1 diet or a Step 1 diet with added monounsaturated fat. N Engl J Med 1990 (Mar 1);322:574–579.

53. Insull W, Henderson MM, Prentice RL, Thompson DJ, Clifford C, Goldman S, Gorbach S, Moskowitz M, Thompson R, Woods M: Results of a randomized feasibility study of a low-fat diet. Arch Intern Med 1990 (Feb);150:421–427.

54. Dreon DM, Vranizan KM, Krauss RM, Austin MA, Wood PD: The effects of polyunsaturated fat vs monounsaturated fat on plasma lipoproteins. JAMA 1990 (May 9);263:2462–2466.

55. Thorogood M, Roe L, McPherson K, Mann J: Dietary intake and plasma lipid levels: Lessons from a study of the diet of health conscious groups. Br Med J 1990 (May 19);300:1297–1301.

56. Blankenhorn DH, Johnson RL, Mack WJ, El Zein HA, Vailas LI: The influence of diet on the appearance of new lesions in human coronary arteries. JAMA 1990 (Mar 23/30);263:1646–1652.

57. Barnard RJ: Short-term reductions in serum lipids through diet and exercise. NEJM 1990 (Oct 18);323:1142–1143.

58. Ornish D, Brown SE, Scherwitz LW, Billings JH, Armstrong WT, Ports TA, McLanahan SM, Kirkeeide RL, Brand RJ, Gould KL: Can lifestyle changes reverse coronary heart disease. Lancet 1990 (July 21);336:129–133.

59. Levin EG, Miller VT, Muesing RA, Stoy DB, Balm TK, Larosa JC: Comparison of psyllium hydrophilic mucilloid and cellulose as adjuncts to a prudent diet in the treatment of mild to moderate hypercholesterolemia. Arch Intern Med 1990 (Sept);150:1822–1827.

60. Reis GJ, Silverman DI, Boucher TM, Sipperly ME, Horowitz GL, Sacks FM, Pasternak RC: Effects of two types of fish oil supplements on serum lipids and plasma phospholipid fatty acids in coronary artery disease. Am J Cardiol 1990 (Nov 15);66:1171–1175.

61. Sullivan JM, Zwaag RV, Hughes JP, Maddock V, Kroetz FW, Ramanathan KB, Mirvis DM: Estrogen replacement and coronary artery disease: Effect on survival in postmenopausal women. Arch Intern Med 1990 (Dec);150:2557–2562.

62. Wysowski DK, Kennedy DL, Gross TP: Prescribed use of cholesterol-lowering drugs in the United States, 1978 through 1988. JAMA 1990 (Apr 25);263:2185–2188.

63. Garg A, Grundy SM: Nicotinic acid as therapy for dyslipidemia in non-insulin-dependent diabetes mellitus. JAMA 1990 (Aug 8);264:723–726.

64. Henkin Y, Johnson KC, Segrest JP: Rechallenge with crystalline niacin after drug-induced hepatitis from sustained-release niacin. JAMA 1990 (July 11);264:241–243.

65. Vega GL, Grundy SM: Management of primary mixed hyperlipidemia with lovastatin. Arch Intern Med 1990 (June);150:1313–1319.

66. Bates MC, Warren SG, Grubb S, Chillag S: Effectiveness of low-dose lovastatin in lowering serum cholesterol: Experience with 56 patients. Arch Intern Med 1990 (Sept);150:1947–1950.

67. Laties AM, Keates EU, Taylor HR, Chremos AN, Shear CL, Lippa EA, Gould AL, Merck Sharp and Dohme Research Laboratories, Hurley DP: The human lens after 48 weeks of treatment with lovastatin. N Engl J Med 1990 (Sept 6);323:683–684.

68. Black DM, Lamkin G, Olivera EH, Laskarzewski PM, Stein EA: Sleep disturbance and HMG CoA reductase inhibitors. JAMA 1990 (Sept 5);264:1105.

69. Brown G, Albers JJ, Fisher LD, Schaefer SM, Lin JT, Kaplan C, Zhao ZQ, Bisson BD, Fitzpatrick VF, Dodge HT: Regression of coronary artery disease as a result of intensive lipid-lowering therapy in men with high levels of apolipoprotein B. N Engl J Med 1990 (Nov 8);323:1289–1298.

70. Pierce LR, Wysowski DK, Gross TP: Myopathy and rhabdomyolysis associated with lovastatin-gemfibrozil combination therapy. JAMA 1990 (July 4);264:71–75.

71. Vega GL, Grundy SM: Primary hypertriglyceridemia with borderline high cholesterol and elevated apolipoprotein B concentrations: Comparison of gemfibrozil vs lovastatin therapy. JAMA 1990 (Dec 5);264:2759–2763.

72. Stein E, Kreisberg R, Miller V, Mangell G, Washington L, Shapiro DR, Multicenter Group I: Effects of simvastatin and cholestyramine in familial and nonfamilial hypercholesterolemia. Arch Intern Med 1990 (Feb);150:341–345.

73. Emmerich J, Aubert I, Bauduceau B, Dachet C, Chanu B, Erlich D, Gauthier D, Jacotot B, Rouffy J: Efficacy and safety of simvastatin (alone or in association with choles-

tyramine). A 1-year study in 66 patients with type II hyperlipoproteinemia. Eur Heart J 1990 (Feb);11:149–155.

74. Reihner E, Rudling M, Stahlberg D, Berglund L, Ewerth S, Bjorkhem I, Einarsson K, Angelin B: Influence of pravastatin, a specific inhibitor of HMG-CoA reductase, on hepatic metabolism of cholesterol. N Engl J Med 1990 (July 26);323:224–228.

75. Manttari M, Romo M, Manninen V, Koskinen P, Huttunen JK, Heinonen OP, Frick MH: Reduction in Q wave myocardial infarctions with gemfibrozil in the Helsinki Heart Study. Am Heart J 1990 (May);119:991–995.

76. Morris JN, Clayton DG, Everitt MG, Semmence AM, Burgess EH: Exercise in leisure time: Coronary attack and death rates. Br Heart J 1990 (June);63:325–334.

77. Williamson DF, Kahn HS, Remington PL, Anda RF: The 10-year incidence of overweight and major weight gain in US adults. Arch Intern Med 1990 (Mar);150:665–672.

78. Manson JE, Colditz GA, Stampfer MJ, Willett WC, Rosner B, Monson RR, Speizer FE, Hennekens CH: A prospective study of obesity and risk of coronary heart disease in women. N Engl J Med 1990 (Mar 29);322:882–889.

79. Anda RF, Williamson DF, Escobedo LG, Mast EE, Giovino GA, Remington PL: Depression and the dynamics of smoking: A national perspective. JAMA 1990 (Sept 26);264:1541–1545.

80. Glassman AH, Helzer JE, Covey LS, Cottler LB, Stetner F, Tipp JE, Johnson J: Smoking, smoking cessation, and major depression. JAMA 1990 (Sept 26);264:1546–1549.

81. Escobedo LG, Anda RF, Smith PF, Remington PL, Mast EE: Sociodemographic characteristics of cigarette smoking initiation in the United States: Implications for smoking prevention policy. JAMA 1990 (Sept 26);264:1550–1555.

82. Nordenberg D, Yip R, Binkin NJ: The effect of cigarette smoking on hemoglobin levels and anemia screening. JAMA 1990 (Sept 26);264:1556–1559.

83. Henningfield JE, Radzius A, Cooper TM, Clayton RR: Drinking coffee and carbonated beverages blocks absorption of nicotine from nicotine polacrilex gum. JAMA 1990 (Sept 26);264:1560–1564.

84. Ending Smoking at the Johns Hopkins Medical Institutions: An evaluation of smoking prevalence and indoor air pollution. JAMA 1990 (Sept 26);264:1565–1569.

85. Bal DG, Kizer KW, Felten PG, Mozar HN, Niemeyer D: Reducing tobacco consumption in California: Development of a statewide anti-tobacco use campaign. JAMA 1990 (Sept 26);264:1570–1574.

86. Yu JJ, Mattson ME, Boyd GM, Mueller MD, Shopland DR, Pechacek TF, Cullen JW: A comparison of smoking patterns in the People's Republic of China with the United States: An impending health catastrophe in the middle kingdom. JAMA 1990 (Sept 26);264:1575–1579.

87. Sullivan L: An opportunity to oppose: Physicians' role in the campaign against tobacco. JAMA 1990 (Sept 26);264:1581–1582.

88. Glass R: Blue mood, blackened lung. JAMA 1990 (Sept 26);264:1583–1584.

89. Haffner SM, Stern MP, Hazuda HP, Mitchell BD, Patterson JK: Cardiovascular risk factors in confirmed prediabetic individuals: Does the clock for coronary heart disease start ticking before the onset of clinical diabetes? JAMA 1990 (June 6);263:2893–2898.

90. Moy CS, LaPorte RE, Dorman JS, Songer TJ, Orchard TJ, Kuller LH, Becker DJ, Drash AL: Insulin-Dependent Diabetes Mellitus Mortality: The Risk of Cigarette Smoking. Circulation 1990 (July);82:37–43.

91. Uusitupa MIJ, Niskanen LK, Siitone O, Voutilainen E, Pyorala, K: 5-Year Incidence of Atherosclerotic Vascular Disease in Relation to General Risk Factors, Insulin Level, and Abnormalities in Lipoprotein Composition in Non-Insulin-Dependent Diabetic and Nondiabetic Subjects. Circulation 1990 (July);82:27–36.

92. Phillips SJ, Whisnant JP, O'Fallon WM, Frye RL: Prevalence of cardiovascular disease and diabetes mellitus in residents of Rochester, Minnesota. Mayo Clin Proc 1990 (Mar);65:344–359.

93. Myers RH, Diely DK, Cupples LA, Kannel WB: Parental history is an independent risk factor for coronary artery disease: The Framingham Study. Am Heart J 1990 (October);120:963–969.

94. Coronary heart disease attributable to sedentary lifestyle—Selected states, 1988. MMWR 1990 (Aug 17);39:541–544.

95. Kannel WB, D'Agostino RB, Wilson PWF, Belanger AJ, Gagnon DR: Diabetes, fibrinogen, and risk of cardiovascular disease: The Framingham experience. Am Heart J 1990 (September);120:672–676.

96. Genest JJ Jr, McNamara JR, Salem DN, Wilson PWF, Schaefer EJ, Malinow MR. Plasma homocyst(e)ine levels in men with premature coronary artery disease. J Am Coll Cardiol 1990 (November);16:1114–9.

97. Tverdal A, Stensvold I, Solvoll K, Foss OP, Lund-Larsen P, Bjartveit K: Coffee consumption and death from coronary heart disease in middle aged Norwegian men and women. Br Med J 1990 (Mar 3);300:566–569.

98. Grobbee DE, Rimm EB, Giovannucci E, Colditz G, Stampfer M, Willett W: Coffee, caffeine, and cardiovascular disease in men. N Engl J Med 1990 (Oct 11);323:1026–1032.

99. Levy D, Garrison RJ, Savage DD, Kannel WB, Castelli WP: Prognostic implications of echocardiographically determined left ventricular mass in the Framingham Heart Study. N Engl J Med 1990 (May 31);322:1561–1566.

Coronary Artery Disease

Prevalence in Massachusetts

Dalen and colleagues[1] from Worcester, Waltham, and Boston, Massachusetts, documented rates of hospitalization, use of various treatment options, and case fatality in the state of Massachusetts during 4 years (1980 through 1984). The data base was that of the Massachusetts Health Data Consortium, covering all hospital discharges in the state, a total of 3.8 million discharge records for this period. Of these, about 190,000 (5%) fell into 2 active symptomatic categories of CAD: chronic active CAD and AMI. Total hospitalization rate for these CAD categories increased by 17%; this was due both to an increased rate of hospital transfers (or readmissions) and to a larger cohort of patients under care. The case fatality rate for hospitalized CAD decreased approximately 16%, from 9.7% (1980) to 8.1 (1984). In chronic active coronary disease the frequency of coronary angiography rose; the use of PTCA increased much faster than the rate of CABG, with a resultant increase in PTCA as a fraction of total interventions. Similar findings were recorded for AMI, but with much more marked changes, the total intervention rate increasing almost 20-fold from 1980 to 1984. The statewide mortality rate for hospitalized CAD patients remained essentially unchanged at 71 to 74 hospital deaths per 100,000 population.

Coronary arteries in acute coronary events during sport

The clinical characteristics and coronary angiographic findings of 42 well-conditioned subjects with an acute ischemic event related to sport are reported in this presentation by Ciampricotti and colleagues[2] from Terneuzen and Eindhoven, The Netherlands. Five patients had unstable angina, 25 had AMI, and 12 were resuscitated victims of sudden ischemic death. Twenty-two events occurred during sport (group A) and 20 after sport (group B). There were 2 women and 40 men. The mean age was 46 years (range 25–65). Twelve (28%) had no identifiable risk factor. Prodromal cardiac symptoms were detected in 3 patients (group A). Two patients had previous AMI (group B). Coronary angiography was performed acutely in 39 patients. The distribution of the ischemia-related coronary artery was comparable in both groups. The lesion morphology of 35 culprit coronary arteries was described as concentric in 6 patients and eccentric with regular borders (type I lesion) in 11 and irregular borders (type II lesion) in 18. Eccentric lesions consistent with ruptured plaques prevailed in both groups. Associated CAD was present in 10 patients. There was no relation between the number of risk factors and the extent of diseased coronary arteries. Clinical characteristics and coronary angiographic findings of patients with unstable angina, AMI, and sudden death either during or after sport are similar and indicate a common pathogenesis. The probable mechanism of a coronary event related to sport is exercise-induced plaque rupture.

Anginal perception in diabetes

Ambepityia and associates[3] in London, UK, studied patients with diabetes mellitus to test the hypothesis that anginal perceptual threshold abnormalities in diabetic patients reflect a specific impairment of the sensory innervation in the heart. This hypothesis was tested in 32 diabetic patients and 36 nondiabetic control patients all of whom had typical exertional angina. Anginal perceptual threshold was defined as the time from onset of 0.1 mV ST depression to the onset of chest pain during treadmill stress electrocardiography. Although ST depression occurred earlier in the diabetic than nondiabetic group (111 ± 82 versus 216 ± 162), the anginal perceptual threshold of the diabetic group was delayed by a mean of 86 s (149 ± 76 versus 63 ± 59) (Figure 2-1). Autonomic function tests were abnormal in the diabetic group, and in both groups, regression analyses showed marked prolongation of anginal perceptual threshold as the heart rate responses to the Valsalva maneuver decreased to below the normal range. There was a similar though less pronounced relation between anginal perceptual threshold and heart rate responses to deep breathing. These data suggest that prolongation of the anginal perceptual threshold may be caused by autonomic neuropathy involving the sensory innervation of the heart. To test sensory function, median nerve conduction studies were performed in 19 patients, and they confirmed that sensory innervation was subclinically impaired in the subgroup with diabetes. Therefore, in patients with diabetes, anginal perceptual threshold is prolonged in association with autonomic and sensory neuropathy. The data suggest that altered perception of myocardial ischemia results from alterations in sensory innervation of the heart.

Coronary arteries in cocaine addicts

Dressler and associates[4] from Bethesda, Maryland, studied 22 cocaine addicts at necropsy to determine the amount of coronary arterial narrowing. The 22 patients were divided into 2 groups: death associated with increased cocaine levels at necropsy (13 patients, aged 23 to 45 years [mean 32], and mean total blood cocaine level, 0.36 mg/dl) and noncocaine-related death (9 patients, aged 15 to 50 years [mean 32]). Of the 22 patients, 17 were men and 5 were women; 19 were black and 3 were white. Gross

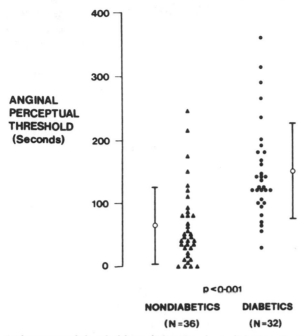

Fig. 2-1. Anginal perceptual thresholds in diabetic and nondiabetic patients. Data points are the time from onset of 0.1 mV ST segment depression to onset of angina in individual patients during treadmill exercise. Points and bars are mean values ±1 SD. Reproduced with permission by Ambepityia, et al.[3]

examination in the 22 patients disclosed that 8 patients (36%) had 1 or more of the 4 major (left main, left anterior descending, left circumflex, and right) coronary arteries narrowed at some point >75% in cross-sectional area by atherosclerotic plaque. In 17 cases, the 4 major epicardial coronary arteries were divided into 805 five-mm long segments and a histologic section was prepared from each segment: of the 12 patients with a cocaine-related death, 41 (8%) of 544 five-mm coronary segments were narrowed 76 to 100% and 106 segments (19%) were narrowed 51–75% in cross-sectional area by plaque. Of the 5 cocaine addicts who did not die from cocaine overdose, 8 (3%) of 261 five-mm coronary segments were narrowed 76–100% and 19 segments (7%) were narrowed 51–75% in cross-sectional area by plaque. The frequency of CAD was greater in patients dying with cocaine in their blood at necropsy compared to those whose death was not cocaine related. Also the frequency of severe coronary arterial narrowing is considerably greater than expected for the entire group of patients whose mean age was only 32 years. Thus, either of 2 possibilities, alone or in combination, may explain the authors' findings: coronary atherosclerosis is accelerated by cocaine addiction for reasons as yet undetermined, or cocaine provides a fatal stress in patients with premature coronary atherosclerosis from other causes.

Lange and associates[5] from Dallas, Texas, in a randomized, double-blind, placebo controlled trial studied 30 clinically stable patient volunteers referred for catheterization for evaluation of chest pain. Heart rate, arterial BP, coronary sinus blood flow and epicardial left coronary arterial dimensions were measured before and 15 minutes after intranasal saline or cocaine administration (2 mg/kg body weight) and again after intracoronary propranolol administration (2 mg in 5 minutes). No variables changed after saline administration. After cocaine administration, arterial pressure and rate-pressure product increased; coronary sinus blood flow fell (139 ± 28 [mean ± SE] to 120 ± 20 mL/min); coronary vascular resistance (mean arterial pressure divided by coronary sinus blood flow) rose (0.87 ± 0.10 to 1.05 ± 0.10 mm Hg/mL · min); and coronary arterial diameters decreased by between 6% and 9%. Subsequently, intracoronary propranolol administration caused no change in arterial pressure or rate-pressure product but further decreased coronary sinus blood flow (to 100 ± 14 mL/min) and increased coronary vascular resistance (to 1.20 ± 0.12 mm Hg/mL · min). Cocaine-induced coronary vasoconstriction is potentiated by beta-adrenergic blockade. Beta-adrenergic blocking agents probably should be avoided in patients with cocaine-associated myocardial ischemia or infarction.

Intracoronary ethanol infusion

To assess the influence of ethanol on coronary arterial blood flow and dimensions, Cigarroa and associates[6] from Dallas, Texas, measured coronary sinus blood flow in 35 individuals (23 men and 12 women, aged 38 to 69 years; 29 with and 6 without CAD) before and during a 15 to 30-minute intracoronary infusion of 1) 5% dextrose in water (n = 15, controls) or 2) 5% ethanol in 5% dextrose in water (n = 20). In the controls, heart rate, arterial pressure, and coronary sinus blood flow were unchanged. In those receiving ethanol at a rate that produced a concentration in coronary sinus blood of 285 ± 102 mg/dl, the product of heart rate × systolic BP was unchanged; coronary sinus blood flow rose 27 ± 36%, and coronary vascular resistance fell 17 ± 22%; arterial-coronary sinus oxygen content difference fell, and epicardial coronary arterial dimensions were unchanged. Thus, intracoronary ethanol increases coronary blood flow and decreases resistance without inducing a change in epicardial coronary dimensions, suggesting that its effect results from dilatation of the intramyocardial resistance vessels.

Effects of acetylcholine on coronary size

Intracoronary acetylcholine produces endothelium-dependent dilation of normal coronary arteries and paradoxical constriction of atherosclerotic vessels. Regional differences in endothelium-dependent vasomotion, however, have not been studied in relation to the nonuniform development of atherosclerosis. McLenachan and co-workers[7] in Boston, Massachusetts, compared the vasomotor response to increasing doses of acetylcholine of angiographically smooth coronary artery segments prone to atherosclerosis (coronary branch points) with segments remote from branch points (straight segments). In patients with entirely smooth coronary arteries and a dilator response to acetylcholine, branch points and straight segments demonstrated equal and significant dose-dependent dilation to acetylcholine. In patients with early atherosclerosis as manifest by luminal coronary irregularities, the lowest dose of acetylcholine produced constriction at branch points and slight dilation at straight segments. At higher doses of acetylcholine, both branch point and straight segments constricted, but constriction remained more pronounced at branch points. Both branch point and straight segments, however, retained the ability to dilate to the non-endothelium-dependent agent, nitroglycerin. In a third group of patients with angiographically entirely smooth coronary arteries but without dilation to acetylcholine, constriction to acetylcholine again occurred first at branch points. Thus, coronary branch points demonstrate increased sensitivity to acetylcholine-induced constriction in patients with angiographic evidence of early coronary atherosclerosis and in middle-aged patients with smooth coronary arteries. These segments, however, retain the ability to dilate to nitroglycerin.

Effects of heart rate on coronary vasomotion

Vasodilation in normal and vasoconstriction in atherosclerotic coronary arteries have been observed in response to complex stimuli such as exercise and the cold pressor test. To study a single parameter that changes during these activities, and to better understand the pathophysiology of ischemia associated with increases in heart rate, Nabel and co-investigators[8] in Boston, Massachusetts, studied coronary vasomotion and blood flow response to increasing heart rate alone, produced by atrial pacing, with quantitative angiographic and Doppler flow-velocity measurements in 15 patients. In 5 patients with angiographically smooth coronary arteries (group 1), tachycardia produced progressive dilation of the epicardial artery with increases in cross-sectional area of 16%, 22%, 29%, and 31%, at 90, 110, 130, and 150 beats/min, respectively. In contrast, in 5 patients with mild angiographic narrowings (group 2), coronary segments failed to dilate with progressive tachycardia (−6%, −8%, −13%, and −11% at 90, 110, 130, and 150 beats/min, respectively), and progressive loss of luminal area was observed in 5 patients with severe angiographic narrowings (group 3) (−34%, −50%, −60% and −73% at 90, 110, 130, and 150 beats/min, respectively). Coronary blood flow significantly increased with tachycardia in group 1 and increased slightly in group 2, but decreased significantly in group 3. The investigators concluded that an isolated increase in heart rate in patients with normal coronary arteries results in a modest increase in flow and vasodilation. In early atherosclerosis, the flow increase is blunted and dilation is replaced with paradoxical loss in luminal size. In patients with stenoses, further loss in luminal size occurs accompanied by a decrease in coronary blood flow. Thus, increasing heart rate alone in the setting of coronary stenoses could produce myocardial ischemia by a reduction in coronary supply, as well as by an increase in oxygen demand.

Effects of atrial natriuretic peptide

Rosenthal and colleagues[9] in Philadelphia, Pennsylvania, and Skokie, Illinois, characterized the direct coronary hemodynamic effects of atrial natriuretic peptide (ANP) in humans and assessed the safety of its administration in patients with CAD using incremental doses of synthetic ANP and nitroglycerin infused into the left coronary arteries of 14 patients, 11 of whom had CAD. Both agents caused dose-related increases in total coronary sinus blood flow. The largest dose of ANP given to all patients (100 μg) increased mean coronary sinus blood flow from 127 ± 7 to 149 ± 9 ml/min and decreased coronary vascular resistance from 0.93 ± 0.07 to 0.81 ± 0.05 mm Hg/ml per min. Mean arterial blood pressures and heart rates were not affected by this dose of ANP. The maximal effects of ANP were similar to those of nitroglycerin and no untoward effects were found. The greatest changes in coronary sinus blood flows and coronary vascular resistances after ANP infusions occurred in patients with CAD. Therefore, ANP is a direct coronary vasodilator in humans and one with similar coronary artery vasodilating properties with nitroglycerin.

Coronary aneurysm

Tunick and associates[10] in New York, New York, evaluated the natural history of discrete atherosclerotic coronary aneurysms in 20 patients with 22 aneurysms representing 0.2% of 8,422 patients referred for coronary angiography (Figure 2-2). Fifteen aneurysms (68%) were in the LAD, 4 (18%) in the LC, 2 (9%) in the right, and 1 (5%) in the LM coronary artery. Aneurysm diameter ranged from 4 to 35 mm (mean 8 mm); 95% of aneurysms were adjacent to the severe obstruction. Seventy-five percent of patients had severe triple vessel CAD that included LM disease in 15%. Total obstruction of 1 or 2 arteries was present in 15 (75%) patients. In patients with wall motion abnormalities, 78% of the abnormalities were

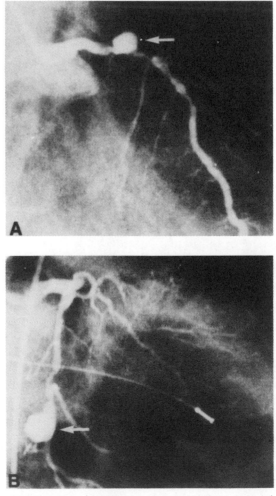

Fig. 2-2. Left coronary angiogram of two patients in the right anterior oblique projection. A, Discrete aneurysm of the left anterior descending coronary artery (arrow). B, Discrete aneurysm of the left circumflex artery (arrow). Reproduced with permission from Tunick, et al.[10]

in the distribution of the aneurysm. Follow-up of a mean of 30 months was available in all 20 patients; there were 2 cardiac deaths and 2 non-cardiac deaths, 12 patients had CABG, and of 16 survivors, 13 were angina-free. Thus, discrete coronary aneurysms are much less common than diffuse ectasia, and they are found in arteries with severe stenosis. They are most common in the LAD and associated CAD is more severe than in patients with diffuse ectasia. Patients with coronary artery aneurysms do not appear to be at increased risk of their rupture and their resection does not appear to be warranted.

Ages of death according to sex

Roberts and associates[11] from Bethesda, Maryland, analyzed 867 necropsy patients >30 years of age with fatal CAD to determine the age of death among 4 subsets of patients, none of whom had PTCA or CABG at any time. The results are displayed in Figures 2-3 and 2-4. The mean age of the 667 men was 60 years and that of the 200 women, 68 years. The group with sudden coronary death had a significantly younger (55 years) mean age than the other 3 groups; the mean age of the AMI group was significantly older (65 years) than that of the other 3 groups. The groups with chronic CHF and unstable angina pectoris had similar and inter-mediate mean ages (62 and 63 years). The sudden coronary death group and the chronic CHF group had the highest percentage of men (90 and 86%).

Medical costs

Wittels and associates[12] from Houston, Texas, and Stanford, California, developed a model to determine the cost of CAD based on the 5 primary events identified in the Framingham Study: AMI, angina pectoris, unstable

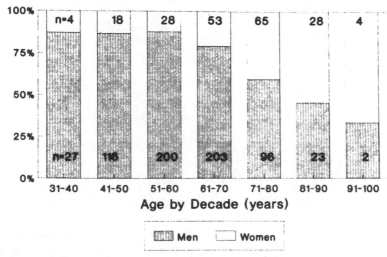

Fig. 2-3. Numbers and percent of patients of each sex by age decade with fatal coronary artery disease. Reproduced with permission from Roberts, et al.[11]

Mean Age at Death in Patients with Fatal Coronary Artery Disease

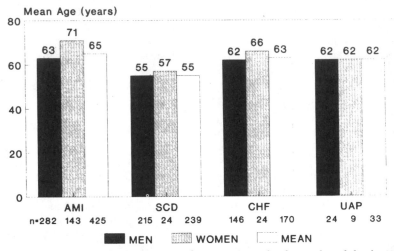

Fig. 2-4. Mean age at death in men and women in each of 4 modes of death. AMI = acute myocardial infarction; CHF = chronic congestive heart failure after healing of acute myocardial infarction; SCD = sudden coronary death; UAP = unstable angina pectoris. Reproduced with permission from Roberts, et al.[11]

angina pectoris, sudden death and nonsudden death. The costs for diagnostic and therapeutic service for patients with CAD were linked to medical decision algorithms outlining the diagnosis and management of patients with CAD. Because CAD is a changing illness not represented by a single event, the algorithm tracked patients for 5 years after the time of diagnosis, or until death, to develop average cost estimates. The estimated 5-year costs (in 1986 United States dollars) of the 5 CAD events were: AMI $51,211, angina pectoris $24,980, unstable angina pectoris $40,581, sudden death $9,078 and nonsudden death $19,697. The costs of major CAD surgical procedures were also calculated because of their impact on health care costs for patients with CAD. These include: CABG per case over 5 years $32,465, and angioplasty per case over 5 years $26,916. The high cost of CAD reflects the improved technology and more effective and expensive therapies now available.

Relation of in-hospital use of cardiac procedures to payer

To investigate the importance of the payer in the utilization of in-hospital cardiac procedures, Wenneker and associates[13] from Boston, Massachusetts, examined the care of 37,994 patients with Medicaid, private insurance, or no insurance who were admitted to Massachusetts hospitals in 1985 with circulatory disorders or chest pain. Using logistic regression to control for demographic, clinical, and hospital factors, the authors found that the odds that privately insured patients received angiography were 80% higher than uninsured patients; the odds were 40% higher for CABG and 28% higher for PTCA. Medicaid patients experienced odds similar to those of uninsured patients for receiving angiography and CABG, but had 48% lower odds of receiving PTCA. In addition, the odds for Medicaid patients were lower than for privately insured patients for all 3 cardiac procedures. These findings suggest that insurance status is associated with the utilization of cardiac procedures.

Early ambulation after cardiac catheterization

Kern and associates[14] of St. Louis, Missouri; New York, New York; Louisville, Kentucky; Los Angeles, California, and Durham, North Carolina, evaluated the influence of earlier ambulation and discharge after cardiac catheterization in a perspective 5 center clinical pilot trial assessing the safety and outcome of early ambulation after routine LV catheterization in 287 patients. Cardiac catheterization routines at each clinical center were unchanged throughout the study. Following the diagnostic cardiac catheterization evaluation using a 5 French catheter and arterial puncture compression times ranging from 5 to 52 minutes with a mean of 15 minutes, 260 patients were ambulated by a physician at a mean time of 2.6 hours and range of 1.8 to 3.1 hours following cardiac catheterization. Follow-up examination or a phone call 24 to 72 hours later was done to obtain further information. The mean age of the patients was 58 years and 58% were men. LVEF was 54 ± 15%. One hundred twenty-seven patients (44%) received intravenous heparin (1,500 to 5,000 U as an intravenous bolus) and 136 (47%) received aspirin. Major complications included a transient ischemic attack in 1 patient and VT requiring cardioversion during ventriculography in 2 patients. A small hematoma (<5.0 cm) after ambulation occurred early from compression to standing in 14 patients (5% of the total) and later after 72 hours in 9 patients. Five patients with a hematoma had studies with a 6F sheath. No patient required surgical intervention for early or late hematoma. Only three patients (1%) needed a 7F or 8F catheter because of suboptimal coronary arteriography with a smaller catheter. Ninety-two percent of patients had a complete coronary arteriographic evaluation with 5F catheters. These results suggest that early ambulation after large lumen 5F femoral left sided heart catheterization is safe with minimal postprocedural complications and without compromising angiographic data quality.

Complications of coronary arteriography

Stewart and associates[15] from London, UK, reviewed the records of the catheter laboratory at St. George's Hospital between 1983–1988 to determine how often emergency CABG was performed because of a complication arising during elective coronary arteriography. A total of 11,216 cardiac procedures were performed; 5781 were confined to LV angiography and coronary arteriography in patients with suspected CAD. Fourteen patients, whose investigation had been considered routine, suffered profound circulatory collapse during the procedure. Emergency cardiac surgery was undertaken in 13, with long term survival in 10. This experience suggests that, even in patients considered to be at low risk, there were major complications requiring emergency CABG in at least 2.4 per 1000 coronary arteriograms performed. Survival after emergency CABG in these patients was 77%. These findings and the access to CABG should be considered when the development of facilities for cardiac catheterization is planned.

VT and VF are recognized complications of cardiac catheterization. Despite numerous reports documenting the frequency of these occurrences, their significance has not been systematically examined. Accordingly, the outcome of 108 patients who experienced either VT or VF during coronary angiography between 1975 and 1979 in the Coronary Artery Surgery Study Registry were examined by Epstein and associates[16] from Birmingham, Alabama, and Seattle, Washington. There were 20,142 patients analyzed. Patients with ventricular tachyarrhythmias had more objective evidence of LV impairment, clinical CHF, and ventricular arrhythmia recorded as a clinical symptom. The overall 5-year survival rates were 83% and 88% for patients with and without ventricular tachyarrhythmias, respectively. When ventricular function, age, gender, angina, and previous AMI were added in a stepwise Cox survival analysis, the presence of arrhythmias was not significant. At 5 years, 80% of the medically treated patients and 82% of the surgically treated patients remained alive. The only statistically significant differences in the patients with ventricular arrhythmias who were treated medically or surgically were age (medically treated patients 52 ± 10 years, surgical patients 57 ± 9 years), and number of diseased vessels. In a stepwise Cox survival analysis, LV functional impairment secondary to CHF was the only significant covariate to affect survival in the medical and surgical groups. Surgical therapy itself was not significant. The incidence of sudden death during 5 years for patients with and without ventricular tachyarrhythmias during catheterization was similar at 5% and 4%, respectively. None of the 29 patients with ventricular tachyarrhythmias who did not have CAD had sudden death. In the 79 patients with CAD, the 5-year incidence of sudden death was 19% in the patients with LV functional impairment due to CHF and 4% in the patient without LV functional impairment due to CHF. For patients with arrhythmias who were candidates for CABG, there were no sudden deaths among the surgical patients. However, 14% of the medically treated patients had sudden death within 5 years. Thus, these data indicate that the occurrence of ventricular tachyarrhythmias occurring in the absence of myocardial infarction during cardiac catheterization does not confer an adverse prognosis. Rather, prognosis is governed by the presence or absence of CAD and the degree of LV dysfunction.

DETECTION

Association with thoracic aortic calcium

The relation between the presence of calcified plaques in the thoracic aorta, as detected on chest x-rays, and the development of cardiovascular disease during 12 years of follow-up of the Framingham cohort (n = 5,209) was reported by Witteman and associates[17] from Rotterdam, The Netherlands, and Boston, Massachusetts. The prevalence of aortic calcified plaques approximately doubled with each decade of age, with only a trivial male predominance. Its presence was associated with a twofold increase in risk of cardiovascular death in men and women younger than age 65, even after other risk factors were taken into account. Similar increases in risk were found for CAD, stroke and intermittent claudication among middle-aged women. In middle-aged men these risks were less marked. The predictive value of aortic calcified plaques generally diminished with age. Risk of sudden coronary death in men with calcified plaques in the thoracic aorta ranged from a 7-fold increase at age 35 to no excess risk at age 70 years. These results support the view that atherosclerosis is a generalized process. The finding of aortic calcified plaques in a relatively young subject on a routine chest x-ray should be regarded as a sign for potential development of clinically manifest atherosclerotic disease in the cardiac, cerebral and peripheral arterial circulation.

Association with carotid artery atherosclerosis

To evaluate the consistency, strength, and independence of the relation of carotid atherosclerosis to coronary atherosclerosis, Craven and colleagues[18] in Winston-Salem, North Carolina quantified CAD risk factors and extend of carotid atherosclerosis in 343 CAD patients and 167 disease-free control patients. In univariable analyses, there was a strong association between coronary status and extent of carotid artery disease in men and women older than and younger than 50 years. The relation remained strong after control for age in men and women older than 50 years and women younger than 50 years, but did not persist after control for age in men younger than 50. Logistic models that included CAD risk factors, as independent variable and presence or absence of CAD as the outcome variable indicated that the extent of carotid atherosclerosis was a strong statistically significant independent variable in models and women older than 50 years of age. Next, the investigators examined the usefulness of a B-mode score as an aid in screening for CAD in men and women older than 50 years. Classification rules, both including and excluding B-mode score, were developed based on logistic regression and, for comparison, recursive partitioning. The performance of these rules and the bias of their performance statistics were estimated. The improved classification of the study sample when B-mode score was incorporated in the rule was statistically significant only for men. The addition of B-mode score was found to 1) increase the median discrimination score for both sex groups based on the logistic model, and 2) yield better sensitivities and specificities for rules based on recursive partitioning. Thus, B-mode score is strongly, consistently, and independently associated with CAD in patients older than 50 and is at least as useful as well-known risk factors for identifying patients with CAD.

ST-segment depression

Lachterman and associates[19] from Long Beach, California, studied 328 men who had had both a sign or symptom-limited treadmill test and coronary angiography. Of the 168 patients who had abnormal ST-segment responses, 26 had such responses only during recovery. The positive predictive value of this pattern for significant angiographic CAD (84%) was not statistically different from the predictive value of ST-depression occurring during exercise (87%). Inclusion of ST-depression during recovery significantly increased the sensitivity of the exercise test from 50% to 59% without a change in predictive value. In addition, ST-segment depression occurring only during exercise was usually associated with less severe angiographically CAD. Thus, the occurrence of ST-segment depression during the recovery period only does not generally represent a "false positive response". The inclusion of findings from this period increases the diagnostic accuracy of the exercise test.

Mirvis and associates[20] from Memphis, Tennessee, evaluated clinical, hemodynamic and coronary angiographic data from 9,801 patients to determine the correlates of ST-segment depression, with or without T-wave inversion, on the resting routine electrocardiogram. The relative risk (RR) of having a measured clinical or angiographic variable was computed whether or not ST-T-wave abnormalities were observed. ST-segment depression was seen significantly more often in subjects >55 years of age (RR = 1.4) who were women (RR = 1.3) or nonwhite (RR = 1.5), were hypertensive (RR = 1.8), had diabetes mellitus (RR = 1.6) or who smoked cigarettes (RR = 1.5). Angiographic findings related to presence of ST-T-wave abnormalities included severe coronary obstruction (<70%), higher number of narrowed vessels, and the presence of obstruction in the LAD descending coronary artery. In a multivariate model, the most significant correlates of ST-T-wave abnormalities were presence of LV contraction abnormality, followed by age, gender, presence of LAD CAD, elevated end-systolic volume index, and a diagnosis of systemic hypertension. Thus, electrocardiographic ST-T abnormalities has specific and significant clinical and pathophysiologic correlates.

Echocardiography in the emergency room

Inappropriate discharge from the emergency room of patients with acute chest pain may have serious consequences. Regional asynergy is one of the first signs of myocardial ischemia and can be detected with 2-dimensional echocardiography (2-DE). Peels and associates[21] from Amsterdam and Utrecht, The Netherlands, determined the value of 2-D echocardiography in the emergency room for immediate detection of myocardial ischemia causing acute chest pain at the time the electrocardiogram was nondiagnostic. Forty-three patients (32 men and 11 women) with a normal or nondiagnostic electrocardiogram during acute chest pain were studied with 2-D electrocardiography. Only patients without a previous AMI and without known CAD were studied. The entire LV wall was examined for presence of regional asynergy. Coronary angiography was performed within 3 weeks. Cardiac enzyme levels were measured serially to establish or rule out an AMI. Sensitivity of 2-D electrocardiography for detection of AMI was 88% (22 of 25), specificity 78% (14 of 18), negative predictive accuracy 82% (14 of 17) and positive predictive accuracy 85% (22 of 26). Sensitivity of 2-D electrocardiography for detection of AMI was 92% (12 of 13), specificity 53% (16 of 30) and negative predictive accuracy 94% (16 of 17). Thus, 2-D electrocardiography during pain and a nondiagnostic electrocardiogram can readily identify patients with CAD in the emergency room, and it can accurately rule out an AMI.

Transesophageal echocardiography

Although transthoracic 2-dimensional echocardiography can detect dilation of the coronary arteries, the reliability of this technique in the detection of CAD is still doubtful. Yoshida and co-workers[22] in Kobe, Japan, performed a study to test the ability of newly developed biplane transesophageal color Doppler and two-dimensional echocardiography in the detection of LM CAD stenosis in 67 patients. Blood flow in the LM coronary artery was detected in 85% of patients by transesophageal color Doppler flow imaging. Using transesophageal two-dimensional echocardiography, adequate images of the full length of the left main coronary artery and identification of the bifurcation were obtained in 90% of patients. Transesophageal echocardiography clearly showed significant narrowing of the coronary lumen in 10 of 11 patients and insignificant narrowing or no abnormalities of the coronary lumen in the other 49 patients. The positive predictive accuracy for left main CAD was 100%, and the negative predictive accuracy was 98%. This preliminary study suggests that biplane transesophageal color Doppler and two-dimensional echocardiography appears to be a feasible noninvasive technique for imaging the LM coronary artery and detecting hemodynamically significant luminal obstruction.

Intravascular ultrasound

Safe and effective clinical application of new interventional therapies may require more precise imaging of atherosclerotic coronary arteries. To determine the reliability of catheter-based intravascular ultrasound as an imaging modality, Potkin and colleagues[23] in Bethesda, Maryland, used a miniaturized prototype ultrasound system to acquire two-dimensional, cross-sectional images in 21 human coronary arteries from 13 patients studies at necropsy who had moderate-to-severe atherosclerosis. Fifty-four atherosclerotic sites imaged by ultrasound were compared with formalin-fixed and fresh histological sections of the coronary arteries with a digital video planimetry system. Ultrasound and histological measurements correlated significantly for coronary artery cross-sectional area, residual lumen cross sectional area, percent cross-sectional area narrowing, and linear wall thickness measured at 0 degree, 90 degree, 180 degree, and 270 degrees. Moreover, ultrasound accurately predicted histological plaque composition in 965 of cases. Anatomic features of the coronary arteries that were easily discernible were the lumen-plaque and media-adventitia interfaces, very bright echoes casting acoustic shadows in calcified plaques, bright and homogeneous echoes in fibrous plaques, and relative echo-lucent images in lipid-filled lesions. These data indicate that intravascular ultrasound provides accurate image characterization of the artery lumen and wall geometry as well as the presence, distribution, and histological type of atherosclerotic plaque. Thus, ultrasound imaging appears to have great potential application for enhanced diagnosis of CAD and may serve to guide new catheter-based techniques in the treatment of CAD.

Thallium-201 scintigraphy

Gibbons and associates[24] from Rochester, Minnesota, studied 391 consecutive patients who had normal resting electrocardiograms and no digoxin therapy within the previous week to determine the incremental value of exercise radionuclide angiography for identification of severe CAD. The exercise electrocardiographic model consisting of magnitude of ST depression, exercise heart rate, and patient gender, was highly predictive of 3 vessel or LM CAD. The model correctly classified 60% of the study group which included 56 patients with and 179 without severe CAD. The addition of radionuclide angiographic variables improved the predictive value of the model. The exercise radionuclide angiographic variables increased the number of patients who were correctly classified by only 11 and the percentage by 3% (to a total of 63% of the study group). This modest additional advantage provided by exercise radionuclide angiography for identification of 3 vessel or LM CAD in patients with normal resting electrocardiograms would not justify its routine use for this purpose.

A fine review of the usefulness of exercise thallium-201 scintigraphy in the diagnosis and prognosis of CAD was reviewed by Kotler and Diamond[25] from Los Angeles, California.

Agati and associates[26] from Rome, Italy, performed 2-dimensional and Doppler echocardiographic studies and a hemodynamic investigation during dipyridamole testing in 42 subjects (29 patients with CAD and 13 control subjects) to evaluate the ability of dipyridamole-Doppler echocardiography in identifying patients with ischemic LV dysfunction. In the control group, after dipyridamole infusion, Doppler-derived parameters increased significantly from baseline. In patients with CAD, peak flow velocity, flow velocity integral and stroke volume failed to increase after dipyridamole infusion (0.89 ± 0.21 to 0.85 ± 0.18 m/s; 14 ± 3 to 12 ± 4 cm; 14 ± 3 to 12 ± 4 cm, and 56 ± 13 to 50 ± 14 ml/beat, respectively). Heart rate, rate-pressure product, systemic vascular resistance and mean RA pressure had similar variations in the 2 groups. Changes in the 3 Doppler-derived parameters are closely related to the variations of peak positive dP/dt, stroke volume (thermodilution) and LV end-diastolic pressure and are closely related to the coronary angiography jeopardy score and to the appearance of wall motion abnormalities. Thus, by combining Doppler and 2-dimensional echocardiography, dipyridamole-induced myocardial ischemia may be detected in a high percentage of CAD patients, providing a sensitive tool for identifying patients with high-risk coronary artery anatomy.

Ranhosky and co-workers[27] in Ridgefield, Connecticut, collected clinical data on 3,911 patients from 64 individual investigators to evaluate the safety of intravenous *dipyridamole*-thallium imaging as an alternative to exercise thallium imaging for the evaluation of CAD. There were two deaths because of AMI, 2 nonfatal AMI and 6 cases of acute bronchospasm. Chest pain occurred in 20% of the patients. Headache and dizziness were reported in 12% of patients. ST-T changes on the electrocardiogram were seen in 8% of patients. Use of parenteral aminophylline to treat adverse events associated with intravenous dipyridamole brought complete relief of symptoms in 97%. There is a potential for increased risk for serious ischemic events in patients with a history of unstable angina who are administered intravenous dipyridamole. In patients with acutely unstable angina or in the acute phase of AMI, use of intravenous dipyridamole in thallium scintigraphy should be avoided. There is also an increased risk of bronchospasm in patients with a history of asthma; acute bronchospasm can be relieved immediately by administration of aminophylline. These results demonstrate that intravenous dipyridamole-thallium scintigraphy is a relatively safe, noninvasive technique for the evaluation of CAD but should be avoided in patients with acutely unstable angina or AMI.

Pharmacological coronary vasodilation induced by dipyridamole is often used in association with thallium-201 myocardial scintigraphy to evaluate the presence and prognostic significance of CAD. Because dipyridamole acts by blocking the cellular uptake of adenosine, Verani and co-workers[28] in Houston, Texas, investigated the usefulness of direct intravenous administration of *adenosine*, a physiological substance with an exceedingly short (<2 seconds) plasma half-life, to induce maximal controlled coronary vasodilation in conjunction with thallium-201 scintigraphy. Investigators studied 89 patients who were unable to perform an exercise test and were referred for evaluation of suspected CAD. The intravenous infusion of adenosine began at an initial rate of 50 microgram/kg/min and was increased by stepwise increments every minute to a maximal rate of 140 micro-gram/kg/min. Thallium-201 was injected intravenously after 1 minute at the highest infusion rate, followed by immediate and delayed 4 hour tomographic imaging. At the highest infusion rate, adenosine induced a significant decrease in systolic (8 mm Hg) and diastolic (7 mm/Hg) blood pressures as well as a significant increase in heart rate. Side effects occurred in 83% of the patients but resolved spontaneously within 1 or 2 minutes after discontinuing the adenosine infusion. Chest, throat, or jaw pain were the most frequent symptoms and occurred in 57% of the patients. Headache (35%) and flush (29%) were also common. Ischemic electrocardiographic changes occurred in 12% of the patients, and transient first-degree atrioventricular block occurred in 10%. The overall sensitivity and specificity for CAD detection were 83% and 94%, respectively. Most false-negative studies occurred in patients with one-vessel CAD. The investigators concluded that maximal controlled pharmacological coronary vasodilation with adenosine, in combination with Thallium-201 scintigraphy appears to be a safe and potentially useful test for the diagnosis of CAD in patients unable to exercise.

The identification of ischemic but viable myocardium by thallium exercise scintigraphy is often imprecise, since many of the perfusion defects that develop in ischemic myocardium during exercise do not "fill in" on subsequent redistribution images. Dilsizian and associates[29] from Bethesda, Maryland, and West Roxbury, Massachusetts, hypothesized that a second injection of thallium given after the redistribution images were taken might improve the detection of ischemic but viable myocardium. The authors studied 100 patients with CAD, using thallium exercise tomographic imaging and radionuclide angiography. Patients received 2 mCi of thallium intravenously during exercise, redistribution imaging was performed three to four hours later, and a second dose of 1 mCi of thallium was injected at rest immediately thereafter. The 3 sets of images (stress, redistribution, and reinjection) were then analyzed. Ninety-two of the 100 patients had exercise-induced perfusion defects. Of the 260 abnormal myocardial regions identified by stress imaging, 85 (33%) appeared to be irreversible on redistribution imaging 3 to 4 hours later. However, 42 of these apparently irreversible defects (49%) demonstrated improved or normal thallium uptake after the second injection of thallium, with an increase in mean regional uptake from 56 ± 12% on redistribution studies to 64 ± 10% on reinjection imaging. Twenty patients were restudied 3 to 6 months after PTCA. Of the 15 myocardial regions with defects on redistribution studies that were identified as viable by reinjection studies before PTCA, 13 (87%) had normal thallium uptake and improved regional wall motion after angioplasty. In contrast, all 8 regions with persistent defects on reinjection imaging before PTCA had abnormal thallium uptake and abnormal regional wall motion after PTCA. These data indicate that the reinjection of thallium improves the detection of ischemic myocardium and that myocardial regions with improved thallium uptake on reinjection imaging represent viable but jeopardized myocardium.

This article was followed by an editorial entitled "The Value of Thallium-201 Imaging" by Gerald M. Pohost and Milena J. Henzlova[30] from Birmingham, Alabama. These authors pointed out that the second injection approach described by Dilsizian and associates would be expected to cost more than the traditional single injection approach.

Right-sided cardiac catheterization

Hill and associates[31] from Gainesville, Florida, assessed the value of right-sided cardiac catheterization prospectively in 200 patients undergoing left-sided catheterization for evaluation of known or suspected CAD. Before catheterization, data from right-sided catheterization was not felt to be necessary for clinical management. There were 6 ± 2 extra minutes of procedure time and 86 ± 63 extra seconds of fluoroscopy time used. Abnormalities were detected in 69 (35%) patients. These findings were unexpected in 37 of these patients and in 3 patients, further evaluation was prompted. Management was altered in only 3 (1.5%) patients as a result of data obtained by right-sided catheterization. In conclusion, this additional procedure rarely adds clinically useful information about patients undergoing left-sided catheterization and angiography for CAD without a clinical indication for right-sided catheterization.

Quantitative coronary angiography

Quantitative coronary angiographic measurements and visual estimates of coronary lesion severity were compared prospectively before, immediately following, and 6 months following PTCA by Goldberg and associates[32] from Houston, Texas. Mean percent diameter stenosis before PTCA was 88 ± 10% by visual analysis and 65 ± 9% by quantitative coronary angiography. Differences between these 2 techniques were also found immediately post-PTCA (visual analysis 30 ± 12%, quantitative coronary angiography 23 ± 12%) and at 6 months (visual analysis 47 ± 27%, quantitative coronary angiography 30 ± 20%). These differences significantly affected the determination of restenosis by 3 definitions. 1) Lesion recurrence with ≥50% stenosis at follow-up: 38 of 92 (41%) by visual analysis versus 20 of 92 (22%) by quantitative coronary angiography. 2) Increase of ≥30% stenosis: 34 of 92 (37%) by visual analysis versus 20 of 92 (22%) by quantitative coronary angiography. 3) Loss of 50% of previous improvement: 31 of 92 (34%) by visual analysis versus 24 of 92 (26%) by quantitative coronary angiography. In addition, determination of success or failure of PTCA was affected by the interpretative technique, but these differences were not statistically significant. It was concluded that visual estimates of narrowing severity are consistently and significantly higher than quantitative measurements. Consequently, restenosis rates, using currently applied definitions, differ considerably depending on the method of analyzing narrowing severity.

Sheikh and associates[33] in Durham, North Carolina, used quantitative measurements of coronary stenoses in comparison with exercise-echocardiography and the evaluation of regional wall motion abnormalities in 34 patients with isolated, single vessel coronary artery stenosis and normal wall motion at rest to determine the clinical utility of exercise echocardiography. Among the 11 patients with a visually estimated stenosis ≥75%, each had an ischemic response and 10 (91%) of the 11 patients with a <25% visually estimated stenosis had a normal response by exercise echocardiography. Among 12 patients with a visually estimated stenosis of 50%, 6 had an ischemic response and the remainder had a normal exercise echocardiogram. Quantitative measurements of stenosis severity distinguished patients with ischemic from normal exercise echocardiographic responses as follows: minimal luminal diameter (mm) in patients with ischemic responses was 1.0 ± 0.4 versus 1.7 ± 0.4 for those with non-ischemic responses; minimal cross-sectional area (mm²) for those with ischemic responses was 0.9 ± 0.6 versus 2.5 ± 1.1 for those without ischemic responses; percent diameter stenosis for those with ischemic responses was 68 ± 14 as compared to 42 ± 12 for those without ischemic responses; and percent area stenosis for those with ischemic responses was 88 ± 8 as compared to 65 ± 16 for those without ischemic responses. These data suggest that exercise echocardiography is useful in identifying patients with coronary stenoses that are physiologically important and that it may be used as a noninvasive means to assess physiologic significance of coronary lesions in many patients.

PROGNOSIS

Type chest pain

In a retrospective 6-year follow-up study, Metcalfe and associates[34] from Aberdeen, UK, obtained data for 536 (95%) of 566 consecutive patients admitted to a coronary care unit with acute chest pain. Their diagnoses were AMI in 290 (54%), myocardial ischemia in 164 (31%), pericarditis in 16 (3%), and non-cardiac in 66 (12%) (Figure 2-5). Six year mortality was 36%, 24%, 0%, and 16% respectively. In patients with AMI a higher mortality rate during follow-up was associated with a higher than average age (Figure 2-6), a higher than average creatine kinase, previous AMI, Q-wave infarction (Figure 2-7), and the presence of reciprocal changes. The presence of reciprocal changes was associated with higher

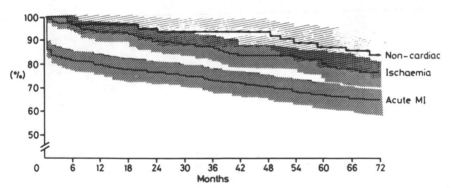

Fig. 2-5. Survival curves for acute myocardial infarction (MI), ischaemic heart disease, and "non-cardiac" pain (95% confidence intervals are shown as shaded areas). Reproduced with permission from Metcalfe, et al.[34]

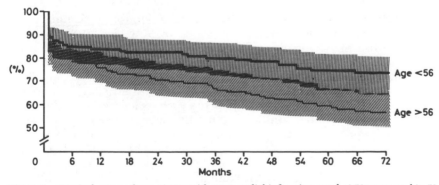

Fig. 2-6. Survival curves for patients with myocardial infarction aged < 56 years and > 56 years (95% confidence intervals are shown as shaded areas). Reproduced with permission from Metcalfe, et al.[34]

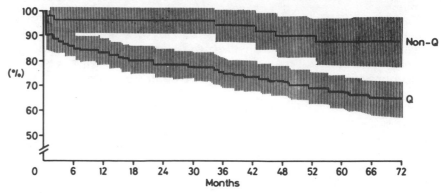

Fig. 2-7. Survival curves for patients with Q wave and non-Q wave infarctions (95% confidence intervals are shown as shaded areas). Reproduced with permission from Metcalfe, et al.[34]

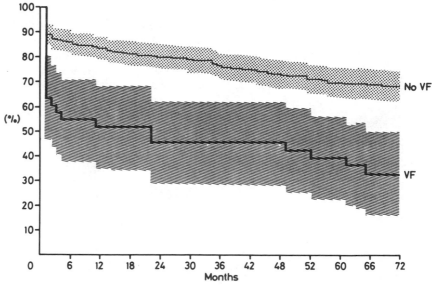

Fig. 2-8. Survival curves for patients without ventricular fibrillation and with ventricular fibrillation (95% confidence intervals are shown as shaded areas). Reproduced with permission of Metcalfe, et al.[34]

than average concentration of serum creatine kinase, indicating more extensive infarction. Infarction complicated by VF or left BBB was associated with a higher death rate (Figure 2-8). The electrocardiogram recorded at the time of AMI contains much useful prognostic information.

White and associates[35] in Boston, Massachusetts; New Haven, Connecticut and Cincinnati, Ohio, compared the natural history of patients with new onset CAD with that of patients with exacerbations of chronic CAD by obtaining short- and long-term outcomes in 3,465 patients seen in the emergency room with acute CAD syndromes of four community and three university hospitals. AMI was diagnosed in 598 (33%) of the 1,835 patients with a prior history of AMI or angina and in 934 (57%) of the 1,630 without such a history. Patients with new onset CAD with AMI were more likely than patients with AMI and exacerbated chronic CAD to have Q wave AMI (57% vs 36%) and to receive thrombolytic therapy

(11% versus 5%). They also had higher maximal serum CK levels. After adjustment for differences in clinical presentation, patients with new onset CAD with AMI were less likely than the comparison group to have CHF (Table 2-1), but they were not less likely to have other complications. In patients with angina without AMI, patients with new onset CAD were less likely to have recurrent ischemic pain and CHF. Multivariate analysis using longer term follow-up data in 457 patients from one hospital demonstrated that patients with new onset CAD had improved cardiovascular survival rates. These data suggest that patients with new onset CAD have a better short- and long-term cardiovascular prognosis than do patients with exacerbations of chronic CAD.

In black patients

Simmons and colleagues[36] from Atlanta, Georgia, reported long-term survival of blacks with angiographically defined CAD was examined in 1233 consecutive patients who underwent cardiac catheterization at a large urban municipal hospital. Vital status information was available at a mean of 86 weeks for the cohort as a whole, and 94 deaths were recorded. As noted in other angiographic series that included blacks, a high proportion of patients in this study had unobstructed coronary arteries (41%), and there was a preponderance of women (56%). Systemic hypertension was present in 82% of the cases, whereas 68% of the sample had LV hypertrophy as revealed by echocardiogram. The cumulative proportion of patients who were surviving at 5 years was 90 ± 1, 79 ± 4, and 70 ± 4 for patients with no obstructive lesions, 1-vessel disease, and multivessel disease, respectively. The survival rate at 3 years for 152 patients who had undergone CABG was only 82%. Noninvasive univariate predictors of mortality included male sex, history of myocardial infarction, Q waves on electrocardiogram, exercise duration on treadmill stress testing, and LV hypertrophy. Angiographic predictors included LV end-

TABLE 2-1. *Clinical outcome during first 72 h in 3,465 patients with acute ischemic heart disease. Reproduced with permission from White, et al.[35]*

	Acute Myocardial Infarction			Angina Without Infarction		
	Ischemic Heart Disease Pattern			Ischemic Heart Disease Pattern		
Outcome	Exacerbated Chronic (n = 598)	New Onset (n = 934)	p Value	Exacerbated Chronic (n = 1,237)	New Onset (n = 696)	p Value
Death in hospital	51 (9%)	47 (5%)	<0.01	3 (0.2%)	2 (0.3%)	NS
≥1 Complication	402 (67%)	575 (62%)	<0.05	444 (36%)	194 (28%)	<0.001
≥1 Arrhythmic complication	74 (12%)	110 (12%)	NS	8 (0.7%)	3 (0.4%)	NS
Ventricular fibrillation	17 (3%)	29 (3%)	NS	4 (0.3%)	3 (0.4%)	NS
Complete heart block	13 (2%)	39 (4%)	<0.05	1 (0.1%)	1 (0.1%)	NS
Cardiac arrest	55 (9%)	51 (5%)	<0.01	4 (0.3%)	2 (0.3%)	NS
Mobitz type II heart block	1 (0.2%)	9 (1%)	NS	0 (0%)	0 (0%)	—
Atrioventricular dissociation	13 (2%)	6 (1%)	<0.01	1 (0.1%)	0 (0%)	NS
≥1 Ischemic complication	311 (52%)	457 (49%)	NS	390 (32%)	177 (25%)	<0.01
Infarct extension	12 (2%)	30 (3%)	NS	0 (0%)	0 (0%)	—
Recurrent ischemic pain	308 (52%)	452 (49%)	NS	390 (32%)	177 (25%)	<0.01
≥1 Congestive complication	180 (30%)	194 (21%)	<0.001	93 (8%)	32 (5%)	<0.05
Congestive heart failure	116 (20%)	137 (15%)	<0.05	74 (6%)	25 (4%)	<0.05
Pulmonary edema	44 (7%)	27 (3%)	<0.001	17 (1%)	6 (1%)	NS
Cardiogenic shock	46 (8%)	56 (6%)	NS	6 (0.5%)	2 (0.3%)	NS
≥1 Major procedure	155 (26%)	233 (25%)	NS	72 (6%)	22 (3%)	<0.01
Cardioversion	31 (5%)	40 (4%)	NS	9 (0.7%)	3 (0.4%)	NS
Intubation	49 (8%)	59 (6%)	NS	6 (0.5%)	2 (0.3%)	NS
Intraaortic balloon pump	34 (6%)	45 (5%)	NS	12 (1%)	6 (1%)	NS
Temporary pacing	49 (8%)	68 (7%)	NS	5 (0.4%)	3 (0.4%)	NS
Pulmonary artery catheter	93 (16%)	168 (18%)	NS	22 (2%)	12 (2%)	NS
Cardiac catheterization leading to surgery	24 (4%)	18 (2%)	<0.05	43 (3%)	10 (1%)	<0.01

diastolic pressure, the number of diseased coronary vessels, EF, and mean PA pressure. Regression analysis showed an independent association for all the angiographic variables noted previously as well as for echocardiographically determined LV hypertrophy. Survival rates for blacks with CAD in this series were considerably lower than those currently reported for whites, particularly for patients who underwent CABG. Over and above the standard angiographic predictors, measures of ventricular hypertrophy and decreased diastolic function that are associated with hypertension appear to be independent correlates of early death and may explain a considerable proportion of the observed excess mortality.

12-lead QRS voltage

It is unclear whether sudden or nonsudden death can be predicted independently from other risk factors for CAD. Lanti and associates[37] from Rome, Italy, measured 12-lead QRS voltage sum, a recently proposed index of LV hypertrophy, and its ability to predict either subsequent sudden (<2 hours) or nonsudden CAD death during 20 to 23 years of follow-up in 1,588 middle-aged men (40 to 61 years old) from 2 cohorts of the Italian section of the 7-country study who were free of demonstrable CAD at entry examination in 1962. The Sokolow-Lyon and the modified Sokolow-Lyon indexes, 2 standard electrocardiographic methods to detect LV hypertrophy were also measured and compared. During follow-up, 67 patients died suddenly and 87 died a nonsudden CAD death. In the Cox proportional-hazards model, age, mean BP, heart rate, body mass index, cholesterol, physical activity, smoking habit, ST-T alterations (Minnesota codes 4.1–4.3 together with 5.1–5.3) and the 3 electrocardiographic indexes, all measured at the time of enrollment into the study, were included. The 12-lead QRS voltage sum retained significant and independent relation to sudden death (t = 2.00); Sokolow-Lyon index entered the Cox solution for nonsudden CAD death but the association was inverse (t = −2.10). ST-T alterations were significantly associated only with nonsudden CAD death (t = 2.19). Thus, in addition to several known risk factors, measurement of 12-lead QRS voltage sum in middle-aged men without clinical evidence of heart disease may help identify subjects at an increased risk of sudden death; nonsudden CAD death is predicted by Sokolow-Lyon index and by ST-T alterations.

Exercise echocardiography

Sawada and colleagues[38] from Indianapolis, Indiana, obtained follow-up information from 148 patients who had normal resting and post-treadmill exercise echocardiograms to determine the prognostic value of a normal exercise echocardiogram in patients evaluated for suspected CAD. There were 77 men and 71 women with a mean age of 53 years and a pretest likelihood of CAD of 39%. Patients were followed for a mean duration of 28 ± 8.5 months. The exercise electrocardiogram was abnormal in 69 patients (47%) including 28 who had ischemic responses. Cardiac events occurred in 6 patients, 3 with normal and 3 with abnormal exercise electrocardiograms. Events occurred only in those patients (6 of 68) who achieved <85% of the age-predicted maximal heart rate. Three patients had CABG for angina from 11 to 23 months after echocardiography. A fourth patient had CABG for mild single-vessel CAD at the time of MVR. Two patients had myocardial infarctions (0.85% per year) at 7.5 and 41 months after echocardiography. There were no deaths. Coronary revascularization is infrequently required in the 28 months after a normal exercise echocardiogram. A normal exercise echocardiogram in a patient with good exercise capacity was predictive of an excellent prognosis, even in those who had abnormal exercise electrocardiograms. AMI and death were rare events, even in patients with decreased exercise capacity.

Radionuclide angiography

To evaluate the usefulness of multiple measures from rest and exercise radionuclide angiography in predicting cardiovascular death and cardiovascular events (death or nonfatal AMI) and to assess the prognostic and catheterization data, Lee and co-workers[39] in Durham, North Carolina, studied 571 stable patients with symptomatic CAD who had upright rest/exercise first-pass angiography within 3 months of catheterization and were medically treated. With a median follow-up of 5.4 years, 90 patients have died from cardiovascular causes, and 147 patients have either died or suggested a nonfatal AMI. Using the Cox regression model and a preselected group of radionuclide angiography variables, the most important angiography predictor of mortality was exercise EF. Neither rest EF nor the change in EF from rest to exercise contributed additional predictive information. Two other radionuclide angiography study variables, the change in heart rate from rest to exercise and rest end-diastolic volume index, did contribute additional prognostic information to the exercise EF. Compared with noninvasive clinical data radionuclide angiography variables were consistently more predictive of mortality. Remarkably, the strength of the relation of radionuclide angiography variables with mortality was equivalent to that of the set of catheterization variables previously demonstrated in the large angiographic population to be prognostically important. Radionuclide angiography contained 84% of the information provided by clinical and catheterization descriptors combined. Furthermore, the radionuclide angiography contributed significant additional prognostic information to the clinical and catheterization data. For cardiovascular events, the relative prognostic usefulness of the radionuclide angiography was similar, although relations with this outcome were generally weaker. Descriptors from the rest/exercise radionuclide angiography exhibit a powerful relation with long-term outcomes and can be useful in defining risk, even when clinical and catheterization data are available.

UNSTABLE ANGINA PECTORIS

Review

An excellent review of unstable angina was published in the March 1990 Mayo Clinic Proceedings.[40]

Composition of coronary plaques

Kragel and associates[41] from Bethesda, Maryland, studied coronary artery plaque morphology in 354 five-mm long segments of the 4 major (LM, LAD, LC and right) spicardial coronary arteries in 10 patients with isolated unstable angina pectoris with pain at rest. The 4 major coronary arteries were sectioned at 5-mm intervals and a drawing of each of the resulting 354 Movat-stained histologic sections was analyzed using a computerized morphometry system. The major component of plaque was a combination of dense acellular and cellular fibrous tissue with much smaller portions of plaque being composed of pultaceous debris, calcium, foam cells with and without inflammatory infiltrates and inflammatory infiltrates without foam cells (Figure 2-9). There were no differences in plaque composition among any of the 4 major epicardial coronary arteries. Plaque composition varied as a function of the degree of luminal narrowing. Linear increases were observed in the mean percent of dense fibrous tissue (from 5–50%), calcific deposits (from 1–10%), pultaceous debris (from 0–10%) and inflammatory infiltrates without significant numbers of foam cells (from 0–5%), and a linear decrease was observed in the mean percent of cellular fibrous tissue (from 94–22%) in sections narrowed up to 25% to more than 95% in cross-sectional area (Figure 2-10). Multiluminal channels were seen in all 10 patients (28 [19%] of the 146 sections narrowed >75% in cross-sectional area and in 36 [10%] of all 354 segments); occlusive thrombi in no patient; nonocclusive thrombi in 2 patients (1 section each of 2 arteries); plaque rupture in 2 patients (4 segments from 2 arteries); and plaque hemorrhages in 6 patients (11 sections from 10 arteries).

Prognosis

To assess the relative value of Holter ST-segment monitoring compared with predischarge exercise thallium tomography, Marmur and associates[42] from Toronto, Canada, studied a cohort of 54 patients with unstable angina who had 6-month follow-up after stabilization on medical therapy. The authors prospectively compared 24-hour Holter ST-segment monitoring at admission, quantitative exercise thallium tomography, and cardiac catheterization 5 ± 2 days after admission, and analyzed their value for predicting a cardiac event in patients with unstable angina within 6 months. When patients with a favorable outcome (n = 40) were compared with patients with an unfavorable outcome (n = 11)

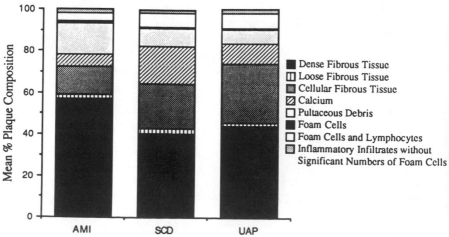

Fig. 2-9. Mean percent plaque composition of sections of coronary artery narrowed > 75% in cross-sectional area. AMI = acute myocardial infarction; SCD = sudden coronary death without left ventricular necrosis; UAP = unstable angina pectoris. Reproduced with permission from Kragel, et al.[41]

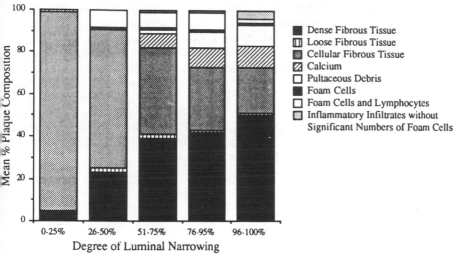

Fig. 2-10. Mean percent plaque composition in each of the 5 categories of cross-sectional-area narrowing. Reproduced with permission from Kragel, et al.[41]

no statistical difference was found in duration of ST shift of ≥ 1 mm on Holter monitoring (51 $\pm$ 119 min compared with 37 $\pm$ 43 min), exercise duration by the standard Bruce protocol (8.0 $\pm$ 3.6 min compared with 7.9 $\pm$ 3.1 min), exercise-induced ST depression (0.6 $\pm$ 0.9 mm compared with 1.0 $\pm$ 1.0 mm), and contrast LVEF (70% $\pm$ 10% compared with 69% $\pm$ 15%). Patients with a favorable outcome were distinguished from those with an unfavorable outcome by a higher maximum rate-pressure product (24 $\times$ 19^3 $\pm$ 6 $\times$ 10^3 $\pm$ 7 $\times$ 10^3), smaller size of the reversible scintigraphic perfusion defect expressed as a percentage of total myocardium imaged (6% $\pm$ 11% compared with 17% $\pm$ 18%) and a smaller number of vessels with stenosis of 50% or more (1.1 $\pm$ 1.2 compared with 2.1 $\pm$ 1.0). On multiple logistic regression analysis, a history of previous AMI was the most powerful predictor of outcome. In patients without AMI, reversible exercise thallium perfusion defect size was the only predictor. After stabilization of an episode of unstable angina, quantitative tomographic exercise thallium scintigraphy has greater value for risk stratification than Holter ST-segment monitoring, particularly in patients who have not had a previous infarction.

C-reactive protein

Unstable angina pectoris occurs most commonly in the setting of atherosclerotic CAD, but little information is available concerning the mechanisms responsible for the transition from clinically stable to unstable coronary atherosclerotic plaque. Recently, increased focal infiltration of inflammatory cells into the adventitia of coronary arteries of patients dying suddenly from CAD and activation of circulating neutrophils in patients with unstable angina have been observed. To characterize the presence of inflammation in "active" atherosclerotic lesions, Berk and associates[43] from Atlanta, Georgia, measured the acute phase reactant C-reactive protein in 37 patients admitted to the coronary care unit with unstable angina, 30 patients admitted to the coronary care unit with nonischemic illnesses, and in 32 patients with stable CAD. C-reactive protein levels were significantly elevated (normal <0.6 mg/dl) in 90% of the unstable angina group compared to 20% of the coronary care unit group and 13% of the stable angina group. The average C-reactive protein values were significantly different for the unstable angina group (2.2 ± 2.9 mg/dl) compared to the coronary care (0.9 ± 0.7 mg/dl) and stable angina (0.7 ± 0.2 mg/dl) groups. There was a trend for unstable angina patients with ischemic ST-T-wave abnormalities to have higher C-reactive protein values (1.6 ± 3.4) than those without electrocardiographic changes (1.3 ± 0.9). The data demonstrate increased levels of an acute phase reactant in unstable angina. These findings suggest that an inflammatory component in "active" angina may contribute to the susceptibility of these patients in vasospasm and thrombosis.

Neutrophil elastase release

Dinerman and associates[44] in Gainesville, Florida, and Uppsala, Sweden, characterized neutrophil activation in patients with CAD using a specific neutrophil elastase-derived fibrinopeptide measured in the plasma of 25 patients with stable angina, 29 patients with unstable angina, 17 patients with AMI, and 22 control individuals. Mean plasma levels ± standard error of the mean of a neutrophil elastase-derived fibrinopeptide measured by specific radioimmunoassay were fivefold higher in patients with AMI and 13-fold higher in patients with unstable angina as compared with control subjects. Mean plasma levels of this peptide in patients with stable angina were higher than in control subjects, but did not approach the levels found in patients with unstable angina or AMI. Total leukocyte counts in patients with unstable angina and AMI were higher than in patients with stable angina and control individuals, but the elevations in the neutrophil elastase-derived fibrinopeptide were independent of the differences in leukocyte counts. These results suggest neutrophil activation in at least some patients with acute myocardial ischemia. The pathophysiologic importance of these observations needs to be established.

Coronary angiographic quantitation

Analysis of lesion morphology is becoming increasingly important in the study of CAD. Lesion irregularity has been shown to be one of the most important predictive features for development of AMI. Most studies have used only qualitative assessments of morphology and thus subject to variability and lack of standardization inherent in subjective visual inspection. Kalbfleisch and colleagues[45] in Ann Arbor, Michigan describe a new approach that allows quantitation of lesion morphology. Fifty-nine patients with unstable angina and 17 patients with stable angina were compared. Five morphometric parameters were tested (peaks/cm, summed maximum error per centimeter, integrated error per cm, number of major features per centimeters, and scaled edge length ratio), 4 of which were significantly different between the 2 groups and indicated greater lesion complexity in unstable compared with stable angina patients. No correlation was found between the parameters tested and the degree of luminal narrowing, showing the method's independence from traditional assessments of lesion severity. Excellent intraobserver and interobserver reproducibility was found for all the parameters. This technique provides a more rigorous approach for analysis of lesion morphology than had previously been available, may provide a method for premorbid detection of high-risk lesions amenable to interventional therapy, and is especially well suited to detect subtle changes in lesion morphology after therapeutic interventions because the parameters are derived on a continuous scale and are not categorical.

Outcome with conservative therapy

Mulcahy and associates[46] from Dublin, Ireland, studied 346 patients admitted to coronary care with unstable angina pectoris. Management was conservative, without the routine use of beta-blockers or calcium antagonists. Mortality was 3.2%, and the nonfatal AMI rate was 10.1% during the first 28 days. After 1 year, coronary mortality was 10.5% with a nonfatal AMI rate of 13.1%. Twenty-six patients were subjected to CABG, 11 during the first 28 days and 15 subsequently. No patient underwent coronary angioplasty. The factors influencing immediate and long-term prognosis in these patients were studied. Persistence of pain in hospital, previous chronic angina, and age had an adverse effect on outcome. A total of 143 patients complained of persistent pain lasting for 24 hours or more. The use of beta blockers or calcium antagonists in patients with persistent pain exceeding 5 days did not appear to influence outcome. The current widespread adherence to "intensive medical treatment," including the routine use of beta blockers and calcium antagonists, is questioned.

Ticlopidine therapy

Balsano and co-workers[47] in Rome, Italy, conducted a controlled multicenter trial with central randomization and evaluation of events under blind conditions involving 652 patients with unstable angina. Patients were treated either with conventional therapy alone or with conventional therapy combined with an inhibitor of platelet aggregation, ticlopidine 250 mg twice daily. Patients were assigned randomly within 48 hours of admission and followed up for 6 months. With the "intention-to-treat" approach, the primary end points, vascular death and nonfatal myocardial infarction, were observed in 14% of the patients in conventional therapy and in 7% of the patients in conventional therapy plus ticlopidine which is a reduction in risk of 46%. Vascular mortality was 5% in patients in conventional therapy and 3% in patients with conventional therapy plus ticlopidine which is a reduction in risk of 47%. The risk of nonfatal myocardial infarction was reduced by 46%, with a frequency of 9% in patients in conventional therapy and 5% in patients treated with ticlopidine. Fatal and nonfatal myocardial infarction was 11% in patients with conventional therapy and 5% in patients with ticlopidine which is a reduction in risk of 53%. These findings confirm the importance of platelets in the pathogenesis of unstable angina and the usefulness of antiplatelet treatment for the prevention of cardiovascular events.

Thrombolytic therapy

Serneri and associates[48] from Florence and Fucecchio, Italy, monitored 399 of 474 in-patients with unstable angina pectoris for 48 hours and 97 of them were found to be refractory to conventional anti-anginal treatments and they were entered into a randomized double-blind study. With the initial protocol heparin infusion or bolus were compared with aspirin; with a modified protocol, heparin infusion, the best of these three treatments, was compared with alteplase. Patients were monitored for 3 days after starting treatment and then observed clinically for 4 more days.

On the first days of treatment heparin infusion significantly decreased the frequency of angina (by 84–94%), episodes of silent ischemia (by 71–77%), and the overall duration of ischemia (by 81–86%). Heparin bolus and aspirin were not effective. Alteplase caused small (non-significant) reductions on the first day only. Only minor bleeding complications occurred.

Because thrombus formation may contribute to coronary obstruction in patients with unstable angina pectoris, Williams and co-investigators[49] in Providence, Rhode Island, performed a pilot investigation to determine whether thrombolytic therapy can relieve coronary narrowing in this acute ischemic syndrome. Sixty-seven patients with rest angina and angiographic evidence of CAD were randomly assigned to receive either low-dose intravenous recombinant tissue-type plasminogen activator (rt-PA) (0.75 mg/kg over 1 hour), high-dose intravenous rt-PA (0.75 mg/kg over 1 hour; total dose, 100 mg over 6 hours), or intravenous placebo followed by repeat coronary angiography at 24–48 hours to assess change in the severity of coronary narrowing. Each patient also received oral aspirin and intravenous heparin. Mean values of coronary stenosis severity declined to a similar extent in each group. Resolution of intracoronary filling defects, increase in antegrade flow grade, or both also occurred equally among the three groups. There was considerable variation in individual patient response. Between 29% and 50% of patients within each group demonstrated a decrease in stenosis severity, whereas 50% to 57% noted either improvement in antegrade flow or resolution of intracoronary thrombus. There was no difference in incidence of major bleeding events among the 3 groups. Thus, a combination of intravenous rt-PA, aspirin, and heparin can reduce the severity of coronary stenosis in patients with unstable angina, but the treatment effect is mild in magnitude, varies among individual patients, and is not clearly superior to that achieved by the combination of aspirin and heparin alone.

Ardissino and associates[50] from Pavia, Italy, examined the incidence of refractory unstable angina in a consecutive series of 103 patients who received conventional medical therapy with nitrates, beta blockers, calcium antagonists, and aspirin. During 48 hours of continuous electrocardiographic monitoring, 24 patients had $\geq$1 anginal attack, 5 of whom had both painful and painless ischemic episodes. In these 24 patients with unstable angina refractory to conventional medical treatment, the short-term efficacy of rt-PA followed by heparin was assessed and compared with heparin alone in a randomized double-blind trial. Recurrences of ischemic attacks during a 72-hour follow-up period were documented in 9 of the 12 patients given heparin alone. All patients experienced at least 1 symptomatic ischemic episode and 1 patient had both painful and painless ischemia. No patient given rt-PA plus heparin had either symptomatic or asymptomatic ischemic attacks during follow-up. Kaplan-Meier curves analysis demonstrated a significantly higher probability of being ischemia free in the group of patients treated with rt-PA followed by heparin than in the group treated with heparin alone. Quantitative coronary arteriography failed to reveal any significant changes of ischemia-related lesions before and after each treatment. This study demonstrates that the combination of rt-PA and heparin has a greater protective effect than heparin alone in treating recurrent ischemic episodes in patients with refractory unstable angina. The clinical benefit of thrombolysis is not persistent and it does not eliminate the need for revascularization but may allow the procedures to be performed under more stable clinical conditions.

STABLE ANGINA PECTORIS

Characteristics of ischemic episodes

To determine the circadian distribution of episodes of myocardial ischemia, Hausmann and associates[51] from Hanover, West Germany, performed studies in 111 patients with chronic stable angina pectoris, positive exercise test results and angiographically proven CAD. During 24 hours of ambulatory electrocardiographic monitoring, 101 symptomatic and 298 asymptomatic ischemic episodes (ST-segment depression >1 mm, duration >1 minute) were observed. The number of ischemic episodes and the cumulative duration of ischemia showed a circadian variation with the highest values between 8 and 10 A.M. and between 4 and 5 P.M. associated with a similar circadian variation of heart rate (Figure 2-11). Mean duration of ischemic episodes, maximal amplitude of ST-segment depression during ischemic episodes and increase in heart rate before the onset of ischemic episodes showed no significant circadian variation. Heart rate at the onset of ischemic episodes and maximal heart rate during ischemic episodes were lower between midnight and A.M. than during other times of the day. The morning and afternoon increase in ischemic activity is not paralleled by changes reflecting a decrease in myocardial oxygen supply during these periods (heart rate at onset of ischemia, heart rate increase before onset of ischemia), but is paralleled by a similar circadian variation of heart rate. The circadian variation in ischemic activity is predominantly based on a comparable variation in myocardial oxygen requirements.

Ischemic threshold

In patients with stable CAD, the ischemic threshold for the production of effort-related angina is often quite variable. Although this feature is commonly attributed to changes in the caliber of coronary arteries at the site of stenosis, it could also be caused by the constriction of distal vessels, collateral vessels, or both. To test this hypothesis, Pupita and associates[52] from London, UK, studied 11 patients with stable angina, total occlusion of a single coronary artery that was supplied by collateral vessels, normal ventricular function, no evidence of coronary artery spasm, and no other coronary stenoses. These conditions precluded the modulation of coronary flow by vasomotion at the site of the coronary stenosis. The ischemic threshold—assessed by multiplying the heart rate by the systolic BP at a 1-mm depression of the ST segment during exercise testing—increased by 19% after the administration of nitroglycerin and decreased by 18% after the administration of ergonovine. Ambulatory electrocardiographic monitoring of the patients when not receiving treatment detected 73 ischemic episodes that, in keeping with the history, showed variations of 25 to 52 beats per minute in the heart rate at a 1-mm depression of the ST segment; 12 episodes of sinus tachycardia exceeded the lowest ischemic heart rate by a mean (±SD) of 22 ± 13 beats per minute without ST-segment depression. Furthermore, 21 ischemic episodes occurred at a heart rate more than 25 beats per minute below that at a 1-mm depression of the ST segment during exercise testing. Delayed and reduced filling of collateral and collateralized vessels associated with depression of the ST segment similar to that observed during ambulatory

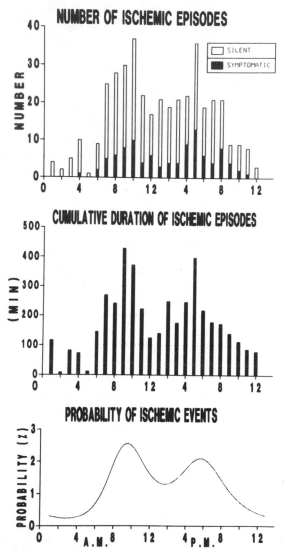

Fig. 2-11. Circadian variation of ischemic episodes in patients with stable coronary artery disease. Top, number of ischemic episodes; middle, cumulative duration of ischemic episodes; bottom, probability of the occurence of ischemic episodes during time intervals of 5 minutes (goodness of fit = 0.326). Reproduced with permission from Hausmann, et al.[51]

monitoring was detected on angiographic evaluation after the intracoronary administration of ergonovine in 3 patients. The authors proposed that the constriction of distal coronary arteries, collateral vessels, or both may cause AMI in patients with chronic stable angina.

Myocardial perfusion with exercise

Mahmarian and colleagues[53] in Houston, Texas, compared the extent of abnormally perfused myocardium in patients with and without chest pain during treadmill exercise from a large, relatively low-risk consecutive patient population referred for quantitative thallium-201 single-photon emission computed tomography. All patients had concurrent coronary angiography. Patients were excluded if they had prior PTCA or CABG. Tomographic images were assessed visually and from computer-generated polar maps. Chest pain during exercise was as frequent in patients with normal coronary arteries as in those with significant CAD. In the 219 patients with significant CAD, silent ischemia was 5-fold more common than symptomatic ischemia. However, there were no differences in the extent, severity, or distribution of coronary stenoses in patients with silent or symptomatic ischemia. A major observation was that the extent of quantified emission computed tomography perfusion defects was nearly identical in patients with and without exertional chest pain. The sensitivity for detecting the presence of CAD was significantly more improved with quantitative emission computed tomography compared with stress electrocardiography. Although streptokinase affords protection against secondary VF most probably by a limitation of infarct size. When the arrhythmia complicates the course of AMI, it is associated with an adverse short-term outcome, whereas the long-term prognosis is not influenced.

Role of adenosine in pathogenesis

The intravenous infusion of adenosine provokes anginalike chest pain. To establish its origin, Crea and co-investigators[54] in London, United Kingdom, administered an intracoronary infusion of increasing adenosine concentrations given to 22 patients with stable angina pectoris. During adenosine infusion, 2 patients had chest pain without electrocardiographic signs of ischemia. They both reported that the chest pain was similar to their usual anginal pain. In ten of the 22 patients adenosine was also infused into the right atrium but it never produced symptoms at the doses that had provoked chest pain during intracoronary infusion. In seven other patients, the intracoronary adenosine infusion was repeated after intravenous administration of aminophylline, an antagonist of adenosine P_1-receptors. Aminophylline decreased the severity of adenosine induced chest pain from 42 to 23 mm. In the remaining 5 of the 22 patients, monitoring of blood oxygen saturation in the coronary sinus during intracoronary adenosine administration showed that maximum coronary vasodilation was achieved at doses lower than those responsible for chest pain. A single-blind, placebo controlled randomized trial of the effects of aminophylline on exercised induced chest pain was also performed in 20 other patients with stable angina. Aminophylline compared with placebo, decreased the severity of chest pain at peak exercise from 67 to 51 mm despite the achievement of a similar degree of ST-segment depression. Finally the effect of intravenous adenosine was compared in 10 patients with predominantly painful myocardial ischemia and in ten patients with predominantly silent ischemia. The latter tolerated a longer period of adenosine infusion and developed significantly less severe chest pain than patients with painful ischemia. Thus, intracoronary adenosine administration provokes chest pain similar to the anginal pain at doses that do not produce symptoms during intra-atrial infusion. Furthermore, aminophylline, an adenosine P_1-receptor antagonist, significantly reduces the severity of both adenosine and exercise induced chest pain. These findings indicate that adenosine is a stimulus adequate to produce cardiac pain and could be partially responsible for the anginal pain during myocardial ischemia. This effect does not seem to be related to adenosine induced coronary dilatation and appears predominately mediated by P_1-receptor stimulation. The fact that the severity of chest pain provoked by intravenous adenosine is less in patients with silent ischemia further supports the hypothesis that adenosine may play an important role in the production of angina.

Coronary prostaglandin modulation

Serneri and associates[55] from Florence and Rome, Italy, investigated whether coronary vasodilating prostaglandins (PGI_2 and PGE_2) have a role in the pathophysiology of myocardial ischemia in 26 patients with angina pectoris and in 23 control individuals (nonischemic patients) studied by assessing coronary hemodynamics and prostaglandin formation in relation to sympathetic stimulation. Following a cold-pressor test, coronary prostaglandin output markedly increased and coronary vascular resistance decreased in all control individuals. In contrast, in anginal patients prostaglandins in the coronary sinus were undetectable and after cold pressor test prostaglandin output did not increase, whereas coronary vascular resistance paradoxically increased. In controls, the inhibition of coronary prostaglandin formation (by ketoprofen [1 mg/kg intravenously] or by aspirin [15 mg/kg intravenously]) caused a paradoxical increase of coronary vascular resistance following cold-pressor test. In anginal patients the inhibition of prostaglandins further exaggerated the increase of coronary vascular resistance after cold-pressor test. These results indicate that coronary vasodilating prostaglandins PGI_2 and PGE_2 play a role in modulating coronary vascular response to sympathetic stimulation induced by cold pressor test. Their defective production in anginal patients may be responsible for the paradoxical increase in coronary vascular resistance following sympathetic stimulation.

SILENT MYOCARDIAL ISCHEMIA

An excellent review on silent myocardial ischemia appeared in the March 1990 issue of the *Mayo Clinic Proceedings*.[56]

Deedwania and Carbajal[57] in San Francisco, California, prospectively examined the prognostic significance of silent myocardial ischemia detected by ambulatory electrocardiogram monitoring during daily life in 107 patients with long-term stable angina who were symptomatically controlled on conventional antianginal agents. Forty-six patients (group 1) demonstrated ≥ 1 episodes (87% silent) of myocardial ischemia; the remaining 61 patients (group 2) had no ischemic ST segment changes. During the mean follow-up period of 23 ± 8 months, 11 cardiac deaths (5 sudden and 6 nonsudden) occurred in group 1, and 5 cardiac deaths (all non sudden) occurred in group 2. Kaplan-Meier survival analysis between the groups confirmed that patients with silent ischemia (group 1) had worse prognoses during the follow-up period. Although the higher incidence of hypertension, smoking, hypercholesterolemia, and diabetes in these patients might reflect a more sickly population of stable angina patients, the multivariate Cox's hazard function analysis of these and other variables including Q waves of electrocardiogram, exercise parameters, and ambulatory electrocardiogram findings revealed presence of silent ischemia during daily life as the most powerful and independent predictor of cardiac mortality. These data indicate that, in such patients with stable angina, silent myocardial ischemia occurs frequently during treatment with conventional antianginal drugs and identifies a subset of patients who are at high risk of cardiac death.

Breitenbücher and associates[58] in Basel, Switzerland, conducted a retrospective 5 year follow-up study in 140 patients with "unequivocal" ischemia during exercise radionuclide ventriculography which consisted of a ≥10% decrease in LVEF or ≥5% decrease in EF with a definite regional wall motion abnormality during exercise. In 84 patients (60%), myocardial ischemia developing during radionuclide ventriculography was silent, whereas 56 patients had angina during the test. Workload and antianginal medication were similar in both groups. Critical cardiac events, including unstable angina, AMI, and cardiac death occurred in 27% of patients in the silent ischemia group and 16% of those in the symptomatic group. AMI or death were more frequent in patients with silent ischemia (22% versus 9%) (Figure 2-12). In the patients with additional exercise-induced ST segment depression, the frequency of critical events was further increased. Thus, these data suggest that patients with documented LV ischemic dysfunction with exercise have an increased incidence of important coronary heart disease events in the future and suggest that more vigorous medical and/or surgical therapy may be necessary in this group.

Deedwania and Carbajal[59] evaluated the prevalence and patterns of silent myocardial ischemia in 105 stable angina patients receiving conventional antianginal drug therapy. During 2,520 hours of electrocardiographic monitoring, silent ischemia was detected in 45 (43%) patients. A total of 188 ischemic episodes was observed; 163 (87%) were silent and accounted for a total ischemic duration of 5,771 minutes. There was no difference in the baseline clinical characteristics between the patients with and without ambulatory silent ischemia. However, patients with silent ischemia on ambulatory electrocardiographic monitoring had earlier onset of ischemia during exercise training. The highest density of silent ischemic events occurred between 6 A.M. and 6 P.M. Comparison of the class or combination of antianginal agents used by the 2 groups revealed no difference. However, in patients with silent ischemia the

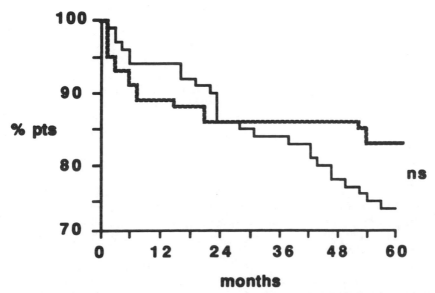

Fig. 2-12. Event-free survival rates in 56 patients with symptomatic (dotted line) and 84 patients with silent (solid line) ischemia during exercise radionuclide angiography. pts = patients. Reproduced with permission from Breitenbücher, et al.[58]

mean duration per event was shorter for those receiving 2 or more antianginal agents compared to those receiving monotherapy. The average duration of silent ischemia per event was significantly less in patients receiving B-blockers. These results demonstrate that silent ischemia during ordinary daily activities occurs frequently despite conventional antianginal drugs prescribed for control of symptoms.

Hausmann and associates[60] in Hanover, Federal Republic of Germany, studied the incidence of ventricular arrhythmias related to episodes of transient myocardial ischemia during ambulatory electrocardiographic monitoring in 97 patients with stable angina pectoris, angiographically proved CAD, and an abnormal exercise test. Five hundred and seventy three episodes with ST depression were documented. In 118 episodes (21%), the patients were symptomatic and in 455 (79%), they were asymptomatic. Ventricular arrhythmias, including >5 PVC/minute, bigeminy, couplets or salvos of PVCs occurred during 27 (5%) of episodes of myocardial ischemia in 10 patients (10%) (group A). The remaining 87 patients (90%) (group B) had myocardial ischemia without ventricular arrhythmias. Comparison of patients in groups A and B showed no differences in hemodynamic, angiographic, exercise testing, and ambulatory electrocardiographic monitoring data. Episodes of myocardial ischemia with and without ventricular arrhythmias showed a similar duration and amplitude of ST segment depression and comparable heart rates at the onset of ischemia. Both types of ischemia, with and without arrhythmias, occurred predominantly during the morning hours between 6:00 A.M. and noon and both types remained asymptomatic to within similar percentages. These data indicate that ventricular arrhythmias may be related to transient myocardial ischemia documented by electrocardiographic monitoring in some patients with stable angina. These arrhythmias appear to be often unrelated to the severity of ischemia as evaluated by ambulatory electrocardiographic monitoring and anginal symptoms.

In a prospective study Wilcox and associates[61] from Camperdown, Australia, evaluated the significance of silent myocardial ischemia in 66 patients with a clinical diagnosis of unstable angina (no requirement for reversible ST-T changes during pain on 12-lead electrocardiograms before entry), and the results of continuous 2-channel electrocardiographic recordings, begun with 24 hours of admission, were compared with other clinical and electrocardiographic predictors of adverse outcome. Ischemic changes were detected in 7 patients (11%) during a mean of 41 hours of recording. There were 37 episodes of transient ST-segment change (16 ST elevation, 21 ST depression) of which 11 (30%) were symptomatic and 26 (70%) were silent. All 7 patients had at least 1 silent episode and 5 also had symptomatic episodes during the recording but only 2 patients had exclusively silent episodes. During a mean follow-up of 13.3 months, 3 patients died, 5 had a nonfatal AMI and 32 required revascularization. Although transient myocardial ischemia during the continuous ECT recording, whether silent or symptomatic, was a specific predictor of subsequent nonfatal AMI or death (specificity 92%), its sensitivity for these events was low (25%). In contrast, recurrent rest pain (≥1 episode) occurred in all patients with these serious adverse events (sensitivity 100%, specificity 49%). Transient ischemia occurs infrequently during continuous ECG recordings in patients with unstable angina not selected by reversible ST-T changes on a 12-lead electrocardiogram at entry. Recurrent rest pain after hospital admission is a more sensitive predictor of serious events in this group.

Deedwania and associates[62] from Fresno and San Francisco, California, examined the predictive value of several exercise test parameters in identifying stable angina pectoris at risk of silent myocardial ischemia during daily life. A total of 97 patients with CAD, stable angina and ambulatory electrocardiographic data were evaluated. Of the 86 patients with a positive exercise test, 39 (group 1) had ≥1 episodes of ST-segment depression and 47 (group 2) did not develop ST changes during ambulatory electrocardiographic monitoring. Comparison of the exercise test parameters between the 2 groups revealed early onset of ischemia during exercise tests as the single most significant predictor of ambulatory silent ischemia. The other exercise test parameters showing significant differences between the 2 groups were the peak exercise heart rate (117 ± 23 vs 126 ± 20 beats/min) and peak systolic BP (160 ± 27 vs 176 ± 27 mm Hg), both of which were significantly lower in the group 1 patients. These data were used to derive simple mathematical formulas for calculating the risk of ambulatory silent ischemia. These results demonstrate that stable angina patients at risk of silent ischemia during daily life can be accurately identified by evaluation of selected exercise test parameters.

Episodes of transient myocardial ischemia during ambulatory activities are common in patients with stable CAD and who are often asymptomatic. Selection of therapy for episodes of asymptomatic ischemia is limited by a lack of direct comparative studies. To determine the most effective monotherapy for patients with stable angina and a high frequency of asymptomatic ischemic episodes, propranolol-LA, diltiazem-SR, nifedipine were compared with placebo, each for 2 weeks, by Stone and co-investigators[63] in Boston, Massachusetts, in a randomized, double-blinded, crossover trial. Entry criteria were a positive exercise treadmill test during placebo therapy characterized by 1.0 mm or more ST-segment depression and angina pectoris, and ≥6 episodes of transient ST-segment depression of 1.0 mm or more on a 48-hour ambulatory electrocardiogram. One hundred ninety-four patients were screened, 63 were eligible and received randomized therapy, of which 56 patients completed at least 2 of the 4 treatment periods and were included in an intent-to-treat analysis. Fifty patients completed all 4 treatment phases and were included in the protocol-completed analysis. Compared with placebo, only propranolol was associated with a marked reduction in all manifestations of asymptomatic ischemia during ambulatory electrocardiographic monitoring. The active agents modestly improved treadmill exercise duration time until 1 mm ST-segment depression and only propranolol and diltiazem had significant effects. Only diltiazem significantly prolonged the total exercise time. Anginal frequency was significantly decreased by both propranolol and diltiazem. The investigators concluded that propranolol is effective for treating episodes of asymptomatic ischemia in patients with stable angina and that the magnitude of improvement in ambulatory asymptomatic ischemia is far greater than the improvement in exercise performance and angina symptoms.

Banai and associates[64] from Jerusalem, Israel, assessed the variations in myocardial ischemic threshold (heart rate at the onset of ischemia) during daily activities in patients with myocardial ischemic episodes on Holter monitoring. Eighty patients from known CAD, positive treadmill stress test results and ≥2 ischemic episodes during a 24-hour period of Holter monitoring were studied. The lowest and the highest ischemic thresholds were determined for each patient. The mean lowest ischemic threshold was 85 beats/min, and the mean highest ischemic threshold was 109 beats/min. The highest ischemic threshold was identical to ischemic threshold values noted during exercise. Of the 895 ischemic episodes, 654 (74%) were preceded by a moderate (>10%) increase in heart rate. The variability of ischemic threshold (difference in percentage between the highest and lowest ischemic thresholds) increased with the number of ischemic episodes (range 2 to 60%). In different patients with a similar number of ischemic episodes, different variability was observed. These differences in ischemic thresholds are probably indirect indicators of the vasomotor activity of the coronary arteries in different patients.

Taki and associates[65] from Boston, Massachusetts, determined the incidence and temporal sequence of LV dysfunction, SD segment depression, and chest pain in 43 ambulatory patients with angina pectoris of increasing frequency who underwent continuous monitoring of LV function for an average of 2.9 ± 1.9 hours. Indicators of ischemia were: a decrease in EF >5% lasting >1 minute; horizontal or down-sloping ST-segment depression of ≥1 mm; or onset of the patient's typical chest pain complex, or a combination of these. During the monitoring interval, subjects performed daily activities such as sitting, walking, climbing stairs and eating. In 11 patients, 22 episodes of chest pain or ST-segment depression, or both, were observed. Eighteen episodes were accompanied by a decrease in EF (9 patients); chest pain accompanied the decrease in EF during 13 episodes, whereas ST-segment changes occurred during 7. In 12 of 13 episodes the decrease in EF began earlier than the onset of chest pain, whereas in 1 patient EF decrease and chest pain onset started at the same time. The average interval from a decrease in EF to the onset of chest pain was 56 ± 41 seconds (range 0 to 120). ST changes occurred after the onset of a decrease in EF in 6 of 7 episodes. The average interval from the onset of EF decrease and the onset of ST change was 99 ± 91 seconds. These data suggest that LV dysfunction manifested by a decrease in EF is an earlier indicator of myocardial ischemia than is angina pectoris or electrocardiographic evidence of ischemia.

VARIANT ANGINA PECTORIS AND CORONARY SPASM

Neglia and co-investigators[66] of Pisa, Italy, assessed the effects of single-vessel CAD on simultaneously evaluated RV and LV performance and compared with LV perfusion patterns in 25 patients with variant angina. Coronary spasms involved the right coronary artery in 15 patients (group 1) and the LAD coronary artery in 10 patients (group 2). Biventricular function was assessed by radionuclide angiography under basal conditions, during spontaneous or ergonovine-induced ischemia, and after resolution of the ischemic attack. Myocardial perfusion was assessed by thallium-201 scintigraphy in 21 patients of this series during superimposable ischemic episodes. In group one, ischemia was caused by RV (fourteen of fifteen patients) and LV (13 of 15 patients) regional dysfunction with significant reduction in RV and LVEF. The ventricular septum was in 6 of 15 patients, causing a more pronounced LV impairment. In group 2, all patients showed septal dyssynergies associated with a reduction of LVEF; absent or trivial RV involvement was observed. In both groups, LV perfusion defects were present in all patients with LV wall motion abnormalities during ischemia, matching the site of regional dyssynergies. Thus, in a group of patients with variant angina and single-vessel CAD, transient occlusion of the right coronary artery directly caused RV and LV impairment; in these patients, the extent of LV but not RV dysfunction appeared related to the presence of septal ischemia. Vasospasm of the LAD coronary artery consistently caused LV dysfunction not associated with secondary effects of RV systolic function.

SYNDROME X (MICROVASCULAR ANGINA)

To ascertain the relative prevalence of abnormalities of coronary flow reserve and esophageal function in patients with chest pain despite angiographically normal coronary arteries, Cannon and associates[67] from Bethesda, Maryland, and Washington, D.C., performed invasive study of coronary blood flow in 87 patients and during the same week esophageal testing. Of the 87 patients, 63 (72%) demonstrated abnormalities of coronary flow reserve, as evidenced by an increase in coronary resistance during the stress of rapid atrial pacing after administration of ergonovine 0.15 mg intravenously (1.33 ± 0.36 mm Hg • minute/mL), compared with pacing at the same heart rate before ergonovine administration (1.10 ± 0.33 mm Hg • minute/mL). This higher coronary vascular resistance occurred in the absence of significant epicardial coronary artery luminal narrowing. Fifty-seven of these 63 patients (90%) with a coronary vasoconstrictor response to ergonovine described their typical chest pain during pacing stress, compared with only 6 of 24 patients (25%) who demonstrated no coronary flow abnormality. After administration of dipyridamole 0.5 to 0.75 mg/kg intravenously to 65 patients, the 48 patients with ergonovine-induced vasoconstriction had a significantly higher minimum coronary resistance, compared with the 17 patients without a coronary vasoconstrictor response to ergonovine (0.65 ± 0.21 vs 0.47 ± 0.13 mm Hg • minute/mL). Twenty of 87 patients (23%) had abnormal esophageal motility [nutcracker esophagus (11), nonspecific motility disorder (7), and diffuse esophageal spasm (2)], including 16 of the 63 patients (25%) with abnormal coronary flow reserve. Twenty-four (28%) of patients experienced their typical chest pain during motility testing, but only five of these patients met criteria for abnormal esophageal motility. Nine of 75 patients tested (12%) had their typical chest pain during Bernstein testing, and 18 of 38 patients (47%) tested had their typical chest pain provoked by intraesophageal balloon distention. The authors concluded that 71 of 87 patients (82%) with anginal-like chest pain and normal epicardial vessels in the series had a disorder of either coronary flow reserve, esophageal motility, and/or reproduction of typical chest pain during acid infusion. Chest pain was commonly encountered during cardiac and esophageal testing (85% of patients), regardless of the ability to demonstrate an abnormality of coronary flow reserve or abnormal esophageal function. This suggests that pain experienced by these patients may be a consequence of myocardial ischemia, esophageal dysfunction, abnormal visceral nociception, or a combination of any or all of these entities.

Since an abnormal shortening of diastolic duration during exercise in patients with CAD has been demonstrated, time course of diastolic period (cardiac cycle minus electromechanical systole) calculated from polycardiographic recording was assessed by Spinelli and associates[68] from Naples, Italy, in patients with X syndrome (angina with normal coronary arteries) and in normal age-matched subjects during supine ergometer exercise. All patients with X syndrome had positive exercise stress response (>0.1 mV of ST segment depression). Duration of diastole expressed as percent of cardiac cycle was significantly shorter at the intermediate steps and at the peak of exercise in patients with X syndrome compared with normal subjects. When the relationship between heart rate and diastolic time was examined, an inverse nonlinear regression was found both in normal subjects and in patients with X syndrome. The exercise values of diastolic time observed in patients with X syndrome were significantly shorter than those predicted as normal diastolic time heart rate relation. Thus patients with X syndrome demonstrated abnormalities in the decrement of diastolic time with exercise. It is speculated that this disproportionate shortening, by reducing subendocardial blood flow, might induce a worsening of ischemic response to exercise.

Geltman and associates[69] in St. Louis, Missouri, used positron emission tomography with oxygen-15-labeled water and oxygen-15-labeled carbon monoxide before and after intravenous dipyridamole to assess regional myocardial perfusion and perfusion reserve in absolute terms in 16 normal subjects and 17 patients with chest pain and angiographically normal coronary arteries. Eight of the 17 patients had a myocardial perfusion reserve <2.5 (the lower limit of normal in studies with positron emission tomography) and 9 of 17 patients had a normal response. In the patients with an impaired perfusion reserve, perfusion at rest was higher than measured in normal subjects and maximal flow and perfusion reserve were significantly reduced. Abnormalities of perfusion and perfusion reserve were homogeneous without detectable regional disparities. Therefore, nearly half of the patients with chest pain and normal coronary arteries angiographically have abnormalities of myocardial perfusion that are detectable noninvasively with positron emission tomography and oxygen-15-labeled water.

To assess whether the time course of ST segment depression differs in patients with CAD and in patients with angina and normal coronary arteries, the exercise tests of 54 patients with documented CAD and 25 patients with syndrome X (angina, positive exercise test, no evidence of coronary artery spasm, and normal coronary arteries) were compared in a study by Pupita and associates[70] from London, UK. All tests were performed with therapy withheld, using the modified Bruce protocol. In each test, time, heart rate and BP were measured at the onset and at 1 mm of ST segment depression, and at peak exercise. Recovery (return of the ST segment to baseline ±0.2 mm) time was also assessed. Peak ST segment depression was similar in CAD and syndrome X patients (1.5 ± 0.3 versus 1.6 ± 0.4 mm). In 42 CAD patients, ST segment depression developed early (≤6 minutes) during exercise; this was associated with a short recovery (≤3 minutes) in 17 (40%) and with a long recovery (>3 minutes) in 25 (60%) patients. In 17 patients with syndrome X, ST segment depression developed early; it was associated with a short recovery in 6 (35%) and with a long recovery in 11 (65%) patients. Late (>6 minutes) onset of ST segment depression was observed in 12 CAD patients; of these, 8 (67%) had a short recovery and 4 (33%) had a long recovery. Late onset of ST segment depression occurred in 8 patients with syndrome X; 6 (75%) had a short recovery and 2 (25%) had a long recovery. Average time, heart rate, and heart rate-BP product were higher in syndrome X than in CAD patients, both at 1 mm of ST segment depression and at peak exercise. One millimeter of ST segment depression developed at a heart rate ≤110 beats/min in 47% of CAD patients but in only 4% of syndrome X patients. Thus the time course of ST segment depression during exercise is similar in syndrome X and in CAD, but the heart rate at which diagnostic ST segment depression develops is significantly different in these 2 conditions.

Anginal chest pain in patients with angiographically normal coronary arteries may be caused by a limited coronary flow response to stress because of abnormal function of the coronary microcirculation (microvascular angina). Studies of forearm arterial function suggested that patients with microvascular angina may have a diffuse disorder of smooth muscle tone. Because dyspnea is common in these patients and seems disproportionate to the severity of myocardial ischemia, Cannon and colleague[71] in Bethesda, Maryland studied air flow (forced expiratory volume in 1 second) in the basal state and after methacholine inhalation to determine whether bronchial smooth muscle is affected in this syndrome. Five of 36 patients with microvascular angina had a basal first expiratory volume of <70% of that predicted and did not receive methacholine. Of the remaining 31 patients, 14 had a more-than-20% reduction in forced expiratory volume after methacholine, a response significantly greater than that of nine patients with heart disease and 24 normal volunteers of similar age and gender distribution. Furthermore, the product of the methacholine dose inhaled and the magnitude of decline in forced expiratory volume from baseline was significantly lower in patients with microvascular angina than in normal volunteers. The investigators concluded that airway hyperresponsiveness is frequently demonstrable in patients with microvascular angina; these findings are consistent with their hypothesis that this syndrome may represent a more generalized abnormality of vascular and nonvascular smooth muscle function.

DRUGS FOR MYOCARDIAL ISCHEMIA

Exercise training

Todd and Ballantyne[72] from Glasgow, UK, studied 40 men less than 60 years of age with stable chronic angina for at least 6 months and no prior AMI. Exercise tolerance testing was carried out all treatment and after atenolol therapy. Atenolol was stopped and the patients were randomized to a control group and a study group of patients who undertook a 1-year high-intensity training program. The groups were then restudied. Submaximum heart rate was reduced by 13 beats per minute by training and by 23 beats per minute by atenolol. Training increased the maximum heart rate by 10 beats per minute and atenolol reduced it by 29 beats per minute. The double produce ST threshold was increased from 183 to 205 by training but reduced to 143 by atenolol. Maximum ST depression was similarly reduced by both training and atenolol. As a result of the effects on maximum heart rate, training produced a greater improvement in exercise tolerance than atenolol with a treadmill time increased from 741 seconds to 1272 seconds with training compared with 974 seconds with atenolol. Other variables were similarly affected. Thus, the antianginal efficacy of exercise training is as good as that achieved by B blockade and represents an alternative to such treatment.

Isosorbide dinitrate and 5-mononitrate

Coster and co-workers[73] in London, UK, compared the effects of isosorbide dinitrate administered by intracoronary and intravenous routes in 10 patients with severe, stable effort angina, and very low exercise tolerance. Supine bicycle ergometer exercise was performed under four conditions: 1) control, 2) after intracoronary administration of 0.4 mg isosorbide dinitrate, 3) 1 hour later (control 2), and 4) after administration of intravenous 4 mg isosorbide dinitrate. At rest, intracoronary isosorbide dinitrate caused no significant hemodynamic effects, whereas intravenous infusion of the agent resulted in a decline in LV systolic pressure, LV end-diastolic volume and LV end-systolic volume. After intracoronary infusion of isosorbide dinitrate ST segment depression and the increase in LV end-diastolic pressure and LV end-systolic volume induced by exercise were significantly less abnormal than during control. When exercise was performed after intravenous infusion of isosorbide dinitrate, the above-mentioned parameters were significantly improved even further: ST segment depression, end-diastolic pressure and LV end-systolic volume as compared to intracoronary isosorbide dinitrate. Thus, in the patients with CAD, it is suggested that intracoronary nitrates increase coronary blood supply during effort-induced ischemia, based on significant improvements in the indirect measures of ST segment depression, LV end-diastolic pressure, and LV volume. More marked effects on these measures were observed after intravenous administration, when coronary and peripheral effects are combined.

Seabra-Gomes and associates[74] from Carnaxide, Portugal, entered 33 men with stable exercise-induced angina pectoris into a randomized, double-blind, crossover study in which controlled-release isosorbide-5-mononitrate 60 mg once daily was compared with conventional isosorbide dinitrate 20 mg 3 times daily. Each drug was given for 2 weeks. Twenty-eight patients completed the study and data on exercise variables are available in 23 patients. Treatment with either drug resulted in significant antianginal effects, when measured 6 hours after a single dose and after 2 weeks of therapy compared with baseline placebo; however, there were significantly fewer signs of myocardial ischemia during treatment with isosorbide-5-mononitrate. There was no evidence of tolerance to either drug treatment but a significant attenuation of resting BP (but not of exercise BP) was observed with both drugs. Headache was the only clinically significant adverse event during therapy and it occurred more frequently in the isosorbide dinitrate treatment group; 3 such patients had to withdraw from the study because of headache. Thus, once-daily, controlled-release isosorbide-5-mononitrate appears as effective as conventional isosorbide dinitrate 3 times daily in patients with stable angina pectoris. The once-daily administration is convenient and improves patient compliance.

Beyerle and associates[75] from Munich, Federal Republic of Germany, in 18 patients with documented CAD and stable angina pectoris investigated using a randomized, double-blind, crossover, placebo controlled protocol the antiischemic effect of 50 and 100 mg isosorbide-5-mononitrate (IS-5-MN) in sustained release form. After the initial administration of both dosages, compared to placebo there were significant reductions in exercise-induced ST-segment depression and significant increases in ischemia-free exercise time at all times of testing. At 12 hours, the 100-mg dosage still amounted to 50% of its maximum and was significantly more marked than the 50 mg dose. Accordingly, the 100-mg dosage can be assumed to confer a longer duration of action. At the end of 3 weeks of long-term treatment, the significant antiischemic effects were not diminished versus those observed after initial administration. There was no evidence of tolerance development with either dosage. The IS-5-MN plasma concentration during long-term administration displayed, within the 24-hour treatment cycle, a clear decrease to low baseline values and a marked 5- to 7-fold increase after the daily dose in accordance with the response known to be prerequisite to successful interval treatment. Thus, the once-daily administration of IS-5-MN SR with dosages of 50 mg and, more markedly, 100 mg, provides effective antiischemic protection throughout the daily period of most physical activities in patients with stable angina pectoris.

Nifedipine ± isosorbide dinitrate

Since not all patients tolerate β-blockers, the efficacy of nifedipine and isosorbide dinitrate was evaluated alone and in combination in patients with stable angina pectoris in a study conducted by Vlay and Olson[76] from Stony Brook, New York. The investigation was a randomized double-blind crossover design with patients titrated to maximally tolerated doses of both drugs. Phases included isosorbide dinitrate alone, nifedipine alone, and isosorbide dinitrate plus nifedipine in combination, with efficacy determined by stress testing. Eleven men and 1 woman patient with a mean age of 60 years and a mean of 5 anginal episodes/week completed the study. Patients were in New York Heart Association classes, I, II, and III. With nifedipine alone compared to isosorbide dinitrate alone, patients had fewer angina attacks/week, exercised longer before experiencing angina, and had less ST segment depression during or after exercise. When patients received isosorbide dinitrate plus nifedipine, only time to onset of angina during exercise was significantly different from the response with isosorbide dinitrate alone. Analysis of variance between nifedipine and isosorbide dinitrate plus nifedipine was not significant. Diastolic BP with isosorbide dinitrate plus nifedipine was lower than with isosorbide dinitrate alone. No significant differences in systolic BP were noted between the treatment groups. The drugs alone and in combination were relatively well tolerated. Nifedipine alone may be superior to isosorbide dinitrate alone. The combination of isosorbide dinitrate plus nifedipine demonstrated no advantage over nifedipine alone compared with isosorbide dinitrate alone.

Betaxolol vs propranolol

Betaxolol is a new, highly cardioselective, once-a-day β-blocker with a long half-life (mean 16 hours). Narahara and associates of the Betaxolol Investigators Group[77] from Los Angeles, California, evaluated the antianginal efficacy of 2 doses of betaxolol (20 and 40 mg) given once daily and compared with propranolol (40 or 80 mg) 4 times daily. Ninety-two patients completed the 10-week double-blind trial. The resting and exercise heart rate, BP and double product were similar for all treatment arms of the study during placebo treatment. Significant decreases in these measures occurred during active drug treatment when compared with placebo. No significant intergroup differences were noted at rest. Maximal exercise heart rate and double product were significantly lower during treatment with betaxolol 40 mg daily than in the propranolol 40 mg 4 times/day treatment group. All patients had chest pain and ≥1 mm of ST-segment depression during the baseline placebo exercise test. After 10 weeks of active treatment, 55% of the patients were free of chest pain during maximal exercise (difference not significant between treatments). In the betaxolol 40 mg/day group, fewer (6 of 19; 32%) of the patients developed ST-segment depression with exercise compared with pro-pranolol 80 mg 4 times daily (21 of 26; 81%). Betaxolol appears to be a useful once-a-day cardioselective β-blocker for the therapy of angina pectoris.

Propranolol intravenously

Bortone and co-investigators[78] in Zurich, Switzerland, studied coro-nary vasomotion at rest and during bicycle exercise with biplane quan-titative coronary arteriography in 28 patients with CAD. Patients were divided into 2 groups; the first 18 patients served as controls (group 1), and the next 10 patients were treated with propranolol 0.1 mg/kg, which was infused intravenously before exercise (group 2). Luminal area of a normal and a stenotic vessel segment was determined at rest, during supine bicycle exercise, and 5 minutes after sublingual administration of 1.6 mg nitroglycerin after exercise. In group 1, the normal vessel showed vasodilation of 16% during exercise, whereas the stenotic vessel segment showed vasoconstriction − 31%. After sublingual administration of nitro-glycerin, there was coronary vasodilation of both normal and stenotic vessel segments. Patients with angina pectoris during supine exercise had significantly more vasoconstriction than patients without angina. In group 2, intravenous administration of propranolol at rest was associated with a decrease in luminal area of both normal and stenotic vessel seg-ments; however, during subsequent exercise, both normal and stenotic vessel segments dilated when compared with the measurements after propranolol. Administration of nitroglycerin further increased luminal area of both vessel segments. The investigators concluded that dynamic exercise in patients with CAD is associated with coronary vasodilation of the normal and vasoconstriction of the stenotic coronary arteries. Patients with exercise-induced angina had significantly more stenosis vasoconstriction than patients without angina although minimal luminal area at rest was similar. Intravenous administration of propranolol is accompanied by a significant decrease in coronary luminal area of both normal and stenotic vessel segments at rest, which is overridden by dynamic exercise and sublingual nitroglycerin. The reduction in myo-cardial oxygen consumption and the prevention of exercise-induced ste-nosis vasoconstriction might explain the beneficial effect of beta-blocker treatment in most patients with CAD.

Theophylline ± atenolol

Crea and associates[79] from London, UK, studied the effects of theo-phylline (400 mg twice a day), atenolol (50 mg twice a day) and their combination on myocardial ischemia in 9 patients with stable angina pectoris in a randomized, single-blind, triple crossover trial. Placebo was administered to the patients during the run-in and the run-off periods. A treadmill exercise test and 24-hour ambulatory electrocardiographic monitoring were obtained at the end of each treatment period. Compared with placebo, theophylline significantly improved the time to onset of myocardial ischemia (1 mm of ST-segment depression) from 7.8 ± 3.7 to 9.5 ± 3.7 minutes and the exercise duration from 9 ± 3.4 to 10.1 ± 3.5 minutes. During atenolol and during combination treatment, the time to the onset of ischemia and the exercise duration were similar (10.8 ± 4.2 and 11.2 ± 3.2 minutes, 11.2 ± 3.6 and 11.5 ± 3.2 minutes, respectively) and longer than during theophylline administration. Ambulatory electrocardiographic monitoring showed that, during theophylline administration, the heart rate was higher than during placebo throughout the 24 hours. During atenolol and during combination treatment the heart rate was similar and in both cases lower than during placebo. Compared with placebo, theophylline decreased the total ischemic time from 97 ± 110 to 70 ± 103 minutes. During combination treatment the total ischemic time (5.6 ± 8.5 minutes) was not statistically different from that during atenolol administration (18 ± 29 minutes), although it was significantly lower than that observed during theophylline administration. Thus, in patients with stable angina pectoris the long-term administration of theophylline improves myocardial ischemia, but to a lesser degree than atenolol. Despite the fact that atenolol abolishes the undesirable chronotropic effect of theophylline and the latter probably reduces the undesirable increase of cardiac volumes caused by atenolol, their combination does not show detectable addictive effects.

MEDICAL VS SURGICAL THERAPY

Changes in the use of CABG and PTCA over the last several years have resulted in a new and different environment for the interventional treatment of CAD. Weintraub and associates[80] from Atlanta, Georgia, explored these changes as applied to the treatment of chronic CAD. The study population comprised 14,078 patients undergoing diagnostic cardiac catheterization between 1981 and 1988. In 1981, 1,704 patients underwent a first known cardiac catheterization at Emory University Hospital or Crawford W. Long Hospital and were found to have significant CAD. Of these patients, 51.7% were treated medically, 44.0% by CABG and 4.3% with PTCA. A similar group comprised 1,719 patients in 1988. Of this group, 41.2% were treated medically, 28.5% with CABG and 30.3% with PTCA. The data reveal a much more complex phenomenon than a simple increase in PTCA for the treatment of CAD at the expense of CABG. The CABG group aged such that the percent of the CABG population more than 65 years old increased from 26.0% of the total in 1981 to 44.9% of the total in 1988. The percent of patients with EF <50% in the CABG population decreased from 24.5% in 1981 to 19.7% in 1988. The PTCA population had less severe disease, was younger and had better LV function. Nonetheless, the percent more than 65 years old increased from 15.4% in 1981 to 35.4% in 1988. The percent of patients with EF <50% increased from 9.6% in 1981 to 15.1% in 1988. Similar changes were noted in the medically treated group. Not surprisingly, the biggest increases in PTCA occurred in 1- and 2-vessel disease patients, with a concomitant decrease in the CABG referrals in these patients. Thus, 2 processes occurred at the same time. The population grew older and had more significant coronary narrowing. At the same time, PTCA was used with increasing frequency as a treatment for 1- and 2-vessel CAD. This has resulted in a marked shift in the CABG population. These changes have significant implications for policy planners, reimbursors and clinical researchers in the treatment of CAD.

Proudfit and associates[81] from Cleveland, Ohio, calculated 10-year survival percentages for groups of 407 initially medically treated patients and for 390 patients who had early CABG; all had either mild angina pectoris or myocardial infarction without subsequent angina pectoris. Uncensored actuarial survival was 77% for medical patients and 83% for the surgical group. For 179 patients who had internal thoracic (mammary) artery grafting as part of their procedures, survival was 91% in contrast to 76% for those who had vein grafts only. A sharp drop of the survival curve for the vein graft group after the seventh year was not shown for those who had internal thoracic artery grafts. Survival was 71% for 280 patients treated medically only.

Allen and associates[82] from Baltimore, Maryland, entered into a perspective comparison study examining functional status and return-to-work during the first year of recovery of 2 cohorts of consecutive patients of comparable age with similar preprocedural cardiac function who underwent either CABG (n = 106) or PTCA (n = 64). Patients were evaluated using standardized functional status instruments for activities of daily living, work performance, social activity, mental health and quality of social interaction at 1, 6 and 12 months after the procedure. Within the CABG group, statistically significant improvements of functional status on every subscale were noted over the 1-year follow-up. Patients undergoing PTCA demonstrated significant improvement in all dimensions except for the quality of interaction at 1 year as compared with baseline. When the 2 groups were compared, the PTCA group demonstrated greater participation than the CABG group in routine daily physical and social activities at 1 and 6 months, but this apparent advantage disappeared by 1 year. Measures of psychological functioning were better after CABG than after PTCA. A reduction in the number of those with employment occurred in both the CABG and PTCA groups, independent of physical functional status measures, which improved in both groups after the procedures. For those with employment, the CABG group reported the greatest improvement in work performance.

Quality of life indexes were assessed by Rogers and co-investigators[83] in Seattle, Washington, in 780 patients 10 years after randomization to medical therapy (n = 390) CABG (n = 390) in the Coronary Artery Surgery Study. At 10 years, mortality was 22% in the medical group and 19% in the surgical group and 37% of the medical group had undergone surgery because of increasing chest pain (Figure 2-13). At study entry, 22% of medical and surgical patients were angina free; at 1 and 5 years after entry, the frequency of asymptomatic patients was 55% and 63% in the surgical group and 30% and 38% in the medical group. However, by 10 years after entry, the proportion of patients free of angina had fallen to 47% in the surgical group and 42% in the medical group. Activity limitation and use of beta-blockers and long-acting nitrates were less in the surgical than the medical group at 1 and 5 years after entry but little different from the medical group at 10 years after entry. Throughout follow-up, recreational status, employment status, frequency of heart failure, use of other medications, and hospitalization frequency were similar between the two groups. Thus, indexes of quality of life such as angina relief, increased activity, and reduction in use of antianginal medications initially appear superior in patients with stable manifestations of CAD assigned to surgery, but by 10 years after entry, these advantages are much less apparent. Although the observed similarities of the medically and surgically assigned group at 10 years reflect return of symptoms in the surgical group to some extent, a more important explanation is performance of late surgery in a large proportion of the medically assigned patients, rendering them asymptomatic.

Time to Initial CABG

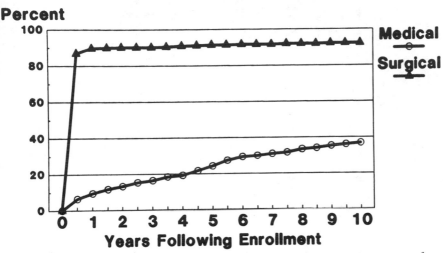

Fig. 2-13. Plot of time to initial coronary artery bypass graft surgery. At 10 years after entry, coronary artery surgery had been performed once or more in 92% of the 390 surgically assigned patients and in 37% of the 390 medically assigned patients. Reproduced with permission from Rogers, et al.[83]

PERCUTANEOUS TRANSLUMINAL CORONARY ANGIOPLASTY

Review

Gary S. Roubin[84] provided a fine review of the status of percutaneous transluminal coronary angioplasty in *Current Problems in Cardiology* (Dec., 1990).

In asymptomatic patients

Anderson and associates[85] from Atlanta, Georgia, performed elective PTCA in 6,545 patients over a 7.5 year period and 114 (1.7%) of them never had symptoms of myocardial ischemia. Exercise-induced silent ischemia was documented before PTCA in 94% of these asymptomatic patients. Angioplasty was successful in 87%, whereas emergency CABG was required in 4%, and a further 2% had AMI after the procedures (Figure 2-14). The remaining 7% had unsuccessful angioplasty procedures but experienced no in-hospital cardiac events. The follow-up period after hospital discharge averaged 43 ± 20 months (range 5–93). There were no deaths. In the group of 99 patients with initially successful angioplasty procedures the follow-up interval ranged from 5–92 months. During that period, 7 patients underwent CABG, 4 patients had AMI and 30 patients had repeat angioplasty procedures for restenosis. The cumulative probability of event-free survival over 5 years for the group with successful angioplasty was: 100% freedom from death, 95% freedom from AMI, 87% freedom from AMI or CABG and 61% freedom from AMI, CABG or repeat angioplasty. Thus, coronary angioplasty performed in 114 asymptomatic

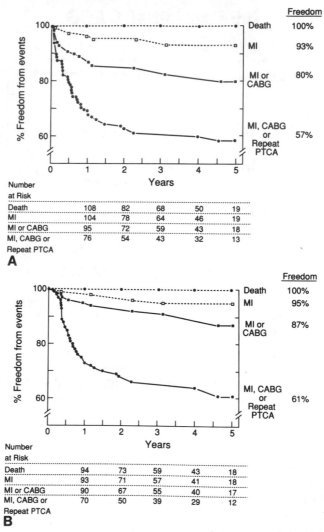

Fig. 2-14. Event-free survival curves after coronary angioplasty for asymptomatic patients with coronary artery disease. A, event-free survival for entire group of 114 asymptomatic patients. B, event-free survival for group of 99 asymptomatic patients with successful angioplasty procedures. The tables below each graph show number of patients at risk for events at end of each year. CABG = coronary artery bypass graft surgery; MI = myocardial infarction; PTCA = percutaneous transluminal coronary angioplasty. Reproduced with permission from Anderson, et al.[85]

patients, most with exercise-induced silent AMI, achieved very good primary success and was accompanied by low cardiac event rates and no deaths over several years of patient follow-up.

With severe left ventricular dysfunction

Kohli and colleagues[86] in Richmond, Virginia, evaluated the short- and long-term effects of PTCA in 61 patients with severely depressed LVEFs ≤35% with unstable or refractory angina in whom revascularization was necessary despite indicators suggesting increased risk. In a retrospective analysis of 1,260 patients undergoing PTCA between January, 1985 through December, 1987, 61 had an LVEF ≤35%. The common clinical presentation was unstable angina (70%) with or without AMI. Mean LVEF was 27 ± 6%. Forty-five patients (74%) had multivessel CAD. Clinical success after PTCA was achieved in 55 patients (90%). Major complications, including death, AMI, and CABG occurred in 5 patients (8%) with death in 2 (3%). During long-term follow-up of 21 ± 11 months study of 55 patients with successful PTCA, 13 (23%) died, including 3 of noncardiac causes, and 11 (20%) had clinically symptomatic recurrences. Continued clinical success occurred in 39 patients (71%) of whom 28 (51%) were event-free patients and 11 (20%) had clinical recurrences. A successful second PTCA procedure was performed in 9 patients because of restenosis. Therefore, in patients with depressed LVEF, PTCA may be performed with a short-term efficacy comparable to that found in patients with a better preserved LVEF undergoing PTCA or CABG. Nevertheless, acute complications are more frequent and the late mortality rates higher than in patients with better preserved LV function.

In chronic renal failure

Accelerated atherosclerosis occurs in chronic renal failure. The role of PTCA in chronic renal failure patients requiring dialysis has not been characterized. Kahn and associates[87] from Kansas City, Missouri, studied 17 chronic dialysis patients requiring PTCA over a 6 year period. Their mean age was 60 years, 4 were diabetic, 8 had severe hypertension, and 7 had unstable angina. Angiographic success was achieved in 47 of 49 (96%) stenoses attempted, including multivessel PTCA in 12 patients. There was 1 procedural death, 2 non-Q wave myocardial infarctions following PTCA, and 1 additional in-hospital noncardiac death. The 15 survivors were asymptomatic on discharge (mean stay 11 days), but recurrent angina developed within 6 months in 12 patients. Angiography in 11 of these 12 patients demonstrated restenosis of 26 of 32 (81%) dilated sites. Repeat PTCA in 6 patients was followed by return of angina in 4 patients with restenosis in 11 of 12 sites. Bypass surgery was ultimately performed in 4 patients with long-term angina relief. During follow-up (mean 20 months), 7 patients died (5 from chronic renal failure, 2 cardiac deaths). Thus although PTCA in chronic dialysis patients is technically feasible and provides relief of angina, aggressive restenosis limits the long-term benefit. CABG may be the preferred therapy for this unique patient group.

For chronic total occlusions

Finci and associates[88] from Geneva, Switzerland, compared results over a 2-year period of successful PTCA in 100 consecutive patients with chronic total coronary occlusion with those in 100 consecutive patients whose PTCA was unsuccessful. The groups were comparable in terms of gender, age and arteries attempted. A control angiography in the group with successful PTCA was performed in 62 patients and showed a restenosis in 28 (45%). Repeat PTCA was performed in 21 versus 1 patient with failed PTCA. At follow-up, in the group with successful PTCA, there were 57 symptom-free patients versus 26 patients in the group with failed PTCA. CABG was performed in 7 versus 37 patients, and there were 5 versus 3 deaths (difference not significant), respectively. In the group with successful PTCA, 27 of 82 patients (33%) had positive stress test results, compared with 49 of 85 patients (58%) in the group with unsuccessful PTCA. The double product (beats/min × mm Hg/100) in patients with successful PTCA improved from 247 ± 57 before PTCA to 277 ± 61 at follow-up, whereas it did not significantly change in patients with failed PTCA. The work load (W) in patients with successful PTCA improved from 95 ± 34 before PTCA to 124 ± 40 at follow-up. In patients with failed PTCA, work load improved less significantly, from 98 ± 37 before PTCA to 108 ± 34 at follow-up. Thus, up to a mean of 2 years, patients with successful coronary angioplasty of chronic total coronary occlusion appeared to fare better than those whose angioplasty was unsuccessful.

In silent ischemia

Tuzcu and associates[89] from Cleveland, Ohio, described short- and long-term outcome of PTCA in 34 patients who had documented CAD without symptoms. Of the 34 patients, 33 had abnormal stress tests before PTCA. PTCA was successful in 31 patients (91%). Follow-up was 100% for a mean period of 36 ± 15 months. Follow-up exercise test was normal or improved in 29 of the 31 patients who had successful PTCA. Follow-up catheterization was performed in 24 of the 31 patients (77%). Restenosis of the previously dilated segment was found in 7 patients. Actuarial cardiac survival at 3 years was 100%. Freedom from AMI, CABG, PTCA for a new lesion, and death was 87%. It was concluded that although the most effective treatment for silent ischemia remains to be determined, these data suggest that PTCA is a therapeutic option.

In patients <40 years old

Webb and colleagues[90] in Vancouver, British Columbia, Canada, and Daly City, California, studied the initial and late outcome of PTCA in 148 patients less than 40 years of age. PTCA was performed on a single vessel in 70% of patients and on multiple vessels in 30%. It was performed on totally occluded vessels in 20%. PTCA was successful in 91% of patients, unsuccessful but uncomplicated in 7.4% and complicated by AMIs in 0.7%, emergency CABGs in 0.7% and death in 0.7%. At late follow-up study after successful PTCA, 94% of patients were alive, 79% were free of angina, and 85% had returned to work. Late AMIs occurred in 4% of the patients. Actuarial survival at 5 years was 95% and 85% of patients free from death, AMIs or CABG procedures (Figure 2-15). A second PTCA was performed in 29 patients and was successful in 27 with no deaths. Elective CABG was performed in 8.5% of patients, with perioperative AMIs in 9% and no deaths. By univariate analysis, late death was more likely to occur in hypertensive (15% vs 2.5%) and diabetic patients (21% vs 4%). Statistical analyses identified hypertension and diabetes as independent time-related predictors of subsequent death. These data indicate that early and late results after PTCA in young adults are favorable, but certain risk factors are important predictors of outcome. Late CABG for restenosis or disease progression are common.

In patients ≥65 years of age

The 1985 to 1986 NHLBI PTCA Registry series of 1,801 initial procedures included 486 patients age ≥65 years (elderly). Kelsey and investigators[91] from the NHLBI PTCA Registry compared these patients to younger ones. In comparison to the younger patients, a greater proportion of elderly patients were women and had unstable angina. Elderly patients had more history of hypertension and more history of congestive heart failure.

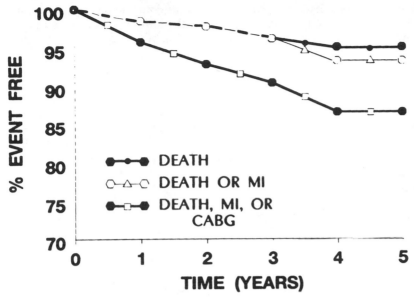

Fig. 2-15. Late outcome (5 years) after successful coronary angioplasty in 130 patients <40 years of age. Life table analysis shows freedom from death, death or myocardial infarction (MI) and death, infarction or elective bypass surgery (CABG). Reproduced with permission from Webb, et al.[90,93]

Although the elderly had more extensive vessel disease, the numbers of lesions and vessels attempted with PTCA were similar in the older and younger cohorts. Angiographic success rates were similar for all age groups. Although complication rates in the catheterization laboratory did not differ, patients ≥65 years were much more likely to require emergency CABG surgery (5.4 vs 2.8%) or elective CABG (3.9 vs 1.6%). The in-hospital death rate was considerably higher among the elderly (3.1 vs 0.2%). At 2-year follow-up, symptomatic status and cumulative rates of myocardial infarction, CABG and repeat PTCA were similar for elderly and younger patients. The death rate after 2 years was higher among elderly patients (8.8% of patients ≥65 years vs 2.9% of patients <65 years). When the relative risk of death for the elderly was adjusted for factors more prevalent among those ≥65 years (history of CHF, multivessel CAD, unstable angina, history of systemic hypertension and female gender), the relative risk remained significant but was substantially reduced (from 3.3–2.4).

In octogenarians

Jeroudi and associates[92] from Houston, Texas, performed PTCA in 54 consecutive octogenarian patients (mean age, 82 years), 91% of whom had severe angina and 59% of whom had unstable angina. Twenty-six patients (48%) had had a previous AMI and 15 (28%) had had previous CABG. Multivessel CAD was present in 44 patients (81%) and follow-up ranged from 1 to 50 months (mean 19). The angiographic success rate was 50 of 54 (93%) and the clinical success rate was 49 of 54 (91%). Two patients had procedure-related AMI and 2 patients died in the hospital. During the follow-up period 4 patients had CABG, 2 had AMI, and 7 died (4 from cardiac causes). Eleven patients (20%) had restenosis, 7 of whom were managed by repeat PTCA, including 1 patient who had PTCA 4 times. At follow-up, 42 of 45 survivors (93%) were asymptomatic or had

Class II angina. Survival was 87% at 1 year and 80% at 3 years. Cumulative freedom from major cardiac events (death, AMI, or CABG) was 81% at 1 year and 78% at 3 years. Thus, results in this older age group were good.

After bypass grafting

Webb and colleagues[93] in Daly City, California, evaluated 422 patients with prior CABG in whom PTCA was performed in the time period 1978–1988. Two hundred sixty-four patients with native coronary artery PTCA and 158 patients with coronary artery graft PTCA were studied. PTCA was successful in 84%, unsuccessful but uncomplicated in 11%, and complicated by one or more major cardiac events in 5%, including AMI in 5%, emergency CABG in 2%, and death in 0.2%. Follow-up data were obtained in 99% of 356 patients with successful PTCA. At a mean of 33 ± 26 months, 92% of patients were alive, 73% had improvement in angina, and 61% were free of angina. One or more of the following late events occurred in 67 patients: AMI in 6%, elective CABG in 13%, and cardiac death in 6%. Repeat PTCA was performed in 27% of patients with a success rate of 89% and no deaths. Initial success rates were equal in native vessel and graft vessel PTCAs, but late outcome was less favorable with graft PTCA because of a higher rate of AMI (11% vs 4%) and need for CABG (19% vs 10%). The initial success rate was higher in vein grafts <1 year old compared with grafts 1 to 4 years or >4 years after operation (92% vs 85% and 83%, respectively) and adverse late events were less frequent after PTCA in recent vein grafts. Initial PTCA success rate was higher with distal anastomotic vein graft sites (89%) than with midshaft (86%) or proximal (80%) anastomotic sites. There was a similar trend for late restenosis. Additional predictors of restenosis included smoking and male sex. Thus, PTCA may be performed with a high success rate, relatively low morbidity and mortality rates in patients with prior CABG, but repeat PTCA for restenosis or disease progression was necessary in 27% of patients. After successful PTCA, life table analysis showed an actuarial 5 year survival rate of 89% and freedom from major complications, including death, AMI or repeat CABG in 71%. Predictors of late death or AMI included prior AMI, unstable angina, multivessel CAD, and LVEF <25%.

With the availability of PTCA, the management of patients who present with recurrent angina following CABG has changed. From January 1987 to December 1988, 149 symptomatic post-CABG patients underwent coronary angiography by Tabbalat and Haft[94] from Newark, New Jersey. Ninety were treated with medical antianginal therapy, 14 had repeat surgery, and 45 underwent PTCA. Complications of repeat CABG included 1 death, 2 perioperative myocardial infarctions, and 4 patients with postoperative supraventricular arrhythmia. PTCA was performed on 42 lesions in 37 native vessels (88% success rate), and on 24 lesions in 23 vein grafts (92% success rate). Complications included acute reocclusion (1 patient), peripheral artery occlusion (1 patient), hematoma formation (1 patient), and periprocedure AMI (1 patient). No deaths occurred. At a mean follow-up of 5.9 ± 3.8 months, 10 patients had recurrent symptoms, 6 of whom were found to have restenosis. Repeat PTCA was successfully accomplished in 4 patients; the other 2 were treated medically. It was concluded that PTCA is a feasible alternative to repeat CABG in selected patients and can be achieved with a high success rate and minimal complications.

In a small number of patients, CABG fails to relieve anginal symptoms. Kahn and associates[95] from Kansas City, Missouri, examined the usefulness of PTCA for the treatment of early (≤90 days) recurrent myocardial ischemia after CABG. Forty-five patients were treated from 2 to 90 days after CABG, including 8 patients studied emergently for prolonged ischemic symptoms. One-, 2- and 3-vessel native disease was found in 4, 10 and 31 patients, respectively. At the time of postoperative angiography, the major anatomic mechanism of recurrent ischemia was complete vein graft occlusion in 12 patients (27%), internal mammary artery occlusion in 3 (7%), vein graft stenoses in 13 (29%), internal mammary artery stenoses in 10 (22%), unbygraft insertion site in 3 (7%). Angioplasty was successful at 91 of 98 sites (93%), including 95% of 41 lesions in native arteries, 89% of 46 lesions in vein grafts and 100% of 11 internal mammary artery lesions attempted. Complete revascularization was achieved in 84% of patients. There were 2 in-hospital deaths and 2 myocardial infarctions. Two additional patients underwent repeat CABG before discharge after uncomplicated but unsuccessful angioplasty. At late follow-up of the 43 survivors (mean 44 months), there were 4 deaths, 2 of which were noncardiac. Repeat CABG was required in only 3 patients and repeat angioplasty was performed in 10. Angina was absent or minimal in 35 patients; 17 patients were employed full time. Thus, PTCA can relieve myocardial ischemia after unsuccessful CABG in most patients.

Surgical standby

To determine patterns of surgical standby for PTCA, Cameron and associates[96] from Baltimore, Maryland, mailed a questionnaire to 196 U.S. institutions in which PTCA and CABG are performed regularly. Eighty-nine responses (46%) were received and comprise this report. Of responding institutions, the mean number of hospital beds was 615. In 1987, these institutions performed a mean of 337 PTCAs and 558 open-heart surgical procedures. The rate of emergency CABG for PTCA complications (occlusion, dissection, or coronary perforation) was 4.4% ± 0.3%, whereas the rate of urgent CABG (within 24 hours) for PTCA failure was 3.7% ± 0.6% (Figure 2-16). The incidence of emergency CABG for PTCA complications was higher (5.1% ± 0.6%) among low-volume PTCA centers (less than 250 cases per year) than at high-volume centers (more than 250 cases per year) (3.7% ± 0.3%). The most common pattern of surgical backup was to maintain an open operating room on standby (57/89, 64%), and the second most common pattern was to make the next open operating room available, allowing operating room access within 1 to 3 hours (21/89, 24%) (Figure 2-17). Nearly a third of institutions (26/89, 29%) maintained a flexible backup arrangement according to PTCA risk. Routine pre-PTCA patient evaluation by surgeon and/or anesthesiologist occurred in 38% (34/89). Fees for standby services were charged by 51% of surgical teams (45/89), 39% of anesthesia teams (35/89), and 38% of operating room facilities (34/89) (Figure 2-18). Thirty-seven percent of surgeons (33/89) were dissatisfied with their present standby arrangements; sources of dissatisfaction included poor communication with cardiologists about high risk or possibly inappropriate PTCA cases, waste of operating room resources, and inadequate compensation. In summary, although PTCA infrequently requires emergent surgical revascularization, many institutions still maintain an open operating room on standby. The economic burden of this support frequently is not compensated. This survey describes current practices of surgical standby for PTCA and encourages closer examination of the total cost of PTCA.

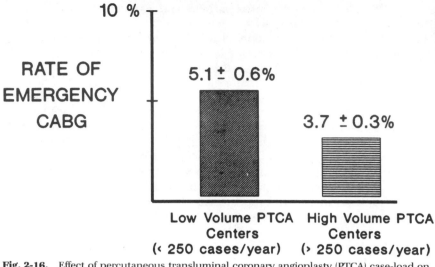

Fig. 2-16. Effect of percutaneous transluminal coronary angioplasty (PTCA) case-load on rate of emergency coronary artery bypass grafting (CABG). Reproduced with permission from Cameron, et al.[96]

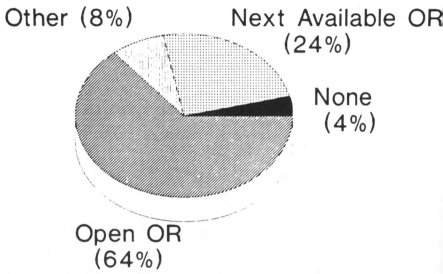

Fig. 2-17. Modes of surgical standby for percutaneous transluminal coronary angioplasty. (OR = operating room). Reproduced with permission from Cameron, et al.[96]

This article was followed by an editorial by Daniel J. Ullyot[97] from Burlingame, California. Ullyot pointed out that the survey by Cameron and co-authors did not attempt to include outcome data to decide which, among the several strategies, is optimal. Given the variety of ways cardiovascular services are provided in the U.S.A., it would be surprising if a consensus existed about an optimal standby strategy.

Pretreatment with aspirin vs aspirin and dipyridamole

It is unknown whether the addition of dipyridamole to aspirin as pretreatment for patients undergoing PTCA decreases acute complica-

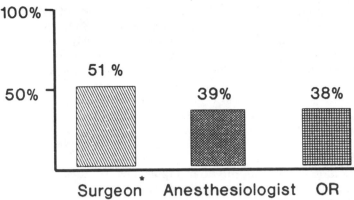

Fig. 2-18. Frequency of billing for percutaneous transluminal coronary angioplasty (PTCA) standby services. (OR = operating room). Reproduced with permission from Cameron, et al.[96]

tions. Lembo and associates[98] from Atlanta, Georgia, prospectively randomized 232 patients to receive either aspirin 225 mg orally 3 times daily (group 1, n = 115) or aspirin 325 mg orally 3 times daily plus dipyridamole 75 mg orally 3 times daily (group 2, n = 117) before elective PTCA. All clinical, angiographic and PTCA-related variables were similar between groups. Angiographic success rate was 93% in both groups. Clinical success was achieved in 107 patients (92%) in group 1 and in 101 patients (88%) in group 2. Q-wave AMI occurred in 2 patients (1.7%) in group 1 and 5 patients (4.3%) in group 2. Emergency CABG was required in 3 patients (2.6%) in group 1 and 7 patients (6.1%) in group 2. There was 1 in-hospital death (in group 2). In this study, the addition of dipyridamole to aspirin as pretreatment of patients undergoing PTCA did not significantly reduce acute complications compared to aspirin alone.

Heparin

Laskey and associates[99] from Philadelphia, Pennsylvania, compared clinical and angiographic outcome of 18 patients with coronary thrombus undergoing PTCA without antecedent heparin therapy to that of 35 patients receiving preprocedural heparin therapy. The former group had a significant reduction in angiographic success (61% vs 95%) and a significant increase in immediate postprocedural thrombotic arterial occlusion (33% vs 6%). This difference existed despite equivalent frequencies of antiplatelet therapy. Prolonged intravenous heparin therapy before angioplasty in the setting of coronary thrombus improves the overall success rate and lessens the likelihood of periprocedural coronary arterial thrombosis.

Rath and Bennett[100] from Manchester, UK, monitored the anticoagulant effect of heparin during PTCA by measurements of the activated clotting time in 2 studies that compared the effects of a single bolus of heparin with those of a bolus of heparin combined with a continuous infusion of the drug. In a preliminary study 40 patients received a single heparin bolus of 10,000 units (protocol I) and a further 40 patients received both a heparin bolus of 10,000 and a continuous infusion of heparin at a rate of 2000 units per hour (protocol II). During the first 45 minutes, 9 patients (23%) in protocol I but only 2 patients (5%) in protocol II were found to be inadequately anticoagulated. For 24 hours after angioplasty both groups received an infusion of heparin at the rate of 2000 units per hour which led to consistent anticoagulation in 73 (91%) of patients. In a subsequent randomized study, 40 patients received heparin according to either protocol I or II. Protocol II was again found to lead to a higher rate of adequate anticoagulation. During the first 60 minutes 11 patients (55%) in protocol I but only 3 patients (15%) in protocol II were inadequately anticoagulated. In addition, the activated clotting time of arterial blood in the first 30 minutes was significantly higher than that of venous blood in 70% of the patients. A bolus of heparin (10,000 units) together with an infusion of 2000 units per hour should be routinely given during coronary angioplasty. The effects of heparin, which can vary considerably from patient to patient, should be monitored by the measurement of the activated clotting time of arterial blood.

Laskey and associates[101] from Philadelphia, Pennsylvania, examined the acute procedural outcome of PTCA in 304 patients with unstable angina with respect to the influence of prolonged pre-procedural intravenous heparin therapy. Clinical and angiographic success in 135 patients receiving heparin therapy for ≥24 hours was 91% while such success was noted in 81% of patients not treated with heparin. The incidence of immediate postprocedural thrombotic vessel occlusion was higher in the nonheparin group than in the heparin-treated group (8.3 vs 1.5%, respectively). In addition, the overall rate of thromboembolic target and branch or distal vessel occlusion was 12.4% in the nonheparin group and 1.5% in the heparin-treated group. Thus, prolonged preprocedural intravenous heparin administration in this well-defined group of patients with unstable angina resulted in an improved procedural success rate and a significant decrease in the risk of abrupt vessel closure. These observations are concordant with current understanding of the pathophysiology of unstable angina.

ST monitoring during the procedure

Mizutani and associates[102] from Sydney, Australia, performed 12-lead electrocardiographic monitoring in 97 patients during PTCA of a single coronary artery to correlate ischemic ST changes with clinical, angiographic and coronary hemodynamic variables and to determine the optimum lead or combination of leads for their detection. Ischemia (chest pain or ST change, group A) occurred in 79 patients (80%), but in only 15 of 23 patients (65%) with collaterals. Ischemia occurred more often in left anterior descending and left circumflex PTCA than right coronary PTCA, but pain was the only manifestation more often in left circumflex and right coronary PTCA. Ischemic ST change was silent in 16% and this proportion did not differ in clinical or angiographic groups except for diabetes with 3 of 5 (60%) having silent ischemia. Patients in group A (ischemia) compared to group B (no ischemia) had less severe lesions (85 ± 9 vs 91 ± 7%), higher transstenotic gradients (62 ± 19 vs 53 ± 9 mm Hg) and lower distal occluded pressures (24 ± 11 vs 33 ± 10 mm Hg), suggesting less collateral flow. Compared with a 12-lead electrocardiogram, the best single lead for detecting ST change during PTCA in each artery had a sensitivity of 80% and this increased to 93% using the best 2 leads. The best 3 leads (V_2/III/V_5 for LAD descending and III/V_2/V_5 for right coronary and left circumflex) increased sensitivity to 100%. In 50 of the patients, the lead showing maximum ST change during PTCA was monitored for a mean of 20 hours after PTCA. Recurrent ST change occurred in 2 patients (4%), both with ST1, which preceded chest pain in both. Thus, ST changes during PTCA may be reliably detected by optimal choice of 3 electrocardiographic leads. The occurrence of ischemia is related principally to the vessel dilated and lesion hemodynamics that probably reflect collateral flow. Recurrent ischemia after PTCA is uncommon and may be detected by ST monitoring of a single lead.

Ninety-second occlusions during procedure

Deutch and co-investigators[103] in Philadelphia, Pennsylvania, examined the clinical, electrocardiographic, and coronary hemodynamic responses to sequential 90-second occlusions of the LAD in 12 patients undergoing elective PTCA. Transmyocardial lactate metabolism was examined in an additional group of seven patients with clinical and hemodynamic features similar to the first group. The investigators noted that in comparison with the initial balloon occlusion the second occlusion was characterized by less subjective anginal discomfort, less ST-segment shift and lower mean pulmonary artery pressure. In addition, for the same heart rate-blood pressure product, cardiac vein flow during the second inflation was significantly lower than that recorded during the first inflation. Finally, there was significantly less myocardial lactate production during the second inflation. The investigators concluded that the lessened clinical, electrocardiographic, hemodynamic, and metabolic evidence of myocardial ischemia during the second of two periods of coronary artery occlusion during PTCA supports the concept of adaptation to myocardial ischemia (ischemic preconditioning).

Granulocyte activation

To determine whether PTCA would lead to neutrophil activation with subsequent discharge of proteolytic enzymes, like elastase, and oxygen free radicals, like superoxide anion, Stefano and co-investigators[104] in Pavia, Italy, took blood samples from the coronary sinus and aorta in 14 patients with stable angina and one-vessel disease who underwent PTCA. Neutrophils were separated by means of the Ficoll-Hypaque system and were stimulated to detect release of elastase and generation of superoxide anion. Plasma levels of elastase were also measured by an immunoenzymatic method. PTCA was successful in all patients. Plasma elastase levels increased significantly at the end of the procedure compared with pre-PTCA values both in the coronary sinus and in the aorta. On the other hand, superoxide anion released in the supernatants after neutrophil stimulation by phorbol-myristate-acetate decreased after PTCA in the coronary sinus, whereas a mild but not significant decrease was observed in the aorta. Similarly, elastase release in the supernatants after neutrophil stimulation by calcium ionophore decreased after PTCA in the coronary sinus whereas no change was observed in the aorta. These results suggest that neutrophil activation occurs during PTCA and leads to higher plasma elastase levels and to a decreased ability of stimulated granulocytes to release their toxic compounds at the end of the procedure. Activation of neutrophils may have potential implication regarding the occurrence of the pathophysiological process occurring after balloon angioplasty in humans.

Buccal nitroglycerin during procedure

Nitroglycerin has the potential to reduce myocardial ischemia during PTCA. Buccal administration of nitroglycerin offers practical advantages compared to intravenous or intracoronary administration. In a double-blind, randomized, placebo-controlled study by Johansson and colleagues[105] from Gothenburg, Sweden, 100 patients were given 5 mg of buccal nitroglycerin or placebo during PTCA. A scoring system for ischemic pain during balloon inflation was defined as pain intensity (0 to 5) multiplied by duration of pain after balloon deflation (1 = 0 to 30 seconds, 2 = 30 to 60 seconds, 3 = 60 to 120 seconds, 4 = >120 seconds but subsiding, and 5 = until next inflation). Fourteen patients were excluded: 12 for vagal reaction (8 nitroglycerin and 4 placebo) requiring atropine, making buccal absorption unreliable, and 2 for inability to dilate. Eighteen patients (9 nitroglycerin and 9 placebo) had no pain during balloon inflation. Sixty-eight patients (32 nitroglycerin and 36 placebo) had ischemic pain with a pain score of 4.8 ± 3.8 for the nitroglycerin group versus 7.1 ± 4.8 for the placebo group. It was concluded that buccal nitroglycerin significantly decreases myocardial ischemia during PTCA.

Supported by cardiopulmonary bypass

Vogel and associates[106] in Baltimore, Maryland, evaluated a cardiopulmonary bypass system capable of providing up to 6 liter/min output prophylactically in 105 patients undergoing supported PTCA who were believed to be high risk as indicated by an LVEF <25% or a target vessel supplying more than half the myocardium or both. The group included 20 patients whose disease was felt to be too severe to permit CABG and 30 patients who had dilation of their only patent coronary vessel. Seventeen patients had stenosis of the left main coronary artery and 15 underwent dilation of that vessel. Chest pain and electrocardiographic changes occurred uncommonly despite prolonged balloon inflations. PTCA success rate was 95% for the 105 patients who underwent an average of 1.7 dilations per patient. Morbidity was frequent, in most cases, due to arterial, venous, or nerve injury associated with cannula insertion, removal, or both. The hospital mortality rate was 7.6% and half of these deaths occurred in patients who were both >75 years of age and had left main coronary artery stenosis. Patients without these two clinical variables had an in-hospital mortality rate of 2.6%. Symptomatic improvement occurred in 91% of the patients surviving hospitalization. During the subsequent follow-up period of 1 to 12 months, 3 patients died of cardiac complications. These data suggest that supported PTCA may be safely performed with an expectation of symptomatic improvement and short-term survival in high risk patients other than elderly patients with LM CAD.

During intraventricular pumping

The 'Hemopump,' an axial flow pump, when inserted in the LV brings about mechanical unloading of the ventricle, thus reducing the risk of cardiac arrest during coronary angioplasty. Loisance and associates[107] from Creteil, France, selected 8 very ill patients with unstable myocardial ischemia and various contraindications for CABG for PTCA with insertion of the hemopump. Anatomical difficulties prevented insertion in 3 patients, but coronary angioplasty was carried out successfully with the pump in place in the other 5. When the pump was working the cardiac index rose by an average of 23% (8–50%) and the pulmonary capillary wedge pressure fell by 17% (0–22%). Though electrocardiographic monitoring showed temporary rhythm instability during angioplasty in 4 of the 5 patients, there was no clinical deterioration. Four of the 5 patients are symptom-free on medical treatment and the other is well after surgical revascularization.

Oxygenated Fluosol

Kent and associates[108] from multiple medical centers examined the effects of perfusion of an oxygen-carrying perfluorochemical emulsion (Fluosol) in alleviating symptoms of myocardial ischemia during balloon occlusion during a multicenter trial of 245 patients. Severe anginal pain occurred less frequently in patients receiving Fluosol perfusion (21%) than in those receiving routine angioplasty (34%). ST-segment changes at balloon deflation in routine angioplasty patients were significantly greater than in patients who received oxygenated Fluosol perfusion (2.2 ± 1.2 vs 1.7 ± 0.9 mm). Profound regional wall dysfunction (−561 ± 224 U) was observed in routine angioplasty patients by 2-dimensional echocardiography. Patients receiving oxygenated Fluosol perfusion, however, maintained near baseline levels of ventricular function (−61 ± 335 U) during occlusion. Mean global LVEF was preserved at baseline levels during balloon inflation in patients perfused with oxygenated Fluosol but decreased significantly during occlusion in routine angioplasty patients. A total of 26 complications (19 routine group; 7 perfusion group) was reported. Adverse responses to the perfusate were infrequent, occurring in 1.6 and 2.0% of patients after the test dose and during perfusion, respectively. Thus, transcatheter perfusion with an oxygen-carrying perfluorochemical emulsion is effective in alleviating myocardial ischemia during angioplasty and can be safely administered in this patient population.

Effects on left ventricular filling patterns

Castello and associates[109] in St. Louis, Missouri, assessed the early effects of successful PTCA on Doppler-derived LV filling patterns and the significance of the extent of revascularization on these variables in 31 patients undergoing PTCA studied within 24 hours before and after coronary artery revascularization procedures. After PTCA, the peak early to late velocity ratio increased from 0.89 ± 0.2 to 1.05 ± 0.3 and the one-third filling fraction increased from 42 ± 10% to 48 ± 10%. The percent atrial contribution to filling decreased from 45 ± 7% to 41 ± 8% and the pressure half-times and isovolumetric relaxation times shortened from 55 ± 15 to 43 ± 13 ms and from 100 ± 14 to 82 ± 17 ms, respectively. When comparing patients with complete (n = 23) and incomplete (n = 8) revascularization, the same changes in the Doppler variables were observed. The mean rate of acceleration of early filling increased significantly after PTCA only in those patients with complete revascularization. Thus, these data suggest that LV diastolic filling patterns are modified as early as 24 hours after successful PTCA. Improvement in the impaired relaxation appears to be an explanation for these findings, although increased myocardial stiffness in patients with incomplete revascularization is also a potential contributing factor.

Effects on wall motion

Broderick and associates[110] in Indianapolis, Indiana, evaluated exercise echocardiography in 36 patients to determine functional alterations after PTCA. Thirty-one patients (86%) had exercise-induced ischemia before PTCA, including 22 with an abnormal exercise electrocardiographic test with angina or ST segment depression, 25 with an abnormal exercise echocardiogram as evidenced by exercise-induced wall motion abnormalities, and 16 with both tests abnormal. Nineteen patients had no inducible myocardial ischemia after PTCA. Seventeen (47%) continued to have myocardial ischemia limited in 12 to exercise-induced wall motion abnormalities detected by echocardiography and which were less severe as compared to the pre-PTCA studies. Fifteen of 23 patients had improvement in rest wall motion abnormalities after PTCA (Figure 2-19). The rest to immediate postexercise change in wall motion score was significantly improved after PTCA. The change in regional wall motion score was significantly improved after PTCA in patients with single vessel right or LC CAD and approached significant improvement in those with single vessel CAD of the LAD. The data obtained in this study suggest exercise echocardiography improves the sensitivity of functional testing

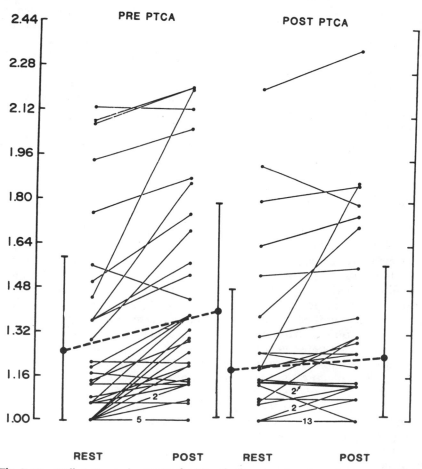

Fig. 2-19. Wall motion index scores depicting both rest and postexercise images with the preangioplasty (PTCA) scores displayed on the left and postangioplasty (PTCA) scores displayed on the right. Bracketed point represents the mean value + SD. Preangioplasty: 1.25 ± 0.34 (rest) to 1.40 ± 0.29 (postexercise); postangioplasty: 1.18 ± 0.28 (rest) to 1.24 ± 0.33 (postexercise). Reproduced with permission from Broderick, et al.[110]

for ischemia, aids in localizing the ischemic zone and helps to document improvement in regional function after PTCA.

Patients with chronic segmental myocardial dysfunction may demonstrate improvement after coronary revascularization. To evaluate the early effects of PTCA on resting LV segmental function, van der Berg and co-investigators[111] in Richmond, Virginia, obtained serial 2-dimensional echocardiograms on day before and three days after elective PTCA in 40 patients. Echocardiograms were reviewed in a blind fashion; LV segmental wall motion was analyzed in four short-axis views, and a score was assigned to each region (0, normal; 1, hypokinetic; and 2, akinetic). Abnormal regional wall motion was present in 20 of the patients before PTCA. Summed segment scores in these 20 patients showed an improvement in regional wall motion from 4.5 to 1.6 after successful PTCA. Similar results were obtained when the patients were divided into those with or without a previous AMI. Improvement occurred in the seven patients without a previous AMI; the summed segment score decreased from 4.2 to 0.86 after PTCA. Ten of the 13 patients with a prior AMI demonstrated improvement in wall motion after PTCA; the summed segment scores decreased 54%. Of the 260 segments analyzed in the study, 180 were normal before and after PTCA. Forty-nine of the 69 hypokinetic segments were normal, and 10 to 12 akinetic segments were hypokinetic after successful coronary revascularization. There was no deterioration in wall motion after PTCA. These data show that 2-dimensional echocardiography was able to detect improvement in abnormal resting LV systolic function after successful PTCA, and they support the hypothesis that patients with CAD recover segmental LV dysfunction after PTCA.

To evaluate the significance of persistent negative T wave during severe ischemia, Renkin and co-investigators[112] in Brussels, Belgium, prospectively studied 62 patients admitted for unstable angina without evidence of recent or ongoing AMI. A critical stenosis of the LAD coronary artery, considered as the culprit lesion, was successfully treated by PTCA. The patients were divided into two groups according to the admission electrocardiogram: T negative group had persistent negative T waves and the T positive group had normal positive T waves on precordial leads. The 2 groups had similar baseline clinical, hemodynamic, and angiographic characteristics. All patients underwent a complete clinical and angiographic evaluation before PTCA and 8 months later. LV anterior wall motion was evaluated by the percent shortening of three areas considered as LAD-related segments on left ventriculograms. Before PTCA there was no significant difference in global EF between the two groups despite a significant depression in anterior mean percent area shortening in the T negative compared to the T positive group. At repeated angiography, the anterior mean percent area shortening improved significantly in the T negative group. This resulted in a reduced end-systolic volume and improved EF compared with baseline. The negative T wave present on the admission electrocardiogram became normalized in 31 patients. There were no differences in any of the data between baseline and follow-up in the T positive group. The investigators concluded that 1) the clinical syndrome of unstable angina with LAD stenosis and persistent negative T waves on a precordial lead is associated with resting anterior hypokinesis that is absent in patients without this electrocardiogram pattern but who are otherwise similar; 2) successful reperfusion by PTCA of LAD can normalize the abnormal regional shortening suggesting that myocardial stunning is present in this syndrome.

Outcome when successful

Samson and associates[113] from Rotterdam, The Netherlands, evaluated the long-term value of performing multiple dilatations according to their procedural (single-vessel multilesion or multivessel dilatations) and anatomic types (single-vessel CAD with multiple dilatations or multivessel CAD dilatations with complete and incomplete revascularization). From 1980 until 1988, 248 patients met the following criteria: 1) ≥2 narrowings dilated (range 2 to 4) and 2) all attempted narrowings successfully dilated. The mean length of follow-up was 33 months. The end points analyzed were death, AMI, redilatation, and CABG. No differences were found for these events between the single-vessel multilesion group (144 patients) and the multivessel group (104 patients). The 4.5-year probability of event-free survival was 68% and 70%, respectively, for the multilesion group and the multivessel group. In the event-free patients, 57% versus 59% were asymptomatic and 45% versus 46% were not taking antianginal drugs. In the anatomic subgroups, there were less event-free patients in the cohort of incompletely revascularized multivessel disease patients (55% of 55 patients) when compared with the cohort of those who were completely revascularized (84% of 79 patients) or when compared with the single-vessel CAD multiple dilatation patients (74% of 107 patients). The 4.5-year event-free survival probability for each group was 44%, 78%, and 74%, respectively. This difference was caused by more infarctions (9% vs 2% vs 4%, respectively) and bypass operations in the multivessel CAD, incomplete revascularization group (20% vs 5% vs 10%, respectively). In event-free patients, improvement of angina was similar and was documented in over 85% of patients in each group. Furthermore, the number of asymptomatic patients at follow-up was similar in all groups except that within the incomplete revascularization group, less patients were free of antianginal drugs (21% vs 51% vs 48%). Finally, 48% of the entire cohort performed an exercise test 4.6 months (mean) after dilatation and no difference was found in any of the variables in any group. About 10% of the patients experienced angina and approximately 30% had a positive exercise test for ischemia by ST segment criteria. The functional performance in every group was >90% of the predicted work load. These results suggest that completeness of revascularization in multivessel CAD patients is an important prognostic variable. The symptomatic improvement after dilatation is very rewarding in all subsets of patients and argues in favor of the continued use of multiple dilatations as a treatment strategy.

Bell and associates[114] in Rochester, Minnesota, evaluated the relative influences of revascularization status and baseline characteristics on long-term outcome in 867 patients with multivessel CAD who had undergone successful PTCA. These patients represented 83% of a total of 1,039 individuals in whom PTCA had been attempted with an in-hospital mortality and AMI rate of 2.5% and 4.8%, respectively. Emergency CABG was needed in 4.9%. Among the 867 patients, 41% (group 1) were thought to have complete revascularization and 59% (group 2) to have incomplete revascularization. Univariate analysis revealed major differences between these 2 groups with patients in group 2 characterized by advanced age, more severe angina, a greater likelihood of previous CABG and AMI, more extensive disease and poorer LV function. During a mean follow-up period of 26 months, the probability of event-free survival was significantly lower for group 2 only with respect to the need for CABG and the occurrence of severe angina. The difference in mortality was of borderline significance, and there were no significant differences between groups 1 and 2 in either the incidence of AMI or the need for repeat PTCA. Multivariate analysis identified independent baseline predictors of late cardiac events that were used to adjust the probabilities of event-free survival. This adjustment removed any significant influence of completeness of revascularization on event-free survival for any of the end points, including the combination of death, AMI and the need for CABG (Figure 2-20). Therefore, 2 year results in similar patients may not be significantly influenced by revascularization status, but appears to depend importantly on baseline patient characteristics.

Shawl and associates[115] in Takoma Park, Maryland, and Nashville, Tennessee, evaluated the impact of semiurgent PTCA on clinical and electrocardiographic variables in 76 patients with unstable angina associated with an isolated severe proximal LAD stenosis. All patients manifested symmetric T wave inversion in two or more anterior electrocardiographic leads. Regional wall motion abnormalities were present in 37 patients on ventriculography before PTCA. PTCA was successful in 70 patients (92%) resulting in a reduction in luminal diameter stenosis from 91 ± 8% to 21 ± 6% with no major acute procedure-related complications. The remaining 6 patients had semiurgent (<48 hours) CABG and 3 patients had an AMI before CABG in 2 of them. Serial electrocardiograms demonstrated complete resolution of ST-T wave changes in 51% of patients by 14 weeks and in 90% of patients by 28 weeks. Prolongation of the corrected QT interval present in 16 patients initially had normalized

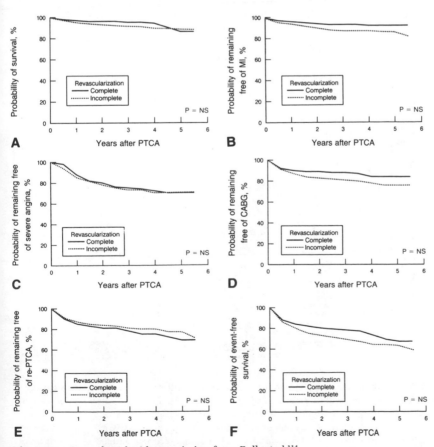

Fig. 2-20. Reproduced with permission from Bell, et al.[114]

within 48 hours of successful PTCA. Twelve of the 16 patients with a prolonged QT interval had nonocclusive thrombus formation and poor collateral circulation on angiography. Patients were followed for 6 to 43 months (mean 23 ± 10 months). Angiographic evidence of restenosis occurred in 34% of patients all of whom underwent a successful second or third procedure. One death occurred at 8 months after successful PTCA. Wall motion abnormalities had completely resolved in 13 of 15 patients who underwent repeat ventriculography at which time they had a normal electrocardiogram. This study demonstrates that electrocardiographic changes may persist for up to 7 months in patients who have successful PTCA for severe LAD disease and unstable angina. Semiurgent PTCA was associated with a high initial success rate although many patients required a second or third PTCA procedure.

Webb and associates[116] in Daly City, California, evaluated 217 symptomatic patients who had PTCA as an alternative to CABG between March 1978 and July 1981. PTCA was successful in 143 patients (66%), unsuccessful but uncomplicated in 65 (30%), and complicated in 9 (4%). Complications included: Q wave AMI (2%); emergency CABG (4%); or death (0.5%). Late follow-up evaluation was obtained in 213 patients at a mean of 9 ± 1 years. Among patients in whom PTCA was successful, 59 (42%) of 140 required another revascularization procedure in the future (repeat PTCA in 26% and CABG in 16%) (Figure 2-21). Actuarial survival rates 5, 9, and 10 years after successful PTCA were 98%, 93% and 92%, respectively. Among the 65 patients with unsuccessful and uncomplicated PTCA, 58 had elective CABG within 2 months and 56 survived. These 56 surgical patients were compared with 140 patients with successful PTCA, and at

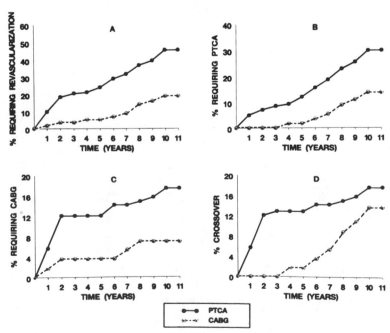

Fig. 2-21. Late revascularization after successful angioplasty and after successful surgery (performed electively within 2 months of an unsuccessful, uncomplicated angioplasty attempt). Life tables show the incidence of late repeat revascularization (surgery or angioplasty) (A), late angioplasty (B), late surgery (C) and treatment crossover (surgery to angioplasty or angioplasty to surgery) (D). Abbreviations as in Figure 2-22. Reproduced with permission from Webb, et al.[116]

late follow-up evaluation, these patients had similar rates of survival and of death or infarction, or both (Figure 2-22). Repeat revascularization was required more frequently after successful PTCA than after surgery (42% vs 18%). Crossover from PTCA to surgery occurred with equal frequency as surgery to PTCA (16% vs 12.5%, p = NS). These data indicate a relatively favorable long-term prognosis for patients with successful PTCA, but a need for some additional revascularization procedures in the future in many of these patients.

O'Keefe and colleagues[117] in Kansas City, Missouri, evaluated 3,186 patients between June 1980 and January 1989 who had PTCA of 2 (2,399 patients) or 3 (787 patients) of 3 major epicardial coronary arteries. A mean of 3.6 narrowings (range 2 to 14) were dilated per patients with a 96% success rate. Acute complications occurred in 94 (3%) and included Q wave infarction in 47 (1%), urgent CABG in 33 (1%), and death in 31 (1%). Multivariate correlates of in-hospital death included impaired LV function, age ≥70 years and female gender. Long-term follow-up data

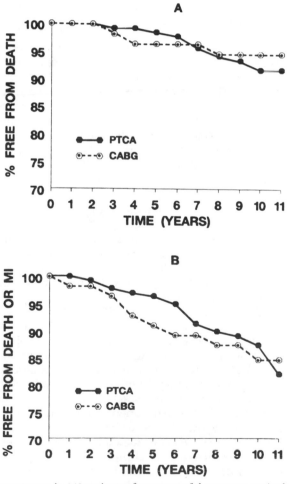

Fig. 2-22. Late outcome in 140 patients after successful coronary angioplasty (PTCA) and 56 patients after successful coronary artery bypass surgery (CABG) (performed electively within 2 months of an unsuccessful but uncomplicated angioplasty attempt). Life tables compare the incidence of survival (A) and freedom from death or myocardial infarction (MI), or both (B). Reproduced with permission from Webb, et al.[116]

were available for the first 700 patients and the follow-up period averaged 54 ± 15 months. Actuarial 1 and 5 year survival rates were 97% and 88%, respectively, and were not different in patients with two or three vessel CAD. By Cox regression analysis, age ≥70 years, LVEF ≤40% and prior CABG were associated with an increased mortality rate during the follow-up period. Repeat revascularization procedures were required in 322 patients (46%). Restenosis resulted in either repeat PTCA or CABG in 227 patients (32%). Repeat PTCA was performed for isolated restenosis in 126 patients (18%), for restenosis and disease progression at new sites in 85 patients (12%), and for new disease progression alone in 54 patients (8%). CABG was required in 110 patients (16%) during the follow-up period. The actuarial 4 year repeat revascularization rate for patients with complete and incomplete revascularization was 24% and 33%, respectively. At follow-up study, 67% of patients were free of angina and 19% had class II angina. Therefore, multivessel PTCA is safe and effective and results in good long-term symptom relief and survival in patients with multivessel CAD.

Outcome when unsuccessful

Stark and associates[118] in Washington, D.C., evaluated 859 patients undergoing PTCA between December 1981 and September 1985 to determine whether emergent CABG after failed PTCA protects the heart. Forty-two patients had emergency CABG for objective evidence of impending AMI. Five patients died. Thirty-six patients were contacted for follow-up; 21 (58%) of 36 had radionuclide ventriculograms performed 39 ± 13 months after CABG. The radionuclide ventriculograms were compared with the patients' PTCA contrast ventriculograms. One patient had an AMI 3 years after CABG. Eleven (55%) of the remaining 20 patients had normal radionuclide ventriculograms at follow-up study with mean LVEFs of 65 ± 9%. Five (25%) of the 20 patients had depressed LVEFs (46 ± 4%) with wall motion abnormalities, but these were unchanged from the previous PTCA studies. Four patients (20%) had significant decreases in their LVEFs over baseline (37 ± 10%) with new wall motion abnormalities. Thus in this series, 1) there was an 80% chance that LVEF will be unchanged during 3 years follow-up in patients surviving emergency CABG for failed PTCA; and 2) early CABG for impending AMI was associated with a good late outcome.

Richardson and associates[119] from Belfast, UK, performed a study to determine whether PTCA may be safely performed in cardiology centers without immediate on site cardiac surgical cover for complications arising at PTCA. A total of 540 PTCA procedures were performed on 512 patients between 1982 and 1988. The indications for PTCA included stable and unstable angina and suitable CAD after coronary angiography after AMI. PTCA was successful in 444 cases (82%). Acute coronary occlusion occurred in 35 cases (6.5%). Twelve patients required urgent revascularization surgery and were transferred safely to the surgical unit; none of these patients died. A mean delay of 268 minutes (range 180–390 minutes) occurred before revascularization compared with 273 minutes (range 108–420 minutes) in the Royal Victoria Hospital, where on site surgical cover was available. The principal cause of delay was the wait for a cardiac operating theater to become available and not the transfer time between hospitals. Five deaths occurred after coronary angioplasty, a mortality of 0.9%. Three deaths were related to acute coronary occlusion. The absence of immediate surgical help did not influence the outcome in any patient.

With careful selection of patients coronary angioplasty may be safely performed in a hospital without on site cardiac surgical facilities, provided that these are available at a nearby center.

Tuzcu and associates[120] from Cleveland, Ohio, analyzed the long-term outcome of 198 patients after successful PTCA. Forty-nine percent underwent emergency CABG, 17% had elective CABG, and 34% were treated medically. The in-hospital mortality rate was 4%, and AMI occurred in 36% of patients. Follow-up was completed in 100% of patients with a mean follow-up period of 35 ± 22 months. Actuarial cardiac survival at 4 years was 97% in the emergency CABG group, 100% in the elective CABG group, and 86% in the medically treated group. Actuarial event-free survival (freedom from AMI, CABG, PTCA, and cardiac death) at 4-year follow-up was 81% in 198 patients, 90% in the emergency CABG group, 85% in the elective CABG group, and 65% in the medically treated group. Results of multivariate analysis showed that emergency or elective CABG after failed PTCA, normal or mildly impaired LV function and male sex were predictors of better outcome at 4 years.

Detre and co-investigators[121] from Pittsburgh, Pennsylvania, reviewed 1,801 patients in the 1985 and 1986 PTCA Registry, and found 122 had periprocedural occlusion (5% in the catheterization laboratory, 2% outside the laboratory). Baseline patient factors independently associated with increased occlusion rates included triple-vessel disease, high risk status for surgery, and acute coronary insufficiency. Lesion characteristics showing significant positive association included severe stenosis before PTCA, diffuse or multiple discrete morphology, thrombus, and collateral flow from the lesion. Intimal tear and dissection were also very strongly associated with occlusion. Sixty patients had a transient occlusion that was reopened with PTCA, 43 patients were not redilated and managed by CABG, and 19 were not redilated and managed medically. In-hospital mortality was 5% in each of these treatment groups, compared with 1% in occlusion-free patients. In-hospital infarction rates ranged from 27% in patients with transient occlusion to 56% in the patients managed with surgery, compared with 2% in patients without occlusion. During 2 years of follow-up, somewhat increased mortality continued in patients with occlusion, whereas follow-up infarction rates were comparable for all patients regardless of occlusion. Patients with an occlusion that was reopened or managed medically had increased rates of surgery during follow-up. Rates of repeat PTCA were comparable in about 23% by 2 years in patients with transient occlusion and those without occlusion. Occlusion remains a serious complication of angioplasty and is associated most strongly with major events and surgical procedures that occur during the in-hospital period.

Gulba and colleagues[122] in Hannover, Federal Republic of Germany, studied 447 patients undergoing single vessel PTCA to evaluate the relation between thrombin activation and abrupt vessel closure. Twenty-seven patients (6%) had acute thrombotic occlusion early after PTCA. They were treated with combined intracoronary and intravenous recombinant tissue-type plasminogen activator and repeat balloon inflations. Reopening of the vessel was achieved in 22 patients (81.5%). Follow-up coronary angiography 24 to 36 hours later revealed reocclusion in 12 patients (54.5%). Thrombin levels measured as thrombin-antithrombin-III complex in patients with successful thrombolysis and persistent patency decreased from 8.5 ± 11.4 µg/L at baseline to 3.5 ± 1.4 µg/L 120 minutes after the start of thrombolysis. These levels increased from 9.4 ± 15.0 µg/L at baseline to 15.7 ± 13.5 µg/L 120 minutes after thrombolysis in patients with unsuccessful thrombolysis or early reocclusion. When a borderline value for thrombin-antithrombin-III complex level of 6 µg/L was selected to separate the two groups of patients, patients with a complicated clinical course subsequently were identified 120 minutes after the start of thrombolysis by levels >6 µg/L. Therefore, after abrupt thrombotic vessel closure during coronary PTCA, the short-term results of thrombolysis may be predicted by measurement of thrombin activation. In two-thirds of patients, the thrombin release may not be suppressed by concomitant aspirin and heparin therapy.

Tally and colleagues[123] in Atlanta, Georgia, performed a study to define the in-house and late clinical outcome at 5-years in 430 patients who had a failed PTCA and underwent CABG during their hospitalization. This group comprised 6% of 7,246 patients undergoing elective PTCA. CABG was performed in 346 patients with ongoing myocardial ischemia and in 84 patients without ischemia. Their mean age was 56 years and 76% were men. One-vessel CAD was present in 72%, and the mean LV EF was 59%. Overall, 1.9 bypass grafts were placed. There was increased use of the internal thoracic artery in the nonischemic group. A new nonfatal postprocedural Q wave AMI occurred in 21% and occurred more frequently in the ischemic than in the nonischemic group. There were 6 in-hospital deaths, an incidence that did not differ between the 2 groups. There were 25 deaths including 16 of cardiac cause. Q wave AMI occurred in 111 patients and freedom from cardiac death or nonfatal AMI at 5 years was 71%. In the group going to CABG with ongoing ischemia, the 5-year cardiac survival was 95% in the group without ischemia, the corresponding survival was 96%. By multivariate analysis, the presence of preoperative myocardial ischemia, pre-PTCA diameter stenosis <90%, and the presence of multiple-vessel CAD correlated with the occurrence of cardiac death or nonfatal AMI at 5 years. At this large-volume center with extensive PTCA operator and surgical experience, the excellent survival and low event rates over 5 years support the concept that despite the failed elective PTCA procedure, there was little effect on long-term survival provided the patients underwent prompt successful surgical revascularization.

Restenosis

To determine the value of a 6-month exercise treadmill test for detecting restenosis after elective PTCA, Bengtson and associates[124] from Durham, North Carolina, studied 303 consecutive patients with successful PTCA and without a recent AMI. Among the 228 patients without interval cardiac events, early repeat revascularization or contraindications to treadmill testing, 209 (92%) underwent follow-up angiography, and 200 also had a follow-up treadmill test and formed the study population. Restenosis (≥75% luminal diameter stenosis) occurred in 50 patients (25%). Five variables were individually associated with a higher risk of restenosis: recurrent angina, exercise-induced angina, a positive treadmill test, more exercise ST deviation and a lower maximum exercise heart rate. However, only exercise-induced angina, recurrent angina and a positive treadmill test were independent predictors of restenosis. Using these 3 variables, patient subsets could be identified with restenosis rates ranging from 11 to 83%. The exercise treadmill test added independent information to symptom status about the risk of restenosis after elective PTCA. Nevertheless, 20% of patients with restenosis had neither recurrent angina nor exercise-induced ischemia at follow-up. For more accurate detection of restenosis, the exercise treadmill test must be supplemented by a more definitive test.

El-Tamimi and associates[125] in London, UK, evaluated the time course of restenosis and used serial treadmill exercise testing in an attempt to identify patients with a risk of restenosis in 31 patients with single vessel CAD who underwent successful PTCA. Exercise tests were performed before PTCA and at 3 days and 1, 3, and 6 months after PTCA. If the test was positive, it was repeated after administration of 10 mg of intravenous verapamil. At arteriography, 6 months after PTCA, 17 patients (group I) showed no restenosis but 14 patients (group II) did. Before PTCA, all 31 patients had a positive exercise test with ST segment depression ≥ 1 mm. Three days after PTCA, 3 patients in group I had a positive exercise test compared with 11 patients in group II. At 1, 3, and 6 months, 1 patient in group I had a positive exercise test compared with 14 patients in group II (Figure 2-23). Heart rate-blood pressure product calculated at 1 mm ST segment depression or at peak exercise if the test was negative was used as an index of the ischemic threshold. In group I without restenosis, the ischemic threshold increased progressively before PTCA to 3 days and 6 months. In the group II patients with restenosis, the ischemic threshold increased from before PTCA to 3 days, but decreased at 6 months. In group II patients, the increase in ischemic threshold afte

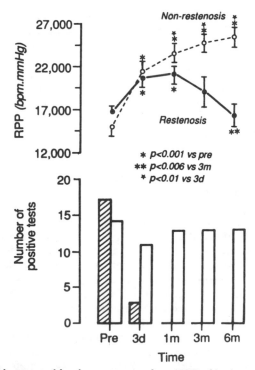

Fig. 2-23. Mean heart rate-blood pressure product (RPP) of both groups and the corresponding number of positive exercise tests at each time interval. The group with no restenosis (group 1) showed a continuous improvement of mean heart rate-blood pressure product up to 6 months after angioplasty and all tests become negative from 1 month onward. The group with restenosis (group 2) showed an initial improvement of mean heart rate-blood pressure product at 3 days after angioplasty but it decreased from 3 months onward and most tests were positive from 1 month onward. Hatched bars = nonrestenosis; open bars = restenosis; Pre = before angioplasty. Reproduced with permission from El-Tamini, et al.[125]

verapamil was greater at 3 and 6 months than before PTCA. Thus, a positive exercise test soon after PTCA is valuable and identifies patients at higher risk of restenosis as early as 3 days to 1 month after PTCA.

Schwartz and colleagues[126] from Toronto, Montreal, and Burlington, Canada, previously reported that a combination of *aspirin* and *dipyridamole* given before, during, and for 6 months following PTCA did not reduce the incidence of restenosis. In that trial, a total of 272 successfully dilated segments in 243 patients reached final quantitative angiography and of these, 86 segments (32%) had restenosed (46 of 130 segments in the group of patients given placebo and 40 of 142 segments in the aspirin-dipyridamole group). A secondary analysis by these investigators of these 86 segments revealed that at follow-up angiography the severity of restenosis was greater in the 46 segments in the placebo group than in the 40 segments in the active treatment group (mean minimal luminal diameter at the stenosis = 0.76 ± 0.52 and 1.03 ± 0.45 mm, respectively). The frequency of total or subtotal occlusions was higher in the placebo group (17%) than in the active treatment group (5.0%), but this observation did not reach statistical significance. Although long-term treatment with aspirin and dipyridamole after successful PTCA does not reduce the incidence of recurrence, this secondary analysis suggests that it is associated with a decreased likelihood of severe restenosis.

To assess the possible progression of CAD after PTCA and its relation to risk factors and restenosis, Benchimol and associates[127] from Bordeaux, France, studied 124 patients who underwent a first successful PTCA. All had routine follow-up angiography 5 to 8 months after PTCA. Restenosis was defined as a 30% decrease in diameter stenosis or a return to >50% stenosis, and progression (in any nondilated site) as a 20% decrease in diameter stenosis, assessed by a video-densitometric computer-assisted technique. Univariate and multivariate analysis with respect to progression was carried out for age, sex, initial unstable angina, previous AMI, diabetes mellitus, hypertension, hypercholesterolemia (≥ 6.2 mmol/L), smoking habits, Jenkins' score, dilated artery and restenosis. Forty-one patients (33%) had restenosis, and 23 (19%) had evidence of progression; 20 (87%) of these latter patients had restenosis and 3 (13%) did not. Univariate correlates of progression were: previous AMI, higher Jenkins' score and restenosis. Restenosis was the only multivariate correlate. Progression at routine angiography after PTCA is not rare, and appears to be related to both the initial extent of CAD and restenosis.

Pepine and co-investigators[128] from Gainesville, Florida, conducted a multicenter, double-blind, placebo-controlled trial to determine if *corticosteroids* influence the development of restenosis after successful PTCA. Either the placebo or 1.0 gram methylprednisolone (steroid) was infused intravenously 2–24 hours before planned PTCA in 915 patients. The PTCA success rate was 87% in the eight centers. There were no differences in clinical or angiographic baseline variables between the two groups. Endpoint analysis (angiographic restenosis, death, recurrent ischemia necessitating early restudy, and coronary artery bypass graft surgery) showed that there was no significant difference comparing placebo- with steroid-treated patients. Angiographic restudy showed the lesion restenosis rate to be 39% after placebo and 40% after steroid treatment. Investigators concluded that pulse steroid pretreatment does not influence the overall restenosis rate after successful PTCA.

Hardoff and associates[129] in Haifa, Israel, examined whether late coronary restenosis may be predicted by abnormalities of myocardial perfusion in the early hours after successful PTCA. A prospective study was done in 90 consecutive patients in whom thallium-201 scintigrams were recorded at rest and during the stress of atrial pacing, and 12 to 24 hours after PTCA. The results were compared with findings at angiography in 70 patients undergoing later cardiac catheterization at 6 to 12 months after PTCA. A reversible thallium-201 perfusion defect was found in 39 (38%) of 104 myocardial regions supplied by the dilated coronary artery and identified a subset at increased risk of late restenosis after PTCA. Late coronary restenosis developed in only 7 (11%) of 65 vessels and in 5 (14%) of 37 patients with a normal thallium-201 scintigram on day 1. Multivariate logistic regression analysis of 14 preangioplasty and periangioplasty clinical and angiographic variables selected reversible perfusion defects on the thallium-201 scintigram on day 1 and immediate post angioplasty residual coronary narrowing as significant independent predictors of late restenosis. Reduced patient age was an additional predictor. These findings suggest that in many patients pathophysiologic events occurring in the early minutes to hours after PTCA may determine and influence the development of restenosis.

Laarman and associates[130] in Rotterdam, The Netherlands, used exercise electrocardiographic testing to follow 141 asymptomatic patients without previous AMI after coronary PTCA to determine whether it might be useful in predicting restenosis. The prevalence of restenosis defined as ≥50% luminal narrowing at the dilation site was 12% in this selected study group. Among 26 patients with an abnormal exercise electrocardiogram, including ST segment depression ≥0.1 mV, only 4 (15%) showed recurrence of restenosis. The sensitivity and specificity for detection of restenosis were 24% and 82%, respectively. One hundred thirty-four patients (95%) were followed for 1 to 64 months (mean 35) after exercise electrocardiographic testing and coronary angiography. Thirty-two patients (24%) had a cardiac event. In 25 patients (78%) the initial event was recurrent angina and in 7 patients (22%), it was AMI, although cardiac death did not occur. The mean interval between exercise electrocardiographic testing and the initial cardiac event was 14 months, but 47% of the initial events took place within 6 months after exercise electrocardiographic testing. An abnormal exercise test result and angiographic restenosis had, respectively, a predictive value of 36% and 41% and a relative risk of 1.7 and 1.9. Gender, age, and extent of ST depression were not related to the occurrence of future cardiac events. Therefore, the exercise electrocardiogram is not the technique of choice to detect silent restenosis after coronary PTCA of single vessel CAD. An abnormal exercise test result and angiographic evidence of restenosis had only limited value in predicting long-term outcome in these patients.

As part of a randomized prospective study designed to investigate the restenosis process after PTCA, Macdonald and associates[131] from multiple North American medical centers examined the relation between patient-related variables and restenosis rate. A total of 722 patients had successful PTCA. Angiographic follow-up was scheduled for 6 ± 2 months after the procedure and achieved in 510 patients (71%), yielding 598 lesions for analysis. The overall restenosis rate was 40%. The rate was higher in patients undergoing early restudy for a clinical event than in those undergoing routinely scheduled follow-up restudy (71% vs 22%). Age, sex, cigarette smoking history, diabetes mellitus and history of previous myocardial infarction were not associated with restenosis rate. Angina duration and severity before PTCA were also unrelated to restenosis rate. In summary, these variables, many of which have been previously implicated in restenosis, were not found to be predictors of restenosis.

Hecht and associates[132] from Daly City, California, evaluated the role of tomographic thallium-201 exercise and redistribution imaging in the detection of restenosis after PTCA in 116 patients: 61 (53%) with 1 and 55 (47%) with multivessel PTCA, with 185 dilated arteries. Complete revascularization was performed in 89 (77%) and partial revascularization in 27 (23%) of the patients. Restenosis was angiographically demonstrated in 69 (60%) of the patients and 85 (46%) of the vessels 6.4 ± 3.1 months after PTCA. Disease progression in previously normal vessels was noted in 11 patients. The results were: 1) for detection of restenosis in the group of patients, single-photon emission computed tomographic (SPECT) versus exercise electrocardiographic sensitivity was 93 versus 52%, specificity 77 versus 64%, and accuracy 86 versus 57%. The results were similar in the complete and partial revascularization groups. 2) SPECT was 86% sensitive, specific and accurate for restenosis detection in specific vessels with comparable results for 1- versus multivessel PTCA and complete versus partial revascularization. Sensitivity, specificity and accuracy were: 89, 95 and 92% for the left anterior descending coronary artery; 88, 79 and 82% for the right coronary artery; and 76, 83 and 85% for the LC coronary artery. Eighty-one percent of the narrowed nondilated arteries were correctly identified. 3) Disease progression to >50% diameter stenosis was detected with 91% sensitivity, 84% specificity and 85% accuracy. SPECT thallium-201 imaging is an excellent tool for the detection of restenosis and disease progression after PTCA in the settings of 1- and multivessel angioplasty and complete and partial revascularization.

ANGIOPLASTY AT OPERATION

Urschel and associates[133] from Dallas, Texas, used operative transluminal coronary artery balloon angioplasty in >3,000 narrowings in 1,000 patients since 1980. Initially it was only used for distal stenoses not accessible to CABG in 200 patients. Recatheterization of patients who had intraoperative transluminal balloon angioplasty of the proximal LAD, right, and LC coronary arteries 3 years previously revealed excellent patency of both the bypass grafts and the dilated native coronary arteries. This observation supports the thesis that with properly constructed bypass anastomoses competitive flow does not significantly mandate graft thrombosis. Subsequently, intraoperative balloon angioplasty has been performed for both proximal and distal stenoses in 800 patients to improve native coronary artery perfusion and maximize revascularization. Follow-up from 1 to 7 years revealed perioperative AMI in 21 patients (2%) and death in 19 patients (2%). Recatheterization from 1 to 7 years after the operation in 51 patients (41 with symptoms) revealed that patency was almost as prevalent in arteries subjected to angioplasty (82%; 137/167) as in bypass grafts (84%; 102/122). Intraoperative balloon angioplasty appears to improve coronary artery perfusion without detrimental competitive flow when used with bypass grafts.

ATHERECTOMY, LASER ANGIOPLASTY, STENTS, AND INTRAARTERIAL ULTRASOUND

During an initial evaluation of transluminal coronary atherectomy, Kaufmann and associates[134] from Rochester, Pennsylvania, performed atherectomy of narrowings in saphenous veins used as aortocoronary bypass grafts in 14 patients (15 grafts). Atherectomy was successful in 13 of 14 patients, decreasing the mean diameter of stenosis from 85 to 15%. In 1 patient, the lesion could not be crossed by the atherectomy device. The following 3 minor complications occurred: 1 embolus of atheromatous material; 1 air embolism; and 1 transient thrombosis leading to subendocardial myocardial infarction. Of the 14 patients, 8 underwent angiography 4 to 6 months after atherectomy; 5 patients had restenosis and 3 had widely patent grafts. Four other patients were clinically evaluated at 3 months after atherectomy. Two were asymptomatic, 1 had class II angina and 1 had class III angina. Transluminal atherectomy achieved excellent immediate results with a low incidence of major complications in the treatment of stenosed saphenous vein bypass grafts. However, preliminary follow-up results suggest a high incidence of restenosis.

Directional coronary atherectomy is a new percutaneous transluminal technique for treating occlusive CAD. In this study, Rowe and associates[135] from Redwood City, California, compared angiographic results (i.e., residual stenosis and angiographic evidence of postprocedure dissection) after directional coronary atherectomy and balloon angioplasty. The atherectomy group consisted of 91 narrowings in 83 consecutive patients who underwent either LAD artery or right coronary artery atherectomy. The angioplasty group consisted of 91 lesions in 84 patients that were matched with the atherectomy lesions with respect to vessel and whether the lesion was a restenosis lesion. The mean preprocedure diameter stenosis was 76% in both groups as measured quantitatively with electronic calipers. After the procedure, the mean residual diameter stenosis of the atherectomy lesions was 13 ± 17%, whereas for the angioplasty lesions it was 31 ± 18%. Success rates in both groups were similar (94.5 and 93.4%, respectively). The incidence of postprocedure dissection was 11% in the atherectomy group and 37% in the angioplasty group. Directional coronary atherectomy results in significantly improved postprocedure angiographic appearances due to significantly less severe residual stenosis and lower incidence of dissection.

Coronary atherectomy and coronary stenting effectively reduce the severity of CAD, but direct comparisons of these interventions with conventional balloon angioplasty have not been performed. To compare the immediate efficacy of these 3 interventions, Muller and associates[136] from Ann Arbor, Michigan, quantitatively evaluated the angiographic morphology and severity of the residual coronary stenosis in 18 patients undergoing coronary atherectomy and in 21 patients treated by endoluminal coronary stenting. Each of these groups of patients was compared with a matched group of coronary angioplasty patients selected from a large, computerized database. The variables matched included patient age and sex, lesions site and severity, and lesion complexity. Both coronary atherectomy and coronary stenting more effectively reduced the severity of the coronary stenosis when compared with balloon angioplasty. The luminal diameter stenosis was reduced from 69 ± 10 to 22 ± 20% in the atherectomy group compared with a reduction from 74 ± 11 to 44 ± 14% in the matched coronary angioplasty population. Similarly, the luminal diameter stenosis was reduced from 77 ± 11 to 26 ± 12% in the stented group compared with a reduction from 81 ± 10 to 42 ± 14% in the matched coronary angioplasty group. In addition, moderate or severe coronary dissections were noted more frequently in the coronary angioplasty groups than in their respective atherectomy and stent groups (0 vs 33% and 5 vs 19%, respectively). These data suggest that, in selected patients, both coronary atherectomy and coronary stenting more effectively reduce the severity of coronary stenoses when compared with conventional balloon angioplasty and that this may be achieved with a lower risk of medial dissection.

Garratt and colleagues[137] in Rochester, Minnesota, evaluated the rates of restenosis after successful directional coronary atherectomy in 70 patients with 74 lesions. The extent of vascular tissue resection was correlated with restenosis rates for coronary (n = 59) and vein (n = 15) lesions. After 6 months, the overall restenosis rate was 50%, including 42% when intima alone was resected, 50% when media was resected, and 63% when adventitia was resected. Subintimal tissue resection increased the restenosis rate for vein grafts (43% with intimal resection and 100% with subintimal resection) but not for coronary arteries. There was no overall difference in restenosis rates after atherectomy between primary lesions and restenosis lesions that occurred after PTCA. Among patients with PTCA restenosis lesions, a higher rate of restenosis after atherectomy was found with subintimal than with intimal resection (78% vs 32%) (Figure 2-24).

A clinical study was conducted by Karsch and colleagues[138] in Tuebingen, Germany, to evaluate the efficacy and safety of percutaneous coronary excimer laser angioplasty in 60 patients with CAD. Forty-nine patients had stable exertional angina, and 11 patients had unstable angina despite medical therapy. A novel 1.4 mm diameter catheter with 20 quartz fibers of 100 micro-meter diameter each arranged concentrically around a central lumen suitable for a 0.014 in. flexible guide wire was coupled to an excimer laser. A commercial excimer laser emitting energy at a wavelength of 308 nm with a pulse duration of 60 nsec was used. In 23 patients with laser ablation alone, percent stenosis decreased from 76% before to 27% after ablation and was 34% at the early follow-up angiogram. In 32 patients, additional balloon angioplasty was performed because of vessel closure after laser ablation in 11 and an insufficient qualitative result in 21 patients. Of the 11 patients with unstable angina, one patient died due to vessel closure 3 hours after intervention, and two patients developed an AMI. In 22 of 47 patients with late follow-up angiography, restenosis within the 6-month follow-up period occurred. Rate of restenosis was higher in patients treated with laser ablation and balloon angioplasty (16 of 28) than in patients treated with laser ablation alone (6 of 19). These results suggest that coronary excimer laser angioplasty for ablation of obstructive lesions is feasible and safe in patients with stable angina.

To determine the efficacy of percutaneous excimer laser coronary angioplasty as an adjunct or alternative to conventional balloon angioplasty, Litvack and associates[139] from Los Angeles, California, Miami, Florida, Indianapolis, Indiana, and Irvine, California, studied in a multi-center trial 55 patients. These patients underwent the procedure using a modification of conventional balloon angioplasty technique. A first-generation, 1.6-mm diameter catheter constructed of 12 individual silica fibers concentrically arranged around a guide wire lumen was used. Catheter tip energy density varied from 35 to 50 mJ/mm^2. The mean number of pulses delivered at 20 Hz was 1,272 ± 1,345. Acute success was defined as a >20% increase in stenotic diameter and a lumen of >1 mm in diameter after laser treatment. Acute success was achieved in 46 of 55 (84%) patients. Adjunctive balloon angioplasty was performed on 41 patients (75%). The percent diameter stenosis as determined by quantitative angiography

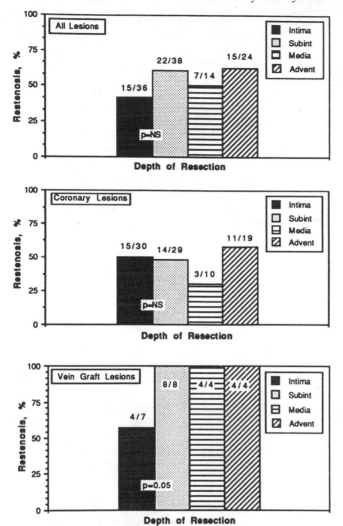

Fig. 2-24. Six month restenosis rates after coronary atherectomy. Restenosis rates are shown for all lesions, coronary artery lesions only and saphenous vein bypass graft lesions only in the top, middle and bottom panels, respectively. Rates are displayed according to the depth of tissue resection. Subintimal (Subint) resection refers to resection of media or adventitia (Advent). Reproduced with permission from Garratt, et al.[137]

decreased from a baseline of 83 ± 14 to 49 ± 11% after laser treatment and to 38 ± 12% in patients undergoing adjunctive balloon angioplasty. The mean minimal stenotic diameter increased from a baseline of 0.5 ± 0.4 to 1.6 ± 0.5 mm after laser treatment and to 2.1 ± 0.5 mm after balloon angioplasty. There were no deaths and no vascular perforations. One patient (1.8%) required emergency coronary bypass surgery. These data suggest that excimer laser energy delivered percutaneously by specially constructed catheters can safely ablate atheroma and reduce coronary stenoses.

Siegel and associates[140] in Los Angeles, California, assessed the potential of intraarterial ultrasound for in vivo recanalization of arterial occlusions. Ultrasound energy at a frequency of 20 kHz was supplied with a prototype solid wire probe to 12 surgically implanted occluded human atherosclerotic arterial xenografts, 9 of which were calcified as well as to the intimal surface of 12 normal canine arteries. In both the normal canine arteries and the atherosclerotic occluded xenografts, there was no angiographic evidence of vasospasm, thrombosis, or arterial dissection. Eleven of the 12 atherosclerotic occlusions were resistant to passage of a conventional guide wire or probe without ultrasound energy. The occlusions were recanalized after administration of 15 s to 14 minutes (mean 1.5 ± 1.3 minutes) of intermittent ultrasound energy. After ultrasound, 8 of the 12 vessels underwent PTCA. Angiographic residual stenosis after ultrasound alone was 62 ± 24% and after combined ultrasound and PTCA, 29 ± 13% (Figure 2-25). Although routine angiography did not reveal arterial emboli, high resolution films demonstrated a few distal nonocclusive thrombi. Histologic studies demonstrated changes similar to those after PTCA with focal cracking of the fibrotic and calcified plaque. These findings demonstrate that ultrasound energy applied through a catheter delivery system may be used in vivo to open obstructed atherosclerotic vessels.

CORONARY ARTERY BYPASS GRAFTING

Comparison with medical therapy

The Coronary Artery Surgery Study by Alderman and co-investigators[141] in Seattle, Washington, randomized 780 patients during an initial strategy of coronary surgery or medical therapy. Of medically randomized patients, 6% had surgery within 6 months and a total of 40% had surgery by 10 years. There was no difference in cumulative survival (medical, 79% vs surgical, 82%) and no difference in percentage free of death and nonfatal AMI (medical, 69% vs surgical, 66%). Patients with an EF of <50% had a better survival with initial surgery treatment (medical, 61% vs sur-

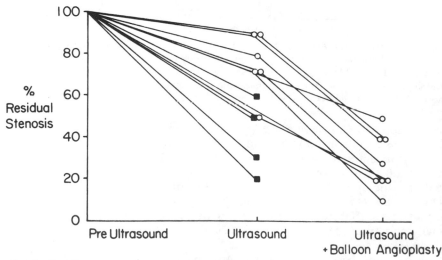

Fig. 2-25. The angiographic residual stenosis after ultrasound ablation without balloon angioplasty (n = 4) was 62 ± 24% (solid squares). When ultrasound was followed by balloon angioplasty (open circles at right), the residual stenosis was 29 ± 13%. In two of the eight cases with combined ultrasound and balloon angioplasty, angiograms were not available for the immediate postultrasound study. Reproduced with permission from Siegel, et al.[140]

gical, 79%). Conversely, patients with an EF ≥50% had a higher proportion free of death and AMI with initial medical therapy (medical, 75% vs surgical, 68%) although long-term survival remained unaffected. There were no significant differences either in survival and freedom from non-fatal AMI, whether stratified on presence CHF, age, hypertension, or number of vessels narrowed. Thus, 10-year follow-up results confirm earlier reports from the Coronary Artery Surgery Study that patients with LV dysfunction exhibit long-term benefit from an initial strategy of surgical treatment. Patients with mild stable angina and normal LV function randomized to initial medical treatment (with an option for later surgery if symptoms progress) have survival equivalent to those patients randomized to initial surgery.

Guidelines for ranking urgency of operation

Naylor and associates[142] for the Revascularization Panel and Consensus Methods Group from Canada developed guidelines for ranking the urgency with which patients with angiographically proven CAD need CABG. Factors that a panel of cardiac specialists agreed were likely to affect the urgency of CABG were incorporated into 438 fictitious case histories. Each panelist then rated the cases on a 7-point scale based on maximum acceptable waiting time for surgery; 1 on the scale represented emergency surgery and 7 delays of up to 6 months (Table 2-2). For only 1% of cases was there agreement on a single rating by at least 12 of 16 panelists. Results of this ranking exercise were used by the panel to draw up triage guidelines. The 3 main urgency determinants were severity and stability of symptoms of angina, coronary anatomy from angiographic studies, and results of non-invasive tests for risk of ischemia (Table 2-3). Together these 3 factors generally gave an urgency rating for any given case to within <0.25 scale points of the value predicted with all factors. A numerical scoring system was derived to permit rapid estimation of the panel's recommended ratings.

TABLE 2-2. *Rating scale accepted by the panel. Reproduced with permission from Naylor, et al.*[142]

	Level	Timing
1	Emergency	Immediate revascularisation
2	Extremely urgent	Within 24 hours
3	Urgent	24–72 hours
4	Semi-urgent	72 hours to 14 days (same admission)
5	Short list	2 weeks to 6 weeks
6	Delayed	6 weeks to 3 months
7	Marked delay	3 months to 6 months

Questionable whether revascularisation should be undertaken.
Inappropriate for revascularisation to be undertaken.

Each urgency rating level represents the period within which the revascularisation procedure is expected to be done; the outer time limit for each level represents the maximum acceptable waiting period for patients assigned that urgency rating.

TABLE 2-3. *Major factors affecting urgency ranking. Reproduced with permission from Naylor, et al.*[142]

A. Presenting pain syndrome and therapeutic response

1. Stable angina on reasonable medical therapy: mild to moderate (Canadian Cardiovascular Society classes I–II).
2. Stable angina on reasonable medical therapy: severe (Canadian Cardiovascular Society class III).
3. Unstable angina, pain resolved with intensified medical therapy, and now stable on oral medication (panel class IV–A).
4. Unstable angina, on oral therapy, symptoms improved but angina with minimal provocation (panel class IV–B).
5. Symptoms not manageable on oral therapy, requires coronary care monitoring and parenteral medication, may be haemodynamically unstable (panel class IV–C).

B. Coronary artery disease defined by angiography (prototypical patterns below or equivalents*)

1. Left mainstem stenosis with or without stenoses of other vessels.
2. Two-vessel or three-vessel disease, including proximal left anterior descending (LAD).
3. Three-vessel disease without significant involvement of the proximal LAD.
4. Single-vessel disease involving the proximal LAD.
5. Single-vessel or two-vessel disease without a proximal lesion of LAD.

C. Reversible ischaemia on non-invasive tests

1. High risk: see text for definitions.
2. Not high risk: any test not meeting high risk criteria.

---

*"Equivalents": anatomical patterns not falling within the five prototypes are rated according to the closest equivalent in terms of viable myocardium at ischaemic risk.

In women

Kahn and associates[143] from Los Angeles, California, analyzed consecutive patients who had isolated CABG between 1982 and 1987: a total of 2,297 patients, 79% men and 21% women were analyzed. The in-hospital mortality was significantly higher for women than for men (4.6% vs 2.6%). Women were older than men (mean 68 years versus 64 years), and a higher percent of women were referred with unstable angina, post AMI angina, CHF, and New York Heart Association Class IV symptoms (66% vs 45%). More men were referred with a history of an abnormal exercise test, and patients referred because of a positive exercise test had a lower mortality. Using multi-variant analysis, adjustment for the higher preoperative functional class of women and for age accounted for all of the difference in mortality between men and women. After correction for functional class alone, there continued to be no significant difference in mortality between men and women. Thus, according to this study, differences in functional class and age account for the higher operative mortality of women compared to men having CABG.

In patients >70 years old

Despite numerous references to the superiority of the internal mammary artery (IMA) over the saphenous vein for CABG, its role in the elderly is still in question. From January 1984 through December 1988, Azariades and associates[144] from Portland, Oregon, performed CABG in 1081 patients

>70 years of age (mean 75), 355 (33%) receiving left IMA grafts based on the surgeon's preference and 727 (67%) receiving saphenous vein grafts only. Selection bias resulted in a higher incidence of known risk factors (such as cardiomegaly, arrhythmias, LV failure, wall motion abnormalities, and preoperative combined New York Heart Association/Canadian Cardiovascular Association functional class IV) in patients in whom the IMA was not used. Unstable angina, acute AMI, LV dysfunction, and LM CAD were not contraindications for using IMA grafts. The operative mortality rate was significantly lower in IMA patients (2.8% vs 7.6%). The actuarial 5-year survival rate was higher in patients with IMA grafts, 89% (3%) versus 78% (2%) (Figure 2-26), and postoperative functional class improved to a greater extent in IMA patients (87% of whom were in classes I and II). Arrhythmias and myocardial infarction were significant causes of late death only in patients with vein grafts. When patients are >70 years, patient selection factors clearly play an important role in the differential results between patients in whom the IMA is used and patients in whom vein grafts are used. As in younger patients, excellent results can be achieved in the elderly.

Use of internal mammary artery

Left IMA grafts have better long-term patency rates than do saphenous vein grafts and result in improved late survival. Gardner and associates[145] from Baltimore, Maryland, reported results of use of the left IMA graft in 723 patients aged ≥70 years who had isolated CABG. During the first 5 years, only 11% of the elderly patients received left IMA grafts, whereas 86% having CABG since 1985 had left IMA grafts. Since 1986, left IMA use in the elderly has become routine, with 92% of patients receiving IMA grafts. During the first 5 years, elderly patients had a hospital mortality rate of 9.3%. Since 1985, the hospital mortality rate fell to 5.5%. In addition,

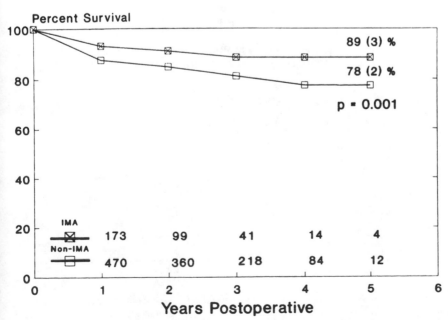

Fig. 2-26. Survival after coronary artery bypass grafting. (IMA = internal mammary artery; Non-IMA = vein grafts only). Reproduced with permission from Azariades, et al.

the occurrence of major surgical complications was either unchanged or reduced in patients receiving left IMA grafts. Furthermore, late follow-up indicates a significantly improved 4-year survival rate in patients with IMA grafts compared with those without: 86 ± 0.02% versus 77 ± 0.03% (Figure 2-27). Analysis of multiple potential risk factors for early mortality was performed using multiple logistic regression and late survival using the Cox proportional hazards model. Although unmeasured predictor variables may confound retrospective analyses, left IMA grafting appears to be an independent predictor both of improved early and late survival.

Fiore and associates[146] from St. Louis, Missouri, compared retrospectively 100 consecutive patients who had CABG using both IMAs and saphenous veins, operated on during a 3-year period between 1972 and 1975 with a series of 100 patients operated on during the same period who had 1 IMA graft along with saphenous vein grafts. The 2 groups were similar with respect to age, sex, risk factors for CAD, angina class, extent of CAD, LV function, number of coronary bypass grafts performed, and completeness of revascularization. Single IMA operative mortality was 2% and double IMA, 9%. The mean follow-up of hospital survivors was 14.4 ± 2.7 years; all but 7 patients had follow-up for at least 10 years. At 13 years, the actuarial patency of the right IMAs was 85% and the left IMAs, 82%. These data strongly suggest a survival benefit for patients with double IMA grafts among hospital survivors (74% vs 59%). Patients receiving 2 IMA grafts had a significant freedom from subsequent AMI (75% vs 59%), recurrent angina pectoris (36% vs 27%), and subsequent total ischemic events (32% vs 18%). These data also suggest improved freedom from coronary artery interventional therapy (PTCA and reoperation) when 2 IMA grafts were used.

Although use of 1 IMA for CABG does not appear to be associated with increased risk, the results with both IMAs are less certain. The potential for high incidence of sternal wound infection as a result of devascularization of the sternum is a major concern. During a 42-month interval ending July 1988, Kouchoukos and associates[147] from St. Louis, Missouri, performed CABG in 1,566 patients alone or in combination with other procedures: 633 received only vein grafts; 687 had unilateral IMA grafting, and 246 had bilateral IMA grafting. The IMA patients were younger, were more often men, had better cardiac function, and underwent fewer

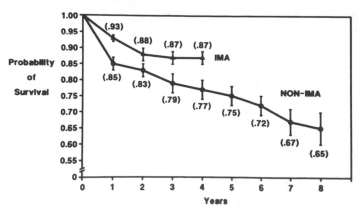

Fig. 2-27. Actuarial Kaplan-Meier survival estimates for coronary bypass patients 70 years and older with internal mammary grafts (IMA) or vein grafts only (NON-IMA). Projected survival for up to 4 years is significantly better for IMA patients. Reproduced with permission from Gardner, et al.[145]

emergent, urgent, or combined procedures than the patients receiving vein grafts. Thirty-day mortality was lower among the IMA patients (unilateral IMA group, 2.8%; bilateral IMA group, 3.7%; and vein graft group, 7.9%). With the exception of sternal wound problems, occurrence rates for postoperative complications among the IMA patients did not differ significantly from or were lower than those among the patients with vein grafts. Sternal infections occurred with greater frequency among bilateral IMA patients (6.9%) than among the unilateral IMA (1.9%) or vein graft (1.3%) patients. By univariate analysis, obesity, diabetes, bilateral IMA grafting, and need for prolonged (>48 hours) mechanical ventilation were associated with a significantly higher incidence of sternal infection. Multivariate logistic regression analysis identified use of bilateral IMA grafts, obesity, and prolonged mechanical ventilation as significant risk factors for the development of sternal infection. The authors concluded that bilateral IMA grafting is an important predictor of sternal infection. It should be used selectively in obese or diabetic patients and in patients who are likely to require prolonged mechanical ventilation postoperatively.

Combined with long arteriotomy, endarterectomy and reconstruction

Sommerhaug and associates[148] from Concord, California, described results of long coronary arteriotomy, endarterectomy and reconstruction (principally LAD coronary artery) and multiple bypass grafting (mean graft rate = 9) performed in 130 of 329 patients (40%) with severe diffuse CAD. Ninety-two percent of the patients who underwent exercise testing had abnormal (>1 mm ST) depression and/or positive results on scintigraphy. Long coronary arteriotomy (5 to 12 cm), endarterectomy and reconstruction of the LAD artery and its branches were performed in 121 patients; of the LC artery and its branches in 13 patients; and of the right coronary artery and its branches beyond the crux in 18 patients. Single endarterectomy and reconstruction was performed in 109 patients, double in 20 and triple in 1. The operative mortality was 2.3% and the perioperative AMI was 1.5%. Twenty-four patients (among them 38% who had undergone >1 previous bypass operation) were randomly selected and studied within 20 days after surgery. This group comprised a total of 69 coronary conduits of which 68 (99%) were patent, and a total of 206 coronary anastomoses of which 202 (98%) were patent. Thirty-two of 33 conduits (97%) to endarterectomized and reconstructed arteries were patent. One hundred and twenty-six of 127 patients were followed up for a mean of 20 months; 120 of the 121 patients (99%) were in angina class I by Canadian Cardiovascular Society classification, and 63 of 71 patients (89%) had a normal treadmill exercise stress test. These data indicate that complete myocardial revascularization can be effectively accomplished by this aggressive surgical approach in patients with severe CAD with low mortality and morbidity; high patency rates of conduits and anastomoses can be achieved with excellent early clinical results on followup.

For failed coronary angioplasty

To assess the frequency and outcome of emergency CABG for failed PTCA in patients with prior CABG, Kahn and associates[149] from Kansas City, Missouri, reviewed 2,136 elective PTCA procedures in prior CABG patients studied over a 10-year period. Emergency surgical revascularization was required in 19 patients (0.9%) with prior CABG, compared with 130 of 6,974 patients (1.9%) without prior CABG. The interval from the most recent CABG to the failed coronary angioplasty was 6.8 years (range 1 to 16). Referral for emergency CABG was made on the basis of an acute closure not responding to repeat dilatation in 12 native coronary arteries and in 7 saphenous vein grafts. Severe hemodynamic instability after acute closure required the placement of an intra-aortic balloon pump in 3 patients, including 2 who required cardiopulmonary resuscitation. A total of 34 saphenous vein grafts and 1 internal mammary artery graft were placed emergently. Three patients with high-risk features (3 prior CABG operations in 1 patient, single remaining vessel to heart in 2 patients) could not be weaned from cardiopulmonary bypass. The remaining 16 patients were discharged after a mean hospital stay of 16 days. Four patients developed new Q waves after CABG. At follow-up (mean 52 months, range 3 to 99), 1 patient died late from an AMI. The 15 survivors had no or mild angina and were free of further CABG. Thus, emergency CABG after failed angioplasty in patients with prior CABG is required infrequently. In patients without extreme high-risk features, emergency repeat CABG can be accomplished with good hospital and long-term results.

Aspirin ± dipyridamole

Sethi and associates[150] from Tucson, Arizona, and Hines, Illinois, studied the perioperative consequences of preoperative aspirin administration in a prospective, cooperative study of 772 patients undergoing CABG. Seven hundred and seventy-two patients were randomized to receive either aspirin (325 mg once per day), aspirin (325 mg 3 times per day), aspirin and dipyridamole (325 mg and 75 mg together 3 times a day) (aspirin group), sulfinpyrazone (267 mg 3 times a day) or placebo (nonaspirin group). Therapy, except in the aspirin groups, was started 48 hours before the operation. In all aspirin subgroups, one 325 mg aspirin dose was given 12 hours before surgery and maintained thereafter. Patients in the aspirin group had significantly more postoperative bleeding and received more packed blood cells and blood products than did patients in the nonaspirin group. Total operative duration and cardiopulmonary bypass duration were not different, but the interval between completion of cardiopulmonary bypass and wound closure was significantly longer in the aspirin group. Thirty-one (6.6%) of 471 patients in the aspirin and 5 (1.7%) of 301 patients in the nonaspirin group required reoperation for control of postoperative bleeding. The site of bleeding found at reoperation was not different among the 2 groups. There was no difference in operative mortality rates, incidence of other bleeding complications, or occurrence of other postoperative complications between the 2 groups. Therefore, antiplatelet regimens involving preoperative initiation of aspirin therapy increase the risk of abnormal postoperative bleeding and the need for reoperation.

Gavaghan and associates[151] in Sydney, Australia, evaluated the therapeutic effects of aspirin on vein graft patency in patients undergoing CABG. Serial beta-thromboglobulin levels were measured in 105 patients randomized to receive aspirin (324 mg/day) or placebo beginning within 1 hour after CABG. Graft patency was assessed angiographically at 1 week and 1 year after CABG. Among 49 patients receiving placebo, 17 (35%) had ≥1 graft occlusions, 6 early, 10 late and 1 with both early and late occlusion. Among 56 patients receiving aspirin, 7 (12.5%) had one or more occlusions, 3 early and 4 late. Plasma beta-thromboglobulin levels remained constant at 3 and 12 months after CABG in the 43 patients who had both samples available. The reduction in beta-thromboglobulin concentration from preoperative levels to 12 months postoperatively was greater in the aspirin-treated groups. Multivariate logistic regression analysis demonstrated a significant association between preoperative beta-thromboglobulin concentrations and graft occlusion and aspirin treatment was effective in preventing occlusion when adjusted for the preoperative beta-thromboglobulin levels. Thus, plasma beta-thromboglobulin concentrations are elevated in patients with CAD suggesting ongoing platelet activation and the risk of coronary artery bypass graft occlusion is greater in patients with higher preoperative levels of beta-thromboglobulin. This increased risk of CABG graft occlusion may be reduced by aspirin therapy begun within 1 hour of surgery and continued for 12 months postoperatively.

To analyze the efficacy of low-dose aspirin in preventing early aortocoronary vein graft occlusion, Sanz and colleagues[152] in Barcelona, Spain, enrolled 1,112 consecutive patients in a multicenter, randomized, double-blind, placebo-controlled trial comparing 50 mg 3 times daily, aspirin, 50 mg aspirin plus 75 mg 3 times daily, dipyridamole, and placebo. All patients received 100 mg 4 times daily, dipyridamole for 48 hours before surgery, and assigned treatment was started 7 hours after surgery. Vein graft angiography was performed in 927 patients within 28 days of surgery. Aspirin plus dipyridamole significantly reduced the occlusion rate of distal anastomoses from 18% to 13%. Occlusion rate in the aspirin group was 14% which approached statistical significance. Furthermore, only aspirin plus dipyridamole reduced the number of patients with occluded grafts (placebo, 33%; aspirin, 27%; aspirin plus dipyridamole, 24%). Mediastinal drainage was slightly higher in the aspirin plus dipyridamole group than in the two other groups, but hospital mortality and early reoperation rates were similar among the three groups. Thus, low-dose aspirin plus dipyridamole safely improves early saphenous vein aortocoronary graft patency; this effect is an added benefit to a preoperative regimen of dipyridamole.

Taggart and associates[153] from Glasgow, UK, recorded the effects of 3 low-dose regimens of preoperative aspirin therapy on post-operative blood loss, transfusion requirements, and length of hospital stay in a prospective cohort study of 202 patients undergoing elective CABG. One hundred one patients had been prescribed daily aspirin by the referring cardiologist (44 at 75 mg, 28 at 150 mg, and 29 at 300 mg); the remaining 101 patients who had not been prescribed aspirin acted as a control group. A median postoperative blood loss at 870 mL in the control group was increased by 280 mL in the 75-mg aspirin group, by 490 mL in the 150-mg aspirin group, and by 230 mL in the 300-mg aspirin group. The median requirement for blood transfusion of 2 U red blood cell concentrates in the control group was increased by 2 U in the 75-mg aspirin group, 2 U in the 150-mg aspirin group, and 1 U in the 300-mg aspirin group. Hemostatic "packs" (fresh frozen plasma, platelets, and cryoprecipitate) were required in 20 patients in the aspirin groups as compared with 5 in the control group. The mean postoperative hospital stay was 8 days for all groups. Regular daily low-dose aspirin therapy produces significant increases in postoperative blood loss, resulting in a substantial increase in blood transfusion and hemostatic pack requirements, but does not prolong postoperative hospital stay.

Atrial fibrillation and/or flutter afterwards

Leitch and associates[154] from Sydney, Australia, sought to identify factors associated with AF and atrial flutter after CABG, by studying 5,807 patients who underwent CABG alone and who were in sinus rhythm preoperatively. AF and flutter were identified during continuous monitoring or by clinical symptoms and signs; they occurred in 17% of the patients. The prevalence of AF and flutter was directly related to age at operation, varying from 4% in patients aged <40 years to 28% in patients aged ≥70 years. In a multivariate analysis, age remained the most important independent predictor of AF and flutter. Other independent predictors of AF and flutter were chronic airflow limitation, preoperative β-adrenergic blockers, and chronic renal failure. Extent of CAD at catheterization, history of a previous AMI, heart size on chest x-ray film, and all operative factors measured, apart from year of operation, were unassociated with AF and flutter. Thus atrial arrhythmias after CABG are most strongly related to advanced age and are unassociated with preoperative LV function and extent of CAD.

Myocardial infarction afterwards

The clinical significance of perioperative AMI after CABG is not known. Therefore, strategies for the risk stratification of these patients do not exist. Force and co-workers[155] in Boston, Massachusetts, undertook a study to define the effect of perioperative AMI prognosis after discharge from the hospital and to develop an approach to the risk stratification of these patients. Fifty-nine patients with and 115 patients without perioperative AMI were observed for 30 months for the development of cardiac events (death, nonfatal AMI, and admission to hospital for unstable angina or CHF). Patients with perioperative AMI were significantly more likely than patients without to have a cardiac event and multiple events. Cox regression analysis identified 2 independent predictors of cardiac events other than perioperative AMI; inadequate revascularization and depressed postoperative EF. Event-free survival rate of patients with perioperative AMI varied markedly depending on the number of their negative prognostic variables present. Patients with perioperative AMI who were adequately revascularized and had a postoperative EF >40% had an event-free survival rate similar to patients without a perioperative AMI. Patients with perioperative AMI who were inadequately revascularized and had depressed postoperative EF had an event-free survival rate of 13%. In conclusion, perioperative AMI adversely affects prognosis. Patients can be stratified into low, high and intermediate risk subsets based on a simple assessment of the adequacy of revascularization and a determination of residual LV function.

Silent myocardial ischemia afterwards

Kennedy and associates[156] from St. Louis, Missouri, prospectively assessed in 94 patients examined early (1 to 3 months) and in 184 patients examined late (12 months) after CABG. The prevalence and characteristics of silent myocardial ischemia as detected by 24-hour electrocardiography ST-segment depression and followed them for a mean of 48 ± 11 months (range 4–62). The relation of ambulatory electrocardiographic silent ischemia to evidence of completeness of revascularization as defined by cardiac angiography performed 1 and 12 months after CABG, and to prognosis by follow-up of adverse clinical events was analyzed. Silent ischemia was detected early in 20% (19 of 95) and late in 27% (50 of 184) of patients, and showed a mean frequency of episodes ranging from 6 to 10 episodes/24 hours with a mean duration ranging from 15 to 23 minutes. The circadian distribution of episodes disclosed a significant peak of ischemic activity during the period of 7 A.M. to noon and a secondary peak between 6 P.M. and midnight. Silent ischemia was not found by univariate analysis to be associated with graft or anastomotic site occlusions, low graft flow rates, grafted arteries with significant distal residual stenoses or ungrafted stenotic native coronary arteries. Kaplan-Meier analysis of time to cardiac event showed that silent ischemia was not predictive of an adverse clinical event in the early years after CABG. Cox regression analysis of 30 covariates only disclosed age (relative risk 1.06) as having an effect on time to adverse clinical event. These data show that ambulatory electrocardiographic-detected silent ischemia during the first year after CABG in patients with predominantly good LV function is not associated with an adverse prognosis.

Repeat operations

During an 18-year period, Salomon and associates[157] from Portland, Oregon, performed primary CABG on 6,591 patients and reoperative CABG on 508 patients. The mean patient age for the reoperative group was identical to that of the primary group, 60 years, but the mean age of initial operation for the reoperative group was 55 years. Mammary grafts were done at initial operation in 59% of patients who have had one operation versus only 46% of patients who subsequently required reoperation. The overall operative mortality rate was 2.0% (134/6591) for primary coronary bypass versus 6.9% (35/508) for reoperations (Figures 2-28 and 2-29). Patients with a reoperative interval of 1 to 10 years had a 6.0% (18/312) mortality rate, compared with 17.6% (13/74) for those in whom the interval between operations was greater than 10 years. Ventricular arrhythmias,

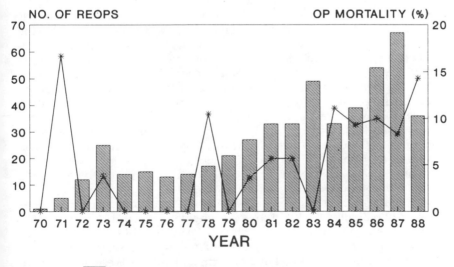

Fig. 2-28. Reoperations by calendar year and operative mortality. Reproduced with permission from Salomon, et al.[157]

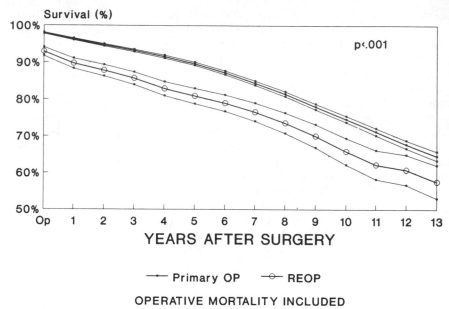

Fig. 2-29. Patient survival, single operation versus reoperation. Reproduced with permission from Salomon, et al.[157]

excessive bleeding, prolonged ventilatory support, intraaortic balloon pump insertion, and perioperative myocardial infarction were all more prevalent after reoperations. Including perioperative mortality, the actuarial survival rate of 5 years was 80% for reoperations versus 90% for primary operations. The corresponding figures at 10 years were 65% and 75%. The probability of undergoing reoperation within 5 and 10 years was 0.034 ± 0.003 and 0.055 ± 0.005, respectively. Ten years postoperatively, 36% of patients having the initial operation had recurrent angina whereas 58% of the reoperative group had significant recurrent angina. Ten years after reoperation, 30% of operative survivors were free of heart-related morbidity and mortality compared with 50% of patients having a primary operation. Univariate analysis of factors increasing the probability of reoperation include the absence of a mammary graft and younger age at operation. Patients undergoing a second bypass operation represent a substantially higher risk subgroup than patients undergoing initial operation in terms of perioperative morbidity, mortality, decreased long-term survival, and decreased relief of recurrent cardiac morbidity.

Owen and associates[158] from Memphis, Tennessee, retrospectively reviewed 21 patients who had CABG for the third time to assess the factors of importance in the management of these patients. The study spanned 6 years and represented 6.2% of CABG reoperations and 0.6% (21/3500) of total bypass operations during that time. The indication for reoperation was disabling angina pectoris not responsive to medical treatment in 20 patients (95%) and unstable angina pectoris in 1 patient (5%). Median sternotomy was used in all and CABG in all but 1 who had an interposition vein graft without cardiopulmonary bypass. Internal mammary artery grafting was used in 86% of patients. There were no operative deaths. One patient died 12 months after his operation. Four patients (19%) required intraaortic balloon pump support postoperatively for up to 6 days. There were no reexplorations for bleeding. One patient required sternal rewiring for an early dehiscence (5%). Respiratory failure occurred in 8 patients (38%). Average stay was 4.4 days in the intensive care unit and postoperative hospital stay was 13.7 days. No new Q waves were noted postoperatively. Detailed follow-up was obtained on 18 of the 20 survivors (90%). The 2 remaining are alive but declined interview efforts. All patients interviewed reported feeling subjectively better than before operation; however 61% of these interviewed continue to have some degree of angina pectoris. One patient has had a late myocardial infarction. This report suggests that the third time CABG can be done with good results.

Blakeman and associates[159] from Maywood, Illinois, retrospectively reviewed 15 patients who had CABG for the third time. These patients were operated on during the period 1985 through 1989. Perioperative mortality was zero and 7 complications occurred in 6 patients. Internal mammary arteries were used in 60% of the group. At follow-up, only 1 patient had died. All patients but 1 were symptomatically improved and 18 patients were angina free at a mean follow-up of 22 months. The authors concluded that a third CABG operation could be beneficial.

Sternal wound complications

Loop and associates[160] from Cleveland, Ohio, described 72 patients (1.1%) of 6,504 consecutive patients undergoing isolated CABG who had sternal wound infections (Table 2-4). Only the patients with negative cultures fared well; of the bacterial culture categories, polymicrobial infection carried the worst prognosis. Effects of recurring infection were seen throughout the first year. Patients, grouped according to conduits received, experienced these wound complication rates: vein grafts only, 11/1,085 (1.0%); one internal thoracic artery, 38/4,073 (0.9%); and bilateral internal thoracic artery grafts, 23/1,346 (1.7%). There were no significant differences in wound complication rates between primary and reoperation patients or among conduit groups. By logistic regression analysis, the relative risk for patients with diabetes and bilateral internal thoracic artery grafting was 5.00. Operation time as a continuous variable increased the relative risk of wound complication 1.47 times per hour (1.3–1.7); obesity, 2.90 times (1.8–4.8); and blood units as continuous variable, 1.05 times per unit (1.01–1.10). Bilateral internal thoracic artery grafting in nondiabetic patients carried no greater risk of wound complication than that in patients with vein grafts only or with one internal thoracic artery graft.

TABLE 2-4. *Incidence of wound complications after coronary artery bypass grafting. Reproduced with permission from Loop, et al.*[160]

Conduit Type	Primary (%)	Reoperation (%)
Vein grafts	6/690 (0.9)	5/395 (1.3)
One internal thoracic artery	30/3480 (0.9)	8/593 (1.3)
Bilateral internal thoracic arteries	19/1199 (1.6)	4/147 (2.7)
Total	55/5369 (1.0)	17/1135 (1.5)

Late morphologic findings

Kalan and Roberts[161] from Bethesda, Maryland, described certain clinical and necropsy findings in 53 patients who died from 13 to 185 months (mean 58) after a single CABG. Of the 53 patients, 32 (60%) died of a cardiac cause and of their 72 saphenous vein aortocoronary conduits, 36 (49%) were narrowed at some point >75% in cross-sectional area by atherosclerotic plaque; the remaining 21 patients (40%) died of a noncardiac cause and of their 50 saphenous vein conduits, 10 (20%) were narrowed at some point >75% in cross-sectional area by plaque. Thus, the noncardiac mode of death in a larger percentage of the patients suggests that the bypass operation prolonged life to a degree sufficient for another condition to develop. The 123 saphenous vein conduits were divided into 5-mm segments, and a histologic section was prepared from each. Of the 1104 five-mm segments in the 32 patients dying as a consequence of myocardial ischemia, 291 (26%) were narrowed >75% in cross-sectional area by plaque; in contrast, of the 761 five-mm segments of veins in the 21 patients with a noncardiac mode of death, 86 (11%) were narrowed >75% by plaque. Of the total 1865 5-mm segments of vein, only 395 (21%) were narrowed ≤25% in cross-sectional area by plaque. Thus, in patients dying late after CABG the atherosclerotic process continues in all segments of the saphenous veins used as aortocoronary conduits. Therapy after the operation must be directed toward prevention of progression of the atherosclerosis in the "new" coronary "arteries."

EFFECTS OF CALCIUM ANTAGONIST ON ATHEROSCLEROTIC PROGRESSION

Lichtlen and associates[162] from Hannover, Federal Republic of Germany, and Rotterdam, The Netherlands, enrolled 425 patients showing mild CAD on angiography in a multicenter trial and randomized to treatment with nifedipine (80 mg/day) or placebo. The 2 groups were well matched for age, sex, and risk factors. Three hundred forty-eight patients (82%) underwent repeat arteriography 3 years later; 282 (134 nifedipine, 148 placebo) had received treatment throughout, but treatment had been stopped in 39 nifedipine-treated and 27 placebo-treated patients after average periods of 354 and 467 days. Computer-assisted measurements of arteriograms from all restudied patients (175 placebo, 173 nifedipine) showed no significant differences in the number or severity of lesions on initial arteriograms, or in the progression or regression of existing lesions over 3 years (Table 2-5). In contrast, the number of new lesions per patient was significantly lower in the nifedipine group than in the placebo group (0.59 vs 0.82 lesions per patient, a 28% reduction). Thus, in patients with mild CAD nifedipine substantially suppresses disease progression as shown by the appearance of new lesions detectable by quantitative coronary arteriography.

To determine whether calcium antagonists influence the progression of coronary atherosclerosis, 383 patients age 65 years or less with 5–75% diameter stenoses in at least 4 coronary artery segments were selected at random by Waters and co-investigators[163] in Montreal, Canada, within 1 month of coronary arteriography to participate in double-blind therapy with a placebo or *nicardipine* 30 mg 3 times daily. Coronary events (5 deaths, 22 AMIs, and 28 unstable anginas) occurred in 28 of 192 nicar-

TABLE 2-5. *Numbers of patients with and without changes in pre-existing stenoses over 3 years. Reproduced with permission from Lichtlen, et al.*[162]

	No (%) of patients	
—	Placebo (n = 175)	Nifedipine (n = 173)
Changes in percent stenosis		
Progression (increase >20%)	42 *(24%)*	48 *(28%)*
Regression (decrease >20%)	25 *(14%)*	17 *(10%)*
Only progression	39 *(22%)*	43 *(25%)*
Only regression	22 *(13%)*	12 *(7%)*
Both	3 *(2%)*	5 *(3%)*
No change	111 *(63%)*	113 *(65%)*
Changes in minimum diameter		
Progression (increase >0·4 mm)	61 *(35%)*	50 *(29%)*
Regression (decrease >0·4 mm)	37 *(21%)*	27 *(16%)*
Only progression	54 *(31%)*	44 *(25%)*
Only regression	30 *(17%)*	21 *(12%)*
Both	7 *(4%)*	6 *(4%)*
No change	84 *(48%)*	102 *(59%)*

dipine patients and 23 of 191 placebo patients. At 24 months coronary arteriography was repeated in 335 patients. Progression, defined as a 10% or more worsening in diameter stenosis, measured quantitatively, was found in 13% of 1,153 lesions in 168 nicardipine patients and in 15% of 1,170 lesions in 167 placebo patients. Ninety-two nicardipine patients and 95 placebo patients had progression at ≥1 site. Regression, that is, an improvement by ≥10% in diameter stenosis, was seen 5% of 2,323 lesions overall, with no significant intergroup difference. Among the 217 patients with 411 stenoses of ≥20% in the first study, such minimal lesions progressed in only 15 of 99 nicardipine patients compared with 32 of 118 placebo patients. In this subgroup, 16 of 178 minimal lesions in nicardipine patients and 38 of 233 minimal lesions in placebo patients progressed. By stepwise logistic-regression analysis, baseline systolic BP and the change in systolic BP between baseline and 6 months correlated with progression of minimal lesions. This suggested BP reduction may account for the beneficial action of nicardipine. These results suggested nicardipine has no effect on advanced coronary atherosclerosis but may retard the progression of minimal lesions.

References

1. Dalen JE, Goldberg RJ, D'Arpa D, Comstock C, Lerner D, Moore FD: Coronary Heart Disease in Massachusetts: The years of change (1980–1984). Am Heart J 1990 (March);119:502–512.
2. Ciampricotti R, El Gamal M, Relik T, Taverne R, Panis J, de Swart J, van Gelder B, Relik-van Wely L: Clinical characteristics and coronary angiographic findings of patients

with unstable angina, acute myocardial infarction, and survivors of sudden ischemic death occurring during and after sport. Am Heart J 1990 (December);120:1267–1278.

3. Ambepityia G, Kopelman PG, Ingram D, Swash M, Mills PG, Timmis AD. Exertional myocardial ischemia in diabetes: A quantitative analysis of anginal perceptual threshold and the influence of autonomic function. J Am Coll Cardiol 1990 (January);15:72–7.

4. Dressler FA, Malekzadeh S, Roberts WC: Quantitative analysis of amounts of coronary arterial narrowing in cocaine addicts. Am J Cardiol 1990 (Feb 1);65:303–308.

5. Lange RA, Cigarroa RG, Flores ED, McBride W, Kim AS, Wells PJ, Bedotto JB, Danziger RS, Hillis LD: Potentiation of cocaine-induced coronary vasoconstriction by beta-adrenergic blockade. An Intern Med 1990 (June 15);112:897–903.

6. Cigarroa RG, Lange RA, Popma JJ, Yurow G, Sills MN, Firth BG, Hillis LD: Ethanol-induced coronary vasodilation in patients with and without coronary artery disease. Am Heart J 1990 (February);119;254–259.

7. McLenachan JM, Vita J, Fish RD, Treasure CB, Cox DA, Ganz P, Selwyn AP: Early Evidence of Endothelial Vasodilator Dysfunction at Coronary Branch Points. Circulation 1990 (October);82:1169–1173.

8. Nabel EG, Selwyn AP, Ganz P: Paradoxical narrowing of atherosclerotic coronary arteries induced by increases in heart rate. Circulation 1990 (March);81:850–859.

9. Rosenthal AD, Moran M, Herrmann HC: Coronary hemodynamic effects of atrial natriuretic peptide in humans. J Am Coll Cardiol 1990 (November);16:1107–13.

10. Tunick PA, Slater J, Kronzon I, Glassman E: Discrete atherosclerotic coronary artery aneurysms: A study of 20 patients. J Am Coll Cardiol 1990 (February);15:279–82.

11. Roberts WC, Kragel AH, Potkin BN: Ages at death and sex distribution in age decade in fatal coronary artery disease. Am J Cardiol 1990 (Dec 1);66:1379–1382.

12. Wittels EH, Hay JW, Gotto AM Jr: Medical costs of coronary artery disease in the United States. Am J Cardiol 1990 (Feb 15);65:432–440.

13. Wenneker MB, Weissman JS, Epstein AM: The association of payer with utilization of cardiac procedures in Massachusetts. JAMA 1990 (Sept 12);264:1255–1260.

14. Kern MJ, Cohen M, Talley JD, Litvack F, Serota H, Aguirre F, Deligonul U, Bashore TM. Early ambulation after 5 french diagnostic cardiac catheterization: Results of a multicenter trial. J Am Coll Cardiol 1990 (June);15:1475–83.

15. Stewart JT, Gray HH, Ward DE, Pumphrey CW, Redwood DR, Parker DJ: Major complications of coronary arteriography: The place of cardiac surgery. Br Heart J 1990 (Feb);63:74–77.

16. Epstein AE, Davis KB, Kay GN, Plumb VJ, Rogers WJ: Significance of ventricular tachyarrhythmias complicating cardiac catheterization: A CASS Registry study. Am Heart J 1990 (March);119:494–502.

17. Witteman JCM, Kannel WB, Wolf PA, Grobbee DE, Hofman A, D'Agostino RB, Cobb JC: Aortic calcified plaques and cardiovascular disease (The Framingham Study). Am J Cardiol 1990 (Nov 1);66:1060–1064.

18. Craven TE, Ryu JE, Espeland MA, Kahl FR, McKinney WM, Toole JF, McMahan MR, Thompson CJ, Heiss G, Crouse JR: Evaluation of the Associations Between Carotid Artery Atherosclerosis and Coronary Artery Stenosis A Case-Control Study. Circulation 1990 (October);82:1230–1242.

19. Lachterman B, Lehmann KG, Abrahamson D, Froelicher VF: "Recovery only" ST-segment depression and the predictive accuracy of the exercise test. An Intern Med 1990 (Jan 1);112:11–16.

20. Mirvis DM, El-Zeky F, Zwaag RV, Ramanathan KB, Crenshaw JH, Kroetz FW, Sullivan JM: Clinical and pathophysiologic correlates of ST-T-wave abnormalities in coronary artery disease. Am J Cardiol 1990 (Sept 15);66:699–704.

21. Peels CH, Visser CA, Kupper AJF, Visser FC, Roos JP: Usefulness of two-dimensional echocardiography for immediate detection of myocardial ischemia in the emergency room. Am J Cardiol 1990 (Mar 15);65:687–691.

22. Yoshida K, Yoshikawa, Hozumi T, Yamaura Y, Akasaka, Fukaya T, Kato H: Detection of Left Main Coronary Artery Stenosis by Transesophageal Color Doppler and Two-Dimensional Echocardiography. Circulation 1990 (April);81:1271–1276.

23. Potkin B, Bartorelli A, Gessert J, Neville R, Almagor Y, Roberts W, Leon M: Coronary Artery Imaging With Intravascular HIgh-Frequency Ultrasound. Circulation 1990 (May);81:1575–1585.

24. Gibbons RJ, Zinsmeister AR, Miller TD, Clements IP: Supine exercise electrocardiography compared with exercise radionuclide angiography in noninvasive identification of severe coronary artery disease. An Int Med 1990 (May 15);112:743–749.

25. Kotler TS, Diamond GA: Exercise thallium-201 scintigraphy in the diagnosis and prognosis of coronary artery disease. An Intern Med 1990 (Nov);113:684–702.

26. Agati L, Arata L, Neja CP, Manzara C, Iacoboni C, Vizza CD, Penco M, Fedele F, Dagianti A: Usefulness of the dipyridamole-Doppler test for diagnosis of coronary artery disease. Am J Cardiol 1990 (Apr 1);65:829–834.

27. Ranhosky A, Kempthorne-Rawson J: The Safety of Intravenous Dipyridamole Thallium Myocardial Perfusion Imaging. Circulation 1990 (April);81:1205–1209.

28. Verani MS, Mahmarian JJ, Hixson JB, Boyce TM, Staudacher RA: Diagnosis of Coronary Artery Disease by Controlled Coronary Vasodilation with Adenosine and Thallium-201 Scintigraphy in Patients Unable to Exercise. Circulation 1990 (July);82:80–87.

29. Dilsizian V, Rocco TP, Freedman MT, Leon MB, Bonow RO: Enhanced detection of ischemic but viable myocardium by the reinjection of thallium after stress-redistribution imaging. N Engl J Med 1990 (July 19);323:141–146.

30. Pohost GM, Henzlova MJ: The value of thallium-201 imaging. N Engl J Med 1990 (July 19);323:190–192.

31. Hill JA, Miranda AA, Keirn SG, Decker MH, Gonzalez JI, Lambert CR: Value of right-sided cardiac catheterization in patients undergoing left-sided cardiac catheterization for evaluation of coronary artery disease. Am J Cardiol 1990 (Mar 1);65:590–593.

32. Goldberg RK, Kleiman NS, Minor ST, Abukhalil J, Riazner AE: Comparison of quantitative coronary angiography to visual estimates of lesion severity pre- and post-PTCA. Am Heart J 1990 (January);119:178–184.

33. Sheikh KH, Bengtson JR, Helmy S, Juarez C, Burgess R, Bashore TM, Kisslo J: Relation of quantitative coronary lesion measurements to the development of exercise-induced ischemia assessed by exercise echocardiography. J Am Coll Cardiol 1990 (April);15:1043–51.

34. Metcalfe MJ, Rawles JM, Shirreffs C, Jennings K: Six year follow up of a consecutive series of patients presenting to the coronary care unit with acute chest pain: Prognostic importance of the electrocardiogram. Br Heart J 1990 (May);63:267–272.

35. White LD, Lee TH, Cook EF, Weisberg MC, Rouan GW, Brand DA, Goldman L, and the Chest Pain Study Group: Comparison of the natural history of new onset and exacerbated chronic ischemic heart disease. J Am Coll Cardiol 1990 (August);16:304–10.

36. Simmons BE, Castaner A, Mar M, Islam N, Cooper R: Survival determinants in black patients with angiographically defined coronary artery diseases. Am Heart J 1990 (March);119:513–519.

37. Lanti M, Puddu PE, Menotti A: Voltage criteria of left ventricular hypertrophy in sudden and nonsudden coronary artery disease mortality: The Italian section of the Seven Countries Study. Am J Cardiol 1990 (Nov 15);66:1181–1185.

38. Sawada SG, Tyan T, Conley MJ, Corya BC, Feigenbaum H, Armstrong WF: Prognostic value of a normal exercise echocardiogram. Am Heart J 1990 (July);120:49–55.

39. Lee KL, Pryor DB, Pieper KS, Harrell FE, Califf RM, Mark DB, Hlatky M, Coleman RE, Cobb FR, Jones RH: Prognostic Value of Radionuclide Angiography in Medically Treated Patients With Coronary Artery Disease: Circulation 1990 (November);82:1705–1717.

40. Munger TM, OH JK: Unstable angina. Mayo Clin Proc 1990 (Mar);65:384–406.

41. Kragel AH, Reddy SG, Wittes JT, Roberts WC: Morphometric analysis of the composition of coronary arterial plaques in isolated unstable angina pectoris with pain at rest. Am J Cardiol 1990 (Sept 1);66:562–567.

42. Marmur JD, Freeman MR, Langer A, Armstrong PW: Prognosis in medically stabilized unstable angina: Early Holter ST-segment monitoring compared with predischarge exercise thallium tomography. An Intern Med 1990 (Oct 15);113:575–579.

43. Berk BC, Weintraub WS, Alexander RW: Elevation of C-reactive protein in "active" coronary artery disease. Am J Cardiol 1990 (Jan 15);65:168–172.

44. Dinerman JL, Mehta JL, Saldeen TGP, Emerson S, Wallin R, Davda R, Davidson A: Increased neutrophil elastase release in unstable angina pectoris and acute myocardial infarction. J Am Coll Cardiol 1990 (June);15:1559–63.

45. Kalbfleisch SJ, McGillem MJ, Simon SB, DeBoe SF, Pinto IMF, Mancini GBJ: Automated Quantitation of Indexes of Coronary Lesion Complexity Comparison Between Patients with Stable and Unstable Angina. Circulation 1990 (August);82:439–447.

46. Mulcahy R, Conroy R, Katz R, Fitzpatrick M: Does intensive medical therapy influence the outcome in unstable angina? Clin Cardiol 1990 (Oct);13:687–689.

47. Balsano F, Rizzon P, Violi F, Scrutinio D, Cimminiello C, Aguglia F, Pasotti C, Rudelli G, the Studio della Ticlopidinia nell'Angina Instabile Group: Antiplatelet Treatment with Ticlopidine in Unstable Angina A Controlled Multicenter Clinical Trial. Circulation 1990 (July);82:17–26.

48. Serneri GGN, Poggesi L, Modesti PA, Margheri M, Rostagno C, Gensini GF, Trotta F, Boddi M, Ieri A, Casolo GC, Bini M, Carnovali M, Abbate R: Effect of heparin, aspirin, or alteplase in reduction of myocardial ischemia in refractory unstable angina. Lancet 1990 (Mar 17);335:615–618.

49. Williams DO, Topol EJ, Califf RM, Roberts R, Mancini J, Joelson JM, Ellis SG, Kleiman NS and Coinvestigators: Intravenous Recombinant Tissue-Type Plasminogen Activator in Patients With Unstable Angina Pectoris Results of a Placebo-Controlled, Randomized Trial. Circulation 1990 (August);82:376–838.

50. Ardissino D, Barberis P, De Servi S, Mussini A, Rolla A, Visani L, Specchia G: Recombinant tissue-type plasminogen activator followed by heparin compared with heparin alone for refractory unstable angina pectoris. Am J Cardiol 1990 (Oct 15);66:910–914.

51. Hausmann D, Nikutta P, Trappe HJ, Daniel WG, Wenzlaff P, Lichtlen PR: Circadian distribution of the characteristics of ischemic episodes in patients with stable coronary artery disease. Am J Cardiol 1990 (Sept 15);66:668–672.

52. Pupita G, Maseri A, Kaski JC, Galassi AR, Gavrielides S, Davies G, Crea F: Myocardial ischemia caused by distal coronary-artery constriction in stable angina pectoris. N Engl J Med 1990 (Aug 23);323:514–520.

53. Mahmarian JJ, Pratt CM, Cocanougher MK, Verani MS: Altered Myocardial Perfusion in Patients with Angina Pectoris or Silent Ischemia During Exercise as Assessed by Quantitative Thallium-201 Single-Photon Emission Computed Tomography. Circulation 1990 (October);82:1305–1315.

54. Crea FC, Pupita G, Galassi AR, El-Tammimi H, Kaski JC, Davies G, Maseri A: Role of adenosine in pathogenesis of anginal pain. Circulation 1990 (Jan);81:164–172.

55. Serneri GGN, Gensini GF, Abbate R, Castellani S, Bonechi F, Carnovali M, Rostagno C, Dabizzi RP, Dagianti A, Arata L, Fedele F, Iacoboni C, Prisco D: Defective coronary prostaglandin modulation in anginal patients. Am Heart J 1990 (July);120:12–21.

56. Hammill SC, Khandheria BK: Silent myocardial ischemia. Mayo Clin Proc 1990 (Mar);65:374–383.

57. Deedwania PC, Carbajal EV: Silent ischemia during daily life is an independent predictor of mortality in stable angina. Circulation 1990 (March);81:748–756.

58. Breitenbücher A, Pfisterer M, Hoffmann A, Burckhardt D: Long-term follow-up of patients with silent ischemia during exercise radionuclide angiography. J Am Coll Cardiol 1990 (April);15:999–1003.

59. Deedwania PC, Carbajal EV: Prevalence and patterns of silent myocardial ischemia during daily life in stable angina patients receiving conventional antianginal drug therapy. Am J Cardiol 1990 (May 1);65:1090–1096.

60. Hausmann D, Nikutta P, Trappe HJ, Daniel WG, Wenzlaff P, Lichtlen PR: Incidence of ventricular arrhythmias during transient myocardial ischemia in patients with stable coronary artery disease. J Am Coll Cardiol 1990 (July);16:49–54.

61. Wilcox I, Freedman B, Kelly DT, Harris PJ: Clinical significance of silent ischemia in unstable angina pectoris. Am J Cardiol 1990 (June 1);65:1313–1316.

62. Deedwania PC, Carbajal EV, Spears K: Exercise test predictors of ambulatory silent ischemia during daily life in stable angina pectoris. Am J Cardiol 1990 (Nov 15);66:1151–1156.

63. Stone PH, Gibson RS, Glasser SP, DeWood MA, Parker JD, Kawanishi DT, Crawford MH, Messineo FC, Shook TL, Raby K, Curtis DG, Hoop RS, Young PM, Braunwald E, and the SIS Study Group: Comparison of Propranolol, Diltiazem, and Nifedipine in the Treatment of Ambulatory Ischemia in Patients with Stable Angina. Circulation 1990 (December) 82:1962–1972.

64. Banai S, Moriel M, Benhorin J, Gavish A, Stern S, Tzivoni D: Changes in myocardial ischemic threshold during daily activities. Am J Cardiol 1990 (Dec 15);66:1403–1406.

65. Taki J, Yasuda T, Tamaki N, Flamm SD, Hutter A, Gold HK, Leinbach R, Strauss HW: Temporal relation between left ventricular dysfunction and chest pain in coronary artery disease during activities of daily living. Am J Cardiol 1990 (Dec 15);66:1455–1458.

66. Neglia D, Parodi O, Marzullo P, Sambuceti G, Marcassa C, Michelassi C, L'Abbate A: Behavior of right and left ventricles during episodes of variant angina in relation to the site of coronary vasospasm. Circulation 1990 (February);81:567–577.

67. Cannon RO III, Cattau EL Jr, Yakshe PN, Maher K, Schenke WH, Benjamin SB, Epstein SE: Coronary flow reserve, esophageal motility, and chest pain in patients with angiographically normal coronary arteries. Am J Med 1990 (Mar);88:217–22.

68. Spinelli L, Ferro G, Genovese A, Cinquegrana G, Spadafora M, Condorelli M: Exercise-induced impairment of diastolic time in patients with X syndrome. Am Heart J 1990 (April);119:829–833.

69. Geltman EM, Henes CG, Senneff MJ, Sobel BE, Bergmann SR: Increased myocardial perfusion at rest and diminished perfusion reserve in patients with angina and angiographically normal coronary arteries. J Am Coll Cardiol 1990 (September);16:586–95.

70. Pupita G, Kaski JC, Galassi AR, Gavrielides S, Crea F, Maseri A: Similar time course of ST depression during and after exercise in patients with coronary artery disease and syndrome X. Am Heart J 1990 (October);120:848–854.

71. Cannon RO, Peden DB, Berkebile C, Schenke WH, Kaliner MA, Epstein SE: Airway Hyperresponsiveness in Patients with Microvascular Angina. Circulation 1990 (December);82:2011–2017.

72. Todd IC, Ballantyne D: Antianginal efficacy of exercise training: a comparison with B blockade. Br Heart J 1990 (July);64:14–19.

73. Coster P, Chierchia S, Davies G, Hackett D, Fragasso G, Maseri A: Combined Effects of Nitrates on the Coronary and Peripheral Circulation in Exercise-Induced Ischemia. Circulation 1990 (June);81:1881–1886.

74. Seabra-Gomes R, Aleixo AM, Adao M, Machado FP, Mendes M, Bruges G, Palos JL: Comparison of the effects of a controlled-release formulation of isosorbide-5-mononitrate and conventional isosorbide dinitrate on exercise performance in men with stable angina pectoris. Am J Cardiol 1990 (June 1);65:1308–1312.

75. Beyerle A, Reiniger G, Rudolph W: Long-acting, marked antiischemic effect maintained unattenuated during long-term interval treatment with once-daily isosorbide-5-mononitrate in sustained-release form. Am J Cardiol 1990 (June 15);65:1434–1437.

76. Vlay SC, Olson LC: Nifedipine and isosorbide dinitrate alone and in combination for patients with chronic stable angina: A double-blind crossover study. Am Heart J 1990 (August);120:303–307.

77. Narahara KA: Double-blind comparison of once daily betaxolol versus propranolol four times daily in stable angina pectoris. Am J Cardiol 1990 (Mar 1);65:577–582.

78. Bortone A, Hess O, Gaglione A, Suter T, Nonogi H, Grimm J, Krayenbuehl H: Effect of Intravenous Propranolol on Coronary Vasomotion at Rest and During Dynamic Exercise in Patients with Coronary Artery Disease. Circulation 1990 (April);81:1225–1235.

79. Crea F, Pupita G, Galassi AR, El-Tamimi H, Kaski JC, Davies GJ, Maseri A: Effects of theophylline, atenolol and their combination on myocardial ischemia in stable angina pectoris. Am J Cardiol 1990 (Nov 15);66:1157–1162.

80. Weintraub WS, Jones EL, King SB III, Craver J, Douglas JS Jr, Guyton R, Liberman H, Morris D: Changing use of coronary angioplasty and coronary bypass surgery in the treatment of chronic coronary artery disease. Am J Cardiol 1990 (Jan 15);65:183–188.

81. Proudfit WL, Kramer JR, Goormastic M, Loop FD: Ten-year survival of patients with mild angina or myocardial infarction without angina: A comparison of medical and surgical treatment. Am Heart J 1990 (April);119:942–948.

82. Allen JK, Fitzgerald ST, Swank RT, Becker DM: Functional status after coronary artery bypass grafting and percutaneous transluminal coronary angioplasty. Am J Cardiol 1990 (Oct 15);65:921–925.

83. Rogers WJ, Coggin J, Gersh BJ, Fisher LD, Myers WO, Oberman A, Sheffield LT, for the CASS Investigators: Ten-Year Follow-up of Quality of Life in Patients Randomized to Receive Medical Therapy or Coronary Artery Bypass Graft Surgery. Circulation 1990 (November);82:1647–1658.

84. Roubin GS: Status of percutaneous transluminal coronary angioplasty. Current Problems in Cardiology 1990 (Dec).

85. Anderson HV, Talley JD, Black ARJ, Roubin GS, Douglas JS Jr, King SB III: Usefulness of coronary angioplasty in asymptomatic patients. Am J Cardiol 1990 (Jan 1);65:35–39.

86. Kohli RS, DiSciascio G, Cowley MJ, Nath A, Goudreau E, Vetrovec GW: Coronary angioplasty in patients with severe left ventricular dysfunction. J Am Coll Cardiol 1990 (October);16:807–11.

87. Kahn JK, Rutherford BD, McConahay DR, Johnson WL, Giorgi LV, Hartzler GO: Short- and long-term outcome of percutaneous transluminal coronary angioplasty in chronic dialysis patients. Am Heart J 1990 (March);119:484–489.

88. Finci L, Meier B, Favre J, Righetti A, Rutishauser W: Long-term results of successful and failed angioplasty for chronic total coronary arterial occlusion. Am J Cardiol 1990 (Sept 15);66:660–662.

89. Tuzcu EM, Nisanci Y, Simpfendorfer C, Dorosti K, Franco I, Hollman J, Whitlow P: Percutaneous transluminal coronary angioplasty in silent ischemia. Am Heart J 1990 (April);119:797–801.

90. Webb JG, Myler RK, Shaw RE, Anwar A, Stertzer SH: Coronary angioplasty in young adults: initial results and late outcome. J Am Coll Cardiol 1990 (December);16:1569–74.

91. Kelsey SF, Miller DP, Holubkov R, Lu AS, Cowley MJ, Faxon DP, Detre KM, Investigators from the NHLBI PTCA Registry: Results of percutaneous transluminal coronary angioplasty in patients ≥65 years of age (from the 1985 to 1986 national heart, lung, and blood institute's coronary angioplasty registry). Am J Cardiol 1990 (Nov 1);66:1033–1038.

92. Jeroudi MO, Kleiman NS, Minor ST, Hess KR, Lewis JM, Winters WL Jr, Raizner AE: Percutaneous transluminal coronary angioplasty in octogenarians. An Intern Med 1990 (Sept 15);113:423–428.

93. Webb JG, Myler RK, Shaw RE, Anwar A, Mayo JR, Murphy MC, Cumberland DC, Stertzer SH: Coronary angioplasty after coronary bypass surgery: Initial results and late outcome in 422 patients. J Am Coll Cardiol 1990 (October);16:812–20.

94. Tabbalat RA, Haft JI: Coronary angioplasty in symptomatic patients after bypass surgery. Am Heart J 1990 (November);120:1091–1096.

95. Kahn JK, Rutherford BD, McConahay DR, Giorgi LV, Johnson WL, Shimshak TM, Hartzler GO: Early postoperative balloon coronary angioplasty for failed coronary artery bypass grafting. Am J Cardiol 1990 (Oct 15);66:943–946.

96. Cameron DE, Stinson DC, Greene PS, Gardner TJ: Surgical standby for percutaneous transluminal coronary angioplasty: A survey of patterns of practice. Ann Thorac Surg 1990 (July);50:35–39.

97. Ullyot DJ: Surgical standby for coronary angioplasty. Ann Thorac Surg 1990 (July);50:3–4.

98. Lembo NJ, Black AJR, Roubin GS, Wilentz JR, Mufson LH, Douglas JS Jr, King SB III: Effect of pretreatment with aspirin versus aspirin plus dipyridamole on frequency and type of acute complications of percutaneous transluminal coronary angioplasty. Am J Cardiol 1990 (Feb 15);65:422–426.

99. Laskey MAL, Deutsch E, Hirshfeld JW, Kussmaul WG, Barnathan E, Laskey WK: Influence of heparin therapy on percutaneous transluminal coronary angioplasty outcome in patients with coronary arterial thrombus. Am J Cardiol 1990 (Jan 15);65:179–182.

100. Rath B, Bennett DH: Monitoring the effect of heparin by measurement of activated clotting time during and after percutaneous transluminal coronary angioplasty. Br Heart J 1990 (Jan);63:18–21.

101. Laskey MAL, Deutsch E, Barnathan E, Laskey WK: Influence of heparin therapy on percutaneous transluminal coronary angioplasty outcome in unstable angina pectoris. Am J Cardiol 1990 (June 15);65:1425–1429.

102. Mizutani M, Freedman SB, Barns E, Ogasawara S, Bailey BP, Bernstein L: ST monitoring for myocardial ischemia during and after coronary angioplasty. Am J Cardiol 1990 (Aug 15);66:389–393.

103. Deutsch E, Berger M, Kussmanul WG, Hirshfeld JW, Hermann HC, Laskey WK: Adaptation to Ischemia During Percutaneous Transluminal Coronary Angioplasty. Circulation 1990 (December);82:2044–2051.

104. DeServi S, Mazzone A, Ricevuti G, Fioravanti A, Bramucci E, Angoli L, Stefano G, Specchia G: Granulocyte Activation After Coronary Angioplasty in Humans. Circulation 1990 (July);82:140–146.

105. Johansson SR, Ekstrom L, Emanuelsson H: Buccal nitroglycerin decreases ischemic pain during coronary angioplasty: A double-blind, randomized, placebo-controlled study. Am Heart J 1990 (August);120:275–281.

106. Vogel RA, Shawl F, Tommaso C, O'Neill W, Overlie P, O'Toole J, Vandormael M, Topol E, Tabari KK, Vogel J, Smith S, Freedman R, White C, George B, Teirstein P: Initial report of the national registry on elective cardiopulmonary bypass supported coronary angioplasty. J Am Coll Cardiol 1990 (January);15:23–9.

107. Loisance D, Dubois-Rande JL, Deleuze PH, Okude J, Rosenval O, Geschwind H: Prophylactic intraventricular pumping in high-risk coronary angioplasty. Lancet 1990 (Feb 24);335:438–440.

108. Kent KM, Cleman MW, Cowley MJ, Forman MB, Jaffe CC, Kaplan M, King SB III, Krucoff MW, Lassar T, McAuley B, Smith R, Wisdom C, Wohlgelernter D: Reduction of myocardial ischemia during percutaneous transluminal coronary angioplasty with oxygenated Fluosol. Am J Cardiol 1990 (Aug 1);66:279–284.

109. Castello R, Pearson AC, Kern MJ, Labovitz AJ, with the technical assistance of Patricia Lenzen: Diastolic function in patients undergoing coronary angioplasty: Influence of degree of revascularization. J Am Coll Cardiol 1990 (June);15:1564–9.

110. Broderick T, Sawada S, Armstrong WF, Ryan T, Dillon JC, Bourdillon PDV, Feigenbaum H: Improvement in rest and exercise-induced wall motion abnormalities after coronary angioplasty: An exercise echocardiographic study. J Am Coll Cardiol 1990 (March);15:591–9.

111. van den Berg E, Popma J, Dehmer G, Snow F, Lewis S, Vetrovec G, Nixon J: Reversible Segmental Left Ventricular Dysfunction After Coronary Angioplasty. Circulation 1990 (April);81:120–1216.

112. Renkin J, Wijins W, Ladha Z, Col J: Reversal of Segmental Hypokinesis by Coronary Angioplasty in Patients with Unstable Angina, Persistent T Wave Inversion, and Left Anterior Descending Coronary Artery Stenosis Additional Evidence for Myocardial Stunning in Humans. Circulation 1990 (September);82:912–921.

113. Samson M, Meester HJ, De Feyter PJ, Strauss B, Serruys PW: Successful multiple segment coronary angioplasty: Effect of completeness of revascularization in single-vessel multilesions and multivessels. Am Heart J 1990 (July);120:1–12.

114. Bell MR, Bailey KR, Reeder GS, Lapeyre AC, Holmes DR: Percutaneous transluminal angioplasty in patients with multivessel coronary disease: How important is complete revascularization for cardiac event-free survival? J Am Coll Cardiol 1990 (September);16:553–62.

115. Shawl RA, Velasco CE, Goldbaum TS, Forman MB: Effect of coronary angioplasty on electrocardiographic changes in patients with unstable angina secondary to left anterior descending coronary artery disease. J Am Coll Cardiol 1990 (August);16:325–31.

116. Webb JG, Myler RK, Shaw RE, Anwar A, Murphy MC, Mooney JF, Mooney MR, Stertzer SH: Bidirectional crossover and late outcome after coronary angioplasty and bypass surgery: 8 to 11 year follow-up. J Am Coll Cardiol 1990 (July);16:57–65.

117. O'Keefe JH Jr, Rutherford BD, McConahay DR, Johnson WL Jr, Giorgi LV, Ligon RW, Shimshak TM, Hartzler GO: Multivessel coronary angioplasty from 1980 to 1989: Procedural results and long-term outcome. J Am Coll Cardiol 1990 (November);16:1097–102.

118. Stark KS, Satler LF, Krucoff MW, Rackley CE, Kent KM: Myocardial salvage after failed coronary angioplasty. J Am Coll Cardiol 1990 (January);15:78–82.

119. Richardson SG, Morton P, Murtagh JG, O'Keeffe DB, Murphy P, Scott ME: Management of acute coronary occlusion during percutaneous transluminal coronary angioplasty: experience of complications in a hospital without on site facilities for cardiac surgery. Br Med J 1990 (Feb 10);300:355–358.

120. Tuzcu M, Simpfendorfer C, Dorosti K, Franco I, Golding L, Hollman J, Whitlow P: Long-term outcome of unsuccessful percutaneous transluminal coronary angioplasty. Am Heart J 1990 (April);119:791–796.

121. Detre MK, Holmes DR, Holubkov R, Cowley MJ, Bourassa MG, Faxon DP, Dorros GR, Bentivoglio LG, Kent KM, Myler RK, and coinvestigators of the National Heart, Lung and Blood Institute's Percutaneous Transluminal Coronary Angioplasty Registry: Incidence and Consequences of Periprocedural Occlusion The 1985–1986 National Heart, Lung, and Blood Institute Percutaneous Transluminal Coronary Angioplasty Registry. Circulation 1990 (September);82:739–750.

122. Gulba DC, Daniel WG, Simon R, Jost S, Barthels M, Amende I, Rafflenbeul W, Lichtlen PR: Role of thrombolysis and thrombin in patients with acute coronary occlusion during percutaneous transluminal coronary angioplasty. J Am Coll Cardiol 1990 (September);16:563–8.

123. Talley JD, Weintraub WS, Roubin GS, Douglas JS, Anderson V, Jones EL, Morris DC, Liberman HA, Craver JM, Guyton RA, King SB: Failed Elective Percutaneous Transluminal Coronary Angioplasty Requiring Coronary Artery Bypass Surgery In-Hospital and Late Clinical Outcome at 5 Years. Circulation 1990 (October);1203–1213.

124. Bengtson JR, Mark DB, Honan MB, Rendall DS, Hinohara T, Stack RS, Hlatky MA, Califf RM, Lee KL, Pryor DB: Detection of restenosis after elective percutaneous transluminal coronary angioplasty using the exercise treadmill test. Am J Cardiol 1990 (Jan 1);65:28–34.

125. El-Tamimi H, Davies GJ, Hackett D, Fragasso G, Crea F, Maseri A, O'Sullivan C: Very early prediction of restenosis after successful coronary angioplasty: anatomic and functional assessment. J Am Coll Cardiol 1990 (February);15:259–64.

126. Schwartz L, Lesperance J, Bourassa MG, Eastwood C, Kazim F, Arafah M, Ganassin L: The role of antiplatelet agents in modifying the extent of restenosis following percutaneous transluminal coronary angioplasty. Am Heart J 1990 (February);119:232–236.

127. Benchimol D, Benchimol H, Bonnet J, Dartigues JF, Couffinhal T, Bricaud H: Risk factors for progression of atherosclerosis six months after balloon angioplasty of coronary stenosis. Am J Cardiol 1990 (Apr 15);65:980–985.

128. Pepine C, Hirshfeld J, Macdonald R, Henderson M, Bass T, Goldberg S, Savage M, Vetrovec G, Cowley M, Taussig A, Whitworth H, Margolis J, Hill J, Bove A, Jugo R: A controlled Trial of Corticosteroids to Prevent Restenosis After Coronary Angioplasty. Circulation 1990 (June);81:1753–1761.

129. Hardoff R, Shefer A, Gips S, Merdler A, Flugelman MY, Halon DA, Lewis BS: Predicting late restenosis after coronary angioplasty by very early (12 to 24 h) thallium-201 scintigraphy: Implications with regard to mechanisms of late coronary restenosis. J Am Coll Cardiol 1990 (June);15:1486–92.

130. Laarman G, Luijten HE, van Zeyl LGPM, Beatt KJ, Tijssen JGP, Serruys PW, de Feyter PJ: Assessment of "silent" restenosis and long-term follow-up after successful angioplasty in single vessel coronary artery disease: The value of quantitative exercise electrocardiography and quantitative coronary angiography. J Am Coll Cardiol 1990 (September);16:578–85.

131. MacDonald RG, Henderson MA, Hirschfeld JW Jr, Goldberg SH, Bass T, Vetrovec G, Cowley M, Taussig A, Whitworth H, Margolis JR, Hill JA, Jugo R, Pepine CJ, M-Heart Group: Patient-related variables and restenosis after percutaneous transluminal coronary angioplasty: a report from the M-Heart Group. Am J Cardiol 1990 (Oct 15);66:926–931.

132. Hecht HS, Shaw RE, Bruce TR, Ryan C, Stertzer SH, Myler RK: Usefulness of tomographic thallium-201 imaging for detection of restenosis after percutaneous transluminal coronary angioplasty. Am J Cardiol 1990 (Dec 1);66:1314–1318.

133. Urschel HC Jr, Razzuk MA, Miller E,, Chung SY: Operative transluminal balloon angioplasty: Adjunct to coronary bypass for extended myocardial revascularization of more than 3000 lesions in 1000 patients. J Thorac Cardiovasc Surg 1990 (Apr);99:581–589.

134. Kaufmann UP, Garratt KN, Vlietstra RE, Holmes DR Jr: Transluminal atherectomy of saphenous vein aortocoronary bypass grafts. Am J Cardiol 1990 (June 15);65:1430–1433.

135. Rowe MH, Hinohara T, White NW, Robertson GC, Selmon MR, Simpson JB: Comparison of dissection rates and angiographic results following directional coronary atherectomy and coronary angioplasty. Am J Cardiol 1990 (July 1);66:49–53.

136. Muller DWM, Ellis SG, Debowey DL, Topol EJ: Quantitative angiographic comparison of the immediate success of coronary angioplasty, coronary atherectomy and endoluminal stenting. Am J Cardiol 1990 (Oct 15);66:938–942.

137. Garratt KN, Holmes DR Jr., Bell MR, Bresnahan JF, Kaufmann UP, Vlietstra RE, Edwards WD: Restenosis after directional coronary atherectomy: Differences between primary atheromatous and restenosis lesions and influence of subintimal tissue resection. J Am Coll Cardiol 1990 (December);16:1665–71.

138. Karsch K, Haase K, Voelker W, Baumbach A, Mauser M, Seipel L: Percutaneous Coronary Excimer Laser Angioplasty in Patients with Stable and Unstable Angina Pectoris Acute Results and Incidence of Restenosis During 6-Month Follow-up. Circulation 1990 (June);18:49–1859.

139. Litvack F, Eigler NL, Margolis JR, Grundfest WS, Rothbaum D, Linnemeier T, Hestrin LB, Tsoi D, Cook SL, Krauthamer D, Goldenberg T, Laudenslager JR, Segalowitz J, Forrester JS: Percutaneous excimer laser coronary angioplasty. Am J Cardiol 1990 (Nov 1);66:1027–1032.

140. Siegel RJ, DonMichael TA, Fishbein MC, Bookstein J, Adler L, Reinsvold T, DeCastro E, Forrester JS: In vivo ultrasound arterial recanalization of atherosclerotic total occlusions. J Am Coll Cardiol 1990 (February);15:345–51.

141. Alderman EL, Bourassa MG, Cohen LS, Davis KB, Kaiser GG, Killip T, Mock MB, Pettinger M, Robertson TL: Ten-Year Follow-up of Survival and Myocardial Infarction in the Randomized Coronary Artery Surgery Study. Circulation 1990 (November);82:1629–1645.

142. Naylor CD, Baigrie RS, Goldman BS, Basinski A: Assessment of priority for coronary revascularization procedures. Lancet 1990 (May 5);335:1070–1073.

143. Kahn SS, Nessim S, Gray R, Czer LS, Chaux A, Matloff: Increased mortality of women in coronary artery bypass surgery: Evidence for referral bias. An Intern Med 1990 (Apr 15);112:561–567.

144. Azariades M, Fessler CL, Floten HS, Starr A: Five-year results of coronary bypass grafting for patients older than 70 years: Role of internal mammary artery. Ann Thorac Surg 1990 (Dec);50:940–945.

145. Gardner TJ, Greene PS, Rykiel MF, Baumgartner WA, Cameron DE, Casale AS, Gott VL, Watkins L, Reitz BA: Routine use of the left internal mammary artery graft in the elderly. Ann Thorac Surg 1990 (Feb);49:188–194.

146. Fiore AC, Naunheim KS, Dean P, Kaiser GC, Pennington G, Willman VL, McBride LR, Barner HB: Results of internal thoracic artery grafting over 15 years: Single versus double grafts. Ann Thorac Surg 1990 (Feb);49:202–209.

147. Kouchoukos NT, Wareing TH, Murphy SF, Pelate C, Marshall WB Jr: Risks of bilateral internal mammary artery bypass grafting. Ann Thorac Surg 1990 (Feb);49:210–219.

148. Sommerhaug RG, Wolfe SF, Reid DA, Lindsey DE: Early clinical results of long coronary arteriotomy, endarterectomy and reconstruction combined with multiple bypass grafting for severe coronary artery disease. Am J Cardiol 1990 (Sept 15);66:651–659.

149. Kahn JK, Rutherford BD, McConahay DR, Johnson WL, Giorgi LV, Shimshak TM, Hartzler GO: Outcome following emergency coronary artery bypass grafting for failed elective balloon coronary angioplasty in patients with prior coronary bypass. Am J Cardiol 1990 (Aug 1);66:285–288.

150. Sethi GK, Copeland JG, Goldman S, Moritz T, Zadina K, Henderson WG, and participants in the Department of Veterans Affairs Cooperative Study on Antiplatelet Therapy: Implications of preoperative administration of aspirin in patients undergoing coronary artery bypass grafting. J Am Coll Cardiol 1990 (January);15:15–20.

151. Gavaghan TP, Hickie JB, Krilis SA, Baron DW, Gebski V, Low J, Chesterman CN: Increased plasma beta-thromboglobulin in patients with coronary artery vein graft occlusion: Response to low dose aspirin. J Am Coll Cardiol 1990 (May);15:1250–8.

152. Sanz G, Pajaron A, Alegria E, Coello I, Cardona M, Fournier JA, Gomez-Recio M, Ruano J, Hidalgo R, Medina A, Oller G, Colman T, Malpartida F, Bosch X, and the Grupo Espano para el Seguimiento del Injerto Coronario (GESIC): Prevention of Early Aortocoronary Bypass Occlusion by Low-Dose Aspirin and Dipyridamole. Circulation 1990 (September);82:765–773.

153. Taggart DP, Siddiqui A, Wheatley DJ: Low-dose preoperative aspirin therapy, post-operative blood loss, and transfusion requirements. Ann Thorac Surg 1990 (Sept);50:425–428.

154. Leitch JW, Thomson D, Baird DK, Harris PJ: The importance of age as a predictor of atrial fibrillation and flutter after coronary artery bypass grafting. J Thorac Cardiovasc Surg 1990 (Sept);100:338–342.

155. Force T, Hibberd P, Weeks G, Kemper AJ, Bloomfield P, Tow D, Josa M, Khuri S, Parisi A: Perioperative Myocardial Infarction After Coronary Artery Bypass Surgery Clinical Significance and Approach to Risk Stratification. Circulation 1990 (September);82:903–912.

156. Kennedy HL, Seiler SM, Sprague MK, Homan SM, Whitlock JA, Kern MJ, Vandormael MG, Barner HB, Codd JE, Willman VL, Lyyski D: Relation of silent myocardial ischemia after coronary artery bypass grafting to angiographic completeness of revascularization and long-term prognosis. Am J Cardiol 1990 (Jan 1);65:14–22.

157. Salomon NW, Page US, Bigelow JC, Krause AH, Okies JE, Metzdorff MT: Reoperative coronary surgery: Comparative analysis of 6591 patients undergoing primary bypass and 508 patients undergoing reoperative coronary artery bypass. J Thorac Cardiovasc Surg 1990 (Aug);100:250–260.

158. Owen EW Jr, Schoettle GP Jr, Marotti AS, Harrington OB: The third time coronary artery bypass graft: Is the risk justified? J Thorac Cardiovasc Surg 1990 (July);100:31–5.

159. Balkeman BP, Thomas NJ, Sullivan HJ, Foy BK, Pifarre R: Myocardial revascularization for the third time: Clinical characteristics and follow-up. Chest 1990 (Nov);98:1099–1101.

160. Loop FD, Lytle BW, Cosgrove DM, Mahfood S, McHenry MC, Goormastic M, Stewart RW, Golding LAR, Taylor PC: Sternal wound complications after isolated coronary artery bypass grafting: Early and late mortality, morbidity, and cost of care. Ann Thorac Surg 1990 (Feb);49:179–187.

161. Kalan JM, Roberts WC: Morphologic findings in saphenous veins used as coronary arterial bypass conduits for longer than 1 year: Necropsy analysis of 53 patients, 123 saphenous veins, and 1865 five-millimeter segments of veins. Am Heart J 1990 (May);119:1164–1184.

162. Lichtlen PR, Hugenholtz PG, Rafflenbeul W, Hecker H, Jost S, Deckers JW: Retardation of angiographic progression of coronary artery disease by nifedipine. Lancet 1990 (May 12);335:1109–1113.

163. Waters D, Lesperance J, Francetich M, Causey D, Theroux P, Chiang Y-K, Hudon G, Lemarbe L, Reitman M, Joyal M, Gosselin G, Dyrda I, Macer J, Havel RJ: A controlled Clinical Trial to Assess the Effect of a Calcium Channel Blocker on the Progression of Coronary Atherosclerosis. Circulation 1990 (December);82:1940–1953.

Acute Myocardial Infarction and Its Consequences

Onset triggers

Recent documentation of a circadian variation in AMI suggests that AMI is not a random event, but may frequently result from identifiable triggering activities. Tofler and associates[1] of the MILIS Study Group analyzed the possible triggers reported by 849 patients enrolled in the Multicenter Investigation of Limitation of Infarct Size. Possible triggers were identified by 48.5% of the population; the most common were emotional upset (18.4%) and moderate physical activity (14.1%) (Figure 3-1). Multiple possible triggers were reported by 13% of the population. Younger patients, men and those without diabetes mellitus were more likely to report a possible trigger than were older patients, women and those with diabetes. The likelihood of reporting a trigger was not affected by infarct size. This study suggests that potentially identifiable triggers may play an important role in AMI.

Circadian variation

Kleiman and the Diltiazem Reinfarction Study Investigators[2] from Houston, Texas, obtained data concerning the time of onset of AMI for 540 of the 544 patients with creatinine kinase MB-confirmed non-Q wave AMI enrolled in the multicenter Diltiazem Reinfarction Study. Data were also collected for 627 patients who were screened but excluded. Among the 1167 patients, no diuranal pattern of onset could be found at either 2 or 6 hour intervals. Among the 540 patients enrolled in the trial, no pattern could be found at these intervals either, although at 8-hour in-

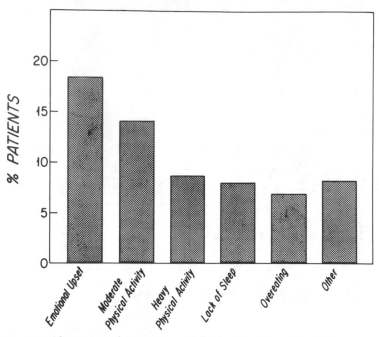

Fig. 3-1. Possible triggers of acute myocardial infarction. A possible trigger was reported by 412 of 849 patients (48.5%); 109 patients (13%) reported 2 or more possible triggers. Reproduced with permission from Tofler, et al.[1]

tervals, 27% of infarctions occurred between midnight and 8 A.M., compared with 37% between 8 A.M. and 4 P.M. and 36% between 4 P.M. and 12 A.M. In contrast to the patterns previously noted for Q wave AMI, there was no preponderance on non-Q wave AMI in the late morning. Circadian rhythm was also absent among patients not treated with beta blockers and among patients presenting with ST segment elevation on their enrollment electrocardiograms. Diabetics, women, and patients with first AMI were more likely to present during the afternoon hours. The study concluded that the late morning preponderance seen for Q-wave AMI is not discernable in patients with non-Q wave AMI. This observation suggests that the pathogenesis of these two infarct subtypes is different or that the process of thrombotic coronary occlusion in Q wave AMI differs from that in non-Q wave AMI.

Several studies have observed an increased occurrence of AMI in the morning based on subject self-reports and objective confirmation. Evidence has also been collected to suggest a circadian variation in the onset of sudden coronary death and silent myocardial ischeamia. No published reports have examined the time of onset of AMI in relation to time after wakening. Goldberg and associates[3] from Worcester, Massachusetts, examined the times of onset of AMI in relation to awakening in 137 patients with confirmed AMI (Figures 3-2 and 3-3).

Increased platelet aggregation in the morning and upon assuming an upright posture may account at least in part for the observed circadian variation in onset of AMI. The Physicians' Health Study, a randomized double-blind, placebo-controlled trial of alternate-day aspirin intake of 325 mg among 22,071 U.S. male physicians, offered Ridker and colleagues[4] in Boston, Massachusetts, the opportunity to assess this circadian pattern and examine whether it is altered by aspirin therapy. During a 5-year

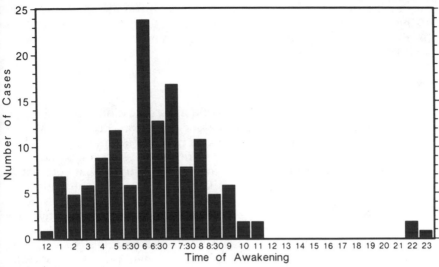

Fig. 3-2. Distribution of time of awakening on day of initial symptoms of acute myocardial infarction. Reproduced with permission from Goldberg, et al.[3,40]

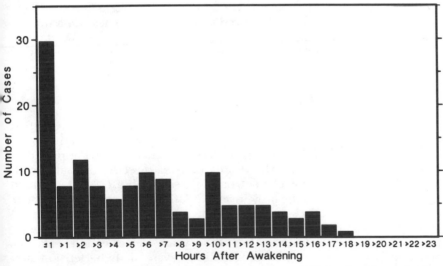

Fig. 3-3. Time of onset of initial symptoms of acute myocardial infarction after awakening. Reproduced with permission from Goldberg, et al.[3,40]

period of follow-up, 342 cases of nonfatal AMI were confirmed of which time of onset was available in 211. The placebo group showed a bimodal circadian variation in onset of AMI with a primary peak between 4:00 A.M. and 10:00 A.M. In the aspirin group, however, this circadian variation was minimal due primarily to a marked reduction in the morning peak of AMI. Specifically aspirin was associated with a 59% reduction in the incidence of AMI during morning waking hours, compared with 34% reduction for the remaining hours of the day. The greater reduction was observed during the 3-hour interval immediately after awakening, a period with a risk of AMI twice that of any other comparable time interval. Aspirin intake was associated with a mean reduction in the incidence of AMI of 45% over the entire 24-hour cycle. These data support the hypothesis that increased platelet aggregability in the morning and upon arising contributes to the occurrence of AMI and that aspirin reduces the risk of AMI by inhibiting platelet aggregation during these critical periods.

Frequency after discontinuing smoking

To assess the relation of cigarette smoking cessation to the risk of a first AMI in women, Rosenberg and associates[5] from Brookline, Massachusetts, compared the cigarette smoking habits of 910 patients who had had their first AMI with those of 2,375 controls in a hospital-based case-controlled study of women aged 25 to 64 years. The estimate of relative risk among current smokers as compared with women who had never smoked was 3.6. Among exsmokers overall, the corresponding estimate of relative risk was 1.2. Among exsmokers, the estimate of relative risk was significantly elevated among women who had stopped smoking <2 years previously. Most of the increase in the risk had dissipated among the women who had stopped smoking 2 to 3 years previously, and the estimate of relative risk among the women who had not smoked for 3 or more years was virtually indistinguishable from that among the women who had never smoked. The same pattern of decline was apparent regardless of the amount smoked, the duration of smoking, the age of the women, or the presence of other predisposing factors. These data suggest that in women, as in men, the increase in the risk of a first AMI among cigarette smokers declines soon after the cessation of smoking and is largely dissipated after 2 or 3 years.

Association with certain foods

Gramenzi and associates[6] from Milan, Italy, examined the relation between selected foods and AMI in 287 women who had had an AMI and in 649 controls with acute disorders unrelated to CAD admitted to hospital during 1983–1989. The risk of AMI was directly associated with frequency of consumption of meat, ham and salami, butter, total fat added to food, and coffee. Significantly inverse relations were observed for fish, carrots, green vegetables, and fresh fruit. The risk was below 1 for moderate alcohol consumption and above 1 for heavier intake. Allowance for major non-dietary covariants including years of education, cigarette smoking, hyperlipidemia, diabetes mellitus, systemic hypertension, and body mass index, did not appreciably alter the estimates of risk for most of the foods; for coffee, however, the odds ratio fell to 1.8 on account of its high correlation with cigarette smoking.

Progression from non-Q to Q-wave infarction

Kleiger and associates[7] for the Diltiazem Reinfarction Study Group analyzed serial 12-lead electrocardiogram and plasma creatine kinase (CK)-MB values from 544 patients with confirmed non-Q-wave AMI to define the rate of progression of non-Q-wave AMI to Q-wave AMI and to examine its relation to CK-MB evidence of extension. The baseline electrocardiogram was obtained 50 ± 10 hours after AMI and compared with subsequent electrocardiograms at 48 and 72 hours after baseline record and at discharge. Plasma CK-MB was assayed every 12 hours after baseline. A total of 76 patients (14%) progressed to Q-wave AMI. Compared to the 468 patients who retained non-Q-wave AMI, those patients who evolved Q-wave AMI were more likely to exhibit ST elevation 1.0 mm in 2 infarct-related leads (49 vs 32%), higher peak CK values with the index AMI (754 ± 625 vs 611 ± 604 IU) and a greater incidence of CK-MB-confirmed extensions (18.5 vs 5.5%). For those patients progressing to Q-wave AMI within 48 hours of baseline electrocardiogram, CK-MB extension occurred in 9.5% (4 of 42) versus 29.4% (10 of 34) of those who progressed after 48 hours. A distinct minority (14%) of patients with non-Q-wave AMI will develop Q waves before discharge. The progression to Q-wave AMI after initial non-Q-wave AMI appears to involve 2 different mechanisms: temporal lag in the electrocardiogram, and actual extension by quantitative CK-MB criteria.

Association with sleep apnea

Hung and associates[8] from Nedlands, Australia, examined the hypothesis that sleep apnea is a risk factor for CAD by performing overnight polysomnography in 101 unselected male survivors of AMI aged <66 years and in 53 male subjects of similar age without evidence of CAD. The apnea index (number of apnea episodes per hour of sleep) was 6.9 in the AMI patients vs 1.4 in the control subjects. After adjustment for age, body mass index, systemic hypertension, smoking, and cholesterol level, multiple logistic regression analysis identified the top quartile of apnea index (>5.3) as an independent predictor of AMI patients. The relative risk for AMI between the highest and lowest quartiles was 23.

After cocaine use

Amin and associates[9] from Bronx, New York, retrospectively evaluated 70 patients hospitalized with chest pain after cocaine use to define the risk and clinical course of AMI. AMI developed in 22 patients (31%) and transient myocardial ischemia was seen in an additional 9 patients (13%). Coronary risk factors did not distinguish those who developed AMI from those who did not. The presenting electrocardiogram was abnormal in 20 of 22 patients who evolved AMI and in 19 of 48 of those who did not. Creatine kinase levels were elevated in 75% of the patients, including 65% of those who did not develop AMI, but creatine kinase-MB elevations were only observed in the AMI group. The route of cocaine administration did not predict AMI and there was no predilection for a particular coronary vascular bed. The length of time between drug use and onset of AMI pain was often quite prolonged (median interval, 18 vs 1 hour in the non-AMI group). Eight patients with AMI underwent cardiac catheterization and 4 had significant CAD.

Late after coronary bypass

Although AMI is usually due to thrombotic occlusion when involving a native coronary artery, the mechanism responsible for AMI in patients with previous CABG is not well understood. Grines and associates[10] from Lexington, Kentucky, reviewed angiograms obtained between 1 hour and 7 days of AMI (median 1 day) in 50 patients >1 year after CABG. The culprit artery was identified by the presence of residual stenosis and/or thrombus in the artery supplying the infarct zone or by reviewing previous angiograms. The infarct artery was identified as a vein graft in 38 (76%) patients, the native vessel in 8 patients (16%) and could not be accurately determined in 4 patients (8%). Among the 38 vein grafts suspected as the infarct artery, unequivocal angiographic evidence of residual thrombus (filling defect/persistent staining) was present in 31 (82%) and was >2 cm in length in 15 patients. Successful reperfusion occurred in only 2 of 8 (25%) grafts after intravenous thrombolytic therapy. Intragraft thrombolysis with or without additional angioplasty was successful at restoring flow in 8 of 10 (80%) grafts. Data indicate that in patients who have undergone previous CABG, AMI is usually caused by thrombotic occlusion of a saphenous vein graft and that conventional intravenous thrombolytic therapy may be inadequate to restore flow. The large mass of thrombus and absent flow in the graft may require subselective drug infusion, a higher thrombolytic dose or a mechanical means of recanalization.

Angiographic progression afterwards

Bissett and associates[11] of the Program on the Surgical Control of Hyperlipidemia (POSCH) assessed the progression of coronary artery stenosis to total occlusion in 413 hyperlipidemic patients with a previous AMI. Coronary angiograms were recorded at baseline, 3 (n = 312), and 5 years (n = 248) after initial study and analyzed by 2 independent readers. There were 177 (43%) patients with 1-, 130 (31%) with 2-, and 61 (15%) with 3-vessel disease (≥50% diameter narrowing), whereas 45 (11%) did not have significant disease within a major coronary vessel at baseline. A new finding of total occlusion occurred in 4% (30 of 748) and 7% (40 of 605) of major coronary artery segments at 3 and 5 years, respectively. The risk of progression to total occlusion was higher if the initial stenosis was >60% compared to narrowings ≤60% both at 3 years (19 of 143 = 13% vs 11 of 605 = 2%) and 5 years (27 of 91 = 30% vs 13 of 514 = 3%). The frequency of occlusion was highest for the right coronary artery by 5 years (18 of 167 = 11 percent for right vs 8 of 225 = 4% for LC vs 14 of 213 = 7% for LAD coronary arteries). Clinical and laboratory data revealed that AMI was associated with a new total occlusion in 23% of patients (7 of 30) at 3 years and in 64% (25 of 39) at 5 years. Serum cholesterol and triglyceride levels were significantly higher in patients with a new finding of total occlusion at 5 years. This prospective serial angiographic study showed that the extent of initial coronary artery narrowing was significantly associated with the risk of progression to total occlusion.

DIAGNOSIS AND EARLY TESTING

Assay of subforms of creatine kinase-MB

Thrombolytic therapy for patients with AMI has produced the need for an accurate early diagnostic marker. Puleo and co-workers[12] in Houston, Texas, had previously developed and evaluated an assay for the creatine kinase in the subforms; assay time is 25 minutes. Plasma MB2 (tissue subform) activity, MB1 (plasma-modified subform) activity, and MB2/MB1 ratio in 56 healthy patients were 0.61 units/1, 0.63 units/1, and 0.94, respectively. Only one individual had both an MB2 activity >1.0 units/1 and an MB2/MB1 ratio of >1.5. Similar results were obtained in 50 hospitalized patients without cardiac disease; 2 of these patients had both an MB2 activity and an MB2/MB1 ratio greater than the cutoff values.

Among 49 patients with AMI, MB2 activity and the MB2/MB1 ratio began to increase 2 hours after AMIs; the ratio reached a plateau of 3.1 by 4–6 hours. The first available plasma sample was abnormal by the subform assay in 67% of patients and by a conventional MB assay in 27% of patients. Assay sensitivities in samples collected at 2–4, 4–6, and 6–8 hours after AMI were 59%, 92%, and 100% for the subform assay and 23%, 50%, and 71% for the conventional assay. False-negative results were obtained by the subform and conventional assays in 15 and 45 samples at a mean of 2.3 and 5.8 hours, respectively. Subform assay provides rapid and reliable diagnosis of AMI within 4–6 hours after the onset of symptoms, which is 6 hours before conventional CK-MB assays are accurate.

Neurohumoral profiles

Neurohumoral activation is readily apparent in patients with symptomatic CHF and in the acute phase of AMI. Vaughan and associates[13] from Boston, Massachusetts, examined the neurohumoral profiles of 36 asymptomatic patients in the early convalescent phase after AMI. All patients in the study had a radionuclide EF ≤45% and underwent cardiac catheterization 11 to 30 days after infarction. Venous blood samples were obtained in the supine state for the measurement of norepinephrine, angiotensin II, plasma renin activity and aldosterone in all patients. Despite the reduced EF and extensive wall motion abnormalities, plasma norepinephrine was not elevated and did not correlate with any measured hemodynamic, angiographic or clinical variables. The renin-angiotensin II aldosterone system was activated, as expected, in the 9 study patients receiving loop diuretics. However, even in the 27 patients not taking diuretics, plasma angiotensin II and renin activity levels were increased in relation to Killip classification, the presence of a LV aneurysm and LVEF. Activation of the renin-angiotensin-aldosterone system can be identified in hemodynamically compensated postinfarction patients not taking diuretics and appears to be related to the extent of LV dysfunction.

Serum myoglobin

Ohman and associates[14] from Dublin, Ireland, and Durham, North Carolina, evaluated the value of the 12 lead electrocardiogram, serum total creatine kinase, creatine kinase MB isoenzyme, and myoglobin for the early detection of AMI within 1 hour of admission to the coronary care unit in 82 consecutive patients with suspected AMI. The 51 patients in whom AMI was diagnosed during the first 24 hours after admission had a higher prevalence of ST elevation (64% vs 11%), higher median serum myoglobin (136 µg/l vs 34 µg/l), higher serum creatine kinase (77 IU/l vs 34 IU/l), and higher MB isoenzyme (7 IU/l vs 4 IU/l) than those in whom it was not. Stepwise logistic regression analysis in 70 patients in whom the electrocardiogram and serum myoglobin were suitable for analysis showed that serum myoglobin was the variable most closely associated with infarction, and contributed additional diagnostic information when ST elevation was entered into the model first. Serum myoglobin remained associated with AMI when patients who had had symptoms for <6 hours were analyzed. An algorithm based on a rapid agglutination test for myoglobin and ST elevation on the electrocardiogram gave an accurate diagnosis in 82% of patients. This approach gave early and rapid recognition of AMI.

Serum myosin heavy chain fragments

To evaluate the correlation between myosin heavy chain release and the necrosis mass, serum levels of myosin heavy chain fragments were determined serially in 55 patients with AMI in a study by Leger and colleagues[15] from Montpellier, Grenoble, and Lyon, France, and Brussels, Belgium. Eight patients were successfully treated with thrombolytic agents; the others were not treated. The same myosin titration was applied to the sera of 25 dogs with an experimental AMI. Six of the dogs were successfully treated with thrombolytic agents. The time courses of the myosin concentrations are typical and monophasic for all patients with a noncomplex AMI. The values for the kinetic parameters of myosin release are comparable to those previously reported. It was determined that cumulative myosin release significantly correlates with cumulative creatine kinase, creatine kinase-MB, and lactate dehydrogenase release, as well as with thallium-201 distribution, as determined for different patient groups. Thrombolytic treatment does not seem to qualitatively upset myosin kinetics. The results obtained in dogs with or without thrombolysis conclusively indicate that myosin release is a quantitative index of the necrosis mass. A few serial determinations of serum levels of myosin heavy chains are enough to estimate the necrotic mass in patients with AMI. More generally, serum myosin titration could be useful in detecting any cardiac disturbance involving myocardial injury resulting in membrane leakage of cardiac cells.

Atrial natriuretic factor

Fontana and associates[16] from Bologna, Italy, determined plasma atrial natriuretic factor (ANF), plasma renin activity (PRA), aldosterone and antidiuretic hormone (ADH) in 16 patients with uncomplicated AMI for 7 days in all patients and in 6 patients for 8 more days. Echocardiograms were performed and central venous pressure was measured on the 2nd, 7th, and 15th days. On admission, plasma ANF was higher in patients with AMI (130 $\pm$ 71 pg ml^{-1}) than in healthy volunteers (51 $\pm$ 10 pg ml^{-1}). Arterial pressure, heart rate, BP, and central venous pressure were normal. LA and LV diameters were increased in 6 patients. EF was reduced in all. A significant inverse relation between ANF and EF was observed. Patients with EF $\leq$45%, high LA and LV dimensions had the highest plasma ANF and showed steady high plasma ANF for 15 days. Patients with EF >45% had normal LA and LV dimensions and elevated ANF levels for 10 days. PRA and ADH values were normal throughout the study. These findings suggest that the reduction in myocardial contractility induced by AMI may account for the rise in ANF secretion via increased LA pressure and LA dilatation.

Use of pulmonary arterial catheters

Zion and associates[17] from the SPRINT Coordinating Center in Tel Hashomer, Israel, analyzed the use of PA catheters in a registry comprising 5,841 hospitalized patients with AMI. A total of 371 patients received a PA catheter. In-hospital mortality was higher in patients with CHF who received a PA catheter where there was no difference in patients with cardiogenic shock or persistent hypotension. Mortality in patients receiving a PA catheter was higher irrespective of the presence or absence of pump failure. A separate analysis of discharge summaries of 364 patients with CHF showed that PA catheters were used more frequently in sicker patients and that when severity of CHF was assessed, no difference in mortality was found in patients with mild or moderate CHF. The authors concluded that while a higher in-hospital mortality was found in patients receiving PA catheters, this excess is likely related to difference in severity of CHF, which has not been assessed in every individual.

This article was followed by an editorial entitled, "Does Pulmonary Artery Catheterization Benefit Patients With Acute Myocardial Infarction?" by James E. Dalen [18] from Tucson, Arizona. Dalen concluded because of potential complications of PA catheterization and its cost that it is still necessary to determine if this procedure is of benefit to patients with AMI. As with other procedures and therapies, Dalen emphasized that the question can only be answered by performing appropriately designed controlled clinical trials even though they may be very difficult.

Ambulatory electrocardiographic monitoring

Ouyang and associates[19] from Baltimore, Maryland, studied the incidence and clinical significance of silent myocardial ischemia occurring in the early period after AMI in 59 patients who had an uncomplicated early course after admission for AMI. Calibrated 2-lead ambulatory electrocardiographic monitoring performed for 39 $\pm$ 2 hours starting 4 $\pm$ 1 days after AMI identified silent myocardial ischemia, defined as $\geq$1 mm ST-segment change lasting $\geq$2 minutes, in 27 patients. These patients had 5 $\pm$ 1 episodes lasting a median of 11 minutes/episode (range 2 to 36 minutes/episode). Patients with and without silent ischemia had comparable baseline demographics, were receiving similar antischemic medications and had similar severity of coronary disease by angiography. No reinfarctions occurred during the in-hospital period. Fourteen of 27 patients (52%) with silent ischemia had $\geq$1 in-hospital clinical ischemic event (pulmonary edema, n = 5, cardiac death, n = 1, and postinfarction angina, n = 11). In contrast, only 7 of 32 patients without silent ischemia (22%) had 1 in-hospital event (pulmonary edema, n = 1, cardiac death, n = 1, and postinfarction angina, n = 6). The frequency of ischemic events was significantly greater in patients with silent ischemia compared to those without silent ischemia. Silent ischemia occurs frequently very early after AMI and identifies a group of patients who are at increased risk for adverse in-hospital clinical outcomes.

Currie and Saltissi[20] from Liverpool, UK, studied the prevalence and characteristics of transient myocardial ischemia in 203 patients with recent AMI by both early (6 days) and late (38 days) ambulatory monitoring of the ST segment. Transient ST segment depression was much commoner during late (32% patients) than early (14%) monitoring. Most transient ischemia (>85% episodes) was silent and 80% of patients had only silent episodes. During late monitoring painful ST depression was accompanied by greater ST depression and tended to occur at a higher heart rate. Late transient ischemia showed a diurnal distribution, occurred at a higher initial heart rate, and was more often accompanied by a further increase in heart rate than early ischemia. Thus in the first 2 months after AMI transient ischemia became increasingly common and more closely associated with increased myocardial oxygen demand. Because transient ischemic episodes during early and late ambulatory monitoring have dissimilar characteristics, they may also have different pathophysiologies and prognostic implications.

Late potentials

In patients with AMI, survival is influenced by the presence or absence of anterograde flow in the infarct artery, and late potentials on signal-averaged electrocardiography identify those at risk for tachyarrhythmias and sudden death. To assess the frequency of late potentials in survivors of first AMI, Lange and associates[21] from Dallas, Texas, performed coronary arteriography and signal-averaged electrocardiography in 109 subjects (64 men, 45 women, aged 30–77 years), 49 with (group I) and 60 without (group II) anterograde flow in the infarct artery. The groups were similar in age, sex, infarct artery, severity of CAD and LV function. Only 4 (8%) of group I had late potentials, whereas 24 (40%) of group II had late potentials. Thus, anterograde flow in the infarct artery after AMI is associated with a low incidence of late potentials on signal-averaged electrocardiography, whereas the absence of anterograde flow is more often associated with late potentials (Figures 3-4 and 3-5).

Echocardiography

To assess the relation between myocardial infarct size and LV diastolic function as measured by radionuclide angiography and Doppler echocardiography, Johannessen and associates[22] from Seattle, Washington, studied 83 patients aged 58 ± 9 years without significant valvular heart disease 8 to 12 weeks after an AMI. AMI size was measured by resting thallium-201 tomography. Peak early filling rate (in end-diastolic volumes/s) was measured by gated blood pool scintigraphy. Doppler measures of mitral inflow were peak early (E) and atrial (A) filling velocities, slopes of E and A, percent E and A filling, E/A ratio and diastolic filling period. In

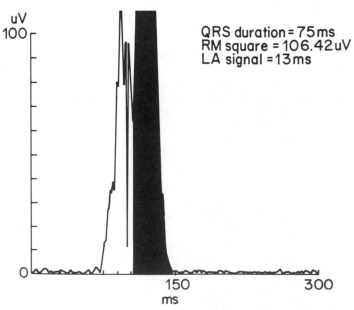

uV
100

QRS duration = 75 ms
RM square = 106.42 uV
LA signal = 13 ms

150   300
ms

Fig. 3-4. The signal-averaged electrocardiogram of a patient with anterograde flow in the infarct artery. Note that all signal-averaged electrocardiographic variables are normal. The darkened area represents the terminal 40 ms of the filtered QRS complex, from which the root mean (RM) square voltage was calculated. LA = low amplitude. Reproduced with permission from Lange, et al.[21]

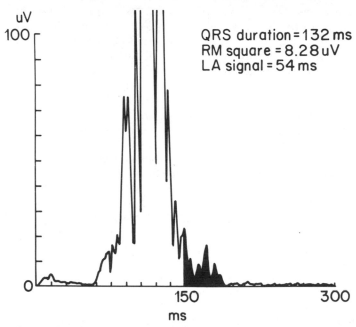

QRS duration = 132 ms
RM square = 8.28 uV
LA signal = 54 ms

Fig. 3-5. The signal-averaged electrocardiogram of a patient without anterograde flow in the infarct artery. Note that all signal-averaged electrocardiographic variables are abnormal. The darkened area represents the terminal 40 ms of the filtered QRS complex, from which the root mean (RM) square voltage was calculated. LA = low amplitude. Reproduced with permission from Lange, et al.[21]

univariate analyses, there was a significant inverse correlation between infarct size and the peak early filling rate, and this remained significant in an analysis that included 2 other determinants of the filling rate, age and diastolic filling period. Infarction size was directly correlated to the peak E velocity, deceleration of E and percent E filling, and was inversely correlated to peak A and percent A filling. The correlation of AMI size with the E/A ratio was $r = 0.43$ and remained significant in a multivariate analysis that included age and diastolic filling period ($r = 0.53$). Thus, a larger AMI size was associated with a reduced peak early filling rate by radionuclide angiography, a higher peak E and a lower peak A velocity, and an increased E/A ratio by Doppler. In addition to the other variables known to influence diastolic measurements, these results suggest that AMI size determines, in part, diastolic function as assessed by either radionuclide or Doppler techniques.

To investigate the natural history of regional dyssynergy and LV size after AMI, Picard and co-workers[23] in Boston, Massachusetts, studied 57 patients with a first Q-wave infarction by 2-dimensional echocardiography and compared with 30 control patients. Measurements from the echocardiograms were used to construct maps of the LV endocardial surface from which the endocardial surface area index and the percent of the endocardial surface area involved by abnormal wall motion were calculated. These maps from entry and 3-month echocardiograms were used to classify patients based on changes in surface area index and abnormal wall motion. Two separate groups of patients were identified at entry—those with a normal surface area index (group 1) and those with an increase surface area index (group 2). Group 1 patients were subdivided at 3 months by changes occurring in surface area index (1A, with 5% increase, 1B, no change, and 1C, 5% decrease). The increase in surface area index in Group 1A was associated with global ventricular function and clinically silent infarct extension. Groups 1B and 1C were composed predominantly of patients with inferior wall AMI and all had either no change or a significant decrease in infarct size. Group 2 patients had a continued increase in surface area index by 3 months. This group comprised only patients with anterior wall AMI, and all had infarct expansion at the LV apex. The changes in LV size and functional size are heterogeneous after AMI and relate to the initial endocardial surface area, infarct location, and functional infarct size.

A variety of experimental studies suggest that diastolic LV function changes after AMI, but limited data exist on these changes in humans. To assess diastolic filling after AMI, Williamson and associates[24] from Ann Arbor, Michigan, performed Doppler echocardiographic examination within 24 hours of AMI in 60 patients. Of 54 patients who also underwent catheterization, 45 (83%) were successfully reperfused. A subgroup of 17 patients underwent a follow-up Doppler examination at 7 days after infarction, whereas 15 patients with stable exertional angina served as control subjects. There was no significant difference in age, gender, incidence of systemic hypertension or diabetes mellitus, heart rate, mean arterial pressure or severity of CAD between the infarct and control groups. The infarct group had a lower velocity time integral total (9.9 ± 0.4 cm vs 12.0 ± 0.9 cm), a lower velocity time integral E (5.8 ± 0.3 cm vs 6.8 ± 0.5 cm) and a lower velocity time integral 0.333 (3.5 ± 0.4 cm vs 6.1 ± 0.5 cm) than the control group. In addition, velocity time integral A/total was significantly greater in the infarction group (0.44 ± 0.03 vs 0.35 ± 0.04) compared to the control group. The follow-up subgroup showed an increase in velocity time integral total, velocity time integral E and velocity time integral 0.333/total over the first 7 days after infarction. The final recovery values at 7 days were not significantly different from those of the CAD group. Patients with initial EF <40% or anterior wall AMI had the greatest recovery during the 7-day period. In conclusion, LV filling is further impaired during AMI compared to patients with stable CAD with the predominant impairment in early diastole. Filling parameters improve over the first 7 days after AMI, suggesting a recovery of diastolic stunning.

Dipyridamole-Thallium 201 imaging

Brown and associates[25] from Burlington, Vermont, tested in 50 patients the ability of dipyridamole—Thallium-201 imaging to predict in-hospital and late cardiac events when performed very early (62 ± 24 hours, range 23–102) after AMI. During hospitalization, 1 patient developed recurrent AMI and 8 patients developed recurrent angina after MI associated with ST-segment depression at 60 ± 42 hours after the dipyridamole-thallium-201 imaging; of these, 6 required urgent coronary revascularization. No patient died in-hospital. There were no serious adverse effects during the dipyridamole protocol. Using stepwise multivariate logistic regression analysis, the best and only statistically significant predictor of in-hospital ischemic cardiac events was the presence of thallium-201 redistribution within the infarct zone. Of 20 patients with infarct zone thallium-201 redistribution, 9 (45%) developed in-hospital ischemic cardiac events compared to 0 of 30 patients without infarct zone thallium-201 redistribution. During a follow-up 12 ± 7 months after discharge, 3 additional patients with infarct zone thallium-201 redistribution developed recurrent AMI or unstable angina, whereas no patient without infarct zone thallium-201 redistribution developed ischemic cardiac events. These data suggest that dipyridamole-thallium-201 imaging performed very early after AMI may identify a subgroup of patients at high risk for in-hospital and late ischemic cardiac events. Such patients may benefit from early cardiac catheterization and revascularization. Patients without infarct zone thallium-201 redistribution appear to be at very low risk for in-hospital and late ischemic cardiac events and may be candidates for early discharge.

Lundgren and associates[26] from Indianapolis, Indiana, assessed regional LV wall motion abnormalities using 2-dimensional echocardiography and contrast ventriculography within 12 hours of onset of chest pain in 20 patients with AMI: 10 patients had anterior wall and 10 had inferior wall infarcts. End-diastolic and end-systolic sinus beats from right anterior oblique contrast ventriculograms were analyzed using the center-line chord technique with both a standard overlap method of chord assignment and a nonoverlap method. Echocardiograms were obtained in parasternal long- and short-axis and apical 2- and 4-chamber views and analyzed using a 16-segment scoring system to derive anterior and inferoposterolateral wall motion indexes using both overlap (10 segments for anterior, 8 inferior) as well as nonoverlap (9 segments anterior, 7 inferior) methods of segment assignment (Figure 3-6). There was a significant inverse correlation between the standard (nonoverlap) echocardiographic analysis and the standard (overlap) angiographic analysis for infarct regions. Fifteen of 18 patients with angiographic infarct regional score ≤ -1 standard deviation/chord had an echocardiographic index ≥ 1.5, while 15 of 16 patients with echocardiographic regional infarct index ≥ 1.5 had an angiographic score ≤ -1 standard deviation/chord. Correlation between the 2 methods for noninfarct territories was poor (r $= -0.34$) because the angiographic method assesses hyperkinesis while the echocardiographic method does not. For noninfarct regions, 13 of 16 patients with an angiographic score > -1 standard deviation/chord had an echocardiographic <1.5, while 13 of 15 patients with an echocardiographic regional index of <1.5 had an angiographic score > -1 standard deviation/chord. In comparing overlap and nonoverlap methods, significant differences were found for noninfarct regions but not for infarct regions for both echocardiographic and angiographic analyses. Data indicate that 2-dimensional echocardiography, which is noninvasive and more easily repeatable for serial studies, yields similar results to contrast angiography for the assessment of regional wall motion abnormalities after AMI.

Nuclear magnetic resonance

Johns and associates[27] in Boston, Massachusetts, used nuclear magnetic resonance (NMR) imaging to evaluate the ability of this noninvasive imaging modality to detect and characterize AMI. The study was performed to evaluate the capability of NMR imaging in the measurement of infarct size in patients with recent AMI. Electrocardiographic-gated spin-echo NMR imaging was performed in 26 patients a mean of 9 ± 3 days (range 5 to 20) after AMI. The imaging technique used provided single-slice, spin-echo imaging of the LV in its true short axis, allowing direct correlation of NMR AMI location and size with a region of severe hypokinesis on left ventriculography. In all 20 patients with complete

REGIONAL WALL SEGMENTS

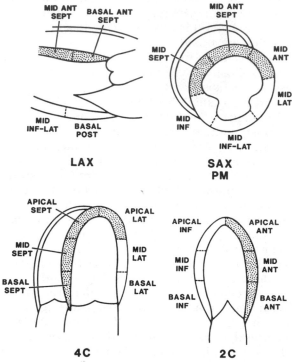

Fig. 3-6. Schematic representation of 16-segment regional wall motion analysis by 2-dimensional echocardiography. Shaded areas represent segments in anterior region (non-overlap), while unshaded segments represent inferoposterolateral region. For overlap method, apical inferior segment is included in anterior region for anterior infarcts and apical lateral segment is included in infero-posterolateral region for inferior infarcts. ANT = anterior; INF = inferior; INFLAT = inferolateral; LAT = lateral; LAX = parasternal long axis; POST = posterior; SAX = parasternal short axis; SEPT = septum; 4C = apical 4-chamber; 2C = apical 2-chamber. Reproduced with permission from Lundgren, et al.[26]

NMR studies, infarct location was correctly identified by using specific, objective criteria and the correlation between mean infarct volume and quantitative left ventricular hypokinetic segment extent was good (Figure 3-7) demonstrating that NMR imaging of the heart may have a role in the noninvasive assessment of AMI in patients.

PROGNOSTIC INDICES

Age

The basis for the excess mortality with age after AMI is not clear, nor is it known whether the mode of death is altered with age. Marcus and associates[28] from several medical centers examined age-related factors predictive of mortality and age-related mechanisms of the 303 deaths in 2,466 patients who were enrolled in a placebo-controlled trial to determine the effect of diltiazem on mortality and reinfarction after AMI. There

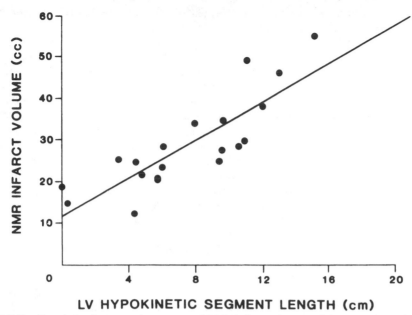

Fig. 3-7. Correlation between the computed NMR infarct volume and the quantitative left ventricular (LV) hypokinetic segment length (y = 2.24x + 12.3, r = 0.84, p = 0.0002). Reproduced with permission from Johns, et al.[27]

were 3 age groups with increasing mortality rates: ages 25 to 49 (n = 499), 50 to 64 (n = 1,228) and 65 to 75 years (n = 739). There was a significant age-related increase in the proportion of patients with baseline risk factors. These baseline characteristics did not differ by treatment (placebo vs diltiazem). However, multivariate survivorship analysis still identified age as an independent risk factor for cardiac death. The proportion of arrhythmic and myocardial failure deaths did not differ by treatment or age group.

Nadelmann and associates[29] from Bronx, New York, assessed in an 8 year prospective study of 390 community-based subjects (aged 75–85 years at entry, mean 79 years) the prevalence, incidence and prognosis of recognized and unrecognized Q-wave AMI. Subjects were studied at baseline and with annual follow-up electrocardiographic examinations. At baseline, 7.9% had a history of AMI without electrocardiographic evidence, 6.4% had electrocardiographic evidence of Q-wave AMI without clinical history, 4.1% had both clinical history and electrocardiographic evidence and 81.5% had neither history nor electrocardiographic evidence (control subjects). After an average follow-up period of 76.1 months, the total mortality rate was 5.9/100 person-years for subjects with some evidence of AMI at baseline versus 3.9 in the control group. The incidence of cardiovascular disease in subjects with evidence of AMI was 8.8/100 person-years versus 4.7 among control subjects. During the follow-up period, 115 new Q-wave AMIs occurred (50 unrecognized, rate 2.4/100; 65 recognized, rate 3.2/100). There was no difference in mortality and morbidity outcome between subjects with recognized and unrecognized AMIs. Those with only a history of AMI at baseline had a three-fold greater risk of a new AMI (recognized and unrecognized) than the control group. Unrecognized Q-wave AMI is a common occurrence in the "old old" with subsequent morbidity and mortality prognosis comparable to that of recognized AMI. History of AMI alone in this age group is also associated with an increased risk of AMI, suggesting the need for better diagnostic markers of AMI in the elderly.

Smith and colleagues[30] in San Diego, California; Vancouver, Canada; and Stockholm, Sweden, evaluated and compared the clinical course and mortality rate for up to 1 year in a large multicenter data base that included 702 patients >75 years of age (mean ± SD 81 ± 4 years) with a less elderly subset of 1,321 patients between 65 and 75 years of age (mean 70 ± 3 years). Postdischarge 1 year cardiac mortality rate was 18% for those >75 years compared with 12% for patients between 65 and 75 years of age. There were differences in the prevalence of several factors, including female sex, history of angina pectoris, history of CHF, smoking habits, and incidence of CHF during hospitalization. Univariate and multivariate analyses of predictors of cardiac death in hospital survivors selected several different factors as important in the 2 age subgroups; age was selected in the 65 to 75 year age group, but it was not an independent predictor in the very elderly (Table 3-1). Survival rates beginning at day 10 for patients 65 to 75 and in those >75 years of age were similar for up to 90 days, but they diverged later. In the very elderly, 63% of late cardiac deaths were sudden or due to new AMI, similar to the causes of 67% of the deaths in the younger age groups (Figure 3-8). These data suggest that elderly patients benefit initially from thrombolytic therapy in a manner similar to those that are less elderly. Future death in

TABLE 3-1. *Comparison of factors related to mortality for the two age groups in 1,335 patients followed up for 1 full year versus 215 dying of cardiac cause after hospital discharge. Reproduced with permission from Smith, et al.[30]*

	Current Study						MILIS
	>75 Years			65–75 Years			65–75 Years
	Survivors	Deaths	RR	Survivors	Deaths	RR	RR
No.	421	90		914	125		
History							
Previous MI	31†	49	1.9	35*	50	1.9	1.9
Cong heart failure	20*	42	2.3	10*	26	2.7	2.1
Angina	46*	71	2.4	42†	56	1.7	1.4
Diabetes	16‡	25	1.6	16*	29	1.9	1.5
Clinical course							
Cong heart failure	56*	73	1.9	45*	75	3.6	1.6
Extension of MI	4	7	1.5	3*	13	3.5	
HR >100 beats/min	27	54	2.5	25*	48	2.4	
Q wave MI	66	62	0.9	74	65	0.7	0.9
QRS duration ≥0.1 s	44‡	58	1.6	33*	56	2.3	
Atrial fib	24	29	1.2	17‡	26	1.6	1.2
Discharge							
S₃ gallop	5‡	11	1.9	3*	19	4.8	
Digitalis	42*	59	1.8	26*	52	2.6	
Diuretic	45*	73	2.8	30*	46	1.8	
Beta-blocker (nonuse)	73	79	1.4	60†	73	1.7	
Special studies							
CTR ≥0.51	61	65	0.8	42‡	54	1.5	
RN LVEF <0.45	43	55	1.5	41*	78	4.1	
Complex VPCs	48‡	64	1.7	46*	70	2.4	

*p < 0.001. †p < 0.01 and ‡p < 0.05, means or proportions. survivors versus deaths. CTR = cardiothoracic ratio: HR = heart rate; RN LVEF = radionuclide left ventricular ejection fraction: RR = risk ratio.

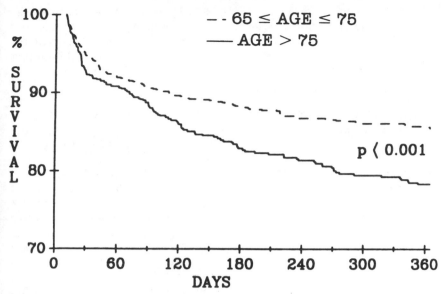

Fig. 3-8. Actuarial survival curves beginning the 10th day after hospital admission for patients between 65 and 75 years of age (dashed line) and patients >75 years of age (solid line). Reproduced with permission from Smith, et al.[30]

the elderly group is delayed and appears to be due primarily to a new ischemic event or sudden death in the convalescent phase after AMI.

Gender

To examine the impact of gender on survival after AMI, Fiebach and associates[31] from New Haven, Connecticut, performed a retrospective cohort study of 332 women and 790 men. Women who had an AMI were older and more often had hypertension, diabetes, previous CHF, and impaired LV function on admission. Cumulative 3-year mortality and in-hospital mortality rates were significantly higher in women than men, but mortality among hospital survivors was similar. After multivariate adjustment for baseline differences, mortality rates were not significantly different between women and men for in-hospital deaths, and mortality at 3 years among hospital survivors tended to be lower among women. The authors concluded that higher observed mortality rates following an AMI in women are related to differences in known risk factors for subsequent mortality and that gender should not be considered an independent risk factor for mortality after AMI.

Type of first infarct

Fox and associates[32] from Birmingham, UK, compared the exercise test characteristics, coronary anatomy, and prognosis of patients discharged after non Q-wave AMI with those with Q-wave AMI. Of the 339 patients studied, all of whom were ≤70 years, 87 (26%) had had a non Q-wave infarction. There were no significant differences in the exercise test characteristics between the 2 groups, and in those 149 patients in whom angiography was performed triple vessel disease was present in 36/114 (32%) of the Q-wave group and 9/35 (26%) of the non Q-wave group. The infarct related artery was more often patent in the non Q-wave group

(27/35 (77%)) than in the Q-wave group (53/224 (46%)). The 1 year mortality and the reinfarction and angina rates were similar in the 2 groups and the exercise test remained a good discriminator for predicting patients at risk of future cardiac events in both groups. In view of the similar outcome and severity of CAD in those aged ≤70 with non Q-wave infarcts, the distinction between Q and non Q-wave infarction need not influence management decisions in patients after AMI.

Schechtman and associates[33] in St. Louis, Missouri; Charlottesville, Virginia; Providence, Rhode Island; Cheyenne, Wyoming; and Houston, Texas, evaluated follow-up data for 515 survivors of acute non-Q wave MI according to mortality: 1) between hospital discharge and 3 months after AMI (early), and 2) between 3 and 12 months after AMI (late). Mortality rate decreased steadily for the first 3 months and was constant thereafter. There were 25 early and 32 late deaths. After adjustment for the longer time associated with the 3 to 12 month period, the relative risk per unit time of earliest compared with late mortality was 2.64. Risk factors for early mortality were different from those that predicted late mortality. Independent predictors of mortality between hospital discharge to 3 months after AMI were ST segment depression that persisted during hospitalization, in-hospital reinfarction, and a history of CHF. Persistent ST depression and in-hospital reinfarction had neither univariate nor an independent association with 3 to 12 month mortality. Age, reinfarction between discharge and 3 months, and diabetes were independently associated with late mortality (Table 3-2). Early mortality was 0.5% in patients with no ST depression at either baseline or discharge,

TABLE 3-2. *Univariate associations with 3 month mortality and mortality between months 3 and 12 in 515 patients. Reproduced with permission from Schechtman, et al.[33]*

	Prevalence (%)	3 Month Mortality			3 to 12 Month Mortality		
		With Factor (%)	Without Factor (%)	p Value	With Factor (%)	Without Factor (%)	p Value
Male gender	77.9	5.4	3.5	0.4670	6.4	5.5	0.6993
Smoking	53.8	5.8	3.8	0.2780	7.7	5.2	0.2908
Obesity	19.3	5.1	4.8	0.9587	3.2	7.3	0.1484
Diltiazem group	49.9	4.3	5.4	0.5368	8.1	4.9	0.1602
Baseline ST ↓	52.8	8.5	.8	0.0001	7.6	5.4	0.2846
Discharge ST ↓	30.2	11.6	2.4	0.0001	9.3	5.2	0.0919
Baseline ST ↑	33.0	7.1	3.8	0.0961	7.0	6.3	0.8038
Discharge ST ↑	30.0	8.3	3.8	0.0386	8.3	5.5	0.2827
T wave inversion	56.9	5.5	4.1	0.4292	6.5	6.6	0.9337
Localizability	79.8	5.8	1.0	0.0399	7.0	4.9	0.4267
LVH	23.1	8.4	3.8	0.0408	8.3	6.0	0.3920
Anterior location	49.9	6.2	3.5	0.1583	7.9	5.2	0.2426
Progression to Q wave MI	12.4	1.4	5.4	0.1341	6.9	6.5	0.8491
In-hospital reinfarction	6.4	18.2	3.9	0.0002	3.7	6.7	0.5572
Angina with ECG changes	17.7	9.9	3.8	0.0112	8.5	6.1	0.3796
Postinfarction angina	41.2	5.7	4.3	0.4440	7.0	6.2	0.7187
Killip class II or III	21.2	8.3	3.9	0.0608	14.0	4.6	0.0007
History of							
Coronary bypass surgery	12.2	9.5	4.2	0.0676	8.8	6.2	0.4659
Previous MI	37.7	7.2	3.4	0.0559	8.9	5.2	0.0997
Hypertension	20.4	5.7	4.6	0.6384	4.0	7.2	0.2574
CHF	21.6	11.7	3.0	0.0001	13.3	4.8	0.0031
Diabetes	19.2	9.1	3.8	0.0280	12.2	5.2	0.0128
Reinfarction–3 months	6.3				24.0	5.3	0.0002

CHF = congestive heart failure; ECG = electrocardiographic; LVH = left ventricular hypertrophy; MI = myocardial infarction; Reinfarction–3 months = discharge to 3 month reinfarction; prevalence computed among 3 month survivors only; ST ↓ = ST segment depression; ST ↑ = ST segment elevation.

4.8% in those with ST segment depression at one time point, and 13.7% in those with ST segment depression at both time points. In-hospital reinfarction was associated with increased early mortality and nonsignificantly associated with decreased late mortality. Thus, these data suggest that 1) in patients with non-Q wave AMI, ST depression that persists throughout hospitalization and in-hospital reinfarction are the major risk factors for mortality at 3 months but not for mortality between 3 and 12 months; 2) after 3 months of decreasing risk, the mortality rate in these patients remained constant for the next 9 months; and 3) with only one early death among 199 patients with non-Q wave AMI and no in-hospital ST segment depression, these patients are at low risk and do not appear to require early angiography.

Benhorin and associates[34] in Rochester and New York, New York and Tucson, Arizona studied the prognostic significance of the first AMI (Q wave versus non-Q wave) and Q wave AMI location (anterior as compared to inferoposterior) from a multicenter data base including 777 placebo-treated patients who were participants in the Multicenter Diltiazem Post-Infarction Trial. There were 224 patients (29%) with a non-Q wave AMI, 326 (42%) with an inferoposterior Q wave AMI, and 227 (29%) with an anterior Q wave AMI. Mean LVEFs were significantly lower in patients with an anterior Q wave AMI than in the other 2 groups, but the total cardiac mortality rate during follow-up of 25 months per patient was only marginally higher in the anterior Q wave group (8.4%) than in the other 2 groups, including 7.1% for inferoposterior Q wave MIs and 6.3% for non-Q wave MIs. The first recurrent cardiac event rate was slightly higher in the anterior Q wave group than in the other two groups (18% vs 11.7% and 15.6%, respectively). Survivorship analyses over 3 years revealed that the electrocardiographic classification of the type of first AMI and Q wave location did not make significant independent contributions to risk of postinfarction cardiac death or first recurrent cardiac event.

Predischarge maximal exercise test

Nielsen and associates[35] from Fredericia, Denmark, performed a maximal exercise test in 54 patients with AMI before discharge and in 49 age-matched control subjects. The long-term prognosis was assessed after an average follow-up of 7.6 years in AMI patients and 5.8 years in control subjects. The maximal work capacity and systolic BP increase in AMI patients was 59% that of control subjects. Seventeen AMI patients had significant ST-segment shifts, 13 with ST depression and 4 with ST elevation. In AMI patients experiencing a cardiac death during follow-up the maximal work capacity and systolic BP increase were significantly lower than in survivors and those who died from noncardiac reasons, with no difference between these groups in the number of patients with ST-segment shifts. The average maximal work capacity of control subjects was 143 watts. A maximal work capacity half this (72 watts) predicted long-term mortality in AMI patients. In addition a low increase in systolic BP (<30 mm Hg) also predicted long-term mortality, whereas ST shifts were of no significant value. In this study maximal work capacity turned out to be the best single exercise variable for identifying groups of AMI patients with very low and relative high risk of cardiac death. When all 3 exercise variables were combined, the predischarge maximal exercise test was of great value in identifying AMI patients at low risk for cardiac death (predictive value of a negative test: 95%).

Postexercise systolic blood pressure

Kato and associates[36] from Nagoya and Hisai Mie, Japan, assessed the prognostic value of an abnormal postexercise response in systolic BP by performing treadmill exercise testing in 217 survivors of AMI at an average of 9.3 weeks after AMI. During the mean follow-up period of 4 years, cardiac events were noted in 34 patients (16%), including cardiac death in 13 (6%), nonfatal reinfarction in 12 (6%), and CABG in 9 (4%). An abnormal postexercise systolic BP response was defined as the ratio of systolic BP at 3 minutes of recovery to peak exercise systolic BP of 0.9 or more, on the basis of the cutoff point with the highest sensitivity and specificity to predict cardiac events. An abnormal postexercise systolic BP response occurred in 90 patients (42%). Patients with an abnormal postexercise systolic BP response had more exercise-induced myocardial ischemia, more LV impairment, and more extensive coronary artery lesions than those without. Cox proportional hazards model demonstrated that the abnormal postexercise systolic BP response was ranked first in ability to predict cardiac death. CABG was associated with an abnormal postexercise systolic BP ratio. Nonfatal reinfarction could not be predicted by any clinical or exercise variables. In conclusion, an abnormal postexercise systolic BP response could be useful for predicting cardiac death and the need for CABG after AMI. This response is probably the result of myocardial ischemia and LV impairment.

Platelet aggregability

Trip and associates[37] from Amsterdam and Leiden, the Netherlands, tested the hypothesis that an increase in spontaneous aggregability of platelets in vitro predicts mortality in coronary events in patients who have survived AMI. A cohort of 129 survivors of AMI entered the study 3 months after the index AMI and was followed for 5 years. At entry and at intervals of 6 months, spontaneous platelet aggregation was tested and graded as positive (aggregation within 10 minutes), intermediate (aggregation after 10–20 minutes), or negative (no aggregation within 20 minutes). During follow-up, 6.4% (6 of 94) of the patients in the spontaneous platelet aggregation-negative group died, as compared with 10.3% (3 of 29) in the spontaneous platelet aggregation-intermediate group and 34.6% (9 of 26) in the spontaneous platelet aggregation-positive group. As compared with the spontaneous platelet aggregation-negative group, the spontaneous platelet aggregation-intermediate group had a relative risk of death of 1.6 (95% confidence interval, 0.5–5.5) and the spontaneous platelet aggregation-positive group had a risk of 5.4. At least 1 cardiac event (cardiac death or recurrent non-fatal AMI) occurred in 14.9% (14 of 94 patients) of the spontaneous platelet aggregation-negative group, 24.1% (7 of 29) of the spontaneous platelet aggregation-intermediate group, and 46.2% (12 of 26) of the spontaneous platelet aggregation-positive group. A positive test result continued to have prognostic value throughout the 5-year study. The authors concluded that spontaneous platelet aggregation in vitro is a useful biologic marker for the prediction of coronary events and mortality in this low-risk group of survivors of an AMI. A causal relation is suggested but not proved by the study.

Precordial ST segment depression

Bates and colleagues[38] in Ann Arbor, Michigan; Durham, North Carolina; and Columbus and Cincinnati, Ohio, evaluated the importance of associated precordial ST segment depression in patients with inferior AMIs on angiographic and clinical outcomes after thrombolytic therapy and selective coronary angioplasty in 583 patients. Anterior AMIs (Group I), inferior AMIs with precordial ST segment depression (Group II) and inferior AMIs without precordial ST segment depression (Group III) were present in 289, 135, and 159 patients, respectively. Precordial ST segment depression was more frequent in patients with circumflex than right coronary AMI-related artery (71% versus 40%). Acute patency rates were not statistically different at day 7 (Group I 88%, Group II 84%, Group III 80%) nor were reocclusion rates (Group I 11%, Group II 10%, Group III 18%). Infarct zone regional wall motion in inferior AMI patients was lower in those with precordial ST segment depression both acutely and on day 7. Precordial ST segment depression was associated with lower LVEFs in inferior AMI patients both acutely (Group I $47 \pm 11\%$, Group II $53 \pm 11\%$, Group III $58 \pm 9\%$) and at day 7 (Group I $49 \pm 12\%$, Group II $53 \pm 10\%$, Group III $58 \pm 8\%$). Complication rates tended to be higher in inferior AMI patients when precordial ST segment depression was present. Mortality rates for patients in Groups I, II and III were 8%, 6%, and 5%, respectively. These data suggest that precordial ST segment depression in patients with inferior AMIs predicts poorer ventricular functional and clinical outcome despite reperfusion therapy.

Heart rate

Elevated heart rate (HR) during hospitalization and after discharge has been predictive of death in patients with AMI, but whether this association is primarily due to associated cardiac failure is unknown. Hjalmarson and associates[39] from multiple medical centers characterized in 1,807 patients with AMI admitted into a multicenter study the relation of HR to in-hospital after discharge and total mortality from day 2 to 1 year in patients with and without CHF. HR was examined on admission of maximum level in the coronary care unit, and at hospital discharge. Both in-hospital and postdischarge mortality increased with increasing admission HR, and total mortality increased with increasing admission HR, and total mortality (day 2 to 1 year) was 15% for patients with an admission HR between 50 and 60 beats/min, 41% for HR >90 beats/min and 48% for HR ≥110 beats/min. Mortality from hospital discharge to 1 year was similarly related to maximal HR in the coronary care unit and to HR at discharge. In patients with severe heart failure (grade 3 or 4 pulmonary congestion on chest x-ray, or shock), cumulative mortality was high regardless of the level of admission HR (range 61 to 68%). However, in patients with pulmonary venous congestion of grade 2, cumulative mortality for patients with admission HR ≥90 beats/min was over twice as high as that in patients with admission HR <90 beats/min (39 vs 18%, respectively); the same trend was evident in patients with absent to mild CHF (mortality 18 vs 10%, respectively). On multivariate analysis HR was independently predictive of 1-year mortality. Elevated HR during hospitalization for AMI is importantly and independently associated with mortality.

Atrial fibrillation

As part of an ongoing community-wide study examining changes over time in the incidence and survival rates of 4108 patients hospitalized with validated AMI in 16 hospitals in the Worcester, Massachusetts, metropolitan area during calendar years 1975, 1978, 1981, 1984, and 1986, Goldberg and associates[40] from Worcester, Massachusetts, examined changes over time in the proportion of patients with AMI developing AF and the impact of AF on in-hospital and long-term survival for up to a 10-year follow-up period. The overall percentage of patients with AF complicating AMI was 16%; this proportion increased over time from 13% in 1975 to 15% in 1978, 15% in 1981, 20% in 1984, and 18% in 1986. Patients with AF experienced consistently higher in-hospital case fatality rates than AMI patients without AF overall (28% versus 17%), as well as during each of the 5 years under study. The independent effect of AF on in-hospital survival was not upheld, however, when a variety of potentially confounding prognostic factors were controlled for in a multivariate analysis. Among discharged hospital patients, while the crude long-term survival rate for patients with AF was poorer than that of patients without AF for the combined as well as for individual study periods, similar to the in-hospital findings the independent effect of AF on long-term prognosis was not upheld after use of a multivariate analysis. The adjusted risk of dying over the 10-year follow-up period for discharged hospital survivors of AF was essentially similar to that for AMI patients without AF. The results of this population-based study suggest that AF is a common complication of AMI and that its potential impact on in-hospital and long-term survival may be mediated through other factors although it remains a marker of underlying ventricular dysfunction and a compromised myocardium.

Supraventricular tachycardia

Berisso and associates[41] from Genova, Italy, assessed the incidence, characteristics and clinical significance of supraventricular tachyarrhythmias occurring in the late hospital phase of AMI in 209 consecutive patients. Arrhythmias were quantified by 24-hour electrocardiographic recording 16 ± 3 days after AMI, and were classified according to the degree of complexity in 5 classes. Class 0 = <5 premature beats/hr; class 1 = between 5 and 100/hr; class 2 = >100/hr or repetitive premature beats; class 3 = atrial-junctional tachycardia; class 4 = atrial flutter-fibrillation. Supraventricular tachyarrhythmias classes 1 to 2 always occurred in the absence of symptoms in 86 patients (41%); supraventricular tachyarrhythmias classes 3 to 4 (paroxysmal, self-limiting, brief) occurred in 27 patients (13%), symptomatically in 6. The presence of supraventricular tachyarrhythmias classes 2 to 3 was related to age >55 years and complex ventricular tachyarrhythmias (>20 premature beats/hr, VT). Increasing complexity of supraventricular tachyarrhythmias was significantly associated with presence and entity of cardiac enlargement and LV dysfunction. Patients with class 4 showed the most severe cardiac deterioration. During the 2 years after AMI, patients with classes 2, 3 and 4 had a higher incidence of acute pulmonary edema, New York Heart Association functional classes III to IV for CAD and a greater need of digitalis and diuretics. In these patients the probability of surviving 2 years was 79% compared to 94% in the remaining population. Cox multiple regression analysis indicated that supraventricular tachyarrhythmia classes 2, 3 and 4 did not predict an increased risk of cardiac death independently from cardiac enlargement and LV dysfunction. Arrhythmia monitoring in the late hospital phase of AMI should take into account complex supraventricular tachyarrhythmias because of their relation to LV dysfunction and subsequent clinical course.

Induced ventricular tachycardia

Iesaka and associates[42] from Tokyo, Japan, evaluated the prognostic significance of sustained monomorphic VT induced by programmed ventricular stimulation using up to 3 extrastimuli in 133 consecutive survivors of AMI at a mean interval of 1.8 ± 1.1 months after onset. This was compared with hemodynamic and angiographic abnormalities shown by cardiac catheterization and ventricular ectopic activity detected by Holter monitoring. Sustained monomorphic VT was induced in 25 (19%) patients, sustained polymorphic VT in 11 (8%) patients, nonsustained monomorphic VT (≥10 beats) in 12 patients (9%) and nonsustained polymorphic VT in 9 patients (7%). Multivariate logistic regression analysis of clinical, angiographic, hemodynamic and electrocardiographic variables showed that the presence of a LV aneurysm and Lown grade 4B ventricular ectopic activity were independent predictors of inducibility of sustained monomorphic VT. During a mean follow-up of 21 ± 13 months, there were 8 (6%) sudden cardiac deaths and 3 (2.3%) spontaneous occurrences of life-threatening sustained VT. The 2-year probability of freedom from sudden cardiac death or sustained VT was 53 ± 13% for patients with inducible sustained monomorphic VT, 70 ± 10% for those with a LVEF <40% and 58 ± 13% for those with Lown grade 4B ventricular ectopic activity. Cox regression multivariate analysis revealed only inducibility of sustained monomorphic VT and lower LVEF as independent predictors of life-threatening cardiac arrhythmic events, and further, the former predictor was relatively stronger than the latter. Programmed ventricular stimulation with an aggressive stimulation protocol and a strict criterion of abnormal response appeared to be useful to predict the high risk of sudden cardiac death or spontaneous sustained VT in survivors of AMI without documented sustained VT.

Electrocardiographic changes 1 year later

The prognostic value of abnormalities on the electrocardiogram present 1 year after initial AMI was examined in relation to reinfarction and coronary death by Wong and colleagues[43] in Boston, Massachusetts, throughout 32 years of the follow-up in the Framingham Heart Study. Resting 12-lead electrocardiograms were available in 251 survivors of clinically recognized Q wave AMI. The electrocardiogram reverted to normal in 31 cases and was abnormal but without Q waves in 37. Q waves persisted without other significant abnormalities in 108 and with other abnormalities in 75 cases. Electrocardiographic abnormalities at follow-up were more common in women and in those persons whose initial AMI was anterior as compared with inferior. Non-specific T wave, ST segment changes, and electrocardiographic LV hypertrophy on the electrocardiogram before and after AMI were powerful predictors of coronary death. The relation of these residual post-AMI electrocardiographic findings to reinfarction and coronary death was assessed by Cox regression analysis. The follow-up electrocardiographic status was unrelated to the risk of subsequent reinfarction. Subjects who lost Q wave evidence of AMI but whose electrocardiogram continued to show evidence of repolarization abnormalities, LV hypertrophy, or blocked intraventricular condition were at a 3.5 fold increased risk of coronary death as compared with those reverting to a normal electrocardiogram. Persons with a persistent Q wave AMI accompanied by these abnormalities were at a 2.7 fold excess risk of coronary death as compared with those with a normalized electrocardiogram. The presence of other electrocardiographic abnormalities without persistence Q waves yielded a worse prognosis than a Q wave persisting alone. The prognostic value of a follow-up electrocardiogram with abnormalities other than a persistent Q wave AMI also remained after considering the effects of left ventricular hypertrophy and cardiac enlargement on x-ray, functional classification, and diuretic usage. Specific electrocardiographic abnormalities present after AMI, however, were potent indicators of long-term prognosis and diminished the importance of the follow-up electrocardiogram. Although survival after initial AMI is improved only if the electrocardiogram reverts to normal, information on electrocardiographic abnormalities before AMI can be especially useful in evaluating long-term risk.

Cycle length variability

Cycle length variability (CLV), defined as the standard deviation of normal cycle length intervals, has been found to be a powerful predictor of subsequent mortality in survivors of AMI. Decreased CLV is associated with a significant increase in mortality. Previous studies CLV remained an independent predictor of outcome, even after adjusting for LVEF, clinical risk factors, heart rate and ventricular arrhythmias. The same population of survivors of AMI, the results of exercise testing also strongly predicted outcome, with those failing to take the test having the worst survival, and those completing the low-level stress test taken before discharge having the best prognosis. Kleiger and associates[44] from St. Louis, Missouri, and New York, New York, tested the hypothesis that the status of stress test (completed; did not complete; failed to take) and CLV were measuring the same factor related to mortality. Although the distribution of CLV was shifted to higher CLV in patients who completed the test and to lower CLV in those who failed to take the test, both predictors of mortality remained independent predictors of long-term mortality (average of 31 months of follow-up) after controlling for each other. Subgroups with an approximate 15-fold difference in mortality were defined using both variables. CLV is a measure of autonomic tone; it is not strongly related to exercise ability and using the results of both stress testing and CLV results in the identification of subgroups of postinfarction patients with markedly disparate risks of mortality.

Periinfarction block

Flowers and associates[45] from Augusta, Georgia, explored the relation of the presence of peri-infarction block to ventricular late potentials in patients with inferior wall myocardial infarction. The hypothesis was that both the gross peri-infarction block pattern and subtle low-level ventricular late potentials are expressions of conduction abnormality associated with infarction. The consequent question arose whether peri-infarction block may have the same association with sustained ventricular arrhythmias that has been demonstrated in postinfarction patients with ventricular late potentials. Seventy patients with documented Q-wave myocardial infarction were divided into those with (n = 23) and those without (n = 47) peri-infarction block. Signal-averaged electrocardiograms were obtained. Analysis of the vectormagnitude complex revealed that the total duration of that complex and the duration of terminal potential <40$_u$V in the peri-infarction group exceeded that in the group without peri-infarction block. The voltage in the last 40 ms of the vectormagnitude complex was also significantly less in the peri-infarction group. There were 13 instances of sustained VT, VF or sudden death occurring subsequent to infarction not associated with the acute ischemic event, 11 of which occurred in the peri-infarction group. The significantly higher incidence of later potentials along with the significantly higher incidence of sustained ventricular arrhythmias in the peri-infarction group suggests that the presence of peri-infarction block on the surface electrocardiogram may provide another marker for identifying persons at increased risk for these arrhythmias subsequent to myocardial infarction.

Reinfarction

Rivers and associates[46] in Auckland, New Zealand, evaluated 456 consecutive patients seen ≤6 hours after the onset of AMI associated with ST segment elevation who received thrombolytic therapy and were followed for 12 months. Intravenous streptokinase was given to 315 patients and recombinant tissue plasminogen activator to 141 patients. Reinfarction rates and risk factors for reinfarction were assessed. Management after thrombolysis was conservative. Revascularization procedures were reserved for patients with symptoms refractory to medical therapy or for those with LM CAD. CABG or PTCA was performed in only 3.7% of patients in the first 30 days after thrombolytic therapy and in 8.6% of patients by 1 year. Most patients (79%) had coronary arteriography. Twenty-six patients (5.7%) had signs of threatened reinfarction at 1 month after thrombolytic therapy and 43 patients (9.4%) had similar signs by 1 year. Reinfarction was apparently prevented in four patients by early readministration of thrombolytic therapy. Multivariate analysis of possible risk factors for reinfarction identified at the time of initial infarction showed current cigarette smoking to be the only predictive risk factor (Table 3-3). Twenty percent of patients who continued to smoke had repeat AMI compared with 5% of those who stopped. Conservative management after thrombolysis with streptokinase or tissue plasminogen activator results in a reinfarction rate of 8.6% at 1 year as evidenced by this study. Cigarette smoking predisposes patients to repeat AMI and cessation of smoking reduces this risk of repeat AMI.

Benhorin and associates[47] in Rochester, New York, evaluated the prognostic significance of nonfatal reinfarction from the multicenter diltiazem trial data base of 1,234 patients treated with placebo followed for 1 to 4 years after AMI. One hundred sixteen patients had at least one fatal reinfarction, 14 (12%) of whom subsequently had cardiac death. Among the remaining 1,118 patients without nonfatal reinfarction, 110 (9.8%) had cardiac death. Compared with event-free patients, patients with nonfatal reinfarction were more likely to be women, to have had an infarction before their index event, and to have had prior cardiac-related symptoms. Cox survivorship analyses revealed that nonfatal reinfarction was associated with a significant and independent risk for subsequent cardiac mortality which was greater than that associated with other significant predictor variables, including New York Heart Association functional class, evidence of CHF on chest x-ray, predischarge Holter-recorded ventricular

TABLE 3-3. *Potential risk factors for reinfarction (defined at time of index infarction) in 456 patients. Reproduced with permission from Rivers, et al.*[46]

	Reinfarction (n = 43)	No Reinfarction (n = 413)	p Value
Smoking	29 (67%)	203 (50%)	0.04
Inferior infarction	28 (65%)	221 (54%)	0.20
Female gender	6 (14%)	99 (24%)	0.20
Non-Q wave infarction	8 (19%)	97 (23%)	0.59
No previous angina	36 (84%)	329 (80%)	0.66
Diabetes	3 (7%)	43 (10%)	0.66
Mean age (yr)	58 ± 9	57 ± 10	0.68
rt-PA therapy	14 (33%)	127 (31%)	0.94
Streptokinase therapy	29 (67%)	286 (69%)	0.94
Hypertension	10 (23%)	103 (25%)	0.95

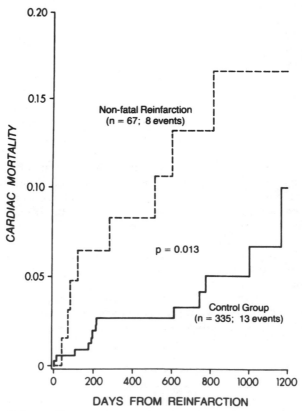

Fig. 3-9. Cumulative cardiac mortality rate in 67 patients after a second nonfatal myocardial infarction and in a 5:1 matched control group (n = 335). See text for details. Reproduced with permission from Benhorin, et al.[34]

premature beats, and radionuclide-determined EF (Figure 3-9). Cardiac mortality risk associated with nonfatal reinfarction was further increased in patients whose index event was their first infarction. These data demonstrate that nonfatal reinfarction is associated with a strong, significant and independent risk for subsequent cardiac death in patients surviving AMI.

COMPLICATIONS

Left ventricular thrombi

Sixty patients (48 men and 12 women; aged 36 to 72 years, mean age 48 ± 9), who survived an AMI and in whom LV thrombus was detected by cross-sectional echocardiography 1 to 2 days before they were discharged from the hospital, were prospectively studied by Kouvaras and associates[48] from Piraeus, Greece. All had evidence of left apical wall motion abnormalities. They were randomly divided into 3 groups of 20 patients each. Group A was given a full dose of oral anticoagulants, group B was given aspirin, 650 mg/day, and group C received no antithrombotic therapy. Echocardiography was performed every 3 months in all patients, and they were followed for 9 to 24 months (mean 16 ± 5 months). Twelve patients in group A had complete resolution of the thrombus and 3 had a significant decrease in the size of the thrombus (≥50% of initial thickness) during the first trimester after AMI. In group B the thrombus resolved in 9 patients and was significantly diminished in 4 during the first trimester of follow-up. In group C the thrombus resolved in 2 patients during the first trimester and showed a significant decrease in size in 2 patients during the second trimester of follow-up. Two patients in group C initially had recurrent transient cerebral ischemic attacks, which did not recur after aneurysmectomy. One patient in group C had a peripheral embolic episode in the femoral artery. It was concluded that anticoagulants and aspirin are equally effective, compared to no treatment, in the resolution of LV thrombosis and prevention of emboli after AMI. Spontaneous resolution of thrombus occurs in very few patients.

To determine whether a positive indium 111 platelet image for a LV thrombus, which indicates ongoing thrombogenic activity, predicts an increased risk of systemic embolization, Stratton and Ritchie[49] in Seattle, Washington, compared the embolic rate in 34 patients with positive indium 111 platelet images with that in 69 patients with negative images during a mean follow-up of 38 months after platelet imaging. The positive and negative image groups were similar with respect to age, prevalence of previous infarction, time from last AMI, EF, long-term or paroxysmal AF, warfarin therapy during follow-up, platelet-inhibitory therapy during follow-up, injected indium dose and latest imaging time. During follow-up, embolic events occurred in 21% of patients with positive platelet images for LV thrombi compared with 3% of patients with negative images. By actuarial methods, at 42 months after platelet imaging, only 86% of patients with positive images were embolus free as compared with 98% of patients with negative images. To determine whether platelet imaging, which detects active thrombosis, offered additional predictive value to 2-dimensional echocardiography, which is less costly and more widely available, the investigators compared the embolic rates in 30 patients with both a positive echocardiogram and a positive platelet image to the rate in 28 patients with a positive echocardiogram but a negative platelet image. Among patients with both studies positive, embolic events occurred in 23% versus 4% in patients with a positive echocardiogram but a negative platelet image. The corresponding actuarial rates at 42 months were 85% and 100%. The investigators concluded that a positive platelet image for a LV thrombus predicts an increased embolic risk and appears more specific for subsequent embolization than a positive echocardiogram. Additionally, in patients with LV thrombus by echocardiography, a negative platelet image predicts a low risk of subsequent embolization.

Right ventricular infarction

Yasuda and colleagues[50] from Boston, Massachusetts, evaluated RV function serially by multigated blood pool imaging in 18 patients with RV dysfunction associated with inferior wall AMI. Radionuclide ventriculograms were performed on all patients within 18 hours of chest pain and again at 10 days. In addition, 15 of 18 patients had rest and exercise radionuclide ventriculogram at 3 months. The mean resting RVEF at admission, 10 days, and 3 months in these patients was 32 ± 13%, 47 ± 11%, and 46 ± 10%, while the LVEF was 56 ± 11%, 58 ± 13%, and 53 ± 11%. The 3-month exercise radionuclide ventriculogram demonstrated an increase in RVEF >5% in 6 of 15 patients. In 8 catheterized patients, neither the location nor the severity of coronary artery narrowing nor the presence of collaterals correlated with the RV exercise response. Improvement in RV function over a 10-day interval following inferior AMI suggests the presence of significant reversible RV dysfunction during the acute phase.

Mavric and associates[51] from Rijeka, Yugoslavia, obtained data in 243 patients with inferior AMI who were admitted to the coronary care unit during the years 1987 and 1988. One hundred and ninety-eight patients had no signs of RV involvement (group I), whereas 45 patients had inferior AMI with RV infarction (group II). Patients were divided into groups depending on the presence or absence of complete AV block during hospital stay (groups Ia and IIa without block and groups Ib and IIb with block). Selected clinical and laboratory variables were compared for each group. It was found that patients with inferior AMI and complete AV block had significantly higher mortality rates only in the presence of RV infarction: 41% mortality rate in group IIb versus 11% mortality rate in group Ib. Patients with RV infarction but without complete AV block (group IIa) had a mortality rate similar to that found in patients with inferior AMI and no AV block (group Ia): 14% versus 11%. In patients with inferior AMI without RV involvement (group I), complete AV block did not influence survival: 14% mortality rate in group Ib versus 11% mortality rate in group Ia. The excessively high mortality rate in patients who have inferior AMI with RV involvement and complete AV block could be the consequence of greater infarct size, but the synergistic influence of RV infarction and complete AV block could be the other factor that influences outcome.

To elucidate determinants of hemodynamic compromise in patients with acute RV infarction, Goldstein and co-investigators[52] in St. Louis, Missouri, studied 16 patients with hemodynamically severe RV infarction by right sided heart catheterization and 2-dimensional ultrasound. Severe RV systolic dysfunction, evident by ultrasound in all patients as RV dilatation and depressed RV free wall motion, was associated with a broad sluggish RV waveform, diminished peak RV systolic pressure and depressed RV stroke work. Paradoxical septal motion was consistently noted. In some cases, the septum bulged into the RV in a pistonlike fashion and appeared to mediate systolic ventricular interaction through which LV septal contraction contributed to RV pressure generation. RV diastolic dysfunction was indicated by elevated RV end-diastolic pressures, RV "dip and plateau," equalization of diastolic filling pressures, and reversal of diastolic septal curvature, toward the volume-deprived LV. A prominent RA X and blunted Y descent, indicative of impairment of RV filling throughout diastole, were confirmed in all patients by their relation to RV systolic events. In eight patients an RA W pattern was evident, characterized by augmented A waves; eight others manifested an M pattern constituted by depressed A waves. Compared with those with an M pattern, patients with a W pattern had higher peak RV pressures, better cardiac output, more favorable response to volume and inotropes, and less frequently required emergency revascularization for refractory shock. Angiography in patients with depressed A waves demonstrated more proximal coronary obstruction leading to ischemic compromise of RA function, whereas in those with augmented A waves, the culprit lesion was proximal to the RV but distal to the RA branches. These results indicate that hemodynamic compromise in patients with RV infarction is exacerbated by deceased preload reserve that is dependent on atrial systole. The amplitude of the RA A wave, an indication of the status of RA function, is an important determinant of RV performance and hemodynamic compromise.

Rupture of left ventricular free wall

Batts and associates[53] from Rochester, Minnesota, reviewed 100 consecutive autopsy cases of rupture of the LV free wall during AMI: 51% deaths were in-hospital and 49% were out-of-hospital. There were 51 men (mean age, 72 years) and 49 women (mean age, 76 years); 81% had multi-vessel CAD. All had severe obstruction of at least 1 major epicardial coronary artery (98 atherosclerotic, 1 thrombotic, and 1 embolic). Acute coronary thrombosis was present in 73 cases and occurred on an atherosclerotic plaque in 72, 49 (68%) of which had associated plaque rupture. In 83 cases, the ruptured infarct represented the subject's first AMI. Despite a history of systemic hypertension in 55 cases, appreciable LV hypertrophy was observed in only 19 cases. By histopathologic age of the infarct, 13 ruptures occurred during the first day, 45 between days 2 and 5, and 22 on days 6 and 7; thus, 58% occurred within 5 days and 80% within 7 days. The mid-ventricle was the most frequent site of rupture (66%). Ruptures most frequently involved the lateral aspect of the LV free wall (44%). In 66 cases, the rupture tract occurred along the interface between viable and necrotic myocardium. Their findings support the observations of others that the risk factors for postinfarction LV free wall rupture include age >60 years, female gender, preexisting hypertension, absence of LV hypertrophy, first AMI, and midventricular or lateral wall transmural infarction.

Rupture of the LV free wall is a major complication of AMI, and it usually leads to hemopericardium with tamponade. During the last 16 years, Roberts[54] from Bethesda, Maryland, studied 138 patients with LV free wall rupture during AMI: 131 (95%) had associated hemopericardium with probable or definite tamponade and 7 (5%) had no blood in the pericardial sac. The 7 patients without hemopericardium had no distinctive features in comparison to the 131 patients who also had LV free wall rupture but with hemopericardium. This report was the first to describe LV free wall rupture during AMI unassociated with either hemopericardium or false LV aneurysm.

Rupture of ventricular septum

Bansal and associates[55] from Loma Linda, California, used 2-dimensional echocardiography, pulsed and continuous wave Doppler techniques for evaluation of 15 consecutive patients aged 51 to 79 years with ventricular septal rupture during AMI. Standard and modified off-axis 2-dimensional echocardiographic views from parasternal, apical and subcostal windows correctly identified this defect in 14 of the 15 patients. Pulsed Doppler echocardiography confirmed the presence of left-to-right-sided shunt by showing a high-velocity, aliased, systolic flow and a low-velocity diastolic flow in the RV in 14 patients. Continuous wave Doppler echocardiography showed a high-velocity systolic and low-velocity diastolic flow signal of left-to-right shunt in 14 patients. Color flow Doppler imaging identified a left-to-right shunt in all 6 patients in whom it was performed. Doppler and 2-dimensional echocardiographic studies missed a small apical septal defect in 1 patient with anteroseptal myocardial infarction. Two-dimensional echocardiography correctly diagnosed RV infarction in all 5 patients with posteroinferior infarction. Ventricular septal rupture and/or left-to-right-sided shunt was confirmed in all 15 patients by the following: surgical inspection in 11, necropsy in 3, LV cineangiography in 5 and right-sided heart catheterization and oximetry data in 13 patients. Data indicate that 2-dimensional echocardiography correctly shows the precise location of septal rupture in most patients after AMI and allows assessment of left and RV infarction and function. Pulsed, continuous wave and color flow Doppler imaging shows the presence and location of left-to-right-sided shunt and differentiates this lesion from acute MR. Complete Doppler and 2-dimensional echocardiographic studies make invasive and potentially hazardous LV cineangiography unnecessary for the majority of patients with ventricular septal rupture.

Doppler color flow mapping in conjunction with 2-dimensional echocardiography was used by Helmcke and co-workers[56] in Birmingham, Alabama, to evaluate ventricular septal rupture after AMI (7 anterior and 8 inferior) in 15 patients and to correlate these findings with cardiac catheterization and surgical or autopsy data. Ventricular septal rupture was diagnosed by turbulent flow traversing the ventricular septum. The direction and velocity of shunt flow was determined by color M-mode and conventional Doppler methods. In all patients, Doppler color flow mapping correctly defined the site of septal rupture, which occurred at areas of discordant septal wall motion or "hinge points". Each of 3 patients with moderate TR and 3 of 4 patients with right-to-left shunting during diastole died, and all had an elevated RV end-diastolic pressure. RV wall motion index was significantly higher in the patients who died compared with those who survived, but there was no difference in LV wall motion index. The rupture size measured by Doppler color flow imaging (1.7 cm) correlated with the size determined during surgery or autopsy (1.8 cm) and the pulmonic-to-systemic shunt flow ratio by cardiac catheterization. Color-guided continuous-wave Doppler estimates of RV systolic pressure correlated with cardiac catheterization measurements. Two dimensional echocardiography combined with Doppler color flow mapping allows detection, evaluation, and prognostication in ventricular septal rupture.

Skillington and associates[57] from Southampton, UK, reviewed results of surgical treatment of post AMI VSD in 101 patients (mean age 65 years) over a 15-year period (1973–1988). The overall early mortality rate was 21%, although the most recent experience with 36 patients (January 1987 to October 1988) has seen this decline to 11% (Figure 3-10). Factors found to influence early death significantly, when analyzed univariately, were as follows: 1) site of infarction (anterior 12%, inferior 33%); 2) time interval between infarction and operation (<1 week 34%, >1 week 11%); 3) cardiogenic shock (present 38%, absent 9%). Nonsignificant variables included preoperative renal function, age, and concomitant CABG, although older age (>65 years) became significant when examined in a multivariate fashion. Of the 80 hospital survivors, 8 were subsequently found to have a recurrent or residual defect necessitating reoperation, with survival in 7. Late follow-up is 99% complete and reveals an actuarial survival rate for 100 patients of 71% at 5 years, and 40% at 10 years. A significant recent change in policy of not using coronary angiography in patients with a VSD caused by anterior wall AMI has not resulted in any increase in either the early mortality or in the late prevalence of angina. The functional status of 38 surviving patients has been analyzed by a graded treadmill exercise protocol, whereas LV functional assessment was by nuclear scan with additional information on MV function by echocardiogram. Most late survivors had limited exercise tolerance related to both cardiac and noncardiac factors. LV function was moderately impaired (mean EF = 0.39). However, many patients were elderly and

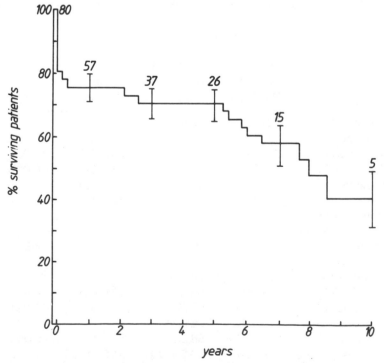

Fig. 3-10. Actuarial survival for all patients (n = 100). Vertical bars refer to ± 1 standard error for each calculation. Numbers above error bars refer to number of surviving patients for each time period. Reproduced with permission from Skillington, et al.[57]

have adapted to their residual symptoms without significant changes in life-style.

Mitral regurgitation

To determine the frequency, natural history and clinical correlates of the murmur of MR detected after AMI, Barzilai and associates[58] from St. Louis, Missouri, analyzed clinical data from 849 patients with AMI. A murmur suggestive of MR was present on admission in 76 patients (9%). Patients with MR on admission were older and more apt to be female and nonwhite (Table 3-4). They also had a significantly greater frequency of prior AMI and signs and symptoms of CHF. There was no difference in the location (anterior or inferior) of the AMI. Patients with MR on admission had a 36% mortality compared to 16% for those who developed MR later in the hospitalization and 15% for those without MR by auscultation. Correction for differences in baseline variables indicated that the presence of MR on admission did not contribute independently to mortality. Thus, the murmur of MR derives its prognostic significance from integration of multiple clinical, radiographic and electrocardiographic characteristics.

Ventricular fibrillation

To determine the prognosis of late VF after AMI, Jensen and associates[59] from Copenhagen, Denmark, extended the length of the monitoring pe-

TABLE 3-4. *Patient characteristics. Reproduced with permission from Barzilai, et al.*[58]

	MR on Admission No. (%)	MR Developing Days 1 to 11 No. (%)	No MR No. (%)	p Value
Female	33 (43)	28 (30)	171 (25)	0.003
Nonwhite	26 (34)	25 (27)	124 (18)	0.001
Previous MI	33 (43)	26 (28)	140 (21)	<0.001
History of CHF	19 (25)	11 (12)	41 (6)	<0.001
S_3 sounds	38 (50)	25 (27)	101 (15)	<0.001
Rales	47 (62)	48 (52)	289 (43)	0.002
Abnormal neck vein distention	25 (33)	20 (22)	84 (12)	<0.001
Infarct extension	5 (7)	9 (10)	58 (9)	NS
ST depression	23 (32)	14 (16)	84 (13)	<0.001
Anterior MI	50 (76)	53 (67)	414 (65)	NS
Transmural MI	34 (48)	53 (63)	418 (64)	0.034
Complex VEA	27 (50)	16 (23)	137 (26)	<0.001
Age (yrs)	61.5 ± 1.8	58.2 ± 1.1	56.2 ± 0.4	<0.001
Karnofsky Score (admission)	8.00 ± 0.15	9.12 ± 0.14	9.05 ± 0.05	<0.001

CHF = congestive heart failure; MI = myocardial infarction; NS = not significant; VEA = ventricular ectopic activity.

riod after AMI. All patients were continuously monitored in a coronary care unit to ensure observation of all VF within 18 days of AMI. From 1977 to 1985, 4,269 patients were admitted with AMI and 413 (9.6%) had in-hospital VF. Of these 281 (6.8%) had early VF (<48 hours after AMI) and 132 (3.2%) had late VF (≥48 hours after AMI). In-hospital mortality was 50 and 54% for early and late VF, respectively. Kaplan-Meier survival analysis showed better survival after discharge for patients with early versus late VF but this difference was fully explained by the presence of heart failure. Survival analysis showed the same prognosis after 1, 3 and 5 years for early and late VF, when VF was not associated with CHF. When VF was associated with heart failure (secondary VF) early VF had a greater mortality than late VF after 2 and 5 years. Logistic regression analysis showed that heart failure (relative risk 1.9) and cardiogenic shock (relative risk 3.9) were significant risk factors for in-hospital death. Late VF compared to early VF had no prognostic implication (relative risk 1.0). For patients discharged from the hospital, risk factors were CHF (1.8) and previous AMI (1.6). Late VF showed a trend (1.2) toward poorer long-term prognosis than early VF.

Willems and associates[60] in Amsterdam, Rotterdam, Nieuwegein, Utrecht and Maastricht, The Netherlands, evaluated 390 patients with sustained symptomatic VT and VF after AMI in a multicenter study. Patients were given standard antiarrhythmic therapy which consisted primarily of drug therapy. During a mean follow-up period of 1.9 years, 133 patients died. Arrhythmic events and CHF were the most common causes of death. Forty-one patients died suddenly, 31 died because of recurrent VT or VF, and 23 died of CHF. One hundred ninety-two patients (49%) had at least 1 recurrent arrhythmic event. Eighty-five percent of first arrhythmic events were nonfatal. Multivariate analysis of data from patients who developed the arrhythmia <6 weeks after AMI identified 5 variables as independent determinants of total mortality, including: 1) age >70 years; 2) Killip class III or IV in the subacute phase of AMI; 3) cardiac arrest during the index arrhythmia; 4) anterior AMI; and 5) multiple previous AMIs. Multivariate analysis of data from patients developing the arrhythmias more than 6 weeks after AMI identified four variables as independently predictive of total mortality, including: 1) Q wave AMI; 2) cardiac arrest during the index arrhythmia; 3) Killip class III or IV in the subacute phase of AMI; and 4) multiple previous AMIs. The two multivariate analyses were used to develop a model for prediction of mortality at one year. The average predicted mortality rate varied according to the model. Among 243 patients (62%) with the lowest predicted risk, it was 13% and corresponded to an observed mortality rate of 12%. In 92 patients (24%) with intermediate risk, it was 27% corresponding to an observed rate of 28%. In the 55 patients (14%) with the highest risk, it was 64% corresponding to an observed rate of 54%. Thus, this study demonstrates that patients with symptomatic VT or VF after AMI who are given standard antiarrhythmic therapy have a relatively high mortality rate. However, models may be developed that identify patients at low, intermediate, and high risk and these may be useful in designing appropriate diagnostic and therapeutic strategies that prolong the lives of these individuals.

The multicenter randomized study of the Gruppo Italiano per lo Studio della Streptochinasi nell'Infarto Miocardico has provided the opportunity to analyze the impact of thrombolytic treatment on secondary VF incidence in a large population of patients (11,712) with AMI. Volpi and co-workers[61] in Milan, Italy, observed a reduction of about 20% in the frequency of secondary VF among patients allocated to thrombolytic treatment (streptokinase, 2.4% versus control, 2.9%). Streptokinase appeared to exert its protective effect specifically in patients treated within 3 hours of onset of symptoms (streptokinase, 2.6% versus control, 3.7%). This protection was essentially due to a reduced incidence of late VF occurring after the first day of hospitalization. The 311 patients with secondary VF represented an overall incidence of 2.7%. Such incidence was not related to infarct location or sex but was significantly more common in patients older than 65 years. The significant excess of in-hospital deaths was found in patients with secondary VF compared with those in the reference group. Conversely, secondary VF was not a predictor of 1-year mortality for hospital survivors. Thrombolytic treatment with intravenous scintigraphic and electrocardiographic evidence of exercise-induced ischemia were comparable in patients with chest pain, emission computed tomography was superior to stress electrocardiography for detecting silent myocardial ischemia. Most patients with CAD who developed ischemia during exercise testing were asymptomatic, although they had an angiographic profile and extent of abnormally perfused myocardium similar to those of patients with symptomatic ischemia.

Behar and other investigators[62] of the Secondary Prevention Reinfarction Israeli Nifedipine Trial (SPRINT) analyzed 5,839 consecutive patients with AMI hospitalized between July, 1981 and July, 1983 in 14 coronary care units in Israel and found incidence of primary VF to be 2.1%. Primary VF was defined as VF complicating a first or recurrent AMI occurring within 48 hours of admission in patients in Killip Class I. Thus, no patient had clinical or x-ray signs of CHF on admission to the coronary care unit and neither CHF, pulmonary edema, cardiogenic shock, or persistent hypotension preceded the occurrence of VF. The patients with primary VF resembled counterparts without VF in terms of age, gender, frequency of previous AMI and past cigarette smoking habits. The hospital course of patients with primary VF revealed increased incidence of primary AF and AV block. Increased serum levels of glutamic oxaloacetic transaminase and lactic dehydrogenase were noted among the patients with primary VF. In-hospital mortality rate was 19% in 122 patients with primary VF compared with 8.5% in 3,707 patients forming the reference group. Adjustment by age using logistic function yielded an estimate of 2.86 for relative mortality odds associated with primary VF, and further adjustment by gender, history of AMI, systemic hypertension, and by enzymatically estimated infarct size slightly reduced the estimated odds, at 2.52. Prognosis after discharge from the hospital was independent of primary VF. In conclusion, primary VF exerts an independent, significant effect on in-hospital mortality.

GENERAL TREATMENT

Therapeutic flow diagram

A superb review on prognosis and management after first AMI was provided by Moss and Benhorin[63] from Rochester, New York. Figure 3-11 provides a flow diagram of the treatment of patients after hospitalization for a first AMI. Moss and Benhorin emphasized a few caveats. First, the rate of progression of CAD is variable and unpredictable. Second, coronary angiography is not indicated as a routine diagnostic procedure

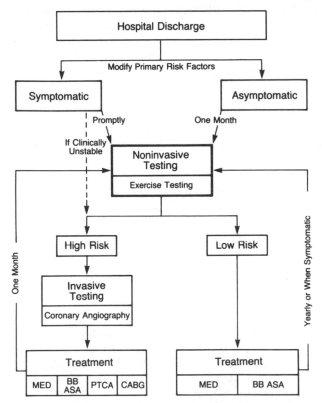

Fig. 3-11. Flow diagram of the treatment of patients after hospitalization for a first myocardial infarction. In patients who become symptomatic early after hospital discharge and are clinically unstable, invasive testing may need to be done immediately (vertical dashed line). In patients at high risk who have undergone invasive testing and treatment, follow-up exercise testing should be done one month later to evaluate the results of treatment. See text for details. ASA denotes acetylsalicylic acid, BB beta blockers, CABG coronary-artery bypass graft surgery, MED medication, and PTCA percutaneous transluminal coronary angioplasty. Reproduced with permission from Moss, et al.[63]

after a first AMI, because it does not provide accurate information about subsequent coronary events. This recommendation applies to all age groups, not withstanding the conventional approach according to which younger patients having their first AMI are usually referred for coronary angiography to evaluate the extent and severity of the CAD. Third, the detection of myocardial ischemia by exercise stress testing is currently the best approach for the identification of asymptomatic patients with myocardial regions supplied by critically narrowed coronary arteries. Nevertheless, non-invasive techniques currently available for detecting jeopardized ischemic myocardium are imperfect. Finally, the appropriate interval for periodic, non-invasive follow-up testing in the asymptomatic patient after a first AMI is not known. On the basis of the reported survivorship studies, the best estimate for periodic testing is at yearly intervals.

Smoking cessation

To determine the effect of a nurse-managed intervention for cigarette smoking cessation in patients who have had an AMI, Taylor and associates[64] from Stanford, California, randomized with a 6-month treatment period and a 6-month follow-up 173 patients 70 years of age or younger who were smoking before hospitalization for AMI. Eighty-six patients were randomly assigned to the intervention and 87 to usual care; 130 patients (75%) completed the study and were available for follow-up. Nurse-managed and focused on preventing relapse to smoking, the intervention was initiated in the hospital and maintained thereafter primarily through telephone contact. Patients were given an 18-page manual that emphasized how to identify and cope with high-risk situations for smoking relapse. One year after AMI, the smoking cessation rate, verified biochemically, was 71% in the intervention group compared with 45% in the usual care group, a 26% difference. Assuming that all surviving patients lost to follow-up were smoking, the 12-month smoking cessation rate was 61% in the intervention group compared with 32% in the usual care group, a 29% difference. Patients who either resumed smoking within 3 weeks after infarction or expressed little intention of stopping in the hospital were unlikely to have stopped by 12 months. A nurse-managed smoking cessation intervention largely conducted by telephone, initiated in the hospital, and focused on relapse prevention can significantly reduce smoking rates at 12 months in patients who have had an AMI.

Lipid lowering

The Program on the Surgical Control of the Hyperlipidemias (POSCH), a randomized clinical trial, was designed to test whether cholesterol lowering induced by the partial ileal bypass operation would favorably affect overall mortality or mortality due to CAD. The study population consisted of 838 patients (417 in the control group and 421 in the surgery group), both men (91%) and women, with an average age of 51 years, who had survived a first AMI. The mean follow-up period was 9.7 years. Buchwald and associates[65] from the POSCH Group found that the surgery group when compared to the control group at 5 years had a total plasma cholesterol level 23% lower (4.71 ± 0.91 vs 6.14 ± 0.89 mmol/l), a LDL cholesterol level 38% lower (2.68 ± 0.78 vs 4.30 ± 0.89 mmol/l) and a HDL cholesterol level 4% higher (1.08 ± 0.26 vs 1.04 ± 0.25 mmol/l) (Figure 3-12). Overall mortality and mortality due to CAD were reduced, but not significantly so (deaths overall [control vs surgery], 62 vs 49; deaths due to CAD, 44 vs 32). The overall mortality in the surgery subgroup with an EF ≥50% was 36% lower (control vs surgery, 39 vs 24). The value for 2 end points combined—death due to CAD and confirmed nonfatal myocardial infarction—was 35% lower in the surgery group (125 vs 82 events) (Figure 3-13). During follow-up, 137 control-group and 52 surgery-group patients underwent CABG. A comparison of base-line coronary arteriograms with those obtained at 3, 5, 7, and 10 years consistently showed less disease progression in the surgery group. The most common side effect of partial ileal bypass was diarrhea; others included occasional kidney stones, gallstones, and intestinal obstruction. Partial ileal bypass produces sustained improvement in the blood lipid patterns of patients who have had a myocardial infarction and reduces their subsequent morbidity due to CAD. These results provide strong evidence supporting the beneficial effects of lipid modification in the reduction of atherosclerosis progression.

Rossouw and associates[66] reviewed relevant data from observational and clinical trials of the value of lowering total and LDL cholesterol levels after AMI. These authors concluded that cholesterol lowering in patients who have had AMI is useful because the already high risk of reinfarction

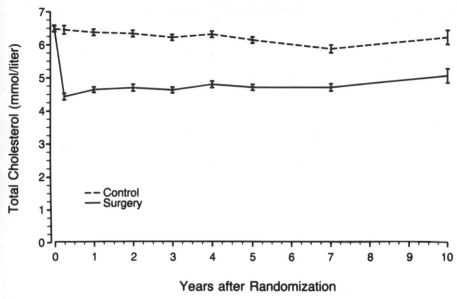

Fig. 3-12. Total plasma cholesterol levels in the control and surgery groups. Values are means with 95 Percent confidence intervals. The difference between the groups at each follow-up interval was significant (P<0.0001). Reproduced with permission from Buchwald, et al.[65]

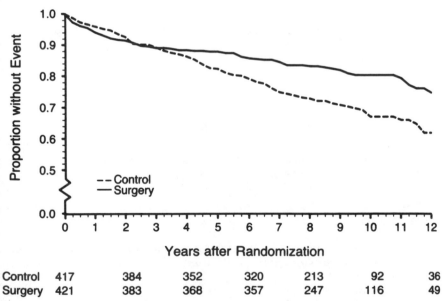

| Control | 417 | 384 | 352 | 320 | 213 | 92 | 36 |
| Surgery | 421 | 383 | 368 | 357 | 247 | 116 | 49 |

Fig. 3-13. Confirmed myocardial infarction and death due to atherosclerotic coronary heart disease as a combined end point ("event") in the study groups. The difference between the groups was significant (P<0.001). The number of patients at risk for an event are shown at two-year intervals. Reproduced with permission from Buchwald, et al.[65]

is aggravated by an elevated serum cholesterol level. The authors summarized secondary prevention trials which in total have demonstrated a 10% reduction in total cholesterol can be expected to reduce the rate of non-fatal reinfarction by 19% and of fatal AMI by 12% (Table 3-5). The

TABLE 3-5. *Rates of myocardial infarction in secondary prevention trials of cholesterol lowering.* Reproduced with permission from Rossouw, et al.[66]

TRIAL	NO. OF PATIENTS RANDOMIZED		NONFATAL INFARCTIONS		FATAL INFARCTIONS		ALL INFARCTIONS	
	TREATED	CONTROL	TREATED	CONTROL	TREATED	CONTROL	TREATED	CONTROL
			percent					
Coronary Drug Project								
Clofibrate	1103	2789	13.1	13.8	17.7	19.2	28.0	30.1
Niacin	1119	2789	10.2	13.8†	18.1	19.2	25.6	30.1‡
Newcastle (clofibrate)	244	253	12.3	18.2	10.2	17.4‡	21.3	32.0†
Edinburgh (clofibrate)	350	367	7.1	11.2	9.7	9.5	15.4	19.6
Stockholm (clofibrate + niacin)	279	276	12.5	18.1	16.8	26.4†	25.8	36.2‡
Oslo (diet)	206	206	11.7	15.0	18.0	24.3	29.6	39.3‡
Medical Research Council								
Low-fat diet	123	129	16.3	14.7	8.1	9.3	24.4	24.0
Soybean oil	199	194	10.1	13.4	12.6	12.9	22.6	26.3
Sum, observed events less expected events§			−63¶		−49†		−98¶	
Odds ratio (95% confidence interval)			0.75 (0.65–0.85)		0.84 (0.74–0.94)		0.78 (0.70–0.86)	

*P values indicate two-sided significance of the differences between the treated and control groups in each trial, as calculated by the Mantel–Haenszel statistic. The meta-analysis of all trials combined was performed as described by Mantel and Haenszel and applied according to the method of Yusuf et al.

†P<0.01.

‡P<0.05.

§Denotes the sum of the differences between the number of events expected in each treated group if there were no treatment effects and the number of events actually observed. If the treated and control groups are equal in size, this number is about half the actual difference in the number of events.

¶P<0.001.

authors point out that two-thirds of patients with symptoms of myocardial ischemia have serum total cholesterol levels >5.17 mmol/l and would thus be subject to lipoprotein analysis under current guidelines, and most would have LDL cholesterol levels >3.36 mmol/l and would thus be considered for therapy under the present guidelines. The authors recommend that the goal for LDL cholesterol lowering should be 2.58 mmol/l.

Beta blocker

Nidorf and associates[67] from Perth, Australia, performed a retrospective analysis collected on patients admitted during 4 years to the hospital with AMI from 1984–1987. The objective was to see whether patients taking an oral β-blocker at the time of admission to hospital with AMI had a reduced risk of death at 28 days. A total of 2,430 consecutive patients were studied. Patients were grouped into those who were and were not taking a β-blocker at the time of admission. Though patients taking a β-blocker were older and more likely to have a history of AMI, angina, or systemic hypertension, the overall mortality at 28 days was similar in the 2 groups. Although the incidence of fatal VF was similar in the 2 groups, mean peak creatine kinase activity was significantly lower in the β-blocker group. A logistic regression model used to adjust for factors predictive of cardiac death at 28 days confirmed that patients taking a β-blocker at the time of admission had a significantly reduced risk of death. These data support the value of long-term use of β-blockers in patients at risk of AMI. They suggest that patients taking these agents before admission to hospital with AMI have a significant survival advantage at 28 days, which may be due to a reduction in infarct size.

Propranolol

Jafri and associates[68] from Detroit, Michigan, studied the effect of propranolol on mortality and reinfarction after AMI in cigarette smokers and nonsmokers in the Beta Blocker Heart Attack Trial. Cigarette smokers (n = 2,332) were 5 years younger than nonsmokers and had a lower incidence of diabetes mellitus, systemic hypertension, previous AMI and cardiomegaly. Among cigarette smokers, the placebo group had a higher total mortality rate than the propranolol group (11.0 vs 7.4%) and more sudden cardiac deaths (7.1 vs 4.6%). In nonsmokers the placebo group had a mortality (7.9 vs 7.1%) similar to the propranolol group. After baseline adjustment, cigarette smokers were estimated to have 1.6 times the risk of dying as compared to nonsmokers. Adjusting for baseline differences, both treatment with propranolol and nonsmoking were predictors of survival. No detectable nonsmoking/propranolol interaction could be identified. In survivors of AMI a beneficial effect of propranolol is observed for cigarette smokers. Nevertheless, cigarette smoking continues to be a risk factor for mortality after AMI even for those receiving propranolol.

Beta-blockers represent the only documented effective long-term prophylactic treatment for patients after AMI. Concern continues to be expressed about the lipid-altering effects of their long-term use, especially β-blockers without intrinsic sympathomimetic activity such as propranolol. Data collected for the Beta-Blocker Heart Attack Trial, the largest long-term clinical trial of β-blocker use in patients after AMI, were analyzed by Byington and associates[69] from Winston-Salem, North Carolina, to address the following questions. To what extent does propranolol alter lipid levels at least 6 months after AMI and initiation of therapy? How predictive of subsequent coronary events and mortality are lipid levels 6 months after AMI? Is there any evidence that altered lipid levels attenuate any of the beneficial effect of propranolol on coronary morbidity and mortality? By the 6-month post-AMI visit, propranolol was shown to raise serum triglyceride levels by about 17% ($\cong$ 35 mg/dl) and to lower serum HDL cholesterol by about 6% ($\cong$ 3 mg/dl). There was no effect on total cholesterol or LDL cholesterol. In other analyses, no lipid measured 6 months after the AMI was strongly predictive of subsequent coronary events or mortality. For example, every 1-mg-lower HDL value was associated with only a 0.7% relative increase in the mortality rate. Theoretically, the estimated relative increase on all-cause mortality associated with propranolol-induced HDL reduction is about 2%. In multivariate analyses adjusting for changes in HDL and serum triglyceride, propranolol-induced beneficial reductions in mortality and morbidity remained on the order of 20%, 10 times the estimated hazard.

Horwitz and associates[70] from New Haven, Connecticut, investigated the relation of treatment adherence to mortality after an AMI among 2,175 participants in the Beta Blocker Heart Attack Trial, which had data for measures of treatment adherence, clinical severity, and the psychological and social features that may influence post-AMI mortality. Overall, patients who did not adhere well to treatment regimen (i.e., who took ≤75% of prescribed medication) were 2.6 times more likely than good adherers to die within a year of follow-up. Poor adherers had an increased risk of death whether they were on propranolol or placebo. Furthermore, this increased risk of death for poor adherers was not accounted for by measures of the severity of AMI, sociodemographic features (e.g., race, marital status, education), smoking, or psychological characteristics (high life-stress or social isolation).

Acebutolol

Acebutolol et Prevention Secondaire de l'Infarctus (APSI), a randomized, placebo-controlled trial, was designed to test long-term acebutolol, 200 mg twice daily, a β-blocker with mild intrinsic sympathomimetic activity, in the prevention of late death in high-risk post-AMI patients. The results of this study were reported by Boissel and associates[71] for the APSI investigators from Lyon, France. APSI was planned because patients with a death rate >20% have not been enrolled in significant numbers in previous trials and in such high-risk patients, it remained to be proven that β-blockers have a beneficial effect. Patients with an expected average risk of >20% were selected based on clinical criteria. At the time of the second interim analysis, the placebo group 1-year mortality was much lower than expected (12%). The ethical board recommended to stop the trial: 309 patients had been allocated to placebo, 298 to acebutolol. The average delay between onset of symptoms and inclusion was 10.5 days. The average follow-up was 318 days after inclusion. About the same number of patients were discontinued from study treatment in both groups. All patients were included in the analysis. There were 17 deaths in the acebutolol group and 34 in the placebo group, a 48% decrease. The vascular mortality decreased by 58%, the highest ever observed with a β-blocker (Figure 3-14). All cardiovascular causes of death, including CAD, were less frequent in the acebutolol group. Although the objective was not achieved, APSI patients were at a higher risk than the average of the 9 previous trials with β-blockers (12% instead of 7%) (Figure

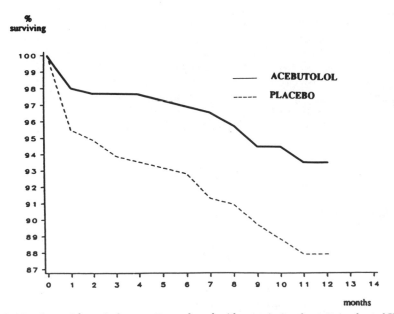

Fig. 3-14. Actuarial survival curve. Reproduced with permission from Boissel, et al.[71]

3-15). In addition, the total mortality reduction did not decrease in 9 subgroups with increasing mortality risk from 2 to 23%. APSI shows that moderately severe post-AMI patients can benefit from a β-blocking treatment and a β-blocker with mild intrinsic sympathomimetic activity can be effective.

Xamoterol

McMurray and associates[72] from Dundee, UK, reported the effects of the new $β_1$ adrenoceptor partial agonist, xamoterol, on neuroendocrine activity after AMI. Fifty-one consecutive patients with AMI were randomized to treatment with xamoterol, 200 mg twice a day, or placebo; patients were also stratified as to whether or not diuretic therapy was given for LV dysfunction. Noradrenalin, plasma renin activity, and atrial natriuretic factor were measured over a 10-day period. Noradrenalin concentrations were higher in patients treated with diuretics at the time of admission and fell over the subsequent 10 days. Treatment with xamoterol did not affect this noradrenalin response to AMI. Plasma renin activity was also significantly higher in the patients treated with diuretics, and there was a nonsignificant trend for xamoterol to blunt the plasma renin activity response in those patients. There was no difference in atrial natriuretic factor levels between those patients who were treated with diuretics and those who were not; xamoterol did not affect atrial natriuretic factor. Thus xamoterol does not further elevate noradrenalin levels as do conventional beta blockers, and it does not activate the renin-angiotensin system as do potent nonselective beta agonists. Furthermore, xamoterol does not increase atrial natriuretic factor levels, probably because it is not negatively inotropic. It was concluded that xamoterol does not cause deleterious neuroendocrine changes in patients with AMI even in those treated for CHF.

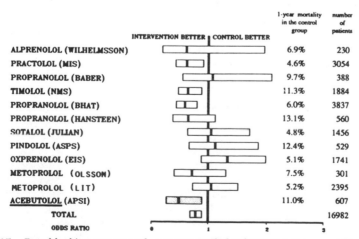

Fig. 3-15. Beta-blocking agents and post-myocardial infarction 1-year mortality. APSI = Acebutolol et Prévention Secondaire de l'Infarctus; ASPS = Australian and Swedish Pindolol Study; BHAT = Beta Blocker Heart Attack Trial; EIS = European Infarction Study; LIT = Lopressor Intervention Trial; MIS = Multicentre International Study; NMS = Norwegian Multicentre Study. Reproduced with permission from Boissel, et al.[71]

Beta blocker vs calcium antagonist

Bekheit and associates[73] from Brooklyn, New York, used spectral analysis of heart rate variability to study the effects of the calcium antagonists *diltiazem* and *nifedipine* and the β-blocker *metoprolol* on the sympathetic nervous system in patients following myocardial infarction. Energy in the low-frequency range (0.04 to 0.12 Hz) in the standing (tilt) position was used as a quantitative index of a sympathetic activity. Twenty-seven male patients, mean age 62 ± 13 years, were studied 2 to 6 weeks after myocardial infarction. Eight patients received metoprolol, 100 mg twice daily; 9 patients received diltiazem, 60 mg 3 times daily; and 10 patients received nifedipine, 10 mg 3 times daily. Heart rate variability and arterial BP were recorded before and 5 to 7 days after initiation of therapy. None of the drugs had significant effects on the systolic BP, and only nifedipine significantly reduced the diastolic BP. Metoprolol and diltiazem reduced the low-frequency heart rate variability in all patients studied, but nifedipine had no consistent effects. These results suggest that diltiazem had a depressant effect on sympathetic activity similar to β-adrenergic blockers. This effect was not observed with nifedipine. The reduction in sympathetic activity by diltiazem may contribute to its therapeutic effects in the post-infarction period.

To test the hypothesis that long-term β- or calcium-antagonist therapy begun before the time of AMI and coronary reperfusion might improve patient in-hospital survival compared with reperfusion alone, Ellis and associates[74] from Ann Arbor, Michigan, retrospectively characterized 424 consecutive patients successfully reperfused with PTCA within 12 hours of AMI symptom onset. Forty-seven patients (11%) were taking β antagonists and 74 patients (17%) were taking calcium antagonists at the time of AMI. Patients receiving β antagonists had a more frequent history of hypertension and prior infarction than those not so treated and patients receiving calcium antagonists had a more frequent history of prior AMI, prior angina, systemic hypertension and diabetes than their nontreated counterparts. Stepwise logistic regression analysis found significant independent correlations between in-hospital death and the following variables: recurrent ischemia, LAD coronary infarct, 3-vessel CAD, patient age; and initial total occlusion of the infarct-related artery. After adjustment for these factors, β antagonist use (mortality = 0 vs 8% without treatment) was still significantly correlated with improved survival, whereas calcium-antagonist therapy made no difference in survival. Heart rate and LV end-diastolic pressure upon presentation were significantly lower in patients treated with β antagonists. Thus, β-antagonist therapy, but probably not calcium-antagonist therapy, taken before reperfusion for AMI, may improve early survival compared to reperfusion alone.

Diltiazem

The a priori hypothesis that diltiazem would reduce the frequency and repetitiveness of ventricular arrhythmias was tested by Bigger and associates and the Multicenter Diltiazem Postinfarction Trial Investigators[75] 3 months after myocardial infarction. After 3 months of follow-up, 1,546 of the 2,466 patients enrolled had a 24-hour continuous electrocardiographic recording that contained ≥12 hours of analyzable data. They were similar to the patients who survived 3 months but chose not to have a 24-hour electrocardiographic recording (i.e., they were representative of the entire group that survived 3 months). After 3 months of follow-up, there were no significant differences between the diltiazem and placebo groups in the prevalence of atrioventricular block, the frequency of atrial arrhythmias or the frequency or repetitiveness of ventricular arrhythmias. Heart rate was significantly lower (67 ± 12 vs 71 ± 12 beats/min) and there was a significantly greater proportion of patients with sinus pauses ≥2 seconds in duration in the diltiazem group (6%) than in the placebo group (3%). Comparison with placebo revealed no evidence either for an anti- or proarrhythmic effect of diltiazem. There was no reduction in sudden or arrhythmic death attributable to diltiazem treatment; the fraction of total deaths that were arrhythmic by the Hinkle classification was 41% in the placebo group and 42% in the diltiazem group. It may be that the lack of effect of diltiazem on ventricular arrhythmias is partially responsible for its lack of effect on mortality after AMI.

Verapamil

The Danish Study Group on Verapamil in Myocardial Infarction[76] studied the effect of verapamil on death and major events, i.e. death or reinfarction, after AMI in a double-blind, randomized, placebo controlled multi-center trial. Eight hundred seventy-eight patients started treatment with verapamil, 360 mg/day, and 897 patients with placebo. Treatment started in the second week after admission and continued for up to 18 months (mean 16 months). Ninety-five deaths and 146 major events occurred in the verapamil group and 119 deaths and 180 major events in the placebo group. The 18-month mortality rates were 11.1 and 13.8%, and major event rates 18.0 and 21.6% in the verapamil and placebo groups, respectively. In patients without heart failure in the coronary care unit the mortality rates were 7.7% in the verapamil group and 11.8% in the placebo group and major event rates 14.6 and 19.7%. In patients with CHF the mortality rates were 17.0 and 17.5% and major event rates 24.9 and 24.9%. Long-term treatment with verapamil after an AMI caused a significant reduction in major events, and the positive effect was found in patients without CHF.

Aspirin—heparin—warfarin

The use of oral anticoagulation in the long-term treatment of survivors of AMI has been highly controversial. Smith and associates[77] from Oslo, Norway, randomly assigned 1,214 patients who had recovered from AMI (mean interval from the onset of symptoms to randomization = 27 days) to treatment with warfarin (607 patients) or placebo (607 patients) for an average of 37 months (range 24–63). At the end of the treatment period, there had been 123 deaths in the placebo group and 94 in the warfarin group—a reduction in risk of 24% (Figure 3-16). A total of 124 patients in the placebo group had reinfarctions, as compared with 82 in the warfarin group—a reduction of 34% (Figure 3-17). Furthermore, the authors observed a reduction of 55% in the number of total cerebrovascular accidents in the warfarin group as compared with the placebo group (44 vs 20). Serious bleeding was noted in 0.6% of the warfarin-treated patients per year. Long-term therapy with warfarin has an important beneficial effect after AMI and can be recommended in the treatment of patients who survive the acute phase.

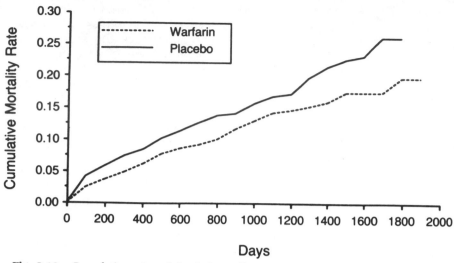

Fig. 3-16. Cumulative rates of death from all causes, according to original treatment assignment. Reproduced with permission from Smith, et al.[77]

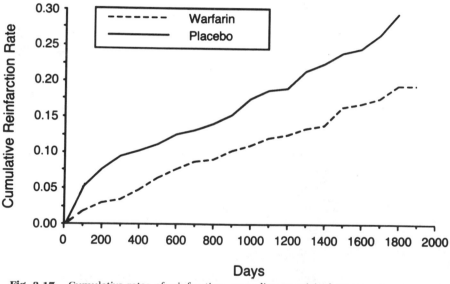

Fig. 3-17. Cumulative rates of reinfarction, according to original treatment assignment. Reproduced with permission from Smith, et al.[77]

Recently, it has been shown that aspirin given early to patients early after onset of AMI improves hospital survival, but the mechanisms involved are unclear. In a perspective, randomized placebo-controlled trial, Verheugt and associates[78] from Amsterdam, The Netherlands, studied the influence of early intervention with low-dose aspirin (100 mg/day) on myocardial infarct size and clinical outcome in 100 consecutive patients with their first anterior wall AMI. Infarct size was calculated by cumulative lactate dehydrogenase release in the first 72 hours after admission and was found to be 1,431 ± 782 U/L in the aspirin group (n = 50) and 1,592 ± 1,082 U/L in the placebo group (n = 50). The study medication was given for 3 months, during which mortality was 10 (20%) in the aspirin patients and 12 (24%) in the placebo patients. However, reinfarction occurred in 2 patients (4%) in the aspirin group and in 9 (18%) in the placebo group. Early intervention with low-dose aspirin showed, in comparison to placebo, a 10% decrease of infarct size, but this difference was not statistically significant. However, early low-dose aspirin effectively decreased the risk of reinfarction. Therefore, the favorable results of early aspirin on mortality in AMI are probably due more to prevention of reinfarction than to decrease of infarct size.

The RISC Group[79], which includes investigators from 8 hospitals in southeast Sweden, randomized 796 men with unstable angina pectoris or non-Q-wave AMI to double-blind, placebo-controlled treatment with oral aspirin 75 mg/day and/or 5 days of intermittent intravenous heparin. The risk of AMI and death was reduced by aspirin (Figure 3-18). After 5 days the risk ratio was 0.43, at 1 month 0.31, and at 3 months 0.36. Aspirin reduced event rate in non-Q-wave AMI and in unstable angina, independently of electrocardiographic abnormalities or concurrent drug therapy. Heparin had no significant influence on event rate, although the group treated with aspirin and heparin had the lowest number of events during the initial 5 days. Treatment had few side-effects and patient compliance was high.

In a prospective pilot trial of antithrombotic therapy in the acute coronary syndromes (ATACS) of resting and unstable angina pectoris or non-Q-wave AMI, Cohen and associates[80] from New York, New York, and Newcastle upon Tyne, UK, compared 3 different antithrombotic regimens in the prevention of recurrent ischemic events. Ninety-three patients were randomized to receive aspirin (325 mg/day), or full-dose heparin followed by warfarin, or the combination of aspirin (80 mg/day) plus heparin and then warfarin. Trial antithrombotic therapy was added to standardized antianginal medication and continued for 3 months or until an end point was reached. Analysis, by intention-to-treat, of the 3- month end points, revealed the following: recurrent ischemia occurred in 7 patients (22%) after aspirin, in 6 patients (25%) after heparin and warfarin, and in 16

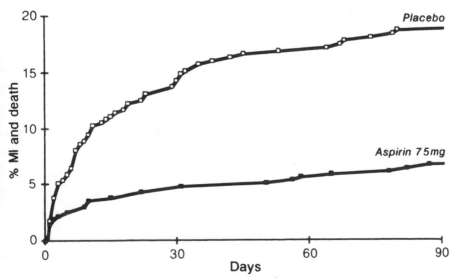

Fig. 3-18. Risk of MI and death during treatment with aspirin or placebo. Reproduced with permission from Wallentin, et al.[79]

patients (43%) after aspirin combined with heparin and then warfarin; coronary revascularization occurred in 12 patients (38%) after aspirin, in 12 patients (50%) after heparin and warfarin, and in 22 patients (60%) after aspirin combined with heparin and then warfarin; AMI occurred in 1 patient (3%) after aspirin, in 3 patients (13%) after heparin and warfarin, and in no patient after aspirin combined with heparin and then warfarin; no deaths occurred after aspirin or after aspirin combined with heparin and then warfarin, but 1 patient (4%) died after warfarin alone; major bleeding occurred in 3 patients (9%) after aspirin, in 2 patients (8%) after heparin and warfarin, and in 3 patients (8%) after aspirin combined with heparin and then warfarin. Recurrent AMI occurred at 3 ± 3 days after randomization. In those who had coronary angioplasty or bypass surgery, revascularization was performed at 6 ± 4 days. During trial therapy, no patient died, had a Q-wave AMI or a major bleed. Most bleeding complications consisted of blood transfusions during or immediately after bypass surgery. Only 25% of patients enrolled were discharged on trial therapy because of revascularization and withdrawals. Thus, irrespective of the antithrombotic regimen used, and even with aggressive combination therapy, a substantial fraction of patients with unstable angina or non-Q-wave AMI have recurrent AMI and are referred for coronary revascularization. Antithrombotic therapy, coupled with early intervention after recurring ischemia, was associated with a low rate of death or AMI within the first 3 months.

Amiodarone

Burkart and colleagues[81] in Basel, Switzerland studied 1,220 survivors of AMI to evaluate the effects of prophylactic antiarrhythmic treatment prospectively in patients with persisting asymptomatic complex arrhythmias after AMI. Among these patients, 312 had Lown class 3 or 4b arrhythmias on 24 hour electrocardiographic recordings before hospital discharge. These patients were randomized to individualized antiarrhythmic therapy (100 patients, Group 1); treatment with low dose amiodarone, 200 mg/day, Group 2 (n = 98); and no antiarrhythmic therapy in Group 3 (n = 114 patients). During the 1 year follow-up period, 10 patients in Group 1, 5 in Group 2 and 15 in Group 3 died. On the basis of an intention to treat analysis, the probability of survival of patients given amiodarone was significantly greater than for control patients. Antiarrhythmic events were also significantly reduced by amiodarone treatment. These effects were less marked and not significant for individually treated patients. These data suggest that low dose amiodarone therapy decreases mortality in the first year after AMI in patients at increased risk for sudden death. (Figures 3-19 and 3-20).

Magnesium sulfate

Shechter and associates[82] from Tel Aviv, Israel, evaluated the effect of magnesium on the incidence of arrhythmias and mortality in 103 patients with AMI in a randomized, double-blind, placebo-controlled study. Fifty patients received a magnesium infusion for 48 hours and 53 received only the vehicle (isotonic glucose) as placebo. The baseline characteristics of the population were similar in the 2 groups. Tachyarrhythmias requiring drug therapy were recorded in 32% of the patients in the magnesium group and in 45% of the placebo group. Conduction disturbances

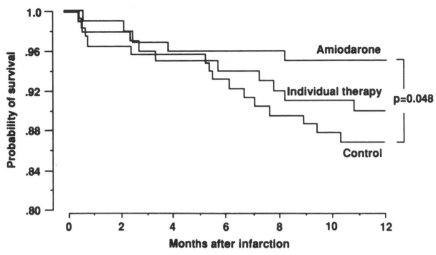

Fig. 3-19. Probability of 12 month survival in the three treatment groups of patients with asymptomatic complex ventricular arrhythmias after myocardial infarction. Reproduced with permission from Burkart, et al.[81]

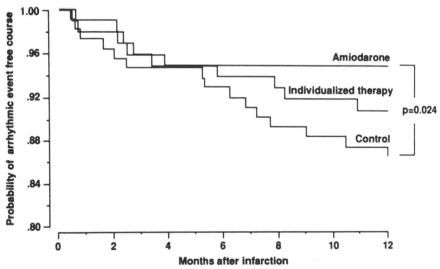

Fig. 3-20. Probability of an arrhythmic event-free course during the 1 year follow-up period in the three treatment groups of patients with asymptomatic complex ventricular arrhythmia after myocardial infarction. Arrhythmic events are sudden death, ventricular fibrillation and symptomatic sustained ventricular tachycardia. Reproduced with permission from Burkart, et al.[81]

were found in 23% of the placebo group as compared to 14% in the magnesium group. The intrahospital mortality was 2% (1 patient) in the magnesium group, compared to 17% (9 patients) in the placebo group. No adverse effects were observed during and after the magnesium infusion. These data support a possible protective role of magnesium in patients with AMI.

THROMBOLYSIS

Eligibility

Muller and Topol[83] provided a superb review of current recommendations regarding the eligibility of patients with AMI for thrombolytic therapy. They also provided a list of common contraindications to thrombolytic therapy (Table 3-6).

Based on the registration of all the 7,157 patients admitted during a 21-month period to the emergency ward of a single hospital in an urban area with chest pain or other symptoms suggestive of AMI, Karlson and co-investigators[84] in Gothenburg, Sweden, studied eligibility for intravenous thrombolysis in suspected AMI. The investigators limited the present analysis to 1,715 patients with a strong suspicion of AMI, and for them calculated the percentages eligible for thrombolysis when various electrocardiographic and delay time criteria were applied, but they did not consider contraindications to thrombolysis. The investigators also calculated the proportions of all infarctions in this group that would thereby receive the treatment, and the proportions of patients treated that would develop a confirmed infarction. Using the criteria ST elevation on the initial electrocardiogram and arrival in hospital within 6 hours from onset of symptoms, 18% of patients would have been given early intravenous thrombolysis, 37% of confirmed infarctions would have been treated, and 91% of all treated patients would have developed a confirmed infarction; with a delay in time criterion of 12 hours, these percentages would have

TABLE 3-6. *Common "contraindications" to thrombolytic therapy. Reproduced with permission from Muller, et al.*[83]

Known bleeding disorders including those secondary to severe hepatic or renal disease

Poorly controlled systolic or diastolic hypertension

Past cerebrovascular event or known intracranial aneurysm, arteriovenous malformation, or neoplasm

Recent trauma including prolonged cardiopulmonary resuscitation within the past 2 weeks

Major surgery within the last 2 months, especially intracranial or spinal surgery

Gastrointestinal or genitourinary bleeding within the preceding 4 weeks

Oral anticoagulant therapy

Childbearing potential

Diabetes with proliferative retinopathy

Likelihood of left atrial or left ventricular thrombus including mitral valve disease and chronic atrial fibrillation

Recent streptococcal infection or treatment with streptokinase (contraindicates further streptokinase therapy)

Previous coronary artery bypass graft surgery

Previous myocardial infarction in the same site

Left bundle-branch block

Cardiogenic shock

been 20%, 41%, and 91%, respectively; with a criterion of 24 hours, they would have been 22%, 45%, and 90%, respectively. By not considering the initial electrocardiogram and applying only the criterion of delay time, these percentages would have been 70%, 72%, and 45%, respectively, for a delay time of 6 hours; 83%, 84%, and 45%, respectively, for a delay time of 12 hours; and 91%, and 92%, and 44%, respectively, for a delay time of 24 hours. The investigators also calculated these percentages for 2 further electrocardiographic criteria, namely, electrocardiogram showing acute ischemia and any form of pathology. The investigators concluded that the percentage of patients with a strong suspicion of AMI, eligible for intravenous thrombolysis varies considerably depending on the electrocardiographic and delay time criteria used. If the delay time is limited to 6 hours and the electrocardiogram is required to show ST elevation, then 37% of patients developing AMI, would receive thromblytic therapy.

Time delay in starting therapy

To evaluate the factors affecting the time between symptom onset and hospital arrival in patients with AMI, Schmidt and Borsch[85] from Morgantown, West Virginia, gave a detailed questionnaire to all who were admitted or transferred with AMI during a 1-year period. In these 126 patients (94 men, 32 women) the mean prehospital time was 5.9 ± 11.0 hours (median 2.0, range 0.4 to 69.0). The time between symptom onset and reaching a decision that medical care should be sought was 62% of the mean prehospital time. In 100 (79%) patients, the prehospital time was ≤6 hours; of these, 61 (61%) were retrospectively judged to have been optimal candidates for lytic therapy. Stepwise multiple regression selected the following variables as independent predictors of prehospital time: slow symptom progression, low income, female gender, and advanced age. All of these variables are predictive of increased prehospital time; absence of prior AMI was of borderline additional significance. Similarly, logistic regression analysis selected slow symptom progression, female gender and low income as significant independent predictors of prehospital time >6 hours. The logistic regression model incorporating these 3 variables had a sensitivity of 54%, a specificity of 95% and a positive predictive value of 72% in identifying patients with prehospital time >6 hours. Thus, these data indicate it is possible to characterize patients likely to experience undue prehospital delay during AMI.

To establish the magnitude of prehospital and hospital delays in initiating thrombolytic therapy for AMI, the time from telephone 911 emergency medical systems activation to treatment and its components in 8 separate ongoing trials, were analyzed by Kereiakes and associates[86] from several centers. This included estimates of ambulance response time, prehospital evaluation and treatment time, and time from admission to the hospital to initiation of thrombolytic therapy. The average time from emergency medical system activation to patient arrival at the hospital was prospectively determined to be 46 ± 8.2 minutes in 3,715 patients from 8 centers. The time from admission to the hospital to initiation of thrombolytic therapy was retrospectively determined to be 84 ± 55 minutes in a separate group of 730 patients from 6 centers. Both the prehospital and hospital time delays were much longer than those perceived by paramedics and emergency department directors. Shorter hospital time delays were observed in patients in whom a prehospital electrocardiogram was obtained as part of a protocol-driven prehospital diagnostic strategy and a diagnosis of AMI made before arrival at the hospital (36 ± 11 minutes in 13 patients) (Figure 3-21). These results show that the magnitude of time required to evaluate, transport, and initiate thrombolytic therapy will preclude initiation of treatment to most patients within the first hour of symptoms. Implementation of a protocol-driven prehospital diagnostic strategy may be associated with a reduction in time to thrombolytic therapy.

Administered in mobile care unit

Roth, and associates[87] in Tel Aviv, Israel, evaluated the effectiveness, feasibility and safety of prehospital thrombolytic therapy in a relatively small study of 118 patients allocated to receive either prehospital treatment with recombinant tissue type plasminogen activator in a mobile intensive care unit (group A, 74 patients) or hospital treatment (group B, 44 patients). A total of 120 mg of tissue plasminogen activator was infused over a period of 6 hours. All patients were heparinized and had radionuclide left ventriculography and coronary angiography during hospitalization. Although group A patients were treated significantly earlier than group B after symptom onset (94 ± 36 vs 137 ± 45 minutes), no significant differences were observed between the groups in 1) extent of myocardial necrosis, 2) global LVEF at hospital discharge, 3) patency of the infarct-related artery, 4) length of hospital stay, and 5) mortality at 60 days. There was a trend toward a lower incidence of CHF at hospital discharge in the prehospital-treated patients compared with the hospital treated group (7% vs 16%). No major complications occurred during

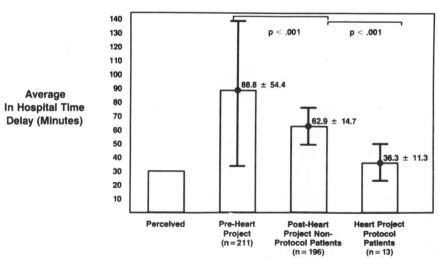

Fig. 3-21. Average (mean ± 1 standard deviation time delay from admission to hospital to initiation of thrombolytic therapy as perceived by interview of 10 emergency room directors (Perceived), retrospectively reviewed from emergency department records before inception of Cincinnati Heart Project (Pre-Heart Project), retrospectively reviewed from emergency department records of nonstudy patients after inception of Cincinnati Heart Project (Post-Heart Project Nonprotocol Patients), and prospectively evaluated by means of prehospital diagnostic strategy (Heart Project Protocol Patients). Most significant reduction in hospital time delay was observed with protocol-driven prehospital diagnostic strategy. Reproduced with permission from Kereiakes, et al.[86]

transportation. These data suggest that AMI may be accurately diagnosed and thrombolytic therapy initiated safely during the prehospital phase by a mobile intensive care unit team.

Streptokinase

Six and associates[88] from Utrecht, The Netherlands, carried out a double-blind randomized trial to *establish the optimal dose of strepto-kinase.* A total of 189 patients who had symptoms of AMI for <4 hours were treated with 200,000, 750,000, 1,500,000 or 3,000,000 IU streptokinase intravenously. At coronary angiography 2.8 ± 2.7 hours after the start of streptokinase infusion, patency of the infarct-related coronary artery was observed in 38, 75, 60 and 82% of the patients, respectively, in the 4 groups. The result of the dosage of 200,000 IU was significantly poorer than that of the other dosages. The result of a dosage of 3,000,000 IU was significantly better than that of 1,500,000 IU, but the differences with 750,000 IU were not significant. Blood transfusion was required in 4 patients (2%), distributed over the 4 groups in 0, 2, 1 and 1 of the patients. One patient had major bleeding; this patient had been treated with 750,000 IU. The 3-month mortality-rate in the whole study population was 5%. Thus, of the 4 doses of streptokinase tested, 750,000 IU is the minimal therapeutic dosage, and the arguments for 1,500,000 IU as standard therapy for comparison with other fibrinolytic drugs are poor. The best results in this study were achieved with 3,000,000 IU, but further research will be needed to establish the efficacy and safety of this new regimen.

Jalihal and Morris[89] from Nottingham, UK, measured *streptokinase neutralization titres* in 25 patients who received streptokinase during AMI. Before treatment, neutralization titres were low (0.3 × 10[6] neutralization units or less) in all patients. Three months after treatment, neutralization titres in 24 were such that a typical therapeutic dose of 1.5 million units of streptokinase would have been fully neutralized. At 4.5–8.5 months, 18 of 20 patients had neutralization titres such that at least 50% of a dose of 1.5 million units of streptokinase would have been neutralized. After 8 months, neutralization titres ranged from 0.4 to 2.0 million units in 8 patients. A decision to readminister streptokinase within 8 months (and probably up to 1 year) of previous thrombolytic treatment should take account of the neutralizing capacity of plasma and the dose should be adjusted accordingly.

In 50 patients receiving thrombolytic treatment for AMI, Davies and associates[90] from London, UK, took peripheral venous blood samples before streptokinase and 2 hours later for *assay of markers of free radical activity.* Coronary arteriography was carried out within 72 hours of thrombolysis. In the 42 patients with patent arteries after thrombolysis, the levels of thiobarbituric-acid-reactive material (TBA-RM), which reflects lipid peroxidation by free radicals, rose after streptokinase by 105 (SD 96) nmol/g albumin, whereas in the 8 whose arteries remained occluded TBA-RM fell by 147 (80) nmol/g albumin. There was no significant change in the 18:2 (9, 11) /18:2 (9, 12) molar ratio, an indicator of lipid isomerization, either between the groups or after streptokinase. Thus, after successful thrombolysis there is a rise in lipid peroxidation, not seen in patients whose arteries remain occluded. This finding suggests free-radical-mediated damage at the time of reperfusion, and provides indirect evidence of reperfusion injury. This study provides evidence associating indicators of free radical activity with documented myocardial reperfusion.

Mahan and associates[91] from Birmingham, Alabama, studied the role of duration of *heparin therapy* in maintaining infarct artery patency retrospectively in 53 consecutive AMI patients who received streptokinase therapy and underwent coronary angiography acutely and at 14 ± 1 days. Of the 39 patients with initial infarct vessel patency, patency at follow-up angiography was observed in 100% (22 of 22) of those who received ≥4 days of intravenous heparin but in only 59% (10 of 17) of those patients who received <4 days of heparin. Of the 14 patients not initially recanalized after streptokinase, patent infarct-related arteries at follow-up angiography were found in 3 of 8 (38%) treated with ≥4 days of heparin therapy but in none of the 6 patients treated for <4 days (difference not significant). No significant difference in hemorrhagic complications was noted between the short- and long-term héparin treatment groups. Thus, ≥4 days of intravenous heparin therapy after successful streptokinase therapy in AMI is more effective in maintaining short-term infarct vessel patency than a shorter duration of therapy and it may maintain the short-term patency of the infarct vessel in those patients who later spontaneously recanalize.

Chew and associates[92] from Belfast, UK, compared the occurrence of *ventricular late potentials* in survivors of AMI treated with intravenous streptokinase with that in a conservatively treated group and the relation between ventricular late potentials and patency of the infarct related artery was examined. Of 115 patients admitted with a first infarct, 55 were treated with intravenous streptokinase (streptokinase group) and 60 were treated conservatively (non-streptokinase group). A signal averaged electrocardiogram was recorded in all patients and coronary angiography was performed in 45 (82%) of the streptokinase group and in 21 (35%) of the non-streptokinase group. At a 40 Hz filter setting ventricular late potentials were significantly less common in patients treated with streptokinase (9 [16%] of 55) than in those who were not (26 [43%] of 60). A total of 66 patients underwent angiography. Of the 26 who had closed infarct-related arteries, 17 had ventricular late potentials at a 40 Hz filter setting (sensitivity 65%, specificity 95%) and 38 of the 40 patients with a patent infarct-related artery did not have ventricular late potentials (sensitivity 81%, specificity 90%). Patients with AMI treated with intravenous streptokinase were significantly less likely to have ventricular late potentials than conservatively treated patients and the absence of ventricular late potentials at 40 Hz filter setting was a good non-invasive predictor that the infarct-related artery was patent.

Davies and colleagues[93] in London, UK, studied coronary artery morphology in 72 patients 1 to 8 days after streptokinase treatment for AMI and compared the findings with lesion morphology in a control group of 24 patients with stable angina. In the streptokinase group, the infarct-related artery was patent in 55 patients (76%). Compared with stenoses in the stable angina group, there were no differences in the stenosis length, severity, calcification or in the proportion located at an acute bend or at a branch point. Lesions in the streptokinase group were more often irregular and eccentric, they had a shoulder, globular-filling or linear filling defects, and contrast staining. Plaque ulceration was higher in the streptokinase than in the stable angina group. Among the 72 streptokinase-treated patients, 35 were maintained on heparin until angioplasty 2 to 10 days later. At repeat angiography before PTCA, globular filling lesion defects found in 8 patients originally had disappeared, whereas linear filling defects persisted in 7 of 14 cases. Fewer lesions were irregular and the ulceration index had decreased. These data demonstrate that the lesion in the infarct-related artery after streptokinase treatment is irregular and often associated with filling defects, probably corresponding to plaque fissuring and intraluminal thrombosis. These findings are at least partially resolved with maintenance heparin therapy for a few days.

Bourke and colleagues[94] in Westmead, Australia, determined whether intravenous streptokinase administered with or without oral aspirin to patients with AMI reduces the *inducibility of VT* at electrophysiologic study and thus the risk of sudden death in infarct survivors. Among 159 patients randomized at Westmead Hospital to the multicenter Second International Study of Infarct Survival (ISIS-2) after streptokinase and aspirin in AMI, 87 underwent electrophysiologic testing 6 to 28 days after their infarcts to determine their risk of subsequent ventricular arrhythmias. This included 20 patients treated with streptokinase; 25 patients treated with aspirin; 21 patients treated with both streptokinase and aspirin; and 21 patients treated with both placebos. Patients who underwent electrophysiologic testing had similar clinical characteristics to those who did not. The stimulation protocol comprised up to and including four extrastimuli applied to the RV apex at twice diastolic threshold. An abnormal result was defined as VT with a cycle length $\geq$230 ms lasting $\geq$10 seconds. VT was inducible at electrophysiologic study in 8 patients who received placebo streptokinase, but in no patient who received active streptokinase. VT was inducible in 4 patients who received aspirin and 4 who did not. During a mean follow-up period of 39 $\pm$ 9 months, there were no spontaneous episodes of VT, VF or witnessed sudden death in the streptokinase-treated group compared with three such events in the placebo-treated group. Thus, these data suggest that the administration of intravenous streptokinase substantially reduces the incidence of inducible VT in AMI survivors.

Midgette and associates[95] from Hanover, New Hampshire, performed a literature search of English-language studies on the use of intravenous streptokinase in the treatment of suspected AMI for the period 1966 to 1989 using Medlars II and the bibliographies of relevant articles. Of 140 originally identified articles, 6 that specifically met their inclusion criteria were selected, randomized trials that used intravenous streptokinase in a dose of 1.5 million units, with or without additional agents, compared with a group that differed only by the absence of streptokinase (Figure 3-22). Among the 9,155 patients with suspected anterior wall AMI, the mortality rate in the control group was 17.4% and in the patients treated with streptokinase, 12.5%. The mean risk of difference was −4.8%. A total of 9,650 patients with suspected inferior wall AMI had a mortality rate in the control group of 7.7%, and in the streptokinase treated patients, 6.6%. The mean risk difference was −0.8%. Thus, intravenous streptokinase clearly confers a protective effect against early mortality in patients with suspected anterior wall AMI. The magnitude of this effect is about 5% absolute reduction in risk of death by 21 to 35 days. For these patients, 21 need to be treated to save 1 additional life. For patients with suspected inferior wall AMI, the benefit of treatment on reducing early mortality is of smaller magnitude and less certain. These patients have an estimated absolute reduction of early mortality of about 1%, which would require treating 125 patients to save 1 additional life.

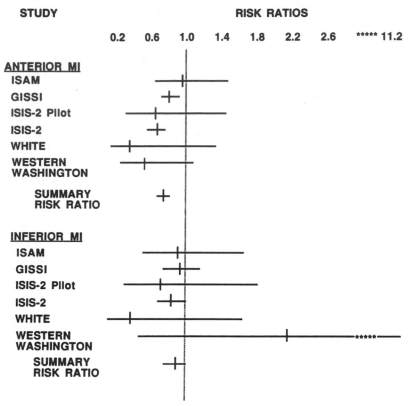

Fig. 3-22. Risk ratios for early mortality by location of myocardial infarction (MI) from randomized trials of intravenous streptokinase. Short vertical lines indicate the point estimates; horizontal lines depict the 95% confidence intervals. Risk ratios less than 1.0 indicate a beneficial effect of intravenous streptokinase on early mortality. Reproduced with permission from Midgette, et al.[95]

Streptokinase vs anistreplase

Hogg and associates[96] from Glasgow, UK, randomized 128 patients with AMI of 6 hour or less duration in a double-blind fashion to receive 30 units anistreplase over 5 minutes of 1.5 MU streptokinase over 1 hour, both intravenously. Angiographic patency was assessed 90 minutes and 24 hours from the start of therapy. Fifty-five percent of patients who received anistreplase and 53% of patients who received streptokinase had patent infarct-related arteries (TIMI grade 2-3) at 90 minutes (95% CI 42–68% and 40–66%, respectively). At 24 hours 81% and 87.5% of arteries were patent respectively (95% CI, 71–91% and 83.5–91.5%). Time to therapy had no significant effect on patency rates. There was one early reocclusion within 24 hours in each treatment group and clinical evidence of reocclusion was recorded between 24 hours and hospital discharge in a further 5 patients (streptokinase 3, anistreplase 2). With these regimens, therefore, anistreplase and streptokinase gave the same patency rates.

Streptokinase vs alteplase

A multicenter, randomized, open trial with a 2 × 2 factorial design was conducted by the collaborators in participating centers in Italy (GISSI-

2) to compare the benefits and risks of 2 thrombolytic agents, streptokinase (SK, 1.5 MU infused intravenously over 30–60 min) and alteplase (tPA, 100 mg infused intravenously over 3 h) in patients with AMI admitted to coronary care units within 6 hours from onset of symptoms[97]. The patients were also randomized to receive heparin (12,500 U subcutaneously twice daily until discharge from hospital, starting 12 hours after beginning the tPA or SK infusion) or usual therapy. All patients without specific contraindications were given atenolol (5–10 mg iv) and aspirin (300–325 mg a day). The end-point of the study was the combined estimate of death plus severe LV damage. Twelve thousand four hundred ninety patients were randomized to 4 treatment groups (streptokinase alone, streptokinase plus heparin, recombinant tissue type plasminogen activator (rtPA) alone, and rtPA plus heparin). No specific differences between the 2 thrombolytic agents were detected as regards the combined end-point (rtPA 23.1%; SK 22.5%), nor after the addition of heparin to the aspirin treatment (hep 22.7%, no hep 22.9%). The outcome of patients allocated to the 4 treatment groups was similar with respect to baseline risk factors such as age, Killip class, hours from onset of symptoms, and site and type of infarct. The rates of major in-hospital cardiac complications (reinfarction, post-infarction angina) were also similar. The incidence of major bleeds was significantly higher in streptokinase and heparin treated patients (respectively, rtPA 0.5%, streptokinase 1.0%, heparin 1.9%, no heparin 0.6%), whereas the overall incidence of stroke was similar in all groups. Streptokinase and rtPA appear equally effective and safe for use in routine conditions of care, in all infarct patients who have no contraindications, with or without post-thrombolytic heparin treatment. The 8.8% hospital mortality of the study population (compared with approximately 13% in the control cohort of the GISSI-1 trial) indicates the beneficial impact of the proven acute treatments for AMI.

In a study with 2 × 2 factorial design, the International Study Group of GISSI[98] randomly allocated to alteplase (recombinant tissue plasminogen activator, rtPA) or streptokinase and to subcutaneous heparin, 20,891 patients with suspected AMI of <6 hours duration (12,490 from the GISSI-2 trial and 8,401 recruited elsewhere) beginning 12 hours after the start of thrombolytic therapy or no heparin. The protocol recommended that, in the absence of specific contraindications, all patients should receive aspirin and intravenous β-blockade as soon as possible. No significant differences in hospital mortality were found between rtPA and streptokinase (8.9% vs 8.5%) or between heparin and no heparin (8.5% vs 8.9%). The incidence of major cardiac complications was also very similar in the different groups. For non-cardiac complications significant differences between the treatment groups were observed: more strokes were reported with rtPA than with streptokinase (1.3% vs 1%) while more major bleeds occurred with streptokinase than with rtPA (0.6% vs 0.9%). Subcutaneous heparin was likewise associated with an excess of major bleeds (1.0% with heparin vs 0.5% without heparin) but did not affect the incidence of stroke or reinfarction.

White[99] from Auckland, New Zealand, provided editorial comment on the GISSI-2 study which showed that streptokinase and alteplase (rtPA) when given for AMI have the same effect on mortality, excluding with 90% power a difference of 1.5%. He asked, does this mean that the superior angiographic 90-minute patency rates achieved with rtPA have not translated into clinical patient benefit? At first glance, he states the answer is yes. The only differences demonstrated were in the frequency of side effects with rtPA patients having 4 extra strokes per 1,000 patients and streptokinase being associated with more allergy and hypotension and an excess of 3 major bleeds per 1,000 patients. Subgroup analysis showed that streptokinase saved more patients with cardiogenic shock. White asked why the 90-minute patency was not a valid endpoint? White concluded that notwithstanding the heparin controversy, the results of GISSI-2 are astounding. Mortality in patients aged <70 years was 5.6%. Whether various thrombolytic agents will have different effects on this already low mortality when given with early intravenous heparin will need to be addressed by further large randomized trials.

Recombinant tissue-type plasminogen activator

In 92 AMI patients treated with tissue plasminogen activator (rt-PA) 2.3 ± 1.2 hours after the onset of chest pain and performed echocardiography 11 ± 14 hours (early) and in 49 patients again at 13 ± 7 weeks (late).[100] *Infarct location* and *LV wall motion score index*—the average score (normal = 1, hypokinetic = 2, akinetic = 3, dyskinetic = 4) for 20 segments—were determined by 2 observers unaware of clinical, angiographic or electrocardiographic data. Concordance between noninvasive infarct location by electrocardiography or echocardiography and infarct-related artery at angiography 4 ± 2 days later (n = 85) was 76 and 81%, respectively. The early wall motion score index was worse for anterior (1.8 ± 0.4) versus inferior (1.3 ± 0.2) or posterior-lateral (1.6 ± 0.2) infarcts. Overall, the wall motion score index improved from early to late echocardiography (n = 49, 1.5 ± 0.3 to 1.3 ± 0.3). However, improvement was confined to those with time to treatment <2 hours (n = 22, 1.4 ± 0.3 to 1.2 ± 0.2), and evidence of reperfusion at angiography (n = 38, 1.5 ± 0.3 to 1.2 ± 0.3). The decrease in the wall motion score index was related to a decrease in the number of adjacent involved segments (5.5 ± 3.0 to 3.7 ± 3.9/patient). Thus, echocardiography early after AMI identifies infarct location. Improvement in regional wall motion is seen after early treatment with intravenous rt-PA.

Controversy exists as to whether and how long heparin treatment is necessary after infarct vessel recanalization during AMI. To determine the role of heparin, Kander and associates[101] from Ann Arbor, Michigan, randomly allocated patients with suitable angiographic features after reperfusion therapy to receive a brief infusion of intravenous heparin for ≤24 hours (group 1), adjusted to a partial thromboplastin time of 2 times control or a prolonged infusion ≥72 hours (group 2), using the same titration mechanism. Patients were excluded for complex intimal dissections, large residual filling defects, less than Thrombolysis in Myocardial Infarction grade 3 flow pattern of >50% residual stenosis. Heparin was sustained except for discontinual, or if significant bleeding (≥2 units blood transfusion) occurred. The primary endpoints were 1-week patency determined by repeat catheterization or recurrent ischemia, or both, and the incidence of bleeding complications. Fifty patients were randomized, 25 in each group. Baseline variables were similar; 14 group 1 and 15 group 2 patients received thrombolytic treatment; 20 patients in each group had coronary angioplasty. Two documented reocclusions occurred in both groups. Significant bleeding complications occurred in 0 of 25 (0%) group 1 versus 6 of 25 (24%) group 2 patients. Thus, in low-risk patients after successful reperfusion, prolonged heparin therapy does not protect against rethrombosis and is associated with a significantly higher rate of bleeding complications. Therefore, prolonged heparin therapy for >24 hours does not appear to be justified in low-risk patients with successful reperfusion.

The Thrombolysis in Myocardial Infarction phase II pilot study enrolled 288 patients with AMI who were treated with rt-PA within 4 hours of symptom onset and who were assigned to PTCA of the infarct-related vessel 18 to 48 hours after rt-PA treatment. In a report by Chaitman and colleagues[102] from Bethesda, Maryland, the patients were followed to ascertain 1) vital status; 2) whether they suffered a recurrent AMI; 3) whether they received PTCA or CABG; and 4) whether they were rehospitalized for a cardiac event. Risk factors for these events or combination of these events were identified and reported. The estimated 6-week, 6-month, and 1-year cumulative event rate of death or AMI was 9.1 ± 1.7%, 13 ± 2.0%, and 14 ± 2.0%, respectively. With the exception of repeat hospital admissions, most of the above cardiac events occurred early during the patients' follow-up course. Cox proportional hazard analyses revealed that continuing chest pain after rt-PA administration, history of CHF, low systolic BP at the time of initial evaluation, and history of hypertension increased the risk of death or recurrent AMI, while a history of chest discomfort at baseline evaluation and older age was predictive of future hospitalization or a revascularization procedure.

The Thrombolysis Early in Acute Heart Attack Trial Study Group[103] from several European Medical Centers randomized 352 patients with suspected AMI to placebo (175 patients) or rt-PA (177 patients). Patients were eligible if evaluated within 165 minutes from onset of chest pain and if age was <75 years. Electrocardiographic criteria were not required. A mobile coronary care unit with a cardiologist present was used to initiate treatment at home in 29% of the patients. Primary endpoints were infarct size (serum lactate dehydrogenase isoenzyme$_1$ activity), LV function (radioangiography) and exercise capacity at 30 days. AMI was diagnosed in 59% of all randomized patients. The incidence was similar in the 2 groups (placebo, 108, rt-PA, 101). Among all randomized patients, rt-PA was associated with significantly decreased infarct size and an increased EF. Among rt-PA-treated patients there were significantly fewer Q-wave infarctions. No difference in exercise capacity could be detected. No benefit was found in subgroups of patients without ST-segment elevation on the initial electrocardiogram. There were 18 (10.3%) and 11 (6.2%) deaths within 30 days in the placebo and rt-PA groups, respectively. Adverse reactions were similar in both groups with no excess of complications in the home-treated group. Very early treatment with rt-PA in patients with a strong suspicion of AMI and ST-segment elevation limits infarct size and improves LV function. The infarct pattern is shifted from Q-wave to non-Q-wave infarcts by rt-PA. The study suggests that thrombolysis can be given before hospital admission without additional risk. Furthermore, electrocardiographic records are useful for selection of patients.

Smalling and associates[104] from Houston, Texas; Indianapolis, Indiana; Atlanta, Georgia; and San Francisco, California, determined whether a *weight-adjusted high dose* (2 mg/kg body weight over 3 hours) rapid infusion of rt-PA was more efficacious than a *weight-adjusted standard dose* (1.25 mg/kg over 3 hours) in leading to reperfusion during AMI in 175 patients entered into a randomized, multicenter trial. Eight-four patients were entered into the high dose group receiving 1.2 mg/kg with 10% given as a bolus injection over 1 hour, followed by 0.8 mg/kg during the next 2 hours. Ninety-one patients were given 0.75 mg/kg with 10% given as a bolus injection in 1 hour followed by 0.5 mg/kg over the next 2 hours.

The median dose in the group that received 2 mg/kg dose was 145 mg compared with 100 mg in the group that received 1.25 mg/kg. A 90 minute patency rate in the group that received 2 mg/kg was 84% compared to 70% in the group that received 1.25 mg/kg. Sixty-four percent of the patients in each group had PTCA at the time of cardiac catheterization. The infarct-related artery patency rate at the end of the catheterization was 91% in the group that received 2 mg/kg compared with 83% in the group that received 1.25 mg/kg. In the patients with a patent infarct-related coronary artery after thrombolytic therapy, the 6 month mortality rate in the group that received 2 mg/kg was 2.9% compared with 9.8% in the group that received 1.25 mg/kg. Bleeding complications in the two groups were similar. Two patients in the group that received 2 mg/kg developed nonfatal intracranial bleeding; in one of these patients, the intracranial bleeding occurred after emergency open heart surgery. Thus, these data suggest that more rapid administration of a higher weight-adjusted dose of tissue plasminogen activator may be more effective in restoring infarct-related artery patency in the setting of AMI than the currently recommended dose of 100 mg during 3 hours.

To evaluate the long-term effects of reperfusion with rt-PA and an aggressive strategy of revascularization with PTCA and CABG, Califf and colleagues[105] from Durham, North Carolina, Ann Arbor, Michigan, and Columbus and Cincinnati, Ohio, obtained 1-year follow-up results from 386 consecutive patients enrolled in the Thrombolysis and Angioplasty in Myocardial Infarction (TAMI I) trial. All patients were treated with 100 to 150 mg of rt-PA intravenously over 6 to 8 hours, and coronary angiography was performed within 90 minutes of initiation of therapy. In 197 patients with suitable anatomic characteristics, PTCA was either performed immediately or was deferred for 7 to 10 days on a randomized basis. The remainder of the patients were treated as considered clinically appropriate. The in-hospital mortality rate was 7%, and only 1.9% of patients died in the first year after discharge from the hospital; 3 patients died of cardiac events and 4 died of noncardiac causes. Ninety-four percent of patients discharged alive from the hospital remained alive and had no AMI during the first 12 posthospital months. Revascularization procedures after discharge from the hospital included PTCA in 8% of patients and CABG in 5%. The high survival rates were evident in high-risk groups defined by age, EF, and extent of CAD. At 1-year follow-up 64% of patients <65 years of age were employed and only 10% reported that they were disabled; 94% of patients were in Canadian Heart Association class I or II. These low rates of follow-up events suggest a change in the "natural history" of the first year after AMI.

To assess the value and timing of PTCA after thrombolytic therapy, Rogers and participants[106] randomized 586 patients in the Thrombolysis in Myocardial Infarction Study Phase II-A among three treatment strategies, one using immediate coronary arteriography followed by PTCA if appropriate (n = 195), a second that deferred angiography and PTCA for 18–48 hours (n = 194), and a third, more conservative approach in which PTCA was used only if ischemia occurred spontaneously or at the time of predischarged exercise testing (n = 197). Predischarged contrast LVEF, the primary study end point, was similar among the patients in all three treatment groups and average 49%. The finding of a patent infarct-related artery at the time of predischarge arteriography was equally common among the patients in the 3 groups (mean, 84%); however, the mean residual infarct artery stenosis was greater in the patients in the conservative strategy group as compared with the patients in the immediate invasive and the delayed invasive groups. Immediate invasive strategy led to a higher rate of CABG after PTCA than delayed invasive and conservative strategies. Furthermore, among patients not undergoing CABG during the first 21 days, blood transfusion of more than 1 unit was used in 14% of the patients in the immediate invasive strategy group, 3% of the patients in the delayed invasive strategy group, and 25 of the patients in the conservative strategy group. At 1-year follow-up, the three treatments groups had similar cumulative rates of mortality (9%), fatal and nonfatal reinfarction (9%), combined death and reinfarction (15%), and CABG (17%), although the cumulative performance rate of PTCA remained higher in invasive group (immediate invasive strategy group 75.8% delayed invasive strategy group, 64%; and conservative strategy group). Thus, because conservative strategy achieves equally good short- and long-term outcome with less morbidity and a lower use of PTCA, this report suggested it as the preferred initial management strategy.

Khan and associates[107] from London, UK, investigated the feasibility and possible advantages of intravenous bolus administration of rt-PA in 26 consecutive patients with early (<6 hours) AMI. Either an intravenous infusion of 40 clot-lysis megaunits (cIMU) double-chain rt-PA over 1.5 hours followed by 20 cIMU over 5 hours (infusion group, n = 12) or 4 intravenous bolus injections of 10 cIMU at 20 minute intervals (bolus group, n = 14) were randomly administered. Coronary arteriography was performed before and at regular predefined intervals up to 90 minutes from the start of rt-PA administration, and at 24 hours. Acute recanalization of the infarct-related coronary artery was demonstrated in 7 of 12 patients (58%; 95% confidence interval 28 to 85%) in the infusion group and 11 of 14 patients (79%; 95% confidence interval 49 to 95%) in the bolus group (difference not significant). Two patients in the bolus group had reoccluded by 24 hours. Mean time from the start of rt-PA to patency of the infarct-related coronary artery was 39 ± 6 (standard error of the mean) minutes in the infusion group and 28 ± 6 minutes in the bolus group. There were no significant differences in the minimum infarct-related coronary artery luminal diameter measured by computerized quantitative arteriography between the infusion group and the bolus group at 90 minutes or at 24 hours. Resolution of ST-segment elevation assessed by continuous electrocardiographic monitoring over the first 24 hours appeared to occur sooner in recanalized patients in the bolus group (2.8 ± 0.5 hours) than in the infusion group (5.5 ± 2.1 hours). The period during which the plasma fibrinogen remained below pretreatment levels was longer in the infusion group (54 ± 7 hours) compared to the bolus group (29 ± 6 hours). Thus, multiple bolus rt-PA appears to result in earlier recanalization of the infarct-related coronary artery and in a shorter duration of acute ischemia compared to an intravenous infusion. The smaller total dose of rt-PA results in less prolonged fibrinogenolysis.

In a randomized, controlled trial, the data of which was collected and reported by Wilcox and associates[108] for the Anglo-Scandinavian Study of Early Thrombolysis, 2,514 patients with suspected AMI were treated with 100 mg intravenous rt-PA plus heparin within 5 hours of onset of symptoms, and 2,499 similar control subjects received placebo plus heparin. At 1 month the overall mortality rates were 7% and 10%, respectively, a relative reduction of 26%. At 6 months the mortality rates were 10% (rt-PA) and 13% (placebo), a relative reduction of 21%. Six-month mortality rates in patients with proven AMI were 13% and 17%, respectively (relative reduction 26%); this effect was similar for anterior (16% vs 21%) and inferior (8% vs 13%) AMI. Six-month mortality rates were lower in those treated with rt-PA irrespective of other recognized cardiac risk factors. However, treatment with rt-PA made no difference to subsequent cardiac events after 1 month (readmissions, reinfarctions, death) nor to treatment for angina or CAD. Product limit estimates of 1 year mortality are 13% with rt-PA and 15% with placebo. The corresponding figures for patients with an index diagnosis of AMI were 16% and 19%, a relative reduction of 17%.

In a double-blind trial of the European Cooperative Study Group by Mortelmans and associates[109] from Leuven, Belgium, and Maastricht, The Netherlands, 721 patients with AMI of <5 hours duration were given either 100 mg rt-PA intravenously over 3 hours of an equivalent placebo infusion. In a subset of 312 patients, *infarct size* was assessed by the cumulative myocardial release of α-hydroxybutyrate dehydrogenase during the first 72 hours and by planar thallium-scintigraphy (index of hypoperfusion) performed 10 to 22 days after the acute event. LVEF was determined by contrast and nuclear angiography. The median values of α-hydroxybutyrate dehydrogenase during the first 72 hours were 20% lower and the median values of thallium-201 28% smaller in the rt-PA group in comparison with controls. A significant but limited improvement of angiographic LVEF (2 absolute percentage points) was also shown in the patients treated with rt-PA activator. A moderate but statistically significant linear association between both measurements of infarct size and LVEF was found.

To examine the sequential *changes in LV volume* after thrombolytic therapy for AMI, Lavie and associates[110] from Rochester, Minnesota, and Kansas City, Missouri, performed gated radionuclide ventriculography within 12 hours of thrombolysis and at 1 and 6 weeks in 34 consecutive patients who received intravenous thrombolytic therapy in the Thrombolysis in Myocardial Infarction Trial. Angiographic confirmation of immediate reperfusion (mean 5.6 hours after onset of symptoms) that persisted at 24 hours was noted in 24 patients; 10 patients were not reperfused. A small (9.5%), but significant, increase in end-diastolic volume index was noted in the reperfused group between 1 and 6 weeks; however, a marked degree of dilatation (35%) was noted in the nonreperfused group. The change in LV volume between 1 and 6 weeks differed in the 2 groups for both end-diastolic volume index and end-systolic volume index. By 6 weeks, both end-diastolic volume index and end-systolic volume index were greater in the nonreperfused group. Between the acute and 6-week studies, definite increases in end-diastolic volume index and end-systolic volume index occurred commonly in the non-reperfused group but rarely in the reperfused group. Compared to the nonreperfused group, the reperfused group also had significantly higher EF at both 1 and 6 weeks. The change in end-diastolic volume index between 1 and 6 weeks correlated significantly and inversely with the EF at 1 week. These results indicate that ventricular dilatation occurs between 1 and 6 weeks after AMI, is proportional to systolic dysfunction and may be largely prevented by successful thrombolytic reperfusion.

Barbash and associates[111] from Tel Aviv, Israel, treated 190 patients with AMI with rt-PA 2.0 ± 0.8 hours after the onset of symptoms. Eighty-seven patients were enrolled via mobile intensive care units and 103 through the emergency ward. Patients who were enrolled via the mobile intensive care units were randomized to immediate, pre-hospital treatment initiation, or to delayed, in-hospital treatment initiation. All 190 patients except 2 underwent delayed coronary angiography and, when indicated, angioplasty at 72 hours after enrollment. Patients treated within

2 hours and those treated 2 to 4 hours after symptom onset had similar preservation of LV function, and similar prevalence of CAD at discharge. Patients treated within 2 hours of symptom onset had significantly lower short- (0.0 vs 6.3%) and long-term (1.0 vs 9.5%) mortality. Prehospital initiation of rt-PA appeared to be safe and feasible and resulted in a 40-minute decrease in the time from symptom onset to treatment initiation.

O'Connor and associates[112] in Durham, North Carolina; Ann Arbor, Michigan; and Columbus and Cincinnati, Ohio, evaluated 708 patients with AMI treated with rt-PA in the Thrombolysis and Angioplasty in Myocardial Infarction (TAMI) I, II, and III trials. Among these patients, 13 (1.8%) developed a *stroke*. Four strokes were hemorrhagic and 9 were nonhemorrhagic. Among five prespecified risk factors for intracranial hemorrhage including age >65 years, history of hypertension, history of prior cerebrovascular disease, aspirin use and acute hypertension, 2 patients had 2 risk factors and 1 patient had 1 risk factor. However, 80% of patients without intracranial hemorrhage had at least 1 risk factor and 31% had 2 risk factors. No patient with a prior stroke or transient ischemic attack >6 months previously had an intracranial hemorrhage. Of the 3 prespecified risk factors for nonhemorrhagic stroke, including AF, prior cerebrovascular disease, and large anterior wall AMI, the occurrence of a large anterior wall AMI with LVEF <45% was a predictor of future stroke with thrombolytic therapy. The in-hospital death rate was 25% for patients with hemorrhagic stroke versus 11% for patients with a nonhemorrhagic stroke and 6% for those patients without a stroke. The hospital stay was >50% longer in patients who had a stroke than in those who did not. Intracranial hemorrhage remains an unpredictable risk in patients treated with thrombolytic therapy. Cerebral infarction is an increased risk for the patient with anterior AMI and reduced LVEF.

To determine the ability of initial ST segment elevation and depression to predict infarct size limitation by thrombolytic therapy, Willems and co-investigators[113] in Leuven, Belgium analyzed data in 721 patients with acute AMI, who were admitted to a randomized, placebo-controlled study of intravenous rt-PA. Patients with QRS duration of ≥120 msec or with previous history of AMI were excluded, leaving 322 in the treatment and 33 in the placebo group. Cumulative 72-hour release of alpha-hydroxy-butyrate dehydrogenase and global EF as well as LV wall motion derived from angiography were used as independent measures of infarct size. Electrocardiograms obtained at admission, 6 hours after start of therapy, and before discharge were analyzed. All ST measurements were made by hand at the J point and 60 msec after the J point. Patients with high ST segment elevation at admission (sum of ST elevation at 60 msec after the J point was 20 mm or more) had significantly larger infarction and higher hospital mortality when compared with those with lower (<29mm) ST elevation. Reciprocal ST segment depression also showed a linear relation within infarct size and mortality, independent from ST elevation, both in anterior and interior AMI. The sum of deviations measured at the J point and 60 msec after the J point differed significantly, especially in anterior wall AMI at admission. The prognostic value of one measurement was not, however, superior over the other. Treatment with rt-PA was most effective in those with large ST deviations at admission, but patients with anterior wall AMI and smaller ST shifts also appeared to benefit from therapy. Results in individual patients were variable, and the overall correlation of initial ST shifts with enzymatic infarct size was rather low. In conclusion, the present study shows that the magnitude of initial ST elevation and also of reciprocal ST depression in the admission electrocardiogram is valuable for the management and assessment of thrombolytic therapy in patients with AMI.

Barbash and associates[114] of the Israeli Study of Early Intervention in Myocardial Infarction infused rt-PA (alteplase) within 4 hours of onset of symptoms in 286 patients with AMI. Delayed coronary angiography was performed 72 hours after admission with coronary angioplasty if indicated. Electrocardiographic monitoring was continuous during the first hour of treatment. The sum of the ST segment elevations (ΣST) was calculated on electrocardiograms recorded at entry and an hour later. ST elevations resolved rapidly within 1 hour of treatment in 189 patients and persisted in 97 patients. Rapid resolution of ST elevation correlated with angiographic coronary patency as determined by coronary angiography 72 hours after admission. The patients with rapid resolution of ΣST had significantly smaller infarcts and a better clinical outcome than the patients with persistent ST elevation. ΣST values at entry and 1 hour after treatment had no additional independent predictive value. Rapid resolution of ST elevations in patients undergoing thrombolysis with alteplase was associated with a significantly smaller release of creatine kinase, better preservation of LV function, lower morbidity, and less short and long term mortality. Rapid resolution of ΣST elevation is an efficient indicator of clinical outcome in groups of patients with AMI undergoing thrombolysis with rt-PA.

Barbash and colleagues[115] in Tel Aviv and Hadera, Israel, studied 52 patients with AMI treated with 1 or 2 additional thrombolytic infusions of rt-PA because of *nonsustained ischemia after initial treatment* with rt-PA or streptokinase. Thirty-five patients received the second infusion within 1 hour of the first and 13 patients received the second infusion 1 to 72 hours after the first. Four patients received it later during their hospitalizations. Bleeding complications occurred in 10 patients (19%). Most of these were minor and included no intracranial bleeding; only 2 patients required blood transfusions. In 14 patients, in whom decreases in systemic fibrinogen and plasminogen levels were measured after the first and second infusions, the decreases were 25% and 63%, respectively. In 44 patients (85%), acute myocardial ischemia resolved completely within 1 hour after initiation of the second infusion. In 23 patients (44%), pain and ST segment elevation did not recur and invasive coronary intervention was avoided. Thus, in patients with AMI, repeat infusions of tissue plasminogen activator after initial thrombolytic therapy may stabilize patients with acute reinfarction and/or myocardial ischemia.

Bonaduce and colleagues[116] in Naples, Italy, evaluated the effects of late thrombolysis on *LV volume and function* in patients with AMI. Two-dimensional echocardiography and radionuclide angiography were performed before discharge and after one year of follow-up in 34 patients with anterior AMIs. Among these patients, 10 were admitted to the coronary care unit within 4 hours from the onset of symptoms and were treated with recombinant tissue type plasminogen activator (Group A) and 24 admitted between 4 and 8 hours after symptom onset were assigned to receive either rt-PA (Group B, n = 12) or conventional therapy (Group C, n = 12). Seven to 10 days after admission, all patients had cardiac catheterization and angiography. Patency of the infarct-related arteries was 70% in Group A, 66% in Group B, and 33% in Group C. At predischarge evaluation, mean LV end-systolic and end-diastolic volumes were higher in patients in Group C than in Groups B and A. Mean LVEFs at rest were lower in Group C than in Groups B and A patients. At 1 year follow-up study, LV end-systolic and end-diastolic volumes were higher in patients in Group C than in Groups B and A. LVEFs at rest were lower in Group C than in patients in Groups A and B and, during exercise, they increased more in patients in Group A than C. Comparison of data obtained before discharge and at the 1 year follow-up study revealed a significant difference in LV end-systolic volumes in Group C patients and in end-diastolic volumes in Group B. The beneficial effect of late thrombolysis with tissue plasminogen activator may be related to a reduction in myocardial expansion and thus a more favorable influence on postinfarction LV remodeling.

Feit and colleagues[117] in Bronx, Valhalla, and New York, New York; Boston, Massachusetts; Baltimore, Maryland and Minneapolis, Minnesota, evaluated the records from 1,461 patients treated with intravenous rt-PA in the conservative strategy arm of phase II of the Thrombolysis in Myocardial Infarction (TIMI) trial to evaluate whether conservative treatment after thrombolysis is feasible. Coronary angiography with angioplasty, if technically possible, was to be performed only for recurrent spontaneous or exercise-induced ischemia. In this study, results in patients treated by this strategy in community and tertiary hospitals were compared. Coronary angiography was performed within 42 days in more patients (542 of 1,155, 48%) initially admitted to a tertiary hospital where on-site coronary angiography/angioplasty was available than in those (94 or 306, 32%) admitted to a community hospital (where transfer to a tertiary hospital for coronary angiography/angioplasty was necessary). This different approach resulted in a greater use of coronary angioplasty (203 [18%] of 1,155 compared to 32 [11%] of 306 patients), CABG (12% vs 8%) and blood transfusion (12% vs 5.5%) in patients admitted to a tertiary hospital. There were no significant differences between the two groups in mortality, recurrent AMI or LV function. These results suggest that a conservative strategy after treatment of AMI with rt-PA is applicable in the community hospital setting.

Althouse and associates[118] from Seattle, Washington, used a registry and an emergency department treatment trial using rt-PA to evaluate currently accepted *criteria for eligibility* for thrombolytic therapy for AMI. During 1 year, 1,028 patients with documented AMI were evaluated for eligibility for thrombolytic therapy. Of these, 221 patients (22%) were eligible for thrombolytic therapy under currently accepted criteria, 175 (79%) of them were correctly identified by emergency department physicians for thrombolytic therapy, and 160 were enrolled in the trial. Only 3 patients (2%) enrolled by emergency department physicians did not subsequently evolve documented AMI. In all, 807 patients (78%) were ineligible for thrombolytic therapy: 335 (33%) because of ≥1 contraindications, 364 (36%) because of nondiagnostic electrocardiograms on presentation, and 105 (10%) because of age >75 years, or >6 hours of chest pain at presentation, or both. Mortality in treated patients at 14 days was 5.6%, and survival at 1 year was 92%. The mean time from hospital arrival to thrombolytic treatment was 55 ± 27 minutes. Initial management of AMI with rt-PA in the emergency department provided rapid and safe treatment comparable to that reported in trials that started treatment in the coronary care unit. The proportions of eligible patients could be increased from 1 in 5 to 1 in 3, if patients currently excluded only because of age >75 years or because of >6 hours of chest pain were offered treatment.

Villari and associates[119] from Naples, Italy, assessed whether administration of rt-PA up to 8 hours after the onset of symptoms of AMI may result in a significant improvement in *LV function*. Sixty patients were classified into 3 groups: group A (n = 21) received rt-PA within 4 hours from symptom onset; the remaining 39 patients, admitted between 4 and 8 hours, were randomized into 2 groups—group B (n = 19) received rt-PA, and group C (n = 21) was treated with conventional therapy. Coronary and LV angiograms were recorded 8 to 10 days after rt-PA administration. The patency rate of the infarct-related artery was 76% in group A, and 63 and 35% in group B and C, respectively. The Thrombolysis in Myocardial Infarction trial perfusion grade was higher in group A and B than in group C (A vs C:; B vs C). LVEF was significantly higher in group A (60 ± 10%) and B (55 ± 12%) compared with group C (44 ± 12%) (A vs C; B vs C). Regional wall motion of the entire ischemic zone was better in group A and B than in group C (A vs C; B vs C). In contrast, the kinesis of the central ischemic zone was significantly better in group A than in both group B and C (A vs B, A vs C). The number of hypokinetic, akinetic and dyskinetic segments were lower in group A and B than in group C (A vs B, B vs C and A vs C and B vs C respectively). Thus, these data confirm the efficacy of early thrombolysis and suggest that late reperfusion may act beneficially in preserving LV volumes and function.

To evaluate whether angiographically determined reperfusion could be predicted from *changes in ST-segment elevation*, Clemmensen and associates[120] from Durham, North Carolina, and Copenhagen, Denmark, compared the sum of ST-segment elevation in affected leads of the electrocardiogram before and after thrombolytic therapy in 53 patients with AMI. Reperfusion status of the infarct-related artery was determined angiographically 8 hours from onset of symptoms. According to the Thrombolysis in Myocardial Infarction trial (TIMI) criteria, 33 patients had successful reperfusion (TIMI grade 2 to 3 flow) after thrombolytic therapy and 20 patients did not (TIMI grade 0 to 1 flow). Logistic multiple regression analysis showed that the proportional value for the shift in the sum of ST elevation, termed the "%ST change," was more strongly associated with reperfusion than the absolute measured difference in millimeters. The entire spectra of sensitivities and specificities were determined to identify a level of the percent ST change with simultaneous high sensitivity and specificity. A 20% decrease in ST elevation provided such a level (88% sensitivity, 80% specificity). The positive and negative predictive values of a 20% decrease in ST elevation were 88 and 80%, respectively. These results suggest that a decrease of only 20% in the sum of ST elevation in the standard electrocardiogram after thrombolytic therapy is a useful non-invasive predictor of reperfusion status in patients with evolving AMI.

Hsia and associates[121] for the Heparin-Aspirin Reperfusion Trial (HART) Investigators from multiple medical centers reported the results of the heparin-aspirin reperfusion trial, a collaborative study comparing early intravenous heparin with oral aspirin as adjunctive treatment when rt-PA was used for coronary thrombolysis during AMI. Two hundred and five patients were randomly assigned to receive either immediate and then continuous intravenous heparin (starting with a 5000-unit bolus; n = 106) or immediate and then daily oral aspirin (80 mg; n = 99) together with rt-PA (100 mg intravenously over a 6-hour period) initiated within 6 hours of the onset of symptoms. The authors evaluated the patency of the infarct-related artery by angiography 7 to 24 hours after beginning rt-PA infusion, the frequency of reocclusion of the artery by repeat angiography on day 7, and ischemic or hemorrhagic complications during the hospital stay. At the time of the first angiogram, 82% of the infarct-related arteries in the patients assigned to heparin were patent, as compared with only 52% in the aspirin group. Of the initially patent vessels, 88% remained patent after 7 days in the heparin group, as compared with 95% in the aspirin group. The numbers of hemorrhagic events (18 in the heparin and 15 in the aspirin group) and recurrent ischemic events (8 in the heparin and 2 in the aspirin group) were similar in the 2 groups. Coronary patency rates associated with rt-PA are higher with early concomitant systemic heparin treatment than with concomitant low-dose oral aspirin. This observation has important implications for clinical practice and should be considered in the design and interpretation of clinical trials involving coronary thrombolytic therapy.

Infarct artery patency rates at 90 minutes after coronary thrombolysis using rt-PA with and without concurrent heparin anticoagulation have been shown to be comparable. The contribution of *heparin* to efficacy and safety after thrombolysis with rt-PA is unknown. In a pilot study, Bleich and associates[122] from 4 medical centers treated 84 patients within 6 hours of onset of AMI (mean 2.7 hours) with a standard dose of 100 mg of rt-PA over 3 hours. Forty-two patients were randomized to receive additionally immediate intravenous heparin anticoagulation (5,000 U of intravenous bolus followed by 1,000 U/hour titrated to a partial thromboplastin time of 1.5 to 2.0 times control) while 42 patients received rt-PA alone. Coronary angiography performed on day 3 (48 to 72 hours, mean 57) after rt-PA therapy revealed infarct artery patency rates of 71 and 43% in anticoagulated and control patients, respectively. Recurrent ischemia or infarction, or both, occurred in 3 (7.1%) anticoagulated patients and 5 (11.9%) control patients (difference not significant). Mild, moderate and severe bleeding occurred in 52, 10 and 2% of the group receiving anticoagulation, respectively, and 34, 2 and 0% of patients in the control group, respectively. These data indicate that after rt-PA therapy of AMI, heparin therapy is associated with substantially higher coronary patency rates 3 days after thrombolysis but is accompanied by an increased incidence of minor bleeding complications.

Gertz and associates[123] from Bethesda, Maryland, and Boston, Massachusetts, and the TIMI Investigators *studied the hearts* of 52 patients aged 61 ± 11 years (34 men) who participated in the Thrombolysis in Myocardial Infarction (TIMI) Study and died from 5 hours to 260 days (median 2.7 days) after onset of chest pain. One heart became available at cardiac transplantation. Of the 52 patients, 38 received rt-PA not followed by PTCA or CABG. Eight had PTCA, and 6 had CABG. The infarcts were hemorrhagic by gross inspection (with histologic confirmation) in 23 patients, nonhemorrhagic in 20, not visible grossly in 2 and, in 7, there was no myocardial necrosis by either gross or histologic examination. Comparisons between the 23 patients with hemorrhagic infarcts and the 20 patients with nonhemorrhagic infarcts showed: (1) similar frequencies of myocardial rupture (LV free wall or ventricular septum) [6 (26%) of 23 vs 5 (25%) of 29], cardiogenic shock [10 (43%) of 23 vs 9 (47%) of 19], and fatal hemorrhage [2 (9%) of 23 vs 2 (10%) of 20]; (2) similar percents of necrotic portions of LV wall among patients surviving >18 hours from onset of chest pain (26 ± 11 vs 23 ± 11%) with the hemorrhage confined to areas of necrotic myocardium in all cases; (3) similar frequencies of thrombi in the infarct-related arteries [7 (32%) vs 7 (37%)], but all thrombi in patients with hemorrhagic infarcts were nonocclusive, and all thrombi in those with nonhemorrhagic infarcts were occlusive; (4) similar degrees of luminal cross-sectional area narrowing over all 5-mm segments of the 4 major (LM, LAD, LC and right epicardial coronary arteries in 27 patients receiving rt-PA alone between patients with hemorrhagic and nonhemorrhagic infarcts; (5) similar numbers of patients in whom the infarct-related artery was narrowed >75% in cross-sectional area at some point by plaque [21 (95%) of 22 vs 16 (84%) of 19], and similar mean percent reduction in cross-sectional area by plaque of the infarct-related arteries calculated by planimetry (67 ± 10 vs 68 ± 9%); (6) similar frequencies of plaque rupture [11 (55%) of 20 vs 12 (75%) of 16] and similar frequencies of hemorrhage into a plaque [13 (65%) of 20 vs 13 (81%) of 16] in patients without PTCA; (7) fewer RV infarcts in patients with hemorrhagic infarcts (2 of 10 posterior hemorrhagic infarcts vs 6 of 9 posterior nonhemorrhagic infarcts); (8) similar percents of plaque with pultaceous debris (13 ± 11 vs 18 ± 9%), calcific deposits (14 ± 12 vs 20 ± 14%) and acellular fibrous tissue (49 ± 14 vs 53 ± 11%). Thus, hemorrhage occurs frequently in the infarcts of patients who receive rt-PA. Hemorrhage into an infarct does not appear to extend the infarct, and patients with hemorrhagic (vs non-hemorrhagic) infarcts have no greater frequency of myocardial rupture or cardiogenic shock, and no significant differences in coronary luminal narrowing, plaque rupture or plaque composition. However, those with hemorrhagic infarcts had only nonocclusive thrombi and fewer RV infarcts.

Gertz and associates[124] from Bethesda, Maryland, and Boston, Massachusetts, *studied the hearts* of 61 patients (39 men aged 64 ± 11 years) who died from 5 hours to 42 days (median 3 days) after fatal first AMI without having undergone PTCA or CABG to compare clinical and cardiac morphologic features of patients receiving thrombolytic therapy with rt-PA to those not receiving thrombolytic therapy. Comparison of findings in the 23 patients who received rt-PA intravenously 3 ± 1 hours after onset of symptoms, with the 38 patients who did not, showed similar baseline characteristics with respect to: age, gender, history of hypertension; location of the infarct; heart weight; severity and numbers of coronary arteries narrowed; and frequencies of plaque rupture, plaque hemorrhage and coronary thrombi. Among the patients receiving rt-PA, however, there was a greater frequency of platelet-rich (fibrin-poor) thrombi in the infarct-related coronary arteries (6 of 11 vs 4 of 25 thrombi), more non-occlusive than occlusive thrombi (6 of 11 vs 4 of 25 thrombi), and a lower frequency of myocardial rupture (LV freewall or ventricular septum) (5 of 23 [22%] vs 18 of 38 [46%]).

Recombinant tissue-type plasminogen activator vs anisoylated plasminogen streptokinase activator complex

An overview by Held and colleagues[125] in Bethesda, Maryland, of 8 randomized controlled trials of rt-PA (Alteplase or Duteplase) and 10 of anisoylated plasminogen streptokinase activator complex (Anistreplase) (APSAC) showed that the odds of early death were reduced by 29% by rt-PA and 45% by APSAC. Although the beneficial effects of both agents are strengthened when all the trials are considered together, the available data do not permit comparisons of the relative efficacy of these 2 agents with each other or with streptokinase.

Anisoylated plasminogen streptokinase activator complex

In a randomized, double-blind study 1,258 patients were allocated by the AIMS Trial Study Group to receive either anistreplase (anisoylated plasminogen streptokinase activator complex [APSAC]) or placebo within 6 hours of onset of suspected AMI[126]. At 30 days, 40 (6%) of 624 patients on anistreplase had died, compared with 77 (12%) of 634 patients on placebo (odds reduction 50.5%). On long-term follow-up a survival benefit was still observed: at 12 months, 69 (11%) patients treated with anistreplase had died, compared with 113 (18%) patients given placebo. This effect on mortality was not related to time between onset of symptoms and treatment or to any patient characteristic. Site of AMI and age were the most important influences on 1-year survival in both treatment groups; tachycardia (>100 beats/min) on admission and previously diagnosed AMI were also associated with increased risk. Major complications of AMI were less frequent in patients treated with anistreplase than in controls. As for other thrombolytic agents, hemorrhage was more common, but usually minor. These findings indicate that anistreplase is an effective and acceptably safe thrombolytic with long-term survival benefits for patients with AMI.

Takens and associates[127] from Groningen, The Netherlands, treated 30 consecutive patients with AMI with anisoylated plasminogen streptokinase activator complex (APSAC) within 4 hours after the onset of symptoms. After 1.5 and 48 hours, patency of the infarct-related vessel and the quantitative degree of residual diameter stenosis were studied by selective coronary angiography. Ventriculograms were made to determine the global LVEF. Patients showing patency at 48 hours were reevaluated angiographically after 3 months. At 1.5 and 48 hours after APSAC administration patent vessels were demonstrated in 65 and 69% of patients, respectively. Mean residual stenosis decreased significantly from 56 ± 11% at 1.5 hours to 46 ± 13% at 48 hours. Patients not responding to thrombolytic therapy showed significant deterioration of the LV function during the first 48 hours after AMI. Side effects were minor and mainly associated with invasive procedures. Despite adequate oral anticoagulation, angiographically documented reocclusion at 3 months amounted to 28%. Reocclusion, however, was neither associated with clinically documented reinfarction, nor with a decrease in the LVEF. The study shows that APSAC is an effective thrombolytic agent in AMI but that late reocclusion may occur.

Urokinase

To determine the outcome of patients after treatment with high-dose intravenous urokinase (3,000,000 U), Wall and associates[128] from Durham, North Carolina, prospectively evaluated 102 patients during AMI. The first 61 patients received intravenous urokinase as a continuous infusion and the last 41 patients were treated with an initial 1.5 million U intravenous bolus. Sixty-two percent of all patients had patent infarct-related arteries by the time of immediate angiography (median time 2.2 hours), which was performed in all patients. There was no significant difference in patency rates between patients treated with or without an initial intravenous bolus. Twenty-eight (28%) patients developed clinical evidence of recurrent ischemia (death, reocclusion, emergency PTCA, urgent CABG) during hospitalization, whereas only 7 (7%) developed angiographically documented reocclusion. Of 28 patients who failed to achieve successful reperfusion at the time of immediate catheterization, rescue angioplasty was technically successful in establishing reperfusion in all but 1 patient. No significant improvement in median global LV function was seen between immediate (48%) and follow-up catheterization (48%). Significant bleeding complications were unusual except in 1 patient who experienced an intracranial hemorrhage. Eight (8%) patients died during hospitalization. Therefore, the use of high-dose intravenous urokinase in patients with AMI is associated with a 62% patency rate, a low incidence of reocclusion and bleeding complications and a high technical success rate with rescue angioplasty at the time of immediate catheterization. This study supports the need for further randomized controlled trials comparing intravenous urokinase directly with other thrombolytic regimens.

Aspirin vs warfarin afterwards

The optimum long-term antithrombolytic strategy for prevention of recurrent cardiac complications after thrombolysis is unknown. To determine whether aspirin or warfarin best prevents postdischarge recurrent cardiac events (unstable angina, reinfarction, pulmonary edema, and/or death), Schreiber and colleagues[129] from Royal Oak, Michigan, and New York, New York, analyzed the long-term course of 203 patients who received intravenous thrombolytic therapy (streptokinase, rt-PA, or urokinase) for AMI. Of these 129 (64%) survived to hospital discharge without PTCA or CABG—92 patients (71%) received aspirin (325 mg/day), whereas 37 (29%) received warfarin. The choice of drug was made by the treating physician. By a mean of 2.5 years of follow-up, 34 of 92 patients receiving aspirin (37%) versus 6 of 37 receiving warfarin (16%) had unstable angina, reinfarction, pulmonary edema, and/or death. No life-threatening hemorrhage occurred in either group. Warfarin appears to be superior to aspirin long-term in patients with postlysis AMI for the prevention of recurrent cardiac complications.

Effects on short-term revascularization rates

Naylor and Jaglal[130] from 3 medical centers sought evidence of the potential impact of intravenous thrombolytic therapy on short-term revascularization rates among patients with AMI. Because nonrandomized comparisons with conventional treatment would be subject to various confounders, a meta-analysis of randomized controlled trials was performed. Seven trials were included, applying standard doses of either rt-PA or streptokinase without an aggressive revascularization protocol. Follow-up ranged from 14 to 30 days. The revascularization rates among treated patients in all trials were lower than in the conservative arm of the Thrombolysis in Myocardial Infarction Phase II trial, which established the current procedural benchmarks for postthrombolysis management. The aggregate volume of CABG and PTCA in patients treated with rt-PA was more than double that of controls, with a smaller but still significant increase for streptokinase-treated patients. Combining all trials, the increase in mechanical revascularization was 80%. Thus, for patterns of practice currently accepted in North America, intravenous thrombolysis for AMI leads to a significant short-term increase in clinical and angiographic indications for revascularization as compared with conventional treatment.

Residual stenosis afterwards

Marshall and associates[131] from Camden, New Jersey, assessed clinical, angiographic, and demographic characteristics of 42 patients with low-grade (<50%) residual stenosis in the infarct related coronary artery after thrombolysis for AMI. The study group (group I) represented 21% of 198 consecutive patients receiving thrombolytic therapy over a 59-

month period. Data on the 156 remaining patients were pooled for comparison (group II). Group I patients were predominantly men (86%) who were cigarette smokers (81%). Group II patients were predominantly men (75%) but were significantly older (52 ± 12 vs 56 ± 10 years). Prior acute AMI or angina was unusual in group I. Sixty percent had no significant (>50%) residual CAD while 25% had residual single CAD. Average significant (>50% diameter stenosis) residual vessel disease was 0.6 ± 1.0 for group I and 1.9 ± 0.9 for group II. In group I, average residual infarct lesion diameter stenosis was 36 ± 7% in the right anterior oblique and 34 ± 8% in the left anterior oblique views. Thirty-nine group I patients were discharged with medical therapy and 100% follow-up was obtained over a mean interval of 18 ± 17 months. Fifteen patients experienced chest pain after acute AMI accounting for 17 discrete events. Fifty-nine percent of group I had a benign course on follow-up. Eight events were classified as unstable angina, 4 as acute AMI and 5 as atypical angina. Documented coronary vasospasm occurred in 3. The infarct narrowing accounted for 58% of documented ischemia and 41% of symptomatic events. Antiplatelet agents, warfarin and residual lesion morphology did not clearly influence frequency of events, whereas data regarding cigarette smoking were suggestive. Events clearly associated with the infarct narrowing occurred earlier (4 ± 4 months) than events not related to (23 ± 15 months). Ischemic events unrelated to the infarct lesion were often related to progressive stenosis or occlusion at the site of previously nonsignificant CAD.

Van Lierde and associates[132] in Leuven, Belgium, evaluated the severity of the infarct-related residual coronary stenosis after spontaneous or therapeutic thrombolysis using quantitative methods in 91 patients with AMIs allocated to treatment in the acute stage with either a thrombolytic agent (100 mg of rt-PA over 3 hours in 49 patients) or placebo (42 patients). Heparin and aspirin were given to both groups until angiography was performed. Digitally subtracted images of the infarct-related coronary arteries were obtained 10 to 14 days after hospital admission. Neither treatment group differed significantly in age, gender or location of the culprit coronary lesion. Median values in the thrombolysis and control groups were 1.95 mm vs 1.7 mm for stenosis lengths; 1.4 mm vs 1.4 mm for minimal luminal diameters; 57% vs 58% for diameter obstructions; 82% and 82% for geometric area obstructions; and 78% and 79% for densitometric area obstructions. No significant differences in anatomy or severity of residual coronary stenosis could be demonstrated at 10 to 14 days after AMI in patients with a recanalized infarct-related vessel, whether or not thrombolytic therapy was given on admission. These results demonstrate that effective antithrombotic treatment, gradual endogeneous fibrinolysis or more rapid lysis induced by the infusion of a thrombolytic agent may result in similar infarct-related coronary lesions at the time of hospital discharge.

Reocclusion after successful reperfusion

To determine the clinical consequences of reocclusion of an infarct-related artery after reperfusion therapy, Ohman and co-workers[133] in Durham, North Carolina, evaluated 810 patients with AMI. Patients were admitted into 4 sequential studies with similar entry criteria in which patency of the infarct-related artery was assessed by coronary arteriography 90 minutes after onset of thrombolytic therapy. Successful reperfusion was established acutely in 733 patients. Thrombolytic therapy included rt-PA in 517, urokinase in 87, and a combination of 2 thrombolytic agents in 129 patients. All patients received aspirin, intravenous heparin and nitroglycerin, and diltiazem during the recovery phase. A repeat arteriogram was performed in 88% of patients at a median of 7 days after onset of symptoms. Reocclusion of the infarct-related artery occurred in 91 patients (12%), and 58% of these were symptomatic. Angiographic characteristics at 90 minutes after thrombolytic therapy that were associated with reocclusion compared with sustained coronary artery patency were right coronary infarct-related artery and Thrombolysis in Myocardial Infarction flow 0 or 1 before further intervention. Median degree of stenosis in the infarct-related artery at 90 minutes was similar between groups. Patients with reocclusion had similar LVEF compared with patients with sustained patency at follow-up period. However patients with reocclusion at follow-up had worse infarct-zone function. The recovery of both global and infarct-zone function was impaired by reocclusion of the infarct related artery to compared with maintain patency. In addition, patients with reocclusion had more complicated hospital courses and higher in-hospital mortality rates (11% vs 5%). The investigators concluded that reocclusion infarct related artery after successful reperfusion is associated with substantial morbidity and mortality rates. Reocclusion is also detrimental to the functional recovery of both global and infarct-zone regional LV function.

Effects on signal-averaged electrocardiogram

Turitto and associates[134] in Rome, Italy, evaluated the prevalence of abnormal signal-averaged electrocardiograms and ventricular arrhythmias on 24-hour ambulatory electrocardiograms in 118 patients 13 ± 2 days after AMI. Group 1 patients (46 patients) underwent intravenous thrombolysis within 6 hours of symptom onset, and group 2 (72 patients) did not receive thrombolytic therapy. An abnormal signal-averaged electrocardiogram was found in 15% of patients in group I and 21% of those in group 2. The number of ventricular premature complexes per hour was lower in group 1 than in group 2 patients, but complex arrhythmias (≥10 VPCs per hour or VT) were equally common among group 1 and 2 patients (20% and 22%, respectively). The prevalence of frequent and complex arrhythmias was similar in patients with and without an abnormal signal-averaged electrocardiogram (29% and 18%, respectively, in group 1 and 27% vs 21%, respectively, in group 2). Comparisons between patients with (n = 26) or without (n = 20) angiographic patency of the infarct-related coronary artery after thrombolysis showed no significance difference in the prevalence of an abnormal signal-averaged electrocardiogram (8% vs 25%, respectively) and complex ventricular arrhythmias (19% vs 20%, respectively). Thus, these data suggest that thrombolysis does not affect the prevalence of complex ventricular arrhythmias and an abnormal signal-averaged electrocardiogram after AMI.

To test the effects of thrombolysis on the incidence and evolution of late potentials, Eldar and associates[135] from Tel Hashomer, Israel, prospectively studied 158 consecutive patients during the first 10 days after AMI. The study population consisted of 2 groups: 93 control patients treated conservatively and 65 patients treated with intravenous thrombolysis. Recordings of signal averaged electrocardiogram were obtained within 2 days and 7–10 days after AMI. The incidence of late potentials in the first 2 days after AMI was not significantly different in the thrombolytic and control groups (14% vs 12%). By 7–10 days the incidence of late potentials among patients who underwent thrombolysis remained unchanged (14%); however, it increased significantly in the control group (11.8%–22.5%). Thus, thrombolysis seems to reduce the evolution of late potentials within 10 days of infarction.

Leor and associates[136] from Tel Hashomer and Tel Aviv, Israel, examined the effects of reperfusion achieved with thrombolytic therapy on the 12-lead signal-averaged electrocardiogram and on ventricular arrhythmias in the early period after AMI. A total of 190 consecutive patients with AMI who fulfilled the inclusion criteria were enrolled. Thrombolysis was attempted in 80 patients and was considered successful in 57 (group I) and unsuccessful in 23 patients (group II); 110 patients were not treated with thrombolytic agents (group III). Signal averaging of 12 electrocardiographic leads was performed within 2 days in all patients and between 7 and 10 days after admission in 163 patients. The filtered QRS complex duration was significantly shorter in group I compared to group III in 7 of 12 electrocardiographic leads at 2 days and in 10 of 12 leads at 7 to 10 days. The root mean square voltage of the terminal 40 msec of the QRS complex did not change between the 2 signal-averaged electrocardiographic recordings in group I, whereas it became lower in 3 electrocardiographic leads in group II and in 7 electrocardiographic leads in group III. There was no correlation between infarct site and significant changes in infarct-related signal-averaged electrocardiographic leads. The occurrence of complex ventricular arrhythmias was not significantly different among the 3 groups. It was concluded that successful reperfusion, compared with failed and nonattempted reperfusion, is associated with fewer abnormalities in the 12-lead signal-averaged electrocardiogram in the early period after AMI. These findings may be related to reduced early and late mortality in patients undergoing successful reperfusion.

Repeat thrombolytic therapy

White and associates[137] from Auckland, New Zealand, assessed the efficacy and safety of repeat thrombolytic treatment in 31 patients treated with streptokinase (n = 13) or rt-PA (n = 18) a median of 5 days (1–716) after the first infusion. The indication for readministration was prolonged chest pain with new ST segment elevation. Efficacy was assessed by infarct artery patency at angiography at a median of 8 days after readministration in 22 patients and by non-invasive criteria in 23 patients (reperfusion was deemed to be likely if serum creatine kinase was not increased or reached a peak 12 hours after infarction). Angiography showed patency of 70% of the infarct arteries after readministration of streptokinase and of 75% after rt-PA. The corresponding patency rates assessed noninvasively were 73% and 75%. Reinfarction was prevented in 9 (29%) patients. Allergic reactions occurred in 4 of 8 patients who received streptokinase twice (plasmacytosis and acute reversible renal failure developed in 1 patient). Two patients had major bleeding and 2 minor bleeding, all after rt-PA, and 1 of them died of cerebral hemorrhage. Repeat thrombolytic treatment results in late patency rates similar to the rates after the initial administration. Allergic reactions were common in those treated twice with streptokinase.

PERCUTANEOUS TRANSLUMINAL CORONARY ANGIOPLASTY

Early after thrombolysis

El Deeb and associates[138] from Eindhoven, The Netherlands, did immediate PTCA after intravenous streptokinase (0.75 to 1.5 million U) in 98 patients with AMI <4 hours after the onset of chest pain. Thirty-four culprit arteries were occluded (group A); 42 arteries were patent with residual stenosis >70% (group B). Twenty-two patients had residual stenosis <70% (group C); 8 of these had severe disease of the remaining vessels. Group C patients were either treated conservatively or underwent CABG. Immediate PTCA was attempted in 74 patients (32 in group A, 42 in group B) and was successful in 68 (92%). Emergency CABG for acute occlusion after PTCA was required in 2 patients. Follow-up averaged 23 months (range 16 to 47 months). Asymptomatic occlusion recurred in 3 patients. Restenosis occurred in 5 patients: 4 had early restenosis (1 in group A, 3 in group B) and 1 had late restenosis (group B). These arteries were successfully redilated. Late reinfarction occurred in 2 patients; they were treated with intravenous urokinase and repeat PTCA. Elective CABG was performed in 3 patients because of recurrent angina; they had severe 3-vessel disease as revealed by control angiography. The mortality rate was 2.7% (2 patients; 1 in group B had early reinfarction, and 1 patient in group A died suddenly after 17 months). Eighty-five percent of patients treated with PTCA alone remain free of symptoms. This approach has a high success rate and low morbidity and mortality rates.

Abbottsmith and colleagues[139] in Cincinnati and Columbus, Ohio; Ann Arbor, Michigan and Durham, North Carolina, evaluated the outcome of 776 patients with patent infarct-related arteries after emergency cardiac catheterization. In the course of 5 Thombolysis and Angioplasty in Myocardial Infarction trials, 607 patients with thrombolysis-mediated patency of the infarct-related artery and 169 with patency achieved by angioplasty were evaluated. Baseline characteristics of the thrombolysis and angioplasty groups were similar except for a higher acute LVEF in the thrombolysis group (51% vs 48%). Seven to 10 day LVEFs were higher (52% vs 48%), infarct zone functional recoveries were greater, and reocclusions of the infarct-related arteries were less frequent (11% vs 21%) in the thrombolysis compared with PTCA groups. Despite these differences, PTCA patency was associated with the same low in-hospital mortality rate (6% vs 5%) and long-term mortality rate (3% vs 2%) as patency achieved by thrombolysis. Reocclusion adversely affected the mortality rate and ventricular functional recovery. Technical failure of rescue PTCA was associated with a higher mortality rate than was technical success (39% vs 6%). Thus, there were early functional benefits of infarct-artery patency achieved by thrombolysis as compared to PTCA in this study in patients with AMI, but both procedures were associated with the same low in-hospital and long-term mortality rates suggesting that rescue PTCA may be beneficial in some patients with failure of infarct-related artery recanalization after thrombolytic therapy.

Early without preceding thrombolysis

Stone and associates[140] in Kansas City, Missouri, performed PTCA as primary therapy in 215 consecutive patients with a mean age of 56 ± 11 years 75% of whom were males with AMI and single vessel CAD. Patency of the infarct-related artery was restored in 212 patients (99%). Complications consisted of one urgent CABG (0.5%). There were no procedural deaths. Recurrent ischemic events before discharge occurred in 8 patients (4%). The in-hospital mortality rate was 1% and 5 of 6 patients presenting with cardiogenic shock were alive at discharge. In 126 patients in whom predischarge angiography was obtained, the EF improved from 55 ± 12% to 61 ± 12% and increased by ≥5% units in 66 patients (52%). Regional wall motion improved in 60 patients. By multivariate analysis, a depressed initial EF, a limited increase in serum creatine kinase, young age and sustained patency of the infarct-related artery were independent predictors of improvement in LV function. Follow-up data were available in 214 patients at a mean interval of 35 months. The actuarial 3 year cardiac survival rate was 92%. By multivariate analysis, only the baseline EF correlated with long-term cardiac survival. Nine patients (4%) sustained a late fatal AMI and 11 patients (5%) underwent CABG. At late follow-up study, 149 (77%) of 194 patients were free of angina. Thus, in patients with AMI and single vessel CAD, PTCA without prior thrombolytic therapy may be performed with a high success rate and few procedural complications. After direct PTCA, regional wall motion and global EF improve in 50% of patients, especially in those with initially depressed LV function.

To compare the results and outcome of different management approaches for AMI, Beauchamp and colleagues[141] from Kansas City, Missouri, analyzed their experience with early (≤6 hours of infarct onset) direct PTCA (group A) vs initial treatment with thrombolytic therapy (group B) followed by PTCA. From 1982 to 1989, a total of 214 patients underwent primary PTCA for AMI. During this time 157 patients underwent initial thrombolytic therapy, 104 with intravenous streptokinase and 53 with intravenous tissue-type plasminogen activator followed by PTCA. Other than age (group A 62 ± 12 years; group B 57 ± 12 years), the clinical characteristics of the groups were similar. In group A, 197 (92%) had successful results, and 17 (7.9%) were failures. Of the group treated with thrombolytic therapy, there was an overall 82% patency rate for patients treated with streptokinase and rt-PA activator with no significant difference between the agents. PTCA success after thrombolytic therapy was 94%. In-hospital and 1-year survival were significantly better in group B patients (96% and 96%, respectively) than in group A patients (92% and 89%, respectively). It was concluded that both direct PTCA and thrombolytic therapy followed by PTCA provide high recanalization rates but that short- and long-term survival are improved when thrombolytic therapy precedes PTCA in AMI patients.

Nath and associates[142] in Richmond, Virginia, evaluated the influence of PTCA of multiple vessels in 105 patients 0 to 15 days after AMI. PTCA was performed at a mean of 5 ± 4 days after AMI. There were 77 men and 28 women with a mean age of 57 years. All patients had severe multivessel CAD, including 68% with 2-vessel and 32% with 3-vessel CAD. Twenty-eight patients (27%) had successful thrombolysis before PTCA and 70 (67%) had postinfarction angina. Mean LVEF was 58 ± 10%, and it was <45% in 13 patients. PTCA was attempted in 319 lesions, mean 3 lesions per patient and a range of 2 to 9, and 252 vessels, mean 2 per patient with success in 302 lesions (95%) and 237 vessels (94%). PTCA was done in two stages in 59 patients (56%). Clinical success occurred in 102 patients (97%). Complications included AMI in six patients (5.7%), need for urgent CABG in two (1.9%) and death in one (0.9%). Seven patients (7%) had a major complication. Follow-up duration for a mean interval of 31 months revealed a clinical recurrence of coronary artery stenoses in 24 patients (23%) of whom 21 had repeat PTCA, 1 had CABG, and 2 were managed medically. Ten patients (9.8%) had a late AMI and 5 (4.9%) died a cardiac death during the follow-up period. Including patients who underwent repeat PTCA, 88 patients (86%) remained improved without need for coronary artery revascularization. Actuarial survival rate was 94% at 24 months and the event-free survival rate was 85% at 2 years. These data suggest that PTCA of multiple vessels can be a safe and effective therapy in selected patients with multivessel CAD after recent AMI when experienced cardiologists perform the procedure.

Lee and associates[143] from Kansas City, Missouri, performed direct PTCA as the primary means of establishing reperfusion during AMI in 105 elderly patients (mean age 75 ± 4 years) at a mean of 5.5 ± 4.0 hours after symptom onset. Fifty-two patients (50%) had anterior infarctions, 70 (67%) had significant narrowing in >1 vessel, and 12 (11%) were in cardiogenic shock. Primary success was achieved in 91% of the infarct-related arteries. Four patients with failed PTCA underwent emergency bypass surgery; 10 had early symptomatic reocclusion of the dilated vessel. There was 1 death acutely in the catheterization laboratory. The overall in-hospital mortality was 18%. Three-vessel CAD and cardiogenic shock on presentation were the strongest predictors of in-hospital death. Global EF improved from 54 ± 13 to 61 ± 15%). The 1- and 5-year survival rates, including in-hospital deaths, were 73 and 67%, respectively. It is concluded that direct PTCA is an effective means of salvaging ischemic myocardium during AMI in the elderly patient. It is associated with a high success rate and low complication rate. The short- and long-term survival in this high-risk group of patients are improved compared with survival rates in historical controls.

The effect of early myocardial reperfusion on patterns of death after AMI is unknown. Kahn and associates[144] from Kansas City, Missouri, determined the mechanism and timing of in-hospital and late deaths among a group of 614 patients treated with PTCA without antecedent thrombolytic therapy for AMI. Death occurred in 49 patients (8%) before hospital discharge. Four patients died in the catheterization laboratory. Death was due to cardiogenic shock in 22 patients, acute vessel reclosure in 5 patients, was sudden in 8 patients, and followed elective CABG in 8 patients. Cardiac rupture was observed in 2 patients after failed infarct angioplasty, and did not occur among the 574 patients with successful infarct reperfusion. Multivariate predictors of in-hospital death included failed infarct angioplasty, cardiogenic shock, 3-vessel CAD and age ≥70 years. During a follow-up period of 32 ± 21 months (range 1 to 87), 55 patients died. The cause of death was cardiac in 36 patients, including an arrhythmic death in 23 patients and was due to circulatory failure in 13 others. One patient died of reinfarction due to late reclosure of the infarct artery. Actuarial survival curves demonstrated overall survival after hospital discharge of 95 and 87% at 1 and 4 years, respectively. Freedom from cardiac death at 1 and 4 years was 96 and 92%. Multivariate predictors of late death included 3-vessel disease, a baseline EF of ≤40%, age >70 years and female gender. Thus, death after PTCA for AMI is related to the status of the LV and the extent of CAD.

Kahn and colleagues[145] in Kansas City, Missouri, used direct PTCA in coronary arteries without antecedent thrombolytic therapy during evolving AMI in 285 patients with multivessel CAD at 5 ± 4 hours after the onset of chest pain. Two vessel CAD was present in 163 patients (57%) and 3-vessel CAD in 122 (43%). An anterior wall AMI occurred in 123 patients (43%), cardiogenic shock in 33 (12%) and age ≥70 years in 59 (21%). PTCA of the infarct-related artery was successful in 256 patients (90%), including 92% with two vessel and 88% with three vessel disease. Emergency CABG was needed in 6 patients. In-hospital death occurred in 33 patients (12%), including 13 with two vessel and 20 with three vessel disease. Morbidity rate was only 4% in the subgroup of 101 patients who met entry criteria for thrombolytic trials. The in-hospital mortality rate was 45% in patients in shock and 7% in patients not in shock. Logistic regression analysis identified shock and age ≥70 years as independently associated with in-hospital death. In 135 patients who underwent pre-discharge left ventriculography, global EF increased from 50% to 57% and regional wall motion in the infarct zone improved in 59% of patients. Follow-up data were available in 251 patients (99%) at a mean of 35 ± 19 months. The actuarial 1 and 3 year survival rates were 92% and 87%, respectively and they were significantly better at both intervals in patients with two vessel disease. Thus, primary PTCA in patients with AMI and multivessel CAD results in a high reperfusion rate, good hospital survival, especially in patients not in shock, and a favorable long-term outcome.

To assess the safety of direct infarct angioplasty without antecedent thrombolytic therapy, Kahn and colleagues[146] in Kansas City, Missouri, assessed catheterization laboratory and hospital events and consecutively treated patients with infarctions involving the LAD (n = 100 patients), right (n = 10), and LC (n = 50) coronary arteries. The groups of patients were similar for age, multivessel CAD and patients with initial grade 0–1 antegrade flow. Cardiogenic shock was present in 16 patients. Major catheterization laboratory events (cardioversion, cardiopulmonary resuscitation, dopamine or intra-aortic balloon pump support for hypotension and urgent surgery) occurred in 22 patients. There was one in-laboratory death in a shock patient. Minor in-laboratory events (brief bolus atropine or pressor, and temporary pacer) occurred in an additional 39 patients. Procedural success was achieved in >90% of the patients. Predischarge angiography demonstrated sustained arterial patency in 95% of 65 patients with LAD angioplasty, 90% of 62 with right angioplasty, and 81% of 26 with LC angioplasty. Hospital survival was 95%. Thus, major catheterization events are infrequent during direct infarct angioplasty. Although minor catheterization laboratory events are common, and should be anticipated, direct infarct angioplasty results in excellent arterial patency and hospital survival.

For non-Q wave infarction

Alfonso and associates[147] from Madrid, Spain, assessed prospectively in 33 consecutive patients the value of PTCA for myocardial ischemia after a non-Q-wave AMI. In 30 patients the indication for the procedure was post-AMI angina and 3 patients underwent PTCA for silent ischemia. A total of 43 lesions were attempted at 63 ± 94 days after the non-Q-wave AMI. Primary PTCA success was obtained in 30 (91%) patients and no major complications occurred. Angiographic evaluation was performed either for symptoms or for protocol (7 ± 1 months after PTCA) in 28 (93%) of the 30 patients with successful PTCA, but 2 patients (7%) who were asymptomatic refused the repeat angiogram. Twenty (71%) had no restenosis and 8 (29%) had restenosis. Of these, 5 patients with restenosis underwent a successful repeat PTCA (6 ± 1 months after the initial procedure). At the last clinical follow-up (17 ± 8 months), 2 of the 30 (7%) patients successfully dilated presented with stable angina despite medical treatment, whereas the rest (93%) remained asymptomatic. During the study period no patient died, had an AMI or required CABG. Thus, selected patients with ischemia after a non-Q-wave AMI, a "high-risk population," can be effectively treated with PTCA with an initial success rate and angiographic restenosis rate similar to that of the general PTCA population and appear to have sustained symptomatic benefit remaining free of subsequent cardiac events.

Suryapranata and associates[148] from Rotterdam, The Netherlands, investigated the effect of PTCA on regional myocardial function of the infarct zone in 36 patients with angina early after a non-Q wave AMI. All had successful PTCA within 30 days of a non-Q wave AMI and sequential LV angiograms of adequate quality were obtained before the initial procedure and at follow-up angiography. The global EF increased significantly from $60 \pm 9\%$ to $67 \pm 6\%$. This significant increase in the global EF was primarily due to a significant improvement in the regional myocardial function of the infarct zone. These results show not only that ischemic attacks early after a non-Q wave AMI may lead to prolonged regional myocardial dysfunction but more importantly that this depressed myocardium has the potential to achieve normal contraction after successful PTCA.

References

1. Tofler GH, Stone PH, Maclure M, Edelman E, Davis VG, Robertson T, Antman EM, Muller JE, Milis Study Group: Analysis of possible triggers of acute myocardial infarction. (The MILIS Study). Am J Cardiol 1990 (July 1);66:22–27.

2. Kleiman NS, Schechtman KB, Young PM, Goodman DA, Boden WE, Pratt CM, Roberts R, Diltiazem Reinfarction study Investigators: Lack of diurnal variation in the onset of non-q wave infarction. Circulation 1990 (February);81:548–555.

3. Goldberg RJ, Brady P, Muller JE, Chen Z, De Groot M, Zonneveld P, Dalen JE: Time of onset of symptoms of acute myocardial infarction. Am J Cardiol 1990 (July 15);66: 14–144.

4. Ridker PM, Manson JE, Buring JE, Muller JE, Hennekens H: Circadian Variation of Acute Myocardial Infarction and the Effect of Low-Dose Aspirin in a Randomized Trial of Physicians. Circulation 1990 (September);82:897–902.

5. Rosenberg L, Palmer JR, Shapiro S: Decline in the risk of myocardial infarction among women who stop smoking. N Engl J Med 1990 (Jan. 25);322:213–217.

6. Gramenzi A, Gentile A, Fasoli M, Negri E, Parazzini F, La Vecchia C: Association between certain foods and risk of acute myocardial infarction in women. Br Med J 1990 (Mar 24);300:771–773.

7. Kleiger RE, Boden WE, Schechtman KB, Gibson RS, Schwartz DJ, Geiger BJ, Capone RJ, Roberts R, Diltiazem Reinfarction Study Group: Frequency and significance of late evolution of Q waves in patients with initial non-Q-wave acute myocardial infarction. Am J Cardiol 1990 (Jan 1);65:23–27.

8. Hung J, Whitford EG, Parsons RW, Hillman DR: Association of sleep apnea with myocardial infarction in men. Lancet 1990 (Aug 4);336:261–264.

9. Amin M, Gabelman G, Karpel J, Buttrick P: Acute myocardial infarction and chest pain syndromes after cocaine use. Am J Cardiol 1990 (Dec 15);66:1434–1437.

10. Grines CL, Booth DC, Nissen SE, Gurley JC, Bennett KA, O'Connor WN, Demaria AN: Mechanism of acute myocardial infarction in patients with prior coronary artery bypass grafting and therapeutic implications. Am J Cardiol 1990 (June 1);65:1292–1296.

11. Bissett JK, Ngo WL, Wyeth RP, Matts JP, Posch Group: Angiographic progression to total coronary occlusion in hyperlipidemic patients after acute myocardial infarction. Am J Cardiol 1990 (Dec 1);66:1293–1297.

12. Puleo PR, Guadagno PA, Roberts R, Scheel MV, Marian AJ, Churchill D, Perryman MB: Early Diagnosis of Acute Myocardial Infarction Based on Assay for Subforms of Creatine Kinase-MB. Circulation 1990 (September);82:759–764.

13. Vaughan DE, Lamas GA, Pfeffer MA: Role of left ventricular dysfunction in selective neurohumoral activation in the recover phase of anterior wall acute myocardial infarction. Am J Cardiol 1990 (Sept 1);66:529–532.

14. Ohman EM, Casey C, Bengtson JR, Pryor D, Tormey W, Horgan JH: Early detection of acute myocardial infarction: Additional diagnostic information from serum concentrations of myoglobin in patients without ST elevation. Br Heart J 1990 (June);63: 355–358.

15. Leger JOC, Larue C, Ming T, Calzolari C, Gautier P, Mouton C, Grolleau R, Louisot P, Puech P, Peperstraete B, Staroukine M, Telerman M, Pau B, Leger JJ: Assay of serum cardiac myosin heavy chain fragments in patients with acute myocardial infarction: Determination of infarct size and long-term follow-up. Am Heart J 1990 (October);120:781–790.

16. Fontana F, Bernardi P, Spagnolo N, Capelli M: Plasma atrial natriuretic factor in patients with acute myocardial infarction. Eur Heart J 1990 (Sept);11:779–787.

17. Zion MM, Balkin J, Rosenmann D, Goldbourt U, Reicher-Reiss H, Kaplinsky E, Behar S, SPRINT Study Group: Use of pulmonary artery catheters in patients with acute myocardial infarction: Analysis of experience in 5,841 patients in the SPRINT registry. Chest 1990 (Dec);98:1331–1335.

18. Dalen JE: Does pulmonary artery catheterization benefit patients with acute myocardial infarction? Chest 1990 (Dec);98:1313–1314.

19. Ouyang P, Chandra NC, Gottlieb SO: Frequency and importance of silent myocardial ischemia identified with ambulatory electrocardiographic monitoring in the early in-hospital period after acute myocardial infarction. Am J Cardiol 1990 (Feb 1);65: 267–270.

20. Currie P, Saltissi S: Transient myocardial ischemia after acute myocardial infarction. Br Heart J 1990 (Nov);64:299–303.

21. Lange RA, Cigarroa RG, Wells PJ, Kremers MS, Hillis LD: Influence of anterograde flow in the infarct artery on the incidence of late potentials after acute myocardial infarction. Am J Cardiol 1990 (Mar 1);65:554–558.

22. Johannessen KA, Cerqueira MD, Stratton JR: Influence of myocardial infarction size on radionuclide and Doppler echocardiogram measurements of diastolic function. Am J Cardiol 1990 (Mar 15);65:692–697.

23. Picard MH, Wilkins GT, Ray PA, Weyman AE: Natural History of Left Ventricular Size and Function After Acute Myocardial Infarction Assessment and Prediction by Echocardiographic Endocardial Surface Mapping. Circulation 1990 (August);82:484–494.

24. Williamson BD, Lim MJ, Buda AJ: Transient left ventricular filling abnormalities (diastolic stunning) after acute myocardial infarction. Am J Cardiol 1990 (Oct 15);66: 897–903.

25. Brown KA, O'Meara J, Chambers CE, Plante DA: Ability of dipyridamole-thallium-201 imaging one to four days after acute myocardial infarction to predict in-hospital and late recurrent myocardial ischemic events. Am J Cardiol 1990 (Jan 15);65:160–167.

26. Lundgren C, Bourdillon DV, Dillon JC, Feigenbaum H: Comparison of contrast angiography and two-dimensional echocardiography for the evaluation of left ventricular regional wall motion abnormalities after acute myocardial infarction. Am J Cardiol 1990 (May 1);65:1071–1077.

27. Johns JA, Leavitt MB, Newell JB, Yasuda T, Leinbach RC, Gold HK, Finkelstein D, Dinsmore RE. Quantitation of myocardial infarct size by nuclear magnetic resonance imaging. J Am Coll Cardiol 1990 (January);15:143–9.

28. Marcus FI, Friday K, Mccans J, Moon T, Hahn E, Cobb L, Edwards J, Kuller L: Age-related prognosis after acute myocardial infarction (The Multicenter Diltiazem Postinfarction Trial) Am J Cardiol 1990 (Mar 1);65:559–566.

29. Nadelmann J, Frishman WH, Ooi WL, Tepper D, Greenberg S, Guzik H, Lazar EJ, Heiman M, Aronson M: Prevalence, incidence and prognosis of recognized and unrecognized myocardial infarction in persons aged 75 years or older: The Bronx aging study. Am J Cardiol 1990 (Sept 1);66:533–537.

30. Smith SC, Gilpin E, Ahnve S, Dittrich H, Nicod P, Henning H, Ross J Jr. Outlook after acute myocardial infarction in the very elderly compared with that in patients aged 65 to 75 years. J Am Coll Cardiol 1990 (October);16:784–92.

31. Fiebach NH, Viscoli CM, Horwitz RI: Differences between women and men in survival after myocardial infarction: Biology or methodology? JAMA 1990 (Feb 23);263:1092–1096.

32. Fox JP, Beattie JM, Salih MS, Davies MK, Littler WA, Murray RG: Non Q-wave infarction: Exercise test characteristics, coronary anatomy, and prognosis. Br Heart J 1990 (Mar);63:151–153.

33. Schechtman KB, Capone RJ, Kleiger RE, Gibson RS, Schwartz DJ, Roberts R, Boden WE, and the Diltiazem Reinfarction Study Group. Differential risk patterns associated with 3 month as compared with 3 to 12 month mortality and reinfarction after non-Q wave myocardial infarction. J Am Coll Cardiol 1990 (April);15:940–7.

34. Benhorin J, Moss AJ, Oakes D, Marcus F, Greenberg H, Dwyer EM, Algeo S, Hahn E, and the Multicenter Diltiazem Post-Infarction Research Group. The prognostic significance of first myocardial infarction type (Q wave versus non-Q wave) and Q wave location. J Am Coll Cardiol 1990 (May);15:1201–7.

35. Nielsen JR, Mickley H, Damsgaard EM, Groland A: Predischarge maximal exercise test identifies risk for cardiac death in patients with acute myocardial infarction. Am J Cardiol 1990 (Jan 15);65:149–153.

36. Kato K, Saito F, Hatano K, Noda S, Tsuzuki J, Yokota M, Hayashi H, Saito H, Sotobata I: Prognostic value of abnormal postexercise systolic blood pressure response: Prehospital discharge test after myocardial infarction in Japan. Am Heart J 1990 (February);119:264–271.

37. Trip MD, Cats VM, Van Capelle FJL, Vreeken J: Platelet hyperreactivity and prognosis in survivors of myocardial infarction. N Engl J Med 1990 (May 31);322:1549–1554.

38. Bates ER, Clemmensen PM, Califf RM, Gorman LE, Aronson LG, George BS, Kereiakes DJ, Topol EJ, and the Thrombolysis and Angioplasty in Myocardial Infarction (TAMI) Study Group. Precordial ST segment depression predicts a worse prognosis in inferior infarction despite reperfusion therapy. J Am Coll Cardiol 1990 (December);16:1538–44.

39. Hjalmarson A, Gilpin EA, Kjekshus J, Schieman G, Nicod P, Henning H, Ross J Jr: Influence of heart rate on mortality after acute myocardial infarction. Am J Cardiol 1990 (Mar 1);65:547–553.

40. Goldberg RJ, Seeley D, Becker RC, Brady P, Chen Z, Osganian V, Gore JM, Alpert JS, Dalen JE: Impact of atrial fibrillation on the in-hospital and long-term survival of patients with acute myocardial infarction: A community-wide perspective. Am Heart J 1990 (May);119:996–1001.

41. Berisso MZ, Carratino L, Ferroni A, Mela GS, Mazzotta G, Vecchio C: Frequency, characteristics and significance of supraventricular tachyarrhythmias detected by 24-hour electrocardiographic recording in the late hospital phase of acute myocardial infarction. Am J Cardiol 1990 (May 1);65:1064–1070.

42. Iesaka Y, Nogami A, Aonuma K, Nitta J, Chun YH, Fujiwara H, Hiraoka M: Prognostic significance of sustained monomorphic ventricular tachycardia induced by programmed ventricular stimulation using up to triple extrastimuli in survivors of acute myocardial infarction. Am J Cardiol 1990 (May 1);65:1057–1063.

43. Wong ND, Levy D, Kannel WB: Prognostic significance of the electrocardiogram after Q wave myocardial infarction. Circulation 1990 (March);81:780–789.

44. Kleiger RE, Miller JP, Krone RJ, Bigger JT Jr, Multicenter Postinfarction Research Group: The independence of cycle length variability and exercise testing on predicting mortality of patients surviving acute myocardial infarction. Am J Cardiol 1990 (Feb 15);65:408–411.

45. Flowers NC, Horan LG, Wylds AC, Crawford W, Sridharan MR, Horan CP, Cliff SF: Relation of peri-infarction block to ventricular late potentials in patients with inferior wall myocardial infarction. Am J Cardiol 1990 (Sept 1);66:568–574.

46. Rivers JT, White HD, Cross DB, Williams BF, Norris RM. Reinfarction after thrombolytic therapy for acute myocardial infarction followed by conservative management: Incidence and effect of smoking. J Am Coll Cardiol 1990 (August);16:340–8.

47. Benhorin J, Moss AJ, Oakes D. Prognostic significance of nonfatal myocardial reinfarction. J Am Coll Cardiol 1990 (February);15:253–8.

48. Kouvaras G, Chronopoulos G, Soufras G, Sofronas G, Solomos D, Bakirtzis A, Pissimissis E, Tzonou A, Cokkinois D: The effects of long-term antithrombotic treatment on left ventricular thrombi in patients after an acute myocardial infarction. Am Heart J 1990 (January);119:73–78.

49. Stratton J, Ritchie J. [111]In Platelet Imaging of Left Ventricular Thrombi Predictive Value for Systemic Emboli. Circulation 1990 (April);81:1182–1189.

50. Yasuda T, Okada RD, Leinbach RC, Gold HK, Phillips H, McKusick KA, Glover DK, Boucher CA, Strauss HW: Serial evaluation of right ventricular dysfunction associated with acute inferior myocardial infarction. Am Heart J 1990 (April);119:816–822.

51. Mavric Z, Zaputovic L, Matana A, Kucic J, Roje J, Marinovic D, Rupcic A: Prognostic significance of complete atrioventricular block in patients with acute inferior myocardial infarction with and without right ventricular involvement. Am Heart J 1990 (April);119:823–828.

52. Goldstein JA, Barzilai B, Rosmond TL, Eisenberg PR, Jaffe AS: Determinants of Hemodynamic Compromise with Severe Right Ventricular Infarction. Circulation 1990 (August);82:359–368.

53. Bates KP, Ackermann DM, Edwards WD: Post-infarction rupture of the left ventricular free wall: Clinicopathologic correlates in 100 consecutive autopsy cases. Hum Pathol 199–(May);21:530–535.

54. Roberts WC: Rupture of the left ventricular free wall during acute myocardial infarction without hemopericardium. Am J Cardiol 1990 (Apr 15);65:1033–1037.

55. Bansal RC, Eng AK, Shakudo M: Role of two-dimensional echocardiography, pulsed, continuous wave and color flow Doppler techniques in the assessment of ventricular septal rupture after myocardial infarction. Am J Cardiol 1990 (Apr 1);65:852–860.

56. Helmcke, F, Mahan E, Nanda N, Jain S, Soto B, Kirklin J, Pacifico A. Two-Dimensional Echocardiography and Doppler Color Flow Mapping in the Diagnosis and Prognosis of Ventricular Septal Rupture. Circulation 1990 (June);81:1775–1783.

57. Skillington PD, Davies RH, Luff AJ, Williams JD, Dawkins KD, Conway N, Lamb RK, Shore DF, Monro JL, Ross JK: Surgical treatment for infarct-related ventricular septal defects: Improved early results combined with analysis of late functional status. J Thorac Cardiovasc Surg 1990 (May);99:798–808.

58. Barzilai B, Davis VG, Stone PH, Jaffe AS, Milis Study Group: Prognostic significance of mitral regurgitation in acute myocardial infarction. Am J Cardiol 1990 (May 15);65:1169–1175.

59. Jensen GVH, Torp Pedersen C, Kober L, Steens-Gaard-Hansen F, Rasmussen YH, Berning J, Skagen K, Pedersen A: Prognosis of late versus early ventricular fibrillation in acute myocardial infarction. Am J Cardiol 1990 (July 1);66:10–15.

60. Willems AR, Tijssen JGP, van Capelle FJL, Kingma JH, Hauer RNW, Vermeulen FEE, Brugada P, van Hoogenhuyze DCA, Janse MJ, on behalf of the Dutch Ventricular Tachycardia Study Group of the Interuniversity Cardiology Institute of The Netherlands. Determinants of prognosis in symptomatic ventricular tachycardia or ventricular fibrillation late after myocardial infarction. J Am Coll Cardiol 1990 (September);16:521–30.

61. Volpi A, Cavalli A, Santoro E, Tognoni G, GISSI Investigators: Incidence and Prognosis of Secondary Ventricular Fibrillation in Acute Myocardial Infarction Evidence for a Protective Effect of Thrombolytic Therapy. Circulation 1990 (October);82:1279–1288.

62. Behar S, Goldbourt U, Reicher-Reiss H, Kaplinsky E, Principal Investigators of the SPRINT Study: Prognosis of acute myocardial infarction complicated by primary ventricular fibrillation. Am J Cardiol 1990 (Nov 15);66:1208–1211.

63. Moss AJ, Benhorin J: Prognosis and management after a first myocardial infarction. N Engl J Med 1990 (Mar 15);322:743–753.

64. Taylor CB, Houston-Miller N, Killen JD, Debusk RF: Smoking cessation after acute myocardial infarction: Effects of a nurse-managed intervention. An Intern Med 1990 (July 15);113:118–123.

65. Buchwald H, Barco RL, Matts JP, Long JM, Fitch LL, Campbell GS, Pearce MB, Yellin AE, Edmiston WA, Smink RD, Sawin HS Jr, Campos CT, Hansen BJ, Tuna N, Karnegis JN, Sanmarco ME, Amplatz K, Castaneda-Zuniga WR, Hunter DW, Bissett JK, Weber FJ, Stevenson JW, Leon AS, Chalmers TC, POSCH Group: Effect of partial ileal bypass surgery on mortality and morbidity from coronary heart disease in patients with

hypercholesterolemia: Report of the program on the surgical control of the hyper-lipidemias (POSCH). N Engl J Med 1990 (Oct 4);323:946–955.

66. Roussouw JE, Lewis B, Path FRC, Rifkind BM: The value of lowering cholesterol after myocardial infarction. N Engl J Med 1990 (Oct 18);323:1112–1119.

67. Nidorf SM, Parsons RW, Thompson PL, Jamrozik KD, Hobbs MST: Reduced risk of death at 28 days in patients taking a β-blocker before admission to hospital with myocardial infarction. Br Med J 1990 (Jan 13);300:71–74.

68. Jafri SM, Tilley BC, Peters R, Schultz LR, Goldstein S: Effects of cigarette smoking and propranolol in survivors of acute myocardial infarction. Am J Cardiol 1990 (Feb 1);65:271–276.

69. Byington RP, Worthy J, Craven T, Furberg CD: Propranolol-induced lipid changes and their prognostic significance after a myocardial infarction: The beta-blocker heart attack trial experience. Am J Cardiol 1990 (June 1);65:1287–1291.

70. Horwitz RI, Vidcoli CM, Berkman L, Donaldson RM, Horwitz SM, Murray CJ, Ransohoff DF, Sindelar J: Treatment adherence and risk of death after a myocardial infarction. Lancet 1990 (Sept 1);336:542–545.

71. Boissel JP, Leizorovicz A, Picolet H, Peyrieux JC, APSI Investigators: Secondary preven-tion after high-risk acute myocardial infarction with low-dose acebutolol. Am J Car-diol 1990 (Aug 1);66:251–260.

72. McMurray JJ, Lang CC, MacLean D, McDevitt DG, Struthers AD: Neuroendocrine changes post myocardial infarction: Effects of xamoterol. Am Heart J 1990 (July);120:56–62.

73. Bekheit S, Tangella M, el-Sakr A, Rasheed Q, Craelius W, El-Sherif N: Use of heart rate spectral analysis to study the effects of calcium channel blockers on sympathetic activity after myocardial infarction. Am Heart J 1990 (January);119:79–85.

74. Ellis SG, Muller DW, Topol EJ: Possible survival benefit from concomitant beta-but not calcium-antagonist therapy during reperfusion for acute myocardial infarction. Am J Cardiol 1990 (July 15);66:125–128.

75. Bigger JT Jr, Coromilas J, Roinitzky LM, Fleiss JL, Kleiger RE, Multicenter Diltiazem Postinfarction Trial Investigators. Effects of diltiazem on cardiac rate and rhythm after myocardial infarction. Am J Cardiol 1990 (Mar 1);65:539–546.

76. Danish Study Group on Verapamil in Myocardial Infarction: Effect of verapamil on mortality and major events after acute myocardial infarction (The Danish verapamil infarction trial II-DAVIT II). Am J Cardiol 1990 (Oct 1);66:779–785.

77. Smith P, Arnesen H, Holme I: The effect of warfarin on mortality and reinfarction after myocardial infarction. N Eng J Med 1990 (July 19);323:147–152.

78. Verheugt FWA, Van Der Laarse A, Funke-Kupper AJ, Sterkman LGW, Galema TW, Roos JP: Effects of early intervention with low-dose aspirin (100 mg) on infarct size, rein-farction and mortality in anterior wall acute myocardial infarction. Am J Cardiol 1990 (Aug 1);66:267–270.

79. RISK Group: Risk of myocardial infarction and death during treatment with low dose aspirin and intravenous heparin in men with unstable coronary artery disease. Lancet 1990 (Oct 6);336:827–830.

80. Cohen M, Adams PC, Hawkins L, Bach M, Fuster V: Usefulness of antithrombotic therapy in resting angina pectoris or non-Q-wave myocardial infarction in preventing death and myocardial infarction (a pilot study from the antithrombotic therapy in acute coronary syndromes study group). Am J Cardiol 1990 (Dec 1);66:1287–1292.

81. Burkart F, Pfisterer M, Kiowski W, Follath F, Burckhardt D, with the technical assistance of Jordi H. Effect of antiarrhythmic therapy on mortality in survivors of myocardial infarction with asymptomatic complex ventricular arrhythmias: Basel Antiarrhythmic Study of Infarct Survival (BASIS). J Am Coll Cardiol 1990 (December);16:1711–8.

82. Schecter M, Hod H, Marks N, Behar S, Kaplinsky E, Rabinowitz B: Beneficial effect of magnesium sulfate in acute myocardial infarction. Am J Cardiol 1990 (Aug 1);66: 271–274.

83. Muller DWM, Topol EJ: Selection of patients with acute myocardial infarction for thrombolytic therapy. An Intern Med 1990 (Dec 15);113:949–960.

84. Karlson BW, Herlitz J, Edvardsson N, Emanuelsson H, Sjolin M, Hjalmarson A: Eligibility for Intravenous Thrombolysis in Suspected Acute Myocardial Infarction. Circulation 1990 (October);1140–1146.

85. Schmidt SB, Borsch MA: The prehospital phase of acute myocardial infarction in the era of thrombolysis. Am J Cardiol 1990 (June 15);65:1411–1415.

86. Kereiakes DJ, Weaver WD, Anderson JL, Feldman T, Gibler B, Aufderheide T, Williams DO, Martin LH, Anderson LC, Martin JS, McKendall G, Sherrid M, Greenberg H, Teichman SL: Time delays in the diagnosis and treatment of acute myocardial infarction: A tale of eight cities. Report from the Pre-hospital Study Group and the Cincinnati Heart Project. Am Heart J 1990 (October);120:773–780.

87. Roth A, Barbash BI, Hod H, Miller HI, Rath S, Modan M, Har-Zahav Y, Keren G, Bassan S, Kaplinsky E, Laniado S. Should thrombolytic therapy be administered in the mobile intensive care unit in patients with evolving myocardial infarction? A pilot study. J Am Coll Cardiol 1990 (April);15:932–6.

88. Six AJ, Louwerenburg HW, Braams R, Mechelse K, Mosterd WL, Bredero AC, Dunselman PHJM, Van Hemel NM: A double-blind randomized multicenter dose-ranging trial of intravenous streptokinase in acute myocardial infarction. Am J Cardiol 1990 (Jan 15);65:119–123.

89. Jalihal S, Morris GK: Antistreptokinase titres after intravenous streptokinase. Lancet 1990 (Jan 27);335:184–185.

90. Davies SW, Ranjadayalan K, Wickens DG, Dormandy TL, Timmis AD: Lipid peroxidation associated with successful thrombolysis. Lancet 1990 (Mar 31);335:741–743.

91. Mahan EF III, Chandler JW, Rogers WJ, Nath HR, Smith LR, Whitlow PL, Hood WP, Reeves RC, Baxley WA: Heparin and infarct coronary artery patency after streptokinase in acute myocardial infarction. Am J Cardiol 1990 (Apr 15);65:967–972.

92. Chew EW, Morton P, Murtagh JG, Scott ME, O'Keeffe DB: Intravenous streptokinase for acute myocardial infarction reduces the occurrence of ventricular late potentials. Br Heart J 1990 (July);64:5–8.

93. Davies SW, Marchant B, Lyons JP, Timmis AD, Rothman MT, Layton CA, Balcon R. Coronary lesion morphology in acute myocardial infarction: Demonstration of early remodeling after streptokinase treatment. J Am Coll Cardiol 1990 (November);16: 1079–86.

94. Bourke JP, Young AA, Richards DA, Uther JB. Reduction in incidence of inducible ventricular tachycardia after myocardial infarction by treatment with streptokinase during infarct evolution. J Am Coll Cardiol 1990 (December);16:1703–10.

95. Midgette AS, O'Connor GT, Baron JA, Bell J: Effect of intravenous streptokinase on early mortality in patients with suspected acute myocardial infarction: A meta-analysis by anatomic location of infarction. An Intern Med 1990 (Dec 15);113:961–968.

96. Hogg KJ, Gemmill JD, Burns JMA, Lifson WK, Rae AP, Dunn FG, Hillis WS: Angiographic patency study of anistreplase versus streptokinase in acute myocardial infarction. Lancet 1990 (Feb 3);335:254–258.

97. GISSI-2: A factorial randomized trial of alteplase versus streptokinase and heparin versus no heparin among 12,490 patients with acute myocardial infarction. Lancet 1990 (July 14);336:65–71.

98. International Study Group: In-hospital mortality and clinical course of 20,891 patients with suspected acute myocardial infarction randomized between alteplase and streptokinase with or without heparin. Lancet 1990 (July 14);336:71–75.

99. White HD: GISSI-2 and the heparin controversy. Lancet 1990 (Aug 4);336:297–298.

100. Otto CM, Stratton JR, Maynard C, Althouse R, Johannessen KA, Kennedy JW: Echocardiographic evaluation of segmental wall motion early and late after thrombolytic therapy in acute myocardial infarction: The western Washington tissue plasminogen activator emergency room trial. Am J Cardiol 1990 (Jan 15);65:132–138.

101. Kander NH, Holland KJ, Pitt B, Topol EJ: A randomized pilot trial of brief versus prolonged heparin after successful reperfusion in acute myocardial infarction. Am J Cardiol 1990 (Jan 15);65:139–142.

102. Chaitman BR, Thompson BW, Kern MJ, Vandormael MG, Cohen MB, Ruocco NA, Solomon RE, Braunwald E, for the TIMI Investigators: Tissue plasminogen activator followed by percutaneous transluminal coronary angioplasty: One-year TIMI phase II pilot results. Am Heart J 1990 (February);119:213–223.

103. The Thrombolysis Early in Acute Heart Attack Trial Study Group: Very early thrombolytic therapy in suspected acute myocardial infarction. Am J Cardiol 1990 (Feb 15);65:401–407.

104. Smalling RW, Schumacher R, Morris D, Harder K, Fuentes F, Valentine RP, Battey LL, Merhige M, Pitts DE, Lieberman HA, Nishikawa A, Adyanthaya A, Hopkins A, Grossbard E. Improved infarct-related arterial patency after high dose, weight-adjusted, rapid

infusion of tissue-type plasminogen activator in myocardial infarction: Results of a multicenter randomized trial of two dosage regimens. J Am Coll Cardiol 1990 (April);15:915–21.

105. Califf RM, Topol EJ, George BS, Kereiakes DJ, Aronson LG, Lee KL, Martin L, Candela R, Abbottsmith C, O'Neill WW, Pryor DB, Stack RS, and the TAMI Study Group: One-year outcome after therapy with tissue plasminogen activator: Report from the Thrombolysis and Angioplasty in Myocardial Infarction Trial. Am Heart J 1990 (April);119:777–785.

106. Rogers W, Baim D, Gore J, Brown G, Roberts R, Williams D, Chesebro J, Babb J, Sheehan F, Wackers F, Zaret B, Robertson T, Passamani E, Ross R, Knatterud G, Braunwald E. Comparison of Immediate Invasive, Delayed Invasive, and Conservative Strategies After Tissue-Type Plasminogen Activator Results of the Thrombolysis in Myocardial Infarction (TIMI) Phase II-A Trial. Circulation 1990 (May);81:1457–1476.

107. Khan MI, Hackett DR, Andreotti F, Davies GJ, Regan T, Haider AW, McFadden E, Halson P, Maseri A: Effectiveness of multiple bolus administration of tissue-type plasminogen activator in acute myocardial infarction. Am J Cardiol 1990 (May 1);65:1051–1056.

108. Wilcox RG, Von Der Lippe G, Olsson CG, Jensen G, Skene AM, Hampton JR: Effects of alteplase in acute myocardial infarction: 6-month results from the ASSET study. Lancet 1990 (May 19);335:1175–1178.

109. Mortelmans L, Vanhaecke J, Lesaffre E, Arnold A, Urbain J-L, Hermens W, De Roo M, De Geest H, Verstraete M, Van de Werf F: Evaluation of the effect of thrombolytic treatment on infarct size and left ventricular function by enzymatic, scintigraphic, and angiographic methods. Am Heart J 1990 (June);119:1231–1237.

110. Lavie CJ, O'Keefe JH, Chesebro JH, Clements IP, Gibbons RJ: Prevention of late ventricular dilatation after acute myocardial infarction by successful thrombolytic reperfusion. Am J Cardiol 1990 (July 1);66:31–36.

111. Barbash GI, Roth A, Hod H, Miller HI, Modan M, Rath S, Zahav YH, Schachar A, Basan S, Battler A, Rabinowitz B, Kaplinsky E, Seligsohn U, Laniado S: Improved survival but not left ventricular function with early and prehospital treatment with tissue plasminogen activator in acute myocardial infarction. Am J Cardiol 1990 (Aug 1);66:261–266.

112. O'Connor CM, Califf RM, Massey EW, Mark DB, Kereiakes DJ, Candela RJ, Abbottsmith C, George B, Stack RS, Aronson L, Mantell S, Topol EJ. Stroke and acute myocardial infarction in the thrombolytic era: Clinical correlates and long-term prognosis. J Am Coll Cardiol 1990 (September);16:533–40.

113. Willems JL, Willems RJ, Willems GM, Arrnold AER, Van de Werf F, Verstraete M for the European Cooperative Study Group for Recombinant Tissue-Type Plasminogen Activator: Significance of Initial ST Segment Elevation and Depression for the Management of Thrombolytic Therapy in Acute Myocardial Infarction. Circulation 1990 (October);82:1147–1158.

114. Barbash GI, Roth A, Hod H, Miller HI, Rath S, Har Zahav Y, Modan M, Seligsohn U, Battler A, Kaplinsky E, Rabinowitz B, Laniado S: Rapid resolution of ST elevation and prediction of clinical outcome in patients undergoing thrombolysis with alteplase (recombinant tissue-type plasminogen activator): Results of the Israeli Study of Early Intervention in Myocardial Infarction. Br Heart J 1990 (Oct);64:241–247.

115. Barbash GI, Hod H, Roth A, Faibel HE, Mandel Y, Miller HI, Rath S, Zahav YH, Rabinowitz B, Seligsohn U, Pelled B, Schlesinger Z, Motro M, Laniado S, Kaplinsky E. Repeat infusions of recombinant tissue-type plasminogen activator in patients with acute myocardial infarction and early recurrent myocardial ischemia. J Am Coll Cardiol 1990 (October);16:779–83.

116. Bonaduce D, Petretta M, Villari B, Breglio R, Conforti G, Montemurro MV, Lanzillo T, Morgano G. Effects of late administration of tissue-type plasminogen activator on left ventricular remodeling and function after myocardial infarction. J Am Coll Cardiol 1990 (December);16:1561–8.

117. Feit F, Mueller HS, Braunwald E, Ross R, Hodges M, Herman MV, Knatterud GL, and the TIMI Research Group. Thrombolysis in Myocardial Infarction (TIMI) phase II trial: Outcome comparison of a "conservative strategy" in community versus tertiary hospitals. J Am Coll Cardiol 1990 (December);16:1529–34.

118. Althouse R, Maynard C, Cerqueira MD, Olsufka M, Ritchie JL, Kennedy JW: The western Washington myocardial infarction registry and emergency department tissue plasminogen activator treatment trial. Am J Cardiol 1990 (Dec 1);66:1298–1303.

119. Villari B, Piscione F, Bonaduce D, Golino P, Lanzillo T, Condorelli M, Chiariello M: Usefulness of late coronary thrombolysis (recombinant tissue-type plasminogen activator) in preserving left ventricular function in acute myocardial infarction. Am J Cardiol 1990 (Dec 1);66:1281–1286.

120. Clemmensen P, Ohman EM, Sevilla DC, Peck S, Wagner NB, Quigley PS, Grande P, Lee KL, Wagner GS: Changes in standard electrocardiographic ST-segment elevation predictive of successful reperfusion in acute myocardial infarction. Am J Cardiol 1990 (Dec 15);66:1407–1411.

121. Hsia J, Hamilton WP, Kleiman N, Roberts R, Chaitman BR, Ross AM, Heparin-Aspirin Reperfusion Trial (HART) Investigators: A comparison between heparin and low-dose aspirin as adjunctive therapy with tissue plasminogen activator for acute myocardial infarction. N Engl J Med 1990 (Nov 22);323:1433–1437.

122. Bleich SD, Nichols TC, Schumacher RR, Cooke DH, Tate DA, Teichman SL: Effect of heparin on coronary arterial patency after thrombolysis with tissue plasminogen activator in acute myocardial infarction. Am J Cardiol 1990 (Dec. 15);66:1412–1417.

123. Gertz SD, Kalan JM, Kragel AH, Roberts WC, Braunwald E, TIMI Investigators: Cardiac morphologic findings in patients with acute myocardial infarction treated with recombinant tissue plasminogen activator. Am J Cardiol 1990 (Apr 15);65:953–961.

124. Gertz SD, Kragel AMH, Kalan JM, Braunwald E, Roberts WC, TIMI Investigators: Comparison of coronary and myocardial morphologic findings in patients with or without thrombolytic therapy during acute myocardial infarction. Am J Cardiol 1990 (Oct 15);66:904–909.

125. Held PH, Teo KK, Yusuf S: Effects of Tissue-Type Plasminogen Activator and Anisoylated Plasminogen Streptokinase Activator Complex on Mortality in Acute Myocardial Infarction. Circulation 1990 (November) 82:1668–1674.

126. AIMS Trial Study Group: Long-term effects of intravenous anistreplase in acute myocardial infarction: Final report of the AIMS study. Lancet 1990 (Feb 24);335:427–431.

127. Takens BH, Brugemann J, Van Der Meer J, Den Heijer P, Lie KI: Reocclusion three months after successful thrombolytic treatment of acute myocardial infarction with anisoylated plasminogen streptokinase activating complex. Am J Cardiol 1990 (June 15);65:1422–1424.

128. Wall TC, Phillips HR III, Stack RS, Mantell S, Aronson L, Boswick J, Sigmon K, Dimeo M, Chaplin D, Whitcomb D, Pasi D, Zawodniak M, Hajisheik M, Hegde S, Barker W, Tenney R, Califf RM: Results of high dose intravenous urokinase for acute myocardial infarction. Am J Cardiol 1990 (Jan 15);65:124–131.

129. Schreiber TL, Miller DH, Silvasi D, McNulty A, Zola BE: Superiority of warfarin over aspirin long term after thrombolytic therapy for acute myocardial infarction. Am Heart J 1990 (June);119:1238–1244.

130. Naylor CD, Jaglal SB: Impact of intravenous thrombolysis on short-term coronary revascularization rates: A meta-analysis. JAMA 1990 (Aug 8);264:697–702.

131. Marshall JC, Waxman HL, Sauerwein A, Gilchrist I, Kurnik PB: Frequency of low-grade residual coronary stenosis after thrombolysis during acute myocardial infarction. Am J Cardiol 1990 (Oct 1);66:773–778.

132. Van Lierde J, De Geest H, Verstraete M, Van de Werf F. Angiographic assessment of the infarct-related residual coronary stenosis after spontaneous or therapeutic thrombolysis. J Am Coll Cardiol 1990 (December);16:1545–9.

133. Ohman EM, Califf RM, Topol EJ, Candela R, Abbottsmith C, Ellis S, Sigmon K, Kereiake D, George B, Stack R, and the TAMI Study Group: Consequences of Reocclusion After Successful Reperfusion Therapy in Acute Myocardial Infarction. Circulation 1990 (September);82:781–791.

134. Turitto G, Risa AL, Zanchi E, Prati PL. The signal-averaged electrocardiogram and ventricular arrhythmias after thrombolysis for acute myocardial infarction. J Am Coll Cardiol 1990 (May);15:1270–6.

135. Eldar M, Leor J, Hod H, Rotstein Z, Truman S, Kaplinsky E, Abboud S: Effect of thrombolysis on the evolution of late potentials within 10 days of infarction. Br Heart J 1990 (May);63:273–276.

136. Leor J, Hod H, Rotstein Z, Truman S, Gansky S, Goldbourt U, Abboud S, Kaplinsky E, Eldar M: Effects of thrombolysis on the 12-lead signal-averaged ECG in the early postinfarction period. Am Heart J 1990 (September);120:495–502.

137. White HD, Cross DB, Williams BF, Norris RM: Safety and efficacy of repeat thrombolytic treatment after acute myocardial infarction. Br Heart J 1990 (Sept);64:177–181.

138. El Deeb F, Ciampricotti R, El Gamal M, Michels R, Bonnier H, Van Gelder B: Value of immediate angioplasty after intravenous streptokinase in acute myocardial infarction. Am Heart J 1990 (April);119:786–791.

139. Abbottsmith CW, Topol EJ, George BS, Stack RS, Kereiakes DJ, Candela RJ, Anderson LC, Harrelson-Woodlief SL, Califf RM. Fate of patients with acute myocardial infarction with patency of the infarct-related vessel achieved with successful thrombolysis versus rescue angioplasty. J Am Coll Cardiol 1990 (October);16:770–8.

140. Stone GW, Rutherford BD, McConahay DR, Johnson WL, Giorgi LV, Ligon RW, Hartzler GO. Direct coronary angioplasty in acute myocardial infarction: Outcome in patients with single vessel disease. J Am Coll Cardiol 1990 (March);15:534–43.

141. Beauchamp GD, Vacek JL, Robuck W: Management comparison for acute myocardial infarction: Direct angioplasty versus sequential thrombolysis-angioplasty. Am Heart J 1990 (August);120:237–243.

142. Nath A, DiSciascio G, Kelly KM, Vetrovec GW, Testerman C, Goudreau E, Cowley MJ. Multivessel coronary angioplasty early after acute myocardial infarction. J Am Coll Cardiol 1990 (September);16:545–50.

143. Lee TC, Laramee LA, Rutherford Bd, McConahay DR, Johnson WL, Giorgi LV, Ligon RW, Hartzler GO: Emergency percutaneous transluminal coronary angioplasty for acute myocardial infarction in patients 70 years of age and older. Am J Cardiol 1990 (Sept 15);66:663–667.

144. Kahn JK, O'Keefe JH, Rutherford BD, McConahay DR, Johnson WL, Giorgi LV, Shimshak TM, Ligon RW, Hartzler GO: Timing and mechanism of in-hospital and late death after primary coronary angioplasty during acute myocardial infarction. Am J Cardiol 1990 (Nov 1);66:1045–1048.

145. Kahn JK, Rutherford BD, McConahay DR, Johnson WL, Giorgi LV, Shimshak TM, Ligon R, Hartzler GO: Results of primary angioplasty for acute myocardial infarction in patients with multivessel coronary artery disease. J Am Coll Cardiol 1990 (November);16:1089–96.

146. Kahn JA, Rutherford BD, McConahay DR, Johnson WL, Giorgi LV, Shimshak TM, Ligon RW, Hartzler G: Catheterization Laboratory Events and Hospital Outcome with Direct Angioplasty for Acute Myocardial Infarction. Circulation 1990 (December) 82:1910–1915.

147. Alfonso F, Macaya C, Iniguez A, Banuelos C, Fernandez-Ortiz A, Zarco P: Percutaneous transluminal coronary angioplasty after non-Q-wave acute myocardial infarction. Am J Cardiol 1990 (Apr 1);65:835–839.

148. Suryapranata H, Serruys PW, Beatt K, De Feyter PJ, van den Brand M, Roelandt J: Recovery of regional myocardial dysfunction after successful coronary angioplasty early after a non-Q wave myocardial infarction. Am Heart J 1990 (August);120:261–269.

Arrhythmias, Conduction Disturbances, and Cardiac Arrest

As a cause of atrial dilatation

To test the hypothesis that atrial dilatation can develop as a consequence of AF, Sanfilippo and co-workers[1] in Boston, Massachusetts, measured LA and RA dimensions echocardiographically at 2 different time points in patients with AF. Patients were selected who initially had normal atrial sizes and who had no evidence of significant structural or functional cardiac abnormalities other than AF either by history or 2-dimensional and Doppler echocardiography. Fifteen patients were studied and the average between studies was 21 months. Three orthogonal LA dimensions and 2 RA dimensions were measured, and all were found to increase significantly between studies. Also, highly significant increases in calculated LA volume and RA volume were observed. The relative extents of LA and RA volume increase did not differ, and LV size did not change significantly between studies. These results indicated that atrial dilatation can occur as a consequence of AF.

Alcohol's inducing recurrences

Koskinen and associates[2] from Helsinki, Finland, assessed the role of alcohol in recurrences of AF in a consecutive series of 98 patients (75 men) aged <65 years. In addition to etiologic assessment using clinical and laboratory methods and echocardiography, the patients' drinking habits were evaluated by recording the amount of alcohol used during the week preceding AF, by responses to the CAGE (Cut, Annoying, Guilt, Eye; see below) questionnaire (a screening test for alcohol abuse) and by selected laboratory tests. Two groups of control subjects were studied: 98 sex- and age-matched patients admitted to the emergency ward for acute illnesses, and 50 subjects selected randomly from the local out-of-hospital population. The mean alcohol consumption among men during the study week was 186 g (median 45 g; range 0 to 2,100 g) among patients, whereas among male hospital and population control subjects it was 86 g (30 g; 0 to 1,050 g) and 94 g (35 g; 0 to 630 g), respectively. When the weekly alcohol consumption was analyzed in 3 categories (0; 1 to 210 g; >210 g), there was a significant difference between AF cases and hospital control patients, but not between AF cases and population control subjects. Multivariate analysis of data of AF cases and population control subjects showed that alcohol intake and a positive response to 1 or more of the CAGE questions were independently related to AF in men. Other independent risk factors were the presence of heart disease, low serum potassium and lack of sleep or experience of excess psychologic stress, or both. These results indicate that alcohol consumption is an independent risk factor for recurrences of AF in men of working age.

Risk factors for emboli

The AFASAK Copenhagen Study involves 1,007 patients with chronic AF. Before inclusion in the trial, all these persons had a physical examination, chest roentgenogram, and echocardiogram with determination of LA size. Petersen and associates[3] from Copenhagen, Denmark, evaluated the importance of cardiovascular risk factors for development of thromboembolic complications. To exclude any treatment effects on occurrence of thromboembolic complications, the authors included only the 336 patients from the placebo group. Using Cox's regression model, previous AMI was a significant risk factor for development of thromboembolic complications. Age, gender, heart failure, chest pain, hypertensive heart disease, diabetes, systolic and diastolic BP, smoking, relative heart volume, and left atrial size were all without statistical importance.

Cabin and associates[4] from New Haven, Connecticut, studied the risk of systemic embolization in 272 patients without MS or prosthetic or bioprosthetic valves who were referred to the echocardiography laboratory with AF. During a mean follow-up period of 33 months (range 1 to 83), 27 (10%) patients had a systemic embolic event, which was cerebral in 23 patients (85%) and peripheral in 4 (15%). In the analysis of individual variables, the risk of embolization was increased by female sex, underlying heart disease and LA size >4.0 cm, but not by age, systemic hypertension or type of AF (paroxysmal vs chronic). In multivariable analysis, LA size >4.0 cm was the single strongest predictor of increased risk for embolization, but female sex and underlying heart disease also contributed. When each of these 3 factors was assigned 1 point in a risk score, embolic events occurred in none (0%) of 24 patients with a risk score of 0, in 2 (3%) of 83 patients with a risk score of 1, in 13 (11%) of 118 patients with a risk score of 2 and in 12 (26%) of 47 patients with a risk score of 3. The score allows patients with AF and without MS to be stratified into high-, medium- and low-risk groups for systemic embolization.

Cerebral infarction

Feinberg and associates[5] from 4 USA medical centers performed unenhanced computed tomographic scans on 141 asymptomatic patients with nonvalvular AF. Thirty-six patients (26%) had hypodense areas consistent with cerebral infarction. Most were small deep infarcts, seen in 29 patients (21%), but 13 patients (9%) had cortical or large deep infarctions. Twelve patients had >1 infarct on computed tomographic scan. Increasing age and increased LA diameter were the only clinical features associated with asymptomatic infarction. Patients >65 years with a LA diameter >5.0 cm (n = 23) had a 52% prevalence of asymptomatic infarction. Patients <65 years with a LA diameter <5.0 cm (n = 38) had an 11% prevalence of silent infarction. Patients with only 1 of these risk factors (n = 72) had a 24% prevalence of silent infarction. Infarction was more common in those with chronic (34%) as opposed to intermittent (22%) nonvalvular AF, but this difference was not significant. Hypertension, diabetes, duration of AF, CHF, history of AMI, and echocardiographic evidence of LV dysfunction were not associated with asymptomatic infarction. A history of hypertension was present in 35% of the patients with small-deep asymptomatic infarction, similar to the percentage in patients without stroke. Thus, asymptomatic cerebral infarction is common in nonvalvular AF.

Digoxin

Rawles and associates[6] from Aberdeen, UK, identified 139 episodes of AF from Holter recordings in 72 patients with paroxysmal AF. Paroxysms occurred more often by day than by night, suggesting that attacks are more closely associated with sympathetic than with vagal activity (Figure 4-1). In 41 patients who were not taking digoxin there were 79 episodes, and in 31 patients who were taking digoxin there were 60 episodes. Significantly more of the episodes that lasted for 30 minutes or more occurred in patients taking digoxin (13/17); the relative risk of a prolonged paroxysm associated with taking digoxin was 4.3. The mean ventricular rate at the onset of the paroxysms was not significantly different in those taking digoxin (140(25) beats/min) and in those who were not (134 (22)

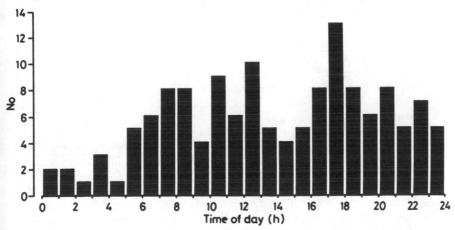

Fig. 4-1. Numbers of paroxysms of atrial fibrillation throughout the day and night. Reproduced with permission from Rawles, et al.[6]

beats/min). In paroxysmal AF, pretreatment with digoxin does not seem to reduce the frequency of paroxysms, or the ventricular rate when paroxysms occur, but it is associated with longer attacks.

Quinidine

Because individual studies evaluating the role of quinidine in the maintenance of sinus rhythm after cardioversion from chronic AF have involved relatively few patients, Coplen and colleagues[7] in Boston, Massachusetts, performed a meta-analysis of randomized control trials. Six trials published between 1970 and 1984 were selected by 2 blind reviewers based on study designed and statistical analysis. Data from these 6 trials involving 808 patients were pooled after testing for homogeneity of treatment effects across trials. Life table estimates of the percent of patients still in sinus rhythm at 3, 6, and 12 months after cardioversion were constructed for quinidine and control groups. The proportion of patients remaining in sinus rhythm in the quinidine group was 69%, 58%, and 50 at 3,6, and 12 months postcardioversion, respectively. The proportion of patients remaining in sinus rhythm in the control group was 45%, 33%, and 25% at the same time intervals. The pooled rate difference, or difference in proportion of patients in sinus rhythm between quinidine and control groups, was 24%, 23%, and 24% at 3, 6, and 12 months of follow-up. The unadjusted total mortality rate in the quinidine-treated patients was 2.9% and in the control group was 0.8%. The odds of dying in the quinidine-treated group were approximately 3 times that of the control group. Thus, quinidine treatment is more effective than no antiarrhythmic therapy in suppressing recurrences of AF but appears to be associated with increased total mortality.

Sotalol vs quinidine

In an open parallel-group study Moller and co-investigators[8] in Malmo, Sweden, compared quinidine and sotalol treatment for maintenance of sinus rhythm after direct current conversion of patients with chronic AF. The patients from 15 centers in Sweden were randomized to sotalol (98 patients) or quinidine (85 patients) after 2 hours of sinus rhythm after direct current conversion. According to primary efficacy assessment, 52% of the patients in the sotalol group and 48% of the patients in the quinidine group remained in sinus rhythm during the following 6-month treatment period. Furthermore, 34% of the patients treated with sotalol and 22% of the patients treated with quinidine relapsed into AF. Heart rate after relapsing into AF was higher in the patients treated with quinidine than in the patients with sotalol. Patients treated with sotalol were found to be less symptomatic at the time of relapse compared with relapsing patients in the quinidine group. In terms of safety, more patients were withdrawn from quinidine than from sotalol, and sotalol was generally better tolerated than quinidine. Twenty-eight of the patients treated with sotalol and 50% of the patients treated with quinidine reported side effects. The difference was primarily a result of early gastrointestinal and skin side effects in the group of patients treated with quinidine. The investigators concluded that sotalol is an effective and well-tolerated alternative for maintenance of sinus rhythm after direct current conversion of chronic AF, and that sotalol has the ability to control ventricular rate in patients with relapse into AF.

Propafenone vs sotalol

Antman and associates[9] in Boston, Massachusetts, studied 109 patients with recurrent episodes of symptomatic AF or flutter, or both who had failed 1–5 previous antiarrhythmic drug trials. These patients were treated with propafenone and, subsequently, sotalol if AF recurred. The clinical profile of the study group was as follows: age 63 ± 13 years, LA anteroposterior dimension 4.4 ± 0.9 cm and LVEF 57 ± 14%. Paroxysmal AF occurred in 56 patients (51%) and chronic AF in 53 patients (49%). After loading and dose titration phases were completed, the maintenance doses of drugs were 450 to 900 mg per day for propafenone and 160 to 90 mg per day for sotalol. The percent of patients free of recurrent symptomatic arrhythmia at 6 months was 39% for propafenone and 50% for sotalol. The cumulative proportion of patients successfully treated with either agent or both by 6 months was 55%, and it remained relatively constant subsequently. The incidence of intolerable side effects requiring discontinuation of therapy was approximately 8%. Therefore, a substantial proportion of patients with recurrent symptomatic AF refractory to conventional therapy may be treated successfully and safely with propafenone and/or sotalol.

Labetalol

Beta-adrenergic blocking agents are useful in controlling excessive ventricular rate in patients with chronic AF but they often reduce exercise capacity. To investigate the advantage of labetalol, a beta blocker with a-blocking property in patients with chronic AF, Wong and associates[10] from Hong Kong studied 10 patients without underlying structural heart disease with treadmill test, 12-minute walk, and 24-hour ambulatory electrocardiographic monitoring. Patients were randomized and crossed over to receive 4 phases of treatment (placebo, digoxin, digoxin with half-dose labetalol, and full-dose labetalol). Exercise durations were 14.1 ± 1.5, 14.2 ± 1.5, 16.1 ± 1.1 and 15.6 ± 1.1 minutes, respectively, indicating that labetalol did not reduce exercise tolerance. Although digoxin had no advantage over placebo in controlling maximal heart rate (177 ± 2 beats per minute and 154 ± 2 vs 177 ± 2 beats per minute respectively). The rate-pressure product was consistently lowered by labetalol at rest and during exercise. At peak exercise, the addition of labetalol to digoxin reduced the maximal rate-pressure product achieved from 30,900 ± 1,300 to 24,000 ± 2,000 mm Hg/min and the maximal heart rate-BP product was lowest with full-dose labetalol (22,300 ± 1,600 mm Hg/min). During submaximal exercise on treadmill or during the 12-minute walk, the combination of labetalol and digoxin produced the best heart rate control, whereas labetalol mono-therapy was comparable to digoxin therapy. During daily activities, digoxin failed to control the maximal ventricular rate (172 ± 5 vs 174 ± 7 beats/min with placebo) but the addition of labetalol was efficacious (141 ± 5 vs 172 ± 5 beats/min). No bradycardia was recorded during labetalol treatment. Thus, labetalol improves heart rate control in chronic AF without decreasing exercise tolerance.

Warfarin

Wipf and Lipsky[11] from Seattle, Washington, reviewed the risk of embolic stroke in patients with AF (Table 4-1) and also the indications for anticoagulant therapy in AF (Figures 4-2 and 4-3). They found that the

TABLE 4-1. *Prevalence of atrial fibrillation (AF) reported in various disease populations.* *Reproduced with permission from Wipf, et al.[11]*

Diagnosis of Population	Prevalence of AF, %
Valvular heart disease	
Mitral stenosis (requiring valve replacement)	41
Mitral regurgitation (requiring valve replacement)	75
Aortic stenosis/aortic insufficiency	1
Coronary artery disease	
Angina	0.8
Immediately after myocardial infarction (transient)	7-16
Immediately after coronary artery bypass grafting (transient)	10
Cardiomyopathy	
Congestive cardiomyopathy	25
Primary hypertrophic cardiomyopathy	8-10
Idiopathic hypertrophic subaortic stenosis	8-10
Pericardial disease	
Acute pericarditis	5
Pericardial constriction	35
Miscellaneous	
Systemic arterial hypertension	5-10
Atrial septal defect (age, >50 y)	53
Hyperthyroidism	12-18

*Derived from data in reference 7.

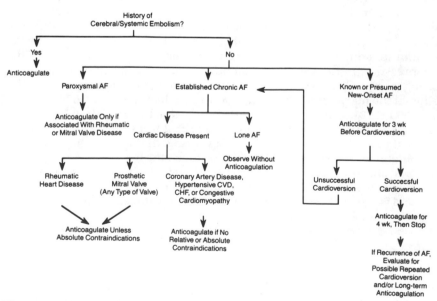

Fig. 4-2. Anticoagulation treatment strategy in atrial fibrillation (AF). See the text for definitions of paroxysmal AF, lone AF, and contraindications. CVD indicates cardiovascular disease; CHF, congestive heart failure. Reproduced with permission from Wipf, et al.[11]

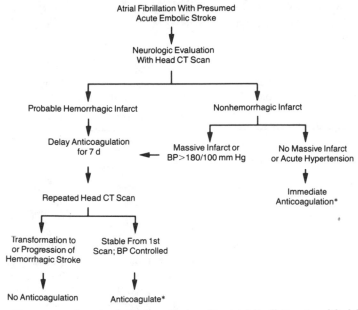

Fig. 4-3. Treatment of acute stroke in patients with atrial fibrillation (modified from Cerebral Embolism Task Force). See the text for further explanation of atrial fibrillation with presumed acute embolic stroke. Asterisk indicates duration unknown, presumed long-term; CT, computed tomographic; and BP, blood pressure. Reproduced with permission from Wipf, et al.[11]

stroke risk was greater with chronic than with paroxysmal AF, was highest in the year after onset of the AF, and was lower in young patients with idiopathic (lone) AF. The decision to anticoagulate a patient with AF should depend on the cause of the AF and the individual's risk from anticoagulation. The authors provided evidence supporting the effectiveness of anticoagulation of most patients with nonvalvular and valvular cardiac disease for the prevention of both primary and recurrent strokes.

Nonrheumatic AF increases the risk of stroke, presumably from atrial thromboemboli. There is uncertainty about the efficacy and risks of long-term warfarin therapy to prevent stroke. The Boston Area Anticoagulation Trial for Atrial Fibrillation Investigators[12] conducted an unblinded, randomized, controlled trial of long-term low-dose warfarin therapy (target prothrombin-time ratio 1.2 to 1.5) in patients with nonrheumatic AF. The control group was not given warfarin but could choose to take aspirin. A total of 420 patients entered the trial (212 in the warfarin group and 208 in the control group) and were followed for an average of 2.2 years. Prothrombin times in the warfarin group were in the target range 83% of the time. Only 10% of the patients assigned to receive warfarin discontinued the drug permanently. There were 2 strokes in the warfarin group (incidence, 0.41% per year) as compared with 13 strokes in the control group (incidence, 2.96% per year), for a reduction of 86% in the risk of stroke (warfarin: control incidence ratio = 0.14). There were 37 deaths altogether. The death rate was markedly lower in the warfarin group than in the control group: 2.25% as compared with 5.97% per year, for an incidence ratio of 0.38. There was 1 fatal hemorrhage in each group. The frequency of bleeding events that led to hospitalization or transfusion was essentially the same in both groups. The warfarin group had a higher rate of minor hemorrhage than the control group (38 vs 21 patients).

Long-term low-dose warfarin therapy is highly effective in preventing stroke in patients with nonrheumatic AF, and can be quite safe with careful monitoring.

SUPRAVENTRICULAR TACHYCARDIA WITH OR WITHOUT SHORT P-R INTERVAL SYNDROME

Wolff-Parkinson-White syndrome

Syncope in patients due to WPW syndrome may be related either to a rapid rate of SVT or to rapid ventricular response over the accessory pathway during AF. From 1982 to 1987 Paul and associates[13] from Houston, Texas, studied 74 patients ≤25 years old (mean age 12.6 years) with the WPW syndrome on electrocardiogram. Of the 74 patients, 14 (19%) had a history of syncope. During electrophysiologic study 9 of 14 patients with syncope had sustained (>5 minutes or requiring termination due to hypotension) AF. Of the remaining 5 patients, 3 had inducible nonsustained AF and 2 had no AF. None of the 60 patients without syncope developed sustained AF; 34 had nonsustained and 26 had no AF. Occurrence of sustained AF had a sensitivity of 64% and specificity of 100% for history of syncope. All patients with syncope and AF (n = 12) had a short RR interval between 2 consecutive preexcited QRS complexes during AF at ≤220 ms, in contrast to 9 of 34 patients without syncope (sensitivity 100%, specificity 74%). No patient with a short RR interval between 2 consecutive preexcited QRS complexes during AF of >220 ms had a history of syncope. Thus, in these young patients with WPW syndrome, occurrence of AF with a rapid ventricular response during electrophysiologic study correlated well with a history of syncope and may be the cause of syncope in most patients.

Beckman and associates[14] in Chicago, Illinois, used invasive electrophysiologic studies to predict future arrhythmic events in patients with minimally symptomatic W-P-W syndrome in 42 patients with evidence of AV pre-excitation on the surface electrocardiogram. These patients underwent electrophysiologic studies and were followed as outpatients taking no medications. The patients were classified into 3 groups, including group I, 15 asymptomatic patients; group II, 10 patients with infrequent symptoms but no documented arrhythmias; and group III, 17 patients with one documented episode of SVT or AF or both. At electrophysiologic study, the number of patients with short anterograde accessory pathway effective refractory periods and rapid ventricular responses during induced AV did not differ among the three groups. During a mean follow-up period of 7.5 ± 4.9 years, 11 of the 42 patients had documented arrhythmias, including 2 patients from group II, 2 patients from group III had SVT, and 7 patients from group III had AF. All 9 patients from group III with subsequent arrhythmias had clinical AF before study. No patient from group I had an arrhythmia during follow-up. There were no episodes of VF or sudden cardiac death during follow-up in any of the patients. The only predischarge variables that correlated with the subsequent occurrence of arrhythmias were a history of documented arrhythmias before electrophysiologic study and inducible SVT at electrophysiologic study. Thus, patients with AV pre-excitation and a single episode of AF are at risk to have recurrent tachyarrhythmias and should be treated. These data suggest the risk of sudden death in adults with AV pre-excitation but no clinical arrhythmias is small and although measurements of the accessory pathway effective refractory period and minimal pre-excitation cycle length during induced AF have an excellent negative predictive value, the positive predictive value may be too low to warrant their routine use as predictors of prognosis.

Perry and Garson[15] from Houston, Texas, reviewed the clinical course of 140 patients with WPW syndrome who had their initial episode of SVT before 18 years of age. Among those whose SVT began at age 0 to 2 months, it disappeared in 93% and persisted in 7%. In 31%, it disappeared and reappeared at an average age of 8 years. Among patients whose tachycardia was present after age 5 years it was persistent in 78% at a mean follow-up period of 7 years. There was no difference in tachycardia onset or recurrence based on accessory connection location. Congenital heart defects were present in 37% of all patients, 23% of whom had Ebstein's anomaly. Among all patients who underwent catheterization, 63% of those with a congenital heart defect had a right-sided connection, whereas 61% of patients with a normal heart had a left-sided connection. Multiple accessory connections were found in 12% of patients with a congenital defect compared with 6% of those without such a defect. These data are helpful to the pediatric cardiologist treating these patients in terms of prognosis and in terms of potential for having a drug free interval after infancy to approximately 8 years of age in patients who may subsequently have recurrence of the problem.

Perry and associates[16] from Houston, Texas, reviewed 66 electrocardiograms in patients with proven WPW, 24 from those with questionable or subtle WPW and 369 electrocardiograms from control patients to identify additional clues that WPW might be present. Three features were notable in WPW: no Q wave in left chest leads in 88%, PR interval <100 ms in 80%, and left axis deviation in 33%. These findings were similar in subtle WPW: 79%, 67%, and 46%, respectively. By comparison, only 5% of control subjects had no Q wave, 16% had a PR interval of <100 ms, and 4% had left axis deviation. The coexistence of 2 of these features was common in WPW (74%) and subtle WPW (63%) but rare in control subjects (2%). A PR interval of <100 ms was less specific before 1 year of age, but 89% of patients with WPW had a QRS duration of >80 ms versus 2% of control subjects in this age group. Obvious WPW disappeared in 11 patients; left axis deviation or lack of Q wave persisted in 8. The diagnosis of WPW in children is sometimes difficult and these features can be helpful in terms of looking closer for this anomaly.

Circadian variation

Kupari and associates[17] from Helsinki, Finland, studied 251 patients ≤65 years of age admitted for treatment of symptomatic SVT to assess whether these arrhythmias begin evenly throughout the day or manifest circadian variation in occurrence. The arrhythmias included 152 episodes of AF, 50 episodes of reentry SVT, 30 episodes of atrial flutter, and 19 cases of ectopic atrial tachycardia. A total of 209 patients could tell the exact time their symptoms had started. In 38 of them (18%), the arrhythmia had begun between midnight and 6 A.M., in 63 (30%) between 6 A.M. and noon, in 46 (22%) between noon and 6 P.M., and in 62 (30%) between 6 P.M. and midnight. This distribution differed significantly from uniform occurrence. Fifty patients were using β-adrenoceptor blocking agents when the arrhythmia occurred. Compared with the other 159 patients, they had no morning surge of arrhythmias (20% vs 33% of episodes between 6 A.M. and noon) but instead a much higher incidence at night (34% vs 13% of episodes between midnight and 6 A.M.). It was concluded that the frequency of onset of sustained SVT varies with the time of day, showing nearly equal peaks in the morning and in the evening and a trough at night. The modifying effect of β-adrenoceptor blockage suggests that many morning arrhythmias are of adrenergic origin while other, probably vagal arrhythmogenic mechanisms, prevail at night.

Intraatrial reentrant tachycardia

Haines and associates[18] in Charlottesville, Virginia, evaluated 19 patients with a clinical history of sustained SVT diagnosed as having intraatrial reentrant tachycardia. Seventeen (89%) patients of the 19 had structural heart disease and 17 had echocardiographic evidence of an enlarged atrium. The mean LVEF was 51 ± 16%. A history of associated AF or flutter was present in 13 patients (68%). The mean atrial cycle length during tachycardia was 326 ± 57 ms. Fourteen patients had 1:1 AV conduction during tachycardia, of whom 50% had an RP'/RR' ratio >0.5. Intravenous adenosine (dose range 37.5 to 150 µg/kg) and verapamil (dose range 5 to 10 mg) had no effect on atrial tachycardia cycle length in 13 of 14 and 9 of 9 patients, respectively, despite induction of second degree AV block. Type 1a antiarrhythmic drugs were associated with long-term suppression of intraatrial reentrant tachycardia in only 6 patients, whereas amiodarone (325 ± 145 mg/day) was successful in 11 patients during a 32 ± 20 month follow-up period. The remaining 2 patients and 1 patient who later developed amiodarone toxicity either progressed to (n=1) or had (n=2) catheter-induced high grade AV block and were treated with long-term ventricular pacing. Thus, intraatrial reentrant tachycardia is associated with underlying heart disease, especially of types that cause atrial abnormalities. Other arrhythmias are also frequently found in these patients and the arrhythmia response to type 1a antiarrhythmic drugs is poor, but good with amiodarone therapy.

Adenosine

Rankin and associates[19] from Glasgow, UK, studied the effects of intravenous adenosine and adenosine triphosphate in a double-blind randomized study during 68 episodes of SVT in 39 patients. Adenosine restored sinus rhythm in 20 patients (25 of 27 episodes) and produced A-V block to reveal atrial arrhythmias in 9. Adenosine triphosphate restored sinus rhythm in 17 patients (22 of 25 episodes) and revealed atrial tachyarrhythmias in 6. In patients receiving both compounds, the effective dosage of adenosine was 3.8 mg and of adenosine triphosphate it was 6.6 mg, suggesting molar equipotency. Transient side effects were common, occurring in 81% of episodes with adenosine and in 94% with adenosine triphosphate. Symptom scores were not significantly different. Adenosine and adenosine triphosphate were equally effective for the diagnosis and treatment of SVT and the incidence and severity of side effects were similar. Adenosine has the advantage of being more stable.

Inappropriate administration of intravenous verapamil to patients with wide QRS complex tachycardia due to VT or AF with WPW syndrome occurs frequently because of misdiagnosis, and may precipitate cardiac arrest. Sharma and associates[20] from London, Canada, evaluated the safety and the diagnostic and therapeutic utility of adenosine triphosphate administered to 34 patients during wide QRS complex tachycardia due to a variety of mechanisms. Patients who had a hemodynamically and electrically stable, monomorphic, wide (>120 msec) QRS complex tachycardia induced during an invasive cardiac electrophysiologic test were studied. Hemodynamic stability was defined by a systolic BP >80 mm Hg and no clinical evidence of cerebral or myocardial ischemia. Adenosine triphosphate, 20 mg, was administered as a rapid intravenous bolus via a peripheral vein during wide QRS complex tachycardia. Five surface electrocardiogram leads, at least 3 intracardiac electrograms, and BP were monitored. VT was present in 14 patients (mean age 51 ± 19 years, cycle length 326 ± 67 msec) and adenosine triphosphate terminated the arrhythmia in 1 case. VT cycle length did not change. Among 10 patients with SVT with mechanisms not involving the AV node (average ventricular cycle length 346 ± 82 msec), 1 case of ectopic atrial tachycardia was terminated. The ventricular rate was transiently increased in patients with WPW syndrome and AF (average R-R interval 351 ± 84 msec in control and 317 ± 82 msec after adenosine triphosphate). Reentrant tachycardias involving the AV node (cycle length 302 ± 52 msec) terminated in 7 of 10 patients. The drug was well tolerated, and no patient developed hemodynamic compromise necessitating cardioversion as a result of adenosine triphosphate. In the setting of electrophysiology testing, adenosine triphosphate is a safe agent, even when administered inappropriately during arrhythmias for which it is relatively ineffective, such as VT, and WPW syndrome with AF. It is an effective agent in terminating SVT involving the AV node. Tachycardia termination following adenosine triphosphate, when used as a diagnostic test to indicate obligatory participation of the AV node, had a sensitivity of 70%, specificity of 92%, and a positive predictive accuracy of 85%.

Amiodarone

To assess the safety and efficacy of intravenous adenosine in terminating acute episodes of paroxysmal SVP, DiMarco and associates[21] from the Adenosine for PSVT Study Group compared 2 prospective, double-blind, randomized, placebo-controlled trials to evaluate dose response in patients receiving adenosine to those receiving verapamil. A total of 359 patients with tachycardia electrocardiographically consistent with paroxysmal SVT were entered into the 2 protocols. Patients subsequently found to have arrhythmias other than paroxysmal SVT were excluded from the efficacy analysis. The first protocol compared sequential intravenous bolus doses of 3, 6, 9, and 12 mg of adenosine to equal volumes of saline. In the second protocol, patients received either 6 mg and, if necessary, 12 mg of adenosine or 5 mg and, if necessary, 7.5 mg of verapamil. When data are expressed in terms of cumulative response in eligible patients, intravenous adenosine terminated acute episodes of paroxysmal SVT in 35%, 62%, and 91% of patients who received maximum doses of 3, 6, 9, and 12 mg, respectively, in a 4-dose sequence, whereas 9%, 11%, 14%, and 16% of patients responded to 4 sequential placebo doses. In the second trial, cumulative response rates after 6 mg followed, if necessary, by 12 mg of adenosine were 57% and 93%, and after 5 mg followed, if necessary, by 8 mg of verapamil were 81% and 91%. The average time after injection to termination of tachycardia by adenosine was 30 seconds. Adenosine caused adverse effects in 36% of patients, but they lasted less than 1 minute and were usually mild. Adenosine in graded doses up to 12 mg rapidly and effectively terminates acute episodes of paroxysmal SVT in which the AV node is an integral part of the re-entrant circuit. The overall efficacy of adenosine is similar to that of verapamil, but its onset of action is more rapid. Adverse reactions to adenosine are common but are minor and brief.

To shorten the delay in the onset of antiarrhythmic effect when using amiodarone for the conversion of refractory atrial tachyarrhythmias to sinus rhythm, 19 patients were given oral amiodarone according to a high-dose loading protocol in this report by Mostow and colleagues[22] from Cleveland, Ohio. In 18 of 19 patients (95%), sinus rhythm was restored 36 hours (range 0 to 96 hours) after starting amiodarone. The conversion occurred as a result of amiodarone therapy alone within 48 hours in 12 patients (63%), and by amiodarone therapy plus electrical cardioversion at 48 to 96 hours in 6 patients (32%). Minor side effects were noted in 8 patients (42%). No major side effects were encountered. The length of hospital stay after initiating amiodarone therapy was 3.6 days (range 2 to 5 days). High-dose oral amiodarone loading is a safe and effective method for the rapid conversion of atrial tachyarrhythmias to sinus rhythm.

Cryosurgery

Atrioventricular node reentry tachycardia is the most common cause of paroxysmal SVT. Available nonpharmacologic therapies include (1) catheter ablation or cryosurgical ablation of the His bundle and insertion of a permanent pacemaker and (2) surgical dissection around the AV node or discrete cryosurgery of the perinodal tissues to divide or ablate only 1 of the dual AV node conduction pathways responsible for the SVT while leaving the other intact. Cox and associates[23] from St. Louis, Missouri, described 23 consecutive patients who underwent the discrete cryosurgical procedure from 1982 to 1989. The first patient in the series, a 38-year-old woman, is the first patient in whom refractory AV node reentry tachycardia was cured surgically by a procedure designed to treat this arrhythmia. The ages of the 13 female and 10 male patients ranged from 12 to 56 years (average 29). Fourteen patients (61%) had the W-P-W syndrome. Other associated arrhythmias included atrial flutter/ AF (n = 2), RA reentrant tachycardia (n = 1), junctional tachycardia (n = 1), and a Mahaim fiber (n = 1). Associated anatomic abnormalities included Ebstein's anomaly in 2 patients and a large RA aneurysm in 1 patient. The perinodal cryosurgical procedure was performed through a right atriotomy in the normothermic beating heart. Multiple 3 mm diameter cryolesions were placed around the borders of the triangle of Koch on the lower right atrial septum to alter the input pathways of the AV node. There were no operative deaths in this series of patients. Postoperatively, all 23 patients had normal AV conduction, and no heart block has occurred in any patients during the follow-up period. All patients have remained free of AV node reentry tachycardia (and of the WPW syndrome) and none has required postoperative antiarrhythmic drugs for either of these arrhythmias. The authors consider this simple, safe, easily performed, and uniformly successful operation to be the procedure of choice for the treatment of medically refractory AV node reentry tachycardia.

VENTRICULAR ARRHYTHMIAS

In children with normal hearts

Characteristics of 18 children with clinical VT and normal hearts documented by physical examination, echocardiography, and angiocardiography were analyzed by Noh and associates[24] from Charleston, South Carolina. There were 13 males and 5 females, aged 1 to 16 years (9.7 ± 4.8 years). Six patients had hemodynamic instability during VT and the other 12 patients were hemodynamically stable. Two patients (11%) presented with sustained VT and 16 (89%) with episodes of nonsustained VT at varying intervals (3 of 16 with repetitive monomorphic VT). Among 14 patients on whom exercise tests were performed, 7 had exercise-induced VT. During electrophysiologic studies, VT was induced in 16 of 18 (89%) (in 13 patients with morphology identical to clinical VT). VT was induced by programmed stimulation (single, double, and burst stimulation of the right atrium or RV apex during sinus rhythm or during pacing for 8 beats) in 5 of 18 (28%) patients; with isoproterenol, VT was aggravated spontaneously in 6 of 15 (40%) patients; and during stimulation VT was induced in 8 of 15 (53%) patients. Among patients whose VT was not induced during programmed stimulation, VT was induced with the addition of isoproterenol in 11 of 12 (92%). All 14 patients in follow-up are in stable condition, 7 patients with medication and 7 without medication. Pediatric patients with normal hearts and clinically detected VT usually have VT induced by programmed stimulation, either with or without isoproterenol stimulation.

Ventricular couplets in children and young adults

Ventricular couplets may be a risk factor for sudden death in adults, but their prognosis in children is unknown. Paul and colleagues[25] from Houston, Texas, and Hannover, West Germany, during the time period from 1981 to 1987 studied 104 patients, mean age 13 years (0.2 to 37 years), with ventricular couplets on a 24-hour electrocardiogram (Holter monitor) and on follow-up with a second Holter (mean, 2.5 years). Of the 104 patients, 22 had a normal heart and 82 had an abnormal heart. Patients with a normal or an abnormal heart did not differ in incidence or severity of symptoms (patients with a normal heart had 17 instances of palpitations and none of syncope; patients with an abnormal heart had 49 instances of palpitations, 6 of dizziness, and none of syncope). Number of ventricular couplets was higher in patients with a normal heart (33 ± 50/day) than in those with an abnormal heart (17 ± 15/day). Of the 22 patients with a normal heart, 11 underwent an electrophysiologic study; none had inducible VT. After mean follow-up of 30 months, all 22 patients with a normal heart were alive without VT; 6 of 22 were treated for palpitations, with complete suppression of couplets in 2. In 11 of 16 untreated patients with a normal heart, ventricular couplets disappeared spontaneously. Of the 82 patients with an abnormal heart, 32 had an electrophysiologic study; 9 (28%) had sustained VT, 16 (50%) had nonsustained VT, and 7 (22%) had no inducible VT. Electrocardiographic criteria and hemodynamic status were of limited value in predicting inducibility of VT. Two of 82 patients with an abnormal heart had sudden death with documented VT/VF; 59 of 82 were treated, with success in 55; 23 were not treated, with spontaneous disappearance of ventricular couplets in 10. As a result of this study, it was concluded that: 1) ventricular couplets appeared benign in patients with a normal heart; 2) in patients with an abnormal heart, inducible VT was common (78%); 3) sudden death occurred in 2 of 82 patients with an abnormal heart within <3 years of detection of couplets; and 4) thus the prognosis of ventricular couplets in the young may be related to the underlying substrate.

Biobehavioral factors

The frequency of VPCs and the degree of impairment of LVEF are major predictors of cardiac mortality in sudden death in the year after AMI. Recent studies have implicated psychosocial factors, including depression, the interaction of social isolation and life stress, and type A-B behavior pattern, as predictors of cardiac events, controlling for known parameters of CAD severity. Results, however, tend not to be consistent and are sometimes contradictory. Ahern and associate CAPS investigators[26] designed an investigation to test the predictive association between biobehavioral factors and clinical coronary events. This evaluation occurred in the context of a prospective clinical trial, the Cardiac Arrhythmia Pilot Study (CAPS). Five-hundred two patients were recruited with ≥10 VPCs/hour or ≥5 episodes of nonsustained VT, recorded 6 to 60 days after an AMI. Baseline behavioral studies, conducted in approximately 66% of patients, included psychosocial questionnaires of anxiety, depression, social desirability and support, and type A-B behavior pattern. In addition, BP and pulse rate reactivity to a portable videogame was assessed. The primary outcome was scored on the basis of mortality or cardiac arrest. Results indicated that the type B behavior pattern, higher levels of depression, and lower pulse rate reactivity to challenge were significant risk factors for death or cardiac arrest, after adjusting statistically for a set of known clinical predictors of disease severity.

Signal averaged electrocardiograms

Lindsay and colleagues[27] in St. Louis, Missouri, have used abnormalities in the fast Fourier transforms of signal-averaged electrocardiograms obtained during sinus rhythm to distinguish patients with CAD and sustained monomorphic VT from those without VT. This study was performed to determine the power of frequency analysis in the detection of patients with a history of VF, to determine the extent to which spectra of signal averaged electrocardiograms from patients with CAD and non-CAD are comparable and to compare results of signal-averaged electrocardiographic analyses in patients with VT with results of programmed ventricular stimulation. Signal-averaged electrocardiograms were obtained during sinus rhythm from 60 patients with sustained VT (Group I) and 34 patients with VF (Group II). Results of signal-averaged electrocardiographic analyses were abnormal in 92% of patients with VT and 85% of patients with VF. Abnormal spectra were detected in the signal-averaged electrocardiograms from 90% of patients with CAD and 86% of patients without CAD. The results of programmed stimulation differed markedly between the two patient groups. Sustained ventricular arrhythmias were induced in 91% of the patients with VT compared with 46% of patients with VF. In addition, VT was inducible in 81% of patients with CAD compared with 50% of those without CAD. Therefore, abnormalities in the spectra of signal-averaged electrocardiograms were found in the majority of patients with VF and were detectable even in patients whose arrhythmia was not inducible. These results provide a broader impetus to use signal-averaged electrocardiograms in the identification of patients with and without CAD prone to VT or VF.

Association with ischemic episodes

Stern and associates[28] from Jerusalem, Israel, investigated in ambulatory patients with stable angina pectoris the association between ventricular ectopic activity (VEA) and ischemic episodes during everyday activities. Seventy-five consecutive patients with proven CAD, ischemic episodes on Holter monitoring and positive treadmill tests, but without known ventricular arrhythmias, were prospectively studied. In these 75 patients, a total of 719 ischemic episodes were recorded during 127 24-hour monitoring periods. Forty-three patients had either no or only very low baseline VEA (14 VPCs/24 hours); none of these patients had increased VEA during any ischemic episode. However, among 32 patients who had 14 VPCs/24 hours (average 243 VPCs/24 hours), increased VEA during ischemic episodes was observed in 11 (31%). These 11 patients had a total of 174 ischemic episodes and the increased VEA appeared in 47 (27%) of the episodes. During 40 of the ischemic episodes the number of single VPCs increased significantly compared to the baseline background VEA: during 4 episodes trigeminy appeared and during another 3 bigeminy was observed. More complex VEA was not observed. Among the 11 patients with increased VEA, only 4 developed VPCs during treadmill testing. No correlation was found between the severity of the ischemic episodes (degree of ST depression and duration of ischemia) and the increased VEA. In 83% of these episodes the increased VEA appeared during the last (possibly reperfusion) phase. No correlation was found between the appearance of ventricular arrhythmias during ischemic episodes and the presence or absence of chest pain at the same time. Thus, in about 33% of chronic stable angina patients without previously known ventricular arrhythmias but with a low-level "background" ectopic activity, increased VEA during ischemic episodes was identified by Holter monitoring, but no malignant ventricular arrhythmias were observed.

Elevated carboxyhemoglobin

Sheps and associates[29] from Chapel Hill, North Carolina, assessed the effects of exposure to 4% and 6% carboxyhemoglobin on ventricular arrhythmias in 41 nonsmokers with documented CAD in a randomized, double-blind, cross-over design study. On day 1, a training session with no exposure, the baseline carboxyhemoglobin level was measured, and a supine bicycle exercise test was done. On days 2 to 4, patients were exposed to room air, 100 ppm carbon monoxide (target, 4% carboxyhemoglobin) or 200 ppm carbon monoxide (target, 6% carboxyhemoglobin), and they then did supine bicycle exercise with radionuclide ventriculography. Ambulatory electrocardiogram recordings were made during the 4 consecutive days to determine the frequency of VPC at various intervals. The frequency of single VPC/h was significantly greater on the 6% carboxyhemoglobin day than on the room air day during the exercise period (168 ± 38 for 6% carboxyhemoglobin compared with 127 ± 28 for room air). During exercise, the frequency of multiple VPC/h was greater on the 6% carboxyhemoglobin day compared with room air (10 ± 4 on the 6% carboxyhemoglobin compared with 3 ± 2 on room air). Patients who developed increased single VPC during exercise on the 6% carboxyhemoglobin day were significantly older than those who had no increased arrhythmia, whereas patients who developed complex arrhythmias were also older and, in addition, exercised longer and had a higher peak workload during exercise. The number and complexity of ventricular arrhythmias increases significantly during exercise after carbon monoxide exposure producing 6% carboxyhemoglobin compared with room air but not after exposure producing 4% carboxyhemoglobin.

Exercise induced

Because there is controversy regarding the clinical relevance of exercise-induced ventricular arrhythmias, Marieb and associates[30] from Charlottesville, Virginia, analyzed their significance in 383 patients who had undergone both exercise thallium-201 stress testing and cardiac catheterization. Two-hundred twenty-one patients (58%) had no exercise-induced ventricular arrhythmias while 162 (42%) did. There was no difference between patients with and without exercise-induced ventricular arrhythmias in terms of previous AMI, incidence of fixed thallium-201 defects (0.06), number of diseased vessels and resting LVEF. In contrast, evidence of provocable ischemia (redistribution on thallium-201 and ST-segment depression on the electrocardiogram) were more likely to be seen in patients with exercise-induced ventricular arrhythmias. Discriminant function analysis revealed that these 2 variables best separated patients with and without exercise-induced ventricular arrhythmias. In a 4- to 8-year follow-up, 89 patients had adverse cardiac events. Of these 89, there were 41 deaths, 9 nonfatal AMIs and 39 coronary revascularization procedures performed later than 3 months after catheterization. Patients with exercise-induced ventricular arrhythmias were more likely to have these events than those without these arrhythmias. Moreover, these arrhythmias provided independent prognostic information beyond that provided by the thallium-201 stress test and coronary angiography. The authors concluded that exercise-induced ventricular arrhythmias are associated with exercise-induced ischemia and provide prognostic information which adds marginally to that provided by other noninvasive and invasive parameters in ambulatory patients being evaluated for chest pain.

After coronary bypass

Exercise-induced ventricular arrhythmias occur often after CABG, but their prognostic significance is unknown. Yli-Mayry and associates[31] from Oulu, Finland, examined 200 patients by exercise electrocardiography and cardiac catheterization before and 3 months after CABG. Exercise-induced ventricular arrhythmias occurred more often after (49 of 200 patients, 24.5%) than before (32 of 200 patients, 16.0%) CABG. There were no differences between the patients with and without ventricular arrhythmias in the prevalence of graft patency (79 vs 80%) or the postoperative EF (57 ± 9 vs 57 ± 12%). Ten cardiac deaths occurred during the mean follow-up time of 61 ± 19 months, 8 of which were witnessed sudden cardiac deaths. All cardiac deaths occurred in patients who did not have exercise-induced ventricular arrhythmias after CABG. The postoperative EF was lower in the cardiac death patients (42 ± 16%) than in the survivors (58 ± 10%). No other clinical or angiographic variable predicted the occurrence of cardiac death. Thus, the prevalence of exercise-induced ventricular arrhythmias increases after CABG, but the occurrence of ventricular arrhythmias does not indicate an increased risk of cardiac death.

Caffeine

Little information is known regarding caffeine's effect on the substrate supporting sustained ventricular arrhythmias. Chelsky and associates[32] from Portland, Oregon, prospectively evaluated the effect of coffee (275 mg of caffeine) on this substrate with programmed ventricular stimulation in 22 patients with a history of symptomatic nonsustained VT, VT, or VF. Patients underwent electrophysiological testing before and 1 hour after coffee ingestion. Mean plasma caffeine level achieved after coffee consumption was 6.2 ± 0.5 mg/L. Mean plasma catecholamine and potassium values were not altered significantly 1 hour following caffeine ingestion. The number of extrastimuli required to induce an arrhythmia was unchanged in 10 patients (46%), increased in 6 (27%), and decreased in 6 (27%). Rhythm severity was unchanged in 17 patients (77%), more severe in 2 (9%), and less severe in 3 (14%). In those patients with clinical ventricular arrhythmias, caffeine did not significantly alter inducibility or severity of arrhythmias, suggesting little effect on the substrate supporting ventricular arrhythmias.

Value of electrophysiologic testing

Manolis and Estes[33] from Boston, Massachusetts, performed programmed ventricular stimulation with up to 3 extra-stimuli at the RV apex in 52 patients with spontaneous nonsustained VT associated with CAD. There were 44 men and 8 women, aged 66 ± 9 years (range 45 to 86). The mean LVEF was $41 \pm 14\%$. Nonsustained VT was asymptomatic in 10 patients (19%), while the arrhythmia was detected during evaluation of palpitations in 5 patients (10%), presyncope in 11 (21%) and syncope in 26 patients (50%). All patients were tested in the drug-free state and were classified as having no inducible arrhythmia (31 patients, group I), or an inducible arrhythmia (21 patients, group II). The age, gender, type of heart disease, symptoms and LVEF were similar in both groups. Group I patients had a higher overall incidence of syncope. Group I patients received no therapy, while group II patients received antiarrhythmic therapy guided by electropharmacologic testing. At 21 ± 17 months there was no sustained VT in either group. There were 3 deaths in group I patients, including 1 sudden, 1 nonsudden cardiac and 1 noncardiac death. In group II patients 6 deaths occurred including 4 nonsudden cardiac and 2 noncardiac deaths. In patients with nonsustained VT and CAD undergoing programmed ventricular stimulation, the incidence of significant arrhythmic events is low in those without therapy with no inducible arrhythmia, and in those with an inducible arrhythmia with therapy guided by electrophysiologic testing.

Previous studies of the value of electrophysiologic studies in patients with nonsustained VT have been hampered by the inclusion of a small number of patients with various types of heart disease. In a retrospective study Kowey and associates[34] of the Philadelphia Arrhythmia Group retrospectively assessed the value of programmed stimulation in 205 asymptomatic patients who had had an AMI >1 month before study. Inclusion was based on 24-hour Holter monitoring during which patients had to manifest ≥3 consecutive ventricular beats at a rate 135 beats/min. Forty-seven (23%) patients had normal, 70 (34%) mildly impaired and 88 (43%) severely impaired LV function. Programmed stimulation, using up to 3 extrastimuli, was used in each. Seventy-five patients (36%) were non-inducible, 59 (29%) had nonsustained VT (<30 seconds), 67 (33%) had sustained monomorphic VT and 4 (2%) had either polymorphic VT or VF. Eighty-two patients were not treated with antiarrhythmic drugs, 57 others were placed on a program selected empirically and 66 had therapy guided by electrophysiologic testing. Satisfactory follow-up information was gathered in 187 of the 205 patients, with a mean follow-up of 18 months. One hundred forty-two patients are alive and well, 39 had sustained VT or sudden death and 6 others had a cardiac death. Only LV function discriminated those who had a sustained arrhythmia or died from those who did not. Thus, programmed stimulation did not have independent predictive value in patients with nonsustained VT.

Hammill and associates[35] from Rochester, Minnesota, evaluated 110 patients with asymptomatic nonsustained VT prospectively to assess the value of electrophysiologic testing. This testing consisted of up to 3 extrastimuli delivered during 3 drive cycle lengths from 2 RV sites. A positive study was defined as monomorphic VT lasting 30 seconds or requiring cardioversion. Patients with a positive study were treated, and serial drug testing was done. An event during follow-up was sustained VT or cardiac arrest. The mean follow-up was 15 months. Of 57 patients with an EF ≥40%, 6 had a positive electrophysiologic test with 1 event. Twenty-eight patients had an EF <40% and CAD; 14 had a positive test with 1 event, and 14 had a negative test with 3 events. Twenty-five patients had an EF <40% and no CAD; 1 had a positive test with no events, and 24 had a negative test with 8 events. Only EF and CAD class were found to be independent predictors of outcome. Patients with an EF >40% had low inducibility (11%), had few events (3.5%) and did not require electrophysiologic testing. In patients with an EF <40% and CAD, inducibility was high (50%) and a negative study was of no value. Patients with an EF <40% and no CAD had low inducibility (4%), had frequent events (33%) and did not benefit from electrophysiologic testing.

Wilber and colleagues[36] in Maywood, Illinois, performed electrophysiological testing in 100 consecutive patients with spontaneous asymptomatic nonsustained VT, chronic CAD, and EF of less than 40%. Fifty-seven patients without inducible sustained ventricular arrhythmias were discharged on no antiarrhythmic therapy. Sustained monomorphic VT was induced in 37 patients, and polymorphic VT or VF was induced in 6 patients. Of the 43 patients with inducible sustained ventricular arrhythmias, three had spontaneous cardiac arrest during serial drug testing and were excluded from further analysis. Twenty patients were discharged on drug therapy, resulting in suppression of inducible sustained ventricular arrhythmias. The remaining 20 patients with persistently inducible sustained arrhythmias were discharged on drug therapy, resulting in maximal rate slowing of the induced tachycardia. During a mean follow-up of 17 months, there were 10 recurrent cardiac arrests or sudden deaths. The 1- and 2-year actuarial incidence of these events was 2% and 6%, respectively, in patients without inducible sustained ventricular arrhythmias; 0% and 11%, respectively, in patients in whom inducible arrhythmias were suppressed; and 34% and 50%, respectively, in patients with persistently inducible sustained arrhythmias. Multivariate Cox analysis identified only the persistence of inducible sustained ventricular arrhythmias as a significant independent predictor of sudden death or recurrent sustained arrhythmias. In this population, therapeutic intervention to prevent sudden death is unnecessary in patients without inducible sustained ventricular arrhythmias. However, electrophysiologically directed drug therapy as the sole treatment strategy in patients with inducible sustained ventricular arrhythmias has important limitations; only 50% of patients are drug responders, and nonresponders remain at high risk for subsequent sudden death.

Silka and associates[37] from Portland, Oregon, systematically evaluated program ventricular stimulation in patients <21 years of age undergoing electrophysiologic testing. A standardized protocol was applied in 55 consecutive patients (mean age 14 years) with the following clinical presentations: sustained VT (n = 17); VF (n = 7); syncope with heart disease (n = 10); nonsustained VT (n = 6); and syncope with an ostensibly normal heart (n = 15). The stimulation protocol consisted of 1 and 2 ventricular extrastimuli during sinus rhythm, followed by 1 to 4 (S_2, S_3, S_4, S_5) extrastimuli during pacing at 2 ventricular sites. Of the 17 patients with sustained VT, 12 had induction of the arrhythmia (sensitivity = 71%). Overall, 18 of 55 patients had inducible sustained VT, with this response significantly enhanced by use of S_4 or S_5 protocols. Although no syncope patient with an ostensibly normal heart had inducible sustained VT, 7 had polymorphic nonsustained VT in response to ventricular stimulation. The mean number of extra-stimuli preceding the induction of nonsustained or sustained VT or VF did not differ. The induction of VF in 5 cases during this study was preceded in each case by extrastimuli intervals ≤ 190 ms. Thus, data indicate that aggressive stimulation protocols appear to be required for induction of sustained VT in most young patients, nonsustained polymorphic VT as a response to aggressive programmed stimulation is of uncertain significance, and that coupling intervals ≤190 ms may correlate with the induction of VF.

Treatment by USA cardiologists

To define the practice habits of USA cardiologists and the treatment of ventricular arrhythmias, Morganroth and associates[38] from 3 medical centers sent a random sample of 12,000 cardiologists a pre-tested questionnaire. After follow-up procedures, 252 responded, of which 18% were academically-based, 29% were hospital-based, and 53% were office-based. Attitudes about antiarrhythmic drug therapy for the treatment of ventricular arrhythmias were influenced by the presence and severity of cardiac disease, the presence of symptoms and the type of ventricular arrhythmias. In this survey, only 1% of cardiologists treated patients with asymptomatic ventricular premature complexes and no heart disease, but 17% treated such patients if unsustained VT was present. The treatment rate among cardiologists increased to 38% when CAD with LV dysfunction was present in patients with asymptomatic ventricular premature complexes. The presence of any cardiac disease and symptomatic ventricular arrhythmias increased the treatment rate to 80 to 100%. Approximately 50% of responding physicians treated patients comparable to the Cardiac Arrhythmia Suppression Trial study population with antiarrhythmic drugs. Beta blockers were the most common antiarrhythmic drug class chosen as the most appropriate initial therapy in new patients with ventricular arrhythmias. Whereas no cardiologists thought that amiodarone was appropriate to initiate in new patients with benign or potentially malignant ventricular arrhythmias, as many as 33 to 43% of cardiologists would use amiodarone for refractory patients with such arrhythmias, a response contradictory to the approved labeling for this drug. Less than one half of cardiologists recognize the high potential organ toxicity for quinidine, procainamide and tocainide. Cardiologists believed that antiarrhythmic agents with class IA and IC action were equally proarrhythmic in patients with potentially malignant ventricular arrhythmias. Antiarrhythmic drugs were initiated only in-hospital by about 25 to 50% of cardiologists. Electrophysiologic testing was always used by 63% of cardiologists for evaluation of sustained ventricular tachycardia; 33% never used such testing for patients with potentially malignant ventricular arrhythmias. There were no differences in these results based on the geographic location of the responding cardiologists. Thus, significant lack of consensus exists on the toxicity of antiarrhythmic drugs, use of electro-physiologic testing and in- versus out-of-hospital drug initiation. At the time of the survey, most cardiologists treated patients with asymptomatic and symptomatic potentially malignant ventricular arrhythmias, although the interim results of the Cardiac Arrhythmia Suppression Trial indicate reconsideration for therapy in such patients.

Effectiveness of different drugs

Salerno and associates[39] from Minneapolis, Minnesota, reports the results of a meta-analysis of the effectiveness of antiarrhythmic drugs for the suppression of VPCs. They analyzed 97 published articles that referred to a total of 27 drugs and contained data from 2989 patient-treatment trials; their goal was to determine the number of patients responding to therapy, defined as ≥80% suppression of VPCs. By means of logistic regression they tested the effect of 10 clinical and experimental variables on the likelihood of response to therapy. The likelihood of a drug response was significantly affected by the following 6 variables: increased by the use of dose titration, increased by the use of a higher daily dose, decreased by older age, decreased by the use of blinding, increased by treating more male patients, and decreased by the presence of cardiovascular disease. Incorporating these 6 variables into a logistic regression model, the response rate was adjusted in each published study and followed by calculation of the mean response and standard error for each drug. Of the drugs tested in at least 100 patients, the most effective were *amiodarone* (estimated response rate 90%), *encainide* (80%), *flecainide* (79%), and *propafenone* (74%). Class IC drugs were significantly more effective than class IB and II drugs. With the exception of lorcainide and moricizine, class IC drugs were also more effective than class IA drugs. Amiodarone was significantly more effective than all drugs except encainide and flecainide. It was found that there were no significant differences among the response rates to class IA, IB, and II drugs. Whereas several patient and study characteristics affect the likelihood of response to antiarrhythmic drugs, class IC drugs and amiodarone are significantly more effective than other drugs in suppressing VPCs.

Griffith and associates[40] from London, UK, assessed the relative safety and efficacy of intravenous administration of *adenosine, lignocaine, disopyramide, flecainide,* and *sotalol* for termination of stable, induced VT in serial trials. VT was terminated by pacing if it persisted 10–15 minutes after the end of drug administration. Twenty-four patients with recurrent VT were studied. VT was terminated by a drug in 35 of 105 trials (Table 4-2). In 6 patients no drug terminated the arrhythmia. Adenosine did not terminate tachycardia or have any serious adverse effect in any patient;

TABLE 4-2. *Drug effects in individuals. Reproduced with permission from Griffith, et al.*[40]

	Adenosine (n=22)	Lignocaine (n=23)	Diso-pyramide (n=24)	Flecainide (n=20)	Sotalol (n=14)
Nil	22 *(100%)*	16 *(69%)*	11 *(46%)*	4 *(20%)*	7 *(50%)*
Termination	0	7 *(30%)*	12 *(50%)*	11 *(55%)*	5 *(36%)*
Arrhythmogenic	0	0	1 *(4%)*	4 *(20%)*	0
Hypotensive	0	0	0	1 *(5%)*	2 *(14%)*

both flecainide and disopyramide were significantly more effective than lignocaine, but flecainide had significantly more severe adverse effects than lignocaine. Lignocaine was the safest drug and should continue to be used as first-line drug therapy for stable VT. Disopyramide should be considered as second-line treatment. DC cardioversion is necessary for unstable VT and its availability must be ensured before attempted pharmacological intervention.

Encainide vs flecainide

An excellent summary of the results of the Cardiac Arrhythmia Suppression Trial (CAST) was summarized by Akhtar and associates[41] of the Task Force of the Working Group on Arrhythmias of the European Society of Cardiology.

To assess the efficacy of encainide and flecainide in treating patients with sustained ventricular arrhythmias, Herre and associates[42] from San Francisco, California, studied 49 patients with spontaneous or inducible sustained VT or VF for whom treatment with at least 1 Class IA antiarrhythmic agent had failed. Patients were treated with encainide, 35 to 50 mg 3 or 4 times daily or flecainide, 100 to 200 mg twice daily. Arrhythmias worsened early in 5 of 16 patients receiving encainide and in 3 of 33 patients receiving flecainide. Patients with poor LV function were more likely to exhibit proarrhythmia. Nine of 11 patients receiving encainide and 23 of 28 patients receiving flecainide who had repeat programmed ventricular stimulation while receiving drug therapy still had inducible, poorly tolerated VT. Encainide and flecainide have a low efficacy rate and a high incidence of worsening of arrhythmia in patients with sustained ventricular arrhythmias, particularly when this condition is associated with poor LV function.

Quinidine vs procainamide

Aronow and associates[43] from New York, New York, performed a prospective study correlating the effects of quinidine or procainamide versus no antiarrhythmic drug on sudden coronary death, total cardiac death, and total death in 406 elderly patients with heart disease and asymptomatic complex ventricular arrhythmias detected by 24-hour ambulatory electrocardiograms. Of 397 patients treated with quinidine, 184 (46%)

developed adverse effects during the first 2 weeks of therapy and were given no further antiarrhythmic therapy. Of 9 patients treated with procainamide, 2 (22%) developed adverse effects during the first 2 weeks of therapy and were given no further antiarrhythmic therapy. Adverse effects developed during long-term therapy in 6 patients (2%) receiving quinidine and in 3 patients (33%) receiving procainamide. Mean follow-up was 24 ± 15 months in both groups. Sudden cardiac death, total cardiac death and total death occurred in 21, 43 and 65% of patients receiving quinidine or procainamide, respectively, and in 23, 44 and 63% of patients receiving no antiarrhythmic drug, respectively (difference not significant). Survival by Kaplan-Meier analysis showed no significant difference between the 2 groups for sudden cardiac death, total cardiac death or total death through 4 years. Patients with abnormal LVEF had a 3.4 times higher incidence of sudden cardiac death, a 2.4 times higher incidence of total cardiac death and a 1.4 times higher incidence of total death than patients with normal LVEF. These data showed no significant difference in sudden cardiac death, total cardiac death or total death between patients treated with quinidine or procainamide or with no antiarrhythmic therapy. The presence or absence of antiarrhythmic therapy did not affect the event risk regardless of LVEF ≥50% vs <50%, presence vs absence of VT, or ischemic vs nonischemic heart disease.

Indecainide vs procainamide

Pratt and associates[44] from Houston, Texas, compared in a placebo controlled, randomized, parallel study indecainide to procainamide. A 24-hour intravenous phase measured and compared invasive hemodynamics, followed by oral administration for assessment of arrhythmia suppression. Thirty-two patients (mean age 61 years) with asymptomatic or mildly symptomatic nonsustained VT were evaluated, 15 while receiving indecainide and 17 while receiving procainamide. A total of 8 patients had serious toxicity during the intravenous phase; 6 receiving indecainide experienced increased LV dysfunction or worsening arrhythmia (sustained VT, arrhythmic death) while 2 receiving procainamide developed serious hypotension. Proarrhythmia developed in 3 of 15 (20%) of the indecainide patients, but in no procainamide patient. In those tolerating indecainide, long-term suppression of VPCs and of runs of VT was more consistent than with procainamide. While indecainide was a potent suppressor of spontaneous VPCs and VT, patients with significant LV dysfunction could not tolerate it. The indecainide patients developing serious toxicity had a common hemodynamic profile: EF <25%, elevated LV filling pressures, low cardiac and stroke volume index and minimal cardiac reserve. Indecainide has a poor risk-benefit ratio in patients similar to the current population, who have potentially lethal ventricular arrhythmias and severe LV dysfunction.

Propranolol

Friehling and associates[45] from Philadelphia, Pennsylvania, prospectively evaluated the effect of adding propranolol to procainamide, quinidine, propafenone or disopyramide in 37 patients, all with prior AMI and inducible VT. After showing that VT remained inducible during therapy with a type I drug, 23 patients received intravenous propranolol. The ventricular effective refractory period, prolonged by the type I agent, was further increased by propranolol. The cycle length of the VT also increased after the type I drug and propranolol exaggerated this effect. Seven of the 23 patients were rendered non-inducible after propranolol and another 10 manifested a >100 ms increase in induced VT cycle length. In the other 14 patients, propranolol was infused immediately after the basal study. If VT remained inducible, testing was repeated after a type I drug was added. The ventricular effective refractory period, as well as the VT cycle length, increased after propranolol and was further prolonged after the addition of a type I agent. Seven of these 14 patients were rendered noninducible, 3 with propranolol alone and 4 others with the combination and in 4, the VT cycle length was prolonged by >100 ms. A total of 17 patients were discharged on either propranolol alone (3 patients) or on an effective combination (14 patients). During a mean follow-up of 20 months, 1 patient died suddenly, 2 had recurrence of well-tolerated VT and 9 remain on therapy. Thus, propranolol has a demonstrable antiarrhythmic effect in the invasive laboratory and may supplement the antiarrhythmic efficacy of conventional type I antiarrhythmic drugs.

Atenolol

Trippel and Gillette[46] from Charleston, South Carolina, reported use of atenolol in 20 children and adolescents treated for chronic paroxysmal VT or long QT syndrome over a 5-year period. Atenolol was effective in each patient whose VT was precipitated or exacerbated by exercise or catecholamines when the patient was receiving a dosage of approximately 1.7 mg/kg/day. In those patients in whom exercise or catecholamines either suppressed or had no effect on the VT none were effectively treated with atenolol. Three of these 4 patients also had structural abnormalities or myocardial dysfunction. Atenolol was effective in treating 4 of 10 patients with long QT syndrome with a dosage of approximately 1.5 mg/kg/day. Cardiovascular side effects included bradycardia in 3 and hypotension in 1. Other side effects included mild fatigue in 4, headache in 2, sleep disturbance in 2 and difficulty concentrating in 1. The observed mortality rate of 2 patients who died suddenly with long QT syndrome raises concern about its use as a single agent in the treatment of this disorder.

Mexiletine

Kerin and associates[47] from Detroit, Michigan, evaluated the antiarrhythmic efficacy of mexiletine hydrochloride in 100 patients with potentially lethal and drug-resistant ventricular arrhythmias. The efficacy of arrhythmia suppression was assessed by Holter monitoring. The overall arrhythmia suppression of VPCs of 70% and greater was low and seen in only 22% of patients, with an additional 16% responding to a combination of mexiletine and an additional antiarrhythmic drug. The suppression of high-grade forms, couplets of 90% and greater, and complete abolition of nonsustained runs of VT was achieved in 22% of patients, with 9% responding to the addition of another antiarrhythmic agent. VPCs, couplets, and nonsustained VT were suppressed in only 16% of the cohort. The drug was poorly tolerated, with intolerable side effects developing in 49% of patients receiving mexiletine alone and in 57% of patients receiving a combination of antiarrhythmic agents. Tolerable adverse effects were relatively common but transient and dose related.

Propafenone

Funck-Brentano and associates[48] from Nashville, Tennessee, provided an excellent review of propafenone in the February 22, 1990, issue of the New England Journal of Medicine. Propafenone is a new antiarrhythmic drug that shares many clinical characteristics with 2 other recently released agents, flecainide and encainide. Like those drugs, propafenone prolongs the PR and QRS intervals and is effective in suppressing nonsustained ventricular arrhythmias in patients with well-preserved LV function. Like encainide and flecainide, propafenone is less effective in patients with sustained ventricular tachyarrhythmias and may exacerbate arrhythmias in such patients. The results of the Cardiac Arrhythmia Suppression Trial indicate that the administration of encainide and flecainide during the early (3 months or less) period after an AMI was associated with increased mortality as compared with placebo, despite the ability of the drugs to suppress nonsustained ventricular arrhythmias. The mechanism that produces this effect is not known. Propafenone has slight β-adrenergic-antagonist properties that might be expected to exert a beneficial effect in these patients. However, in the absence of data demonstrating that propafenone can reduce mortality in this group, it should not be used. In other patients, the use of propafenone, like that of all antiarrhythmic agents, should be predicated on the assumption that the potential and real benefits outweigh any risks of therapy.

Shen[49] from Honolulu, Hawaii, also provided a fine review on propafenone.

Amiodarone

In this report by Myers and associates[50] from Los Angeles, California, the experience with amiodarone therapy in 145 consecutively referred patients with medically refractory sustained VT and/or VF treated for at least 3 years was reviewed. Ninety-seven had sustained VT; the remaining 48 patients were survivors of sudden cardiac death. The patients had a mean of 3.7 ± 1.4 unsuccessful antiarrhythmic drug trials before initiation of amiodarone. The initial doses of amiodarone averaged 845 ± 258 mg for the first 2 weeks and 56% of all patients received a type I antiarrhythmic drug in addition to amiodarone during the initial phase of therapy. The average maintenance dose of amiodarone was 410 ± 187 mg per day. All patients were followed for a minimum of 3 years or until death or withdrawal from therapy. The maximum follow-up was a period of 8 years. Thus, the average duration of amiodarone therapy was 39 ± 26 months, representing 472 patient-years of therapeutic time on amiodarone. The incidence of deaths either caused by a documented ventricular tachyarrhythmia or presumed to result from an arrhythmic cause was 5.5% in the first year and 3.4% in each of the second and third years of follow-up. During the entire period of follow-up, 56 patients died of all causes (39% of the study population). Survival over the follow-up period was influenced significantly by LV function, as judged by either New York Heart Association Functional Class or objective assessment of LVEF, which was available in 102 patients. Seventeen percent of the patients had to be withdrawn from the study because of side effects to amiodarone, including 6% caused by pulmonary toxicity. In conclusion, amiodarone was found to be highly effective in prophylaxis of arrhythmic deaths in a high-risk population of patients referred for refractory life-threatening ventricular arrhythmias.

High-dose intravenous amiodarone was given to 35 patients with recurrent life-threatening VT refractory to conventional antiarrhythmic drugs by Mooss and associates[51] from Omaha, Nebraska. Intravenous amiodarone was given as a 5 mg/kg dose over 30 minutes followed by 20 to 30 mg/kg/day as a constant infusion for 5 days. Twenty-two (63%) patients responded to intravenous amiodarone. All 22 responders received oral amiodarone. Thirteen (59%) continue to receive oral amiodarone after an average follow-up of 19 months, 4 (18%) had sudden cardiac death on oral amiodarone, 2 (9%) died while receiving amiodarone, secondary to LV failure, and 3 (14%) discontinued amiodarone because of side effects. Of the 13 (37%) nonresponders, 10 died in the hospital while receiving intravenous amiodarone, secondary to lethal arrhythmia. Three nonresponders were discharged from the hospital; 2 with automatic cardioverter/defibrillators and 1 receiving a combination of antiarrhythmic agents. Serious adverse events occurred in 13 (37%) patients during intravenous amiodarone therapy. These included hypotension in 8 patients, symptomatic bradycardia in 4 patients and sinus arrest with bradycardia and hypotension in 1 patient. Minor side effects occurred in 23 (66%) patients. In conclusion, high dose intravenous amiodarone is effective in most patients with recurrent, sustained VT but is associated with an unacceptably high incidence of serious adverse events. The optimal dose and duration of intravenous amiodarone for patients with recurrent, refractory sustained VT remain unknown.

Guccione and associates[52] from Rome, Italy, Hanover, West Germany, and Houston, Texas, reported long-term data on 95 young patients with a mean age of 12 years who received amiodarone. Minimal follow-up time was 1.5 years and a mean duration of therapy was 2.3 years with a maximum of 6.5 years. The mean maintenance dosage was 7.7 mg/kg/day with a range of 1.5 to 25. Initial success based on symptoms and 24 hour electrocardiogram was achieved in 23 of 34 patients with VT, and 32 of 33 with atrial flutter and in 21 of 28 with SVT. However, in 7 of 33 patients with atrial flutter, the arrhythmia returned after 6 months. Patient growth continued in the same percentiles achieved before amiodarone in all but 8 patients, improving in 6 and worsening in 2 with severe underlying disease. Proarrhythmia occurred in 3 patients: 1 had torsade de pointes that disappeared when amiodarone was stopped; 2 with severe anatomic heart disease died suddenly during the loading period (1 with atrial flutter and 1 with VT). Side effects occurred in 29% with keratopathy in 11, abnormal thyroid function test in 6, chemical hepatitis in 3, rash in 3, peripheral neuropathy in 2, hypertension in 1 and vomiting in 1. All side effects disappeared when amiodarone was discontinued or the dose reduced. These authors show good results from treatment of severe arrhythmia when no other medications proved useful. Side effects were relatively common but not severe and no pulmonary side effects were found.

The incidence and clinical predictors of amiodarone pulmonary toxicity were examined by Dusman and co-investigators[53] in Indianapolis, Indiana in 573 patients treated for amiodarone for recurrent ventricular or supraventricular tachyarrhythmias. Amiodarone pulmonary toxicity was diagnosed in 33 of the 573 patients (6%), based on symptoms and new chest radiographic abnormalities and supported by pulmonary biopsy, low pulmonary diffusion capacity and/or abnormal gallium lung scan. Toxicity occurred between 6 days and 60 months of treatment for a cumulative risk of 9% with the highest incidence occurence in the first 12 months. Older patients developed a toxicity more frequently (63 vs 57 years) with no cases diagnosed in patients who started therapy at less than 40 years of age. Gender, underlying heart disease arrhythmia, and pretreatment chest radiographic, spirometric, or lung volume abnormalities did not predict development of amiodarone pulmonary toxicity whereas pretreatment low pulmonary diffusing capacity was lower in the group developing toxicity. There was a high mean daily amiodarone maintenance dose in the pulmonary toxicity group but no difference in loading dose. No patient receiving a mean daily dose less than 305 mg developed pulmonary toxicity. Patients who developed toxicity had higher plasma desethylamiodarone but not amiodarone concentrations during maintenance therapy. Death due to pulmonary toxicity occurred in three of 33 patients (9%). In conclusion: 1) amiodarone pulmonary toxicity occurred in 6% of patients and was more common with a higher amiodarone maintenance dose, advanced age, pretreatment low pulmonary diffusing capacity and higher plasma desethylamiodarone concentrations; and 2) pretreatment chest radiographic, spirometric, and lung volume abnormalities were not predictive for development of amiodarone pulmonary toxicity.

Epicardial laser photocoagulation

Svenson and associates[54] in Charlotte, North Carolina, used electrical activation-guided laser photocoagulation intraoperatively to terminate VT in patients with CAD. During VT, laser irradiation was delivered to mapped sites with local diastolic activation. In 30 long-term survivors, 85 VT configurations were terminated by ablation; 72 (85%) were terminated by endocardial photocoagulation. Thirteen required epicardial photocoagulation, but these thirteen VTs occurred in 10 (33%) of the 30 patients. A ventricular aneurysm was present in 70% of patients with successful endocardial photocoagulation, but in only 10% of patient requiring epicardial photocoagulation for at least one VT configuration. Ninety percent of all patients requiring epicardial laser photocoagulation had no aneurysm and had either a right or a left circumflex coronary artery-related AMI. In these patients, epicardial activation data were similar to those described for VT of an "endocardial" origin and included 1) delayed potentials during sinus rhythm, 2) presystolic or pandiastolic activation sequences during VT, and 3) regions of block near the presumed region of reentry during VT. These data suggest that the critical anatomic substrates supporting reentry in VT occurring after AMI are at intramural or epicardial sites, especially in patients with right or circumflex coronary artery-related AMI and no ventricular aneurysm.

Operative therapy

Landymore and associates[55] in Halifax, Canada, used endocardial resection in 26 patients with sustained drug-resistant VT. The early mortality rate within 30 days of operation was 12%. Two deaths were the result of reduced cardiac output and a third death was related to recurrent VSD after septal endocardial resection. Survivors of endocardial resection were followed for a mean of 43 months (range 6 to 92). There were no recurrences of ventricular arrhythmias and these patients did not require antiarrhythmic drug therapy. The late mortality rate after endocardial resection was 19%. There were 2 late cardiac-related deaths unrelated to arrhythmias and three late deaths from noncardiac causes. Complete endocardial resection ablates drug-resistant VT, but it is associated with an increased perioperative mortality in those patients with severely depressed LV function and without a well defined LV aneurysm.

Bourke and associates[56] at Newcastle upon Tyne, UK, evaluated 27 patients with a mean age of 57 ± 7 years who had surgery for control of recurrent drug-refractory ventricular tachyarrhythmias. These arrhythmias included uniform ventricular tachycardia alone in 9 patients, VT and VF in 15, and VF alone in 3 patients. These patients were operated on within 2 months of AMI. The mean number of major arrhythmic episodes per patient was 15 with a range of 2 to 200 and of drug failures 4 ± 2. LV function was severely impaired in most patients with a mean LVEF of 29% (range 14% to 47%). Eighteen patients (66%) had an LV aneurysm. Endocardial resection guided by a combination of endocardial activation mapping during tachycardia and fragmentation mapping during sinus rhythm was performed in all patients. All electrically abnormal LV endocardium was excised. Eight patients (30%) died within 30 days of surgery. Death was not related to age, time of surgery after AMI, ventricular function, bypass time or type of arrhythmia. Patients undergoing emergency surgery had a higher early post-operative mortality rate than those undergoing elective surgery i.e., 43% versus 15%, respectively. During a follow-up period of 32 ± 20 months there were no arrhythmic deaths and only three patients (16%) required antiarrhythmic drug therapy. Thus, these data suggest that surgery for ventricular arrhythmias offers a relatively high cure rate for patients at risk, but it is associated with a substantial mortality risk, especially when performed as an emergency procedure.

CARDIAC ARREST

Non-fatal arrest

Few if any prearrest or intraarrest variables have been identified as highly predictive of in-hospital mortality following cardiopulmonary arrest. Roberts and associates[57] from Winnepeg, Canada, reviewed 310 consecutive patients requiring advanced cardiac life support during 1985 and 1986 with respect to 8 specific variables. These included age, diagnosis, location, mechanism of the event, duration of resuscitation, whether the event was witnessed or unwitnessed, the initial observed rhythm and medications administered. A total of 37% of the patients were successfully resuscitated, but only 10% survived until discharge. Factors strongly associated with in-hospital mortality included unwitnessed events, the need for epinephrine, identification of electromechanical dissociation or asystole as initial rhythms, and cardiac vs respiratory mechanism of arrest.

Moosvi and associates[58] from Detroit, Michigan, examined the effect of empiric antiarrhythmic therapy with quinidine and procainamide on long-term mortality in 209 patients with CAD resuscitated after out-of-hospital cardiac arrest. The antiarrhythmic agent used was determined by the patient's private physician without knowledge of the study ambulatory electrocardiogram. Of the 209 patients, procainamide was prescribed in 45 (22%), quinidine in 48 (23%) and no antiarrhythmic therapy in 116 (55%). Digoxin therapy was initiated in 101 patients. The 2-year total survival rate for the quinidine, procainamide and nontreated patients was 61, 57 and 71%, and for sudden death was 69, 69 and 89%, respectively. These observations suggest that empiric antiarrhythmic therapy in survivors of out-of-hospital cardiac arrest did not affect total mortality and was associated with an increased frequency of sudden death.

Poole and associates[59] in Seattle, Washington; Portland, Oregon and Palo Alto, California evaluated the long-term outcome of 241 survivors of out of hospital VF who underwent programmed electrical stimulation. Patients were categorized according to the rhythm induced at baseline drug-free electrophysiologic testing. VF was induced in 39 patients (16%)(Group 1), sustained VT in 66 patients (27%)(Group 2) and nonsustained VT in 34 patients (14%)(Group 3). One hundred two patients (42%)(Group 4) did not have an arrhythmia inducible at baseline electrophysiologic testing. Antiarrhythmic drugs were administered over the long term to 92% of patients in Group 2, 91% of patients in Group 1, and 47% of patients in Group 4. During a mean follow-up time of 30 months, recurrent sudden cardiac death or nonfatal VF occurred in 11 (28%) of 39 patients with inducible VF (Group 1), 14 (21%) of 66 patients with inducible sustained VT (Group 2), 4 (12%) of 34 patients with inducible nonsustained VT (Group 3) and 16 (16%) of 102 patients without inducible arrhythmias (Group 4). Actuarial survival analysis revealed a 2 year cumulative arrhythmia-free survival rate of 65% for patients in Group 2, 71% for patients in Group 1, 79% for patients in Group 3, and 81% for patients in Group 4. Actuarial survival of patients with inducible sustained VT or VF suppressed by electrophysiologically guided drug therapy was not significantly different from that in patients in whom arrhythmias were not suppressed. Multivariate regression analysis revealed that only the presence of CHF was an independent predictor of outcome in these patients. The prognostic significance of inducibility at baseline electrophysiologic testing in survivors of VF is dependent on the status of their LV function. Patients with inducible sustained VT or VF that was subsequently rendered noninducible by electrophysiologically guided drug therapy with class I antiarrhythmic drugs did not have an improved survival rate compared with that found in patients whose tachyarrhythmia could not be suppressed. These data are different from previous observations made in other laboratories where suppression of arrhythmias induced at the time of electrophysiologic study by antiarrhythmic agents chosen on the basis of electrophysiologic testing have appeared to reduce mortality in patients resuscitated from sudden death.

One hundred ninety-nine patients with out-of-hospital cardiac arrest persisted in VF after the first defibrillation attempt, Weaver and colleagues[60] in Seattle, Washington, randomly assigned patients to receive either epinephrine or lidocaine before the next 2 shocks. The resulting electrocardiographic rhythms and outcomes for each group of patients were compared for each group and also compared with results during the prior 2 years, a period when similar patients primarily received sodium bicarbonate as initial adjunctive therapy. Asystole occurred after defibrillation with 3-fold frequency after repeated injection of lidocaine compared with patients treated with epinephrine. There was no difference in the proportion of patients resuscitated after treatment with either lidocaine or epinephrine and in the proportion surviving, respectively. Resuscitation not survival rates were higher during the prior 2-year period in which initial adjunctive drug treatment for persistent VF primarily consisted of a continuous infusion of sodium bicarbonate. The negative effect of lidocaine or epinephrine treatment was explained in part by their influence on delaying subsequent defibrillation attempts. Survival rates were highest in a subset of patients who received no drug therapy between shocks. The investigators concluded that currently recommended doses of epinephrine and lidocaine are not useful for improving outcome in patients who persist in VF. Lidocaine administration is commonly associated with asystole, and any possible attribute of initial adjunctive drug therapy is outweighed by its detrimental effect on delaying successive shocks for persistent VF.

The long-term prognosis of patients successfully resuscitated from cardiac arrest who do not have acute precipitating factors and in whom ventricular arrhythmias cannot be induced during baseline electrophysiologic testing is controversial. Sager and associates[61] from Los Angeles, California, evaluated the long-term risk of recurrent sudden death and determined the clinical, angiographic, hemodynamic, and electrophysiologic predictors of recurrent cardiac arrest in such patients. Twenty-six (37%) of 71 consecutive patients with a single episode of aborted sudden death did not have inducible ventricular arrhythmias (<7 intraventricular responses) during baseline drug-free electrophysiologic study and they form the basis of this report. Their mean age was 54 ± 13 years and the LVEF was 0.47 ± 0.2. After a mean follow-up period of 16 months, 11 patients (42%) had a recurrent cardiac arrest (fatal in 10 patients). The actuarial incidence of recurrent cardiac arrest was 30 ± 10% at 1 year and 55 ± 13% at 3 years. Patients with LVEF ≤0.40 had a significantly higher occurrence of recurrent cardiac arrest than those with LVEF >0.40 (1-year actuarial incidence of 57 ± 17% vs 13 ± 19%). Patients with recurrent sudden death had a significantly greater incidence of dilated cardiomyopathy (55% vs 7%) and baseline frequent VPCs (64% vs 17%) or nonsustained VT (36% vs 0%) than patients without these characteristics. The latter results were obtained despite the treatment of most patients (6 of 8) who manifested frequent ectopy with an antiarrhythmic agent that significantly suppressed VPC frequency and eliminated salvos of nonsustained VT. All 6 patients with frequent ectopy and LVEF ≤0.40 developed recurrent arrest compared with 5 of 20 patients without these characteristics. Thus specific subgroups of patients with aborted sudden cardiac death without inducible ventricular arrhythmias during baseline drug-free electrophysiologic study are still at significant risk for recurrent cardiac arrest and 24-hour ambulatory electrocardiographic guided therapy was ineffective in preventing recurrent cardiac arrest. Those patients with LV systolic dysfunction, dilated cardiomyopathy, and frequent baseline ventricular ectopic activity have a high likelihood of recurrent sudden death and should be considered for aggressive therapeutic interventions.

Cardiopulmonary resuscitation

Coronary perfusion pressure, the aortic-to-RA pressure gradient during the relaxation phase of cardiopulmonary resuscitation, was measured by Paradis and associates[62] from Detroit, Michigan, in 100 patients with cardiac arrest. Coronary perfusion pressure and other variables were compared in patients with and without return of spontaneous circulation. Twenty-four patients had return of spontaneous circulation. Initial coronary perfusion pressure (mean ± SD) was 1.6 ± 8.5 mm Hg in patients without return of spontaneous circulation and 13.4 ± 8.5 mm

Hg in those with return of spontaneous circulation. The maximal coronary perfusion pressure measured was 8.4 ± 10.0 mm Hg in those without return of spontaneous circulation and 26 ± 8 mm Hg in those with return of spontaneous circulation. Differences were also found for the maximal aortic relaxation pressure, the compression-phase aortic-to-right atrial gradient, and the arterial Po_2. No patient with an initial coronary perfusion pressure less than 0 mm Hg had return of spontaneous circulation. Only patients with maximal coronary perfusion pressures of 15 mm Hg or more had return of spontaneous circulation, and the fraction of patients with return of spontaneous circulation increased as the maximal coronary perfusion pressure increased. A coronary perfusion pressure above 15 mm Hg did not guarantee return of spontaneous circulation, however, as 18 patients whose coronary perfusion pressures were 15 mm Hg or greater did not resuscitate. Of variables measured, maximal coronary perfusion pressure was most predictive of return of spontaneous circulation, and all coronary perfusion pressure measurements were more predictive than was aortic pressure alone. The study substantiates animal data that indicate the importance of coronary perfusion pressure during cardiopulmonary resuscitation.

Longstreth and associates[63] from Seattle, Washington, examined the relation between age and outcomes in patients treated for out-of-hospital cardiac arrest in Seattle, Washington. Considering all out-of-hospital cardiac arrests treated by paramedics over a recent 5-year period, 386 (27%) of 1405 consecutive patients aged 70 years or older were resuscitated and admitted to a hospital vs 474 (29%) of 1624 younger patients; 140 elderly patients (10%) were discharged alive vs 223 younger patients (14%). Of the 140 elderly patients, 112 went home and 28 went to a nursing home. Considering only patients whose initial rhythms were VF, the percent of patients discharged alive was substantially higher: 120 (24%) of 493 for elderly patients and 194 (30%) of 639 for younger patients. Elderly patients can benefit from attempted resuscitation from out-of-hospital cardiac arrest.

Geographic variation

To describe geographic variations in an indicator of sudden coronary death, data from the National Center for Health Statistics were examined for deaths occurring out of hospital or in emergency rooms in 1984 to 1986 in 42 states by Gillum[64] from Hyattsville, Maryland. In white males aged 55 to 64 years, the percent of CAD deaths coded as occurring out of hospital or in the emergency room ranged from 50% to 70%. The percents tended to be higher in mountain states and around Lake Michigan. However, neighboring states sometimes had very different percents. Within regions, percents were higher in nonmetropolitan than in metropolitan areas. Standard mortality ratios for white males of all ages revealed that several states had relatively high rates of death out of hospital or in the emergency room. These included New York, Michigan, and Wisconsin. High rates of coronary death out of hospital or in the emergency room may be due to high overall coronary death rates, high percent of coronary deaths occurring out of hospital or in the emergency room, or both. Further studies are needed of geographic variation in sudden coronary death and cardiac arrest and factors that might explain the variation such as emergency medical services. Place of death data from death certificates may be useful in monitoring efforts to prevent sudden coronary death.

In young vs in old

To obtain further information concerning differences in the mechanism of out-of-hospital cardiac arrest between elderly and younger patients, Tresch and associates[65] from Milwaukee, Wisconsin, studied 381 consecutive patients with out-of-hospital cardiac arrest and whose arrest was witnessed by paramedics. In 91% the arrest occurred at the time the patient's cardiac rhythm was monitored. Patients were divided into 2 age groups: elderly patients were >70 years (187) and younger patients were <70 years (194). Elderly patients more commonly had a past history of heart failure (25 vs 10%) and were more commonly taking digoxin (40 vs 20%) and diuretics (35 vs 25%). Before the cardiac arrest, elderly patients were more likely to be complaining of dyspnea (53 vs 40%), whereas younger patients were more likely to complain of chest pain (27 vs 13%). Forty-two percent of younger patients demonstrated VF as the initial out-of-hospital rhythm associated with the arrest, compared to only 22% of elderly patients. Besides patient age, initial cardiac rhythm varied according to the patient's complaint preceding the arrest. Sixty-eight percent of patients with chest pain demonstrated VF, whereas only 21% of patients with dyspnea demonstrated VF. Elderly patients could be as successfully resuscitated as younger patients; however, 24% of younger patients survived, compared to only 10% of elderly patients. Survival was not only dependent on the patient's age, but was dependent on the patient's complaint preceding arrest and the initial cardiac rhythm associated with the arrest. Sixty-five percent of younger patients complaining of chest pain and demonstrating ventricular fibrillation survived. Even in the elderly patients, 58% survived if their complaint was chest pain and if VF was their initial out-of-hospital rhythm associated with the cardiac arrest.

Signal-averaged late potentials

Dolack and associates[66] from Seattle, Washington, evaluated the results of signal-averaged electrocardiography and programmed electrical stimulation in 25 patients with recurrent sustained VT and in 46 patients with a history of out-of-hospital VF to characterize the electrophysiologic substrate responsible for these different clinical arrhythmia presentations. Patients with VT had a higher incidence of late potentials (VT 83%, VF 50%). Significant differences between these groups were also noted in response to programmed electrical stimulation. A sustained ventricular arrhythmia was induced in 24 of 25 (96%) patients with a history of VT but in only 27 of 46 (59%) of VF patients. In addition, VF was induced in 11 (24%) patients in the VF group but in none of the patients in the VT group. When the 2 groups were compared on the basis of select clinical characteristics, no significant difference in age, sex, presence of CAD or EF was noted. The frequency of prior AMI was significantly higher in the VT group (VT 20 of 25, 80%; VF 24 of 46, 52%). Finally, no significant relation between the presence of late potentials and induced arrhythmias was noted in either group. The inability of signal averaged electrocardiography to predict inducibility in VF patients may represent a significant limitation of this technique in identifying patients at risk for sudden cardiac death.

In competitive athletes

Corrado and associates[67] from Padova, Italy, studied at necropsy 22 patients who died suddenly and they were all young competitive athletes in the Veneto region of northern Italy. They died during the period January 1979 to December 1989. The athletes included 19 males and 3 females aged 11 to 35 years (mean 23). In 18 cases, sudden death occurred during (16 cases) or immediately after (2 cases) a competitive sport activity. In 10 subjects, sudden death was apparently the first sign of disease. Postmortem examination disclosed that this fatality was due to arrhythmic cardiac arrest in 17 cases; among these, RV cardiomyopathy, also known as "RV dysplasia," was the most frequently encountered cardiovascular disease (6 cases), followed by atherosclerotic CAD (4 cases), conduction system pathology (3 cases), anomalous origin of right coronary artery from the wrong aortic sinus (2 cases), and mitral valve prolapse (2 cases). In 2 athletes, the abrupt lethal complication was "mechanical" and consisted of pulmonary embolism and rupture of the aorta; in 3 athletes, death was due to a cerebral cause. All athletes with RV cardiomyopathy died during effort, and most had a history of palpitations and/or syncope. Whenever available, electrocardiographic tracings showed inverted T waves in precordial leads and/or left BBB ventricular arrhythmias. Clinicopathologic correlations indicate that in the Veneto region of Italy, RV cardiomyopathy is not so rare among the cardiovascular diseases associated with the risk of arrhythmic cardiac arrest, and seems to account for most cases of sudden death in young athletes; this disorder can be suspected during life on the basis of prodromal symptoms and echocardiographic signs.

From natural disease in drivers

Antecol and Roberts[68] studied the heart in 30 persons who died suddenly from natural causes in the driver's seat of an automobile, truck, or bus. Twenty had cardiac arrest while driving and the other 10 while sitting in the driver's seat of a parked vehicle. Of the 20 drivers, 16 died from atherosclerotic CAD: 12 (75%) had minor collisions and 4 did not. Of the 16 with fatal CAD, an average of 2.3 ± 0.8 of the 4 major coronary arteries were narrowed >75% in cross-sectional area (CSA) by plaque; of 668 five-mm segments of the 4 major (right, left main, left anterior descending, left circumflex) coronary arteries in 13 of these 16 cases, 27 (4%) were narrowed 96 to 100% and 127 (19%) were narrowed 76 to 95% in CSA by plaque. The remaining 4 drivers died from noncoronary conditions: aortic rupture associated with the Marfan syndrome in 1; cardiac sarcoidosis in 1; thoracic aortic dissection in 1; and severe mitral regurgitation from infective endocarditis, which had healed in 1. The other 10 persons were found dead in the driver's seat of a parked vehicle and 8 of them had fatal CAD. Of the 8 CAD victims, an average of 2.5 ± 1.2 of the 4 major coronary arteries was narrowed >75% by plaque; of the 283 five-mm segments of coronary arteries in 7 of the 8 cases, 44 (16%) were narrowed 96 to 100% and 69 (24%) were narrowed 76 to 95% in CSA by plaque. Victims dying suddenly from CAD while driving are similar to other out-of-hospital sudden coronary death victims with respect to mean age, gender, heart weight, frequency of healed AMI, number of major epicardial coronary arteries severely narrowed, and the percentge of 5-mm-long segments of the major arteries severely narrowed by atherosclerotic plaque. Most drivers stopped the vehicle without injury to themselves or to others.

Coronary bypass in survivors

Kelly and associates[69] in Boston, Massachusetts, studied 450 survivors of cardiac arrest to determine the value of CABG on inducible arrhythmias, arrhythmia recurrence and long-term survival. The effects of several clinical, angiographic and electrophysiologic variables on arrhythmia recurrence and survival were analyzed. All patients had a prehospital cardiac arrest and severe operable CAD and underwent CABG. Preoperative electrophysiologic study was performed in 41 patients among whom 33 (80%) had inducible ventricular arrhythmias. Of the 42 patients studied off antiarrhythmic drugs postoperatively, 19 (45%) had inducible ventricular arrhythmias. Thirty patients with inducible arrhythmias preoperatively underwent postoperative testing off antiarrhythmic drugs and arrhythmia induction was suppressed in 14 (47%). Using multivariate analysis, the induction of VF at the postoperative electrophysiologic study was the only significant predictor of inducible ventricular arrhythmia suppression by CABG. Inducible VF was not present postoperatively in any of the 11 patients who manifested the arrhythmia preoperatively, but inducible VT persisted in 80% of patients in whom preoperative testing indicated this arrhythmia. Patients were followed for 39 ± 29 months. There were 4 arrhythmia recurrences and one was fatal. There were 3 nonsudden cardiac deaths and 3 cardiac deaths. Analysis by life table analysis of 5 year survival, cardiac survival, and arrhythmia-free survival rates were 88%, 98%, and 88%, respectively. Depressed LVEF and advanced age were predictors of subsequent premature death. Thus, in a selected subgroup of survivors of cardiac arrest, CABG abolished inducible arrhythmias in a substantial proportion, especially when the arrhythmia induced was VF. Long-term prognosis in these patients was good.

SICK SINUS SYNDROME

Santini and associates[70] from Rome, Italy, analyzed a large population of sick sinus syndrome (SSS) patients to determine whether age of patients, presence of conduction disturbances, and mode of permanent pacing are related to the occurrence of supraventricular tachyarrhythmias, cerebral embolism and cardiac mortality. Three hundred thirty-nine patients permanently paced (135 AAI, 79 DDD, 125 VVI) because of SSS were followed for a mean period of 5 years (range 2 to 10). Patients were divided into 4 groups according to age (<70 or >70 years) and the presence or absence of an associated conduction disturbance. Sixty-eight percent of VVI, 55% of AAI and 40.5% of DDD patients were >70 years of age. In the VVI and DDD groups a conduction disturbance was present in 67 of 204 (33%) patients; conduction disturbances were more common in patients >70 years old (46 of 111, 41%) than in those <70 years old (21 of 93, 22%). The Wenckebach threshold (>140 beats/min) remained unchanged during the follow-up period in 82% of AAI patients. In 9% of these patients, the Wenckebach threshold showed some degree of deterioration, but only in 2 patients was it <100 beats/min (1.5%). Spontaneous second-degree atrioventricular block was observed in 7 patients

(5%); it disappeared in 6 of these patients when drug therapy was discontinued. The incidence of AF was higher in the VVI group (47%) than in the DDD (13%) and the AAI (4%) patients without conduction disturbance. It was still higher in VVI patients with conduction disturbance (44%) compared to that of DDD patients with conduction disturbance (11.5%). A higher incidence of stable AF in the VVI group was also observed, regardless of age or conduction disturbance. Overall mortality rates were 30% in VVI, 16% in DDD and 13% in the AAI mode. Cardiac mortality was significantly higher in the VVI group (13%) compared to that of the AAI group (3%) regardless of age. It was also higher in the VVI group >70 years old (15%) than in the DDD group >70 years. The presence of conduction disturbance did not influence cardiac mortality. The stroke mortality rates were 8% in the VVI, 2% in the AAI and 2.5% in the DDD group (difference not significant). The difference in stroke mortality became statistically significant in the subgroup of patients >70 years old between the VVI (17%) and AAI (3%) modes. Our data indicate that the AAI and DDD modes should always be preferred to the VVI mode in treatment of SSS, particularly in patients >70 years of age.

LONG QT INTERVAL SYNDROME

Weintraub and associates[71] from Melbourne, Australia, studied 23 children and young persons with congenital long QT syndrome; the median age at time of referral was 10 years with a range of 4 days to 19 years. Family history of the syndrome was present in 14 of 23. Among the 19 patients with symptoms, the initial symptom was syncope in 69%, aborted sudden death in 26% and near drowning in 5%. There were 3 deaths during a combined follow-up period of 67 patient years with an annual mortality rate of 4.5%. Patients who did not respond to therapy with a beta-adrenergic blocker and those who died were significantly younger than the remaining patients at the time of diagnosis. Congenital long QT syndrome was associated with a significant mortality rate in childhood despite the use of conventional therapy in symptomatic patients. Ambulatory holter monitoring and treadmill exercise test may be helpful in confirming the diagnosis and monitoring the adequacy of treatment. Children with sustained ventricular arrhythmias merit early consideration of beta blockade plus cardiac pacemaker or left cardiac sympathectomy.

SYNCOPE

Manolis and associates[72] from Boston, Massachusetts, provided a comprehensive review of the causes, current diagnostic evaluation, and treatment of syncope. New data and knowledge in this evolving field were critically analyzed by doing a MEDLINE search on syncope supplemented by selective review of English language literature citations in the Index Medicus before 1980. The authors reviewed approximately 200 published articles on syncope and closely related topics as well as using their own clinical experience. The articles were selected if they addressed the pathophysiology of syncope, classification and causes, differential diagnosis, noninvasive and invasive evaluation, and current therapy. Syncope is a common clinical problem, occurring in 30% to 50% of the adult population. The prognosis for syncope depends on its cause. Cardiac syncope has the worst prognosis and therefore mandates thorough evaluation and prompt treatment. Diagnostic evaluation is made difficult by the transient nature of the episodes and the many causes. Noninvasive testing reveals the cause of syncope in approximately 50% of cases. More extensive evaluation, including invasive electrophysiologic studies, has assumed a larger role in defining the cause of syncope in selected patients with structural heart disease in whom a noninvasive evaluation has been nondiagnostic. Recently tilt-table studies have been proposed as a clinically useful noninvasive test for vagally mediated syncope. A rational stepwise diagnostic and therapeutic approach to patients with syncope can be developed by initially doing a careful history and physical examination followed by a noninvasive evaluation and selective use of additional, more specialized or invasive tests. Future research should focus on defining the validity and utility of current diagnostic testing in syncope and on exploring further the pathophysiology of patients with recurrent, unexplained syncope.

To determine the incremental yield of ambulatory monitoring in the evaluation of syncope, Bass and associates[73] from Pittsburgh, Pennsylvania, obtained 3 serial 24-hour Holter recordings in a consecutive series of 95 patients with syncope, the cause of which was not explained by history, physical examination, or 12-lead electrocardiogram. The mean age of patients was 61 years and 41% were men. Major electrocardiographic abnormalities were found in 26 patients (27%), including unsustained VT (19 patients), pauses of at least 2 seconds (8 patients), profound bradycardia (1 patient), and complete heart block (1 patient). The first 24-hour Holter recording had at least 1 major abnormality in 14 patients (15%). Of the 81 patients without a major abnormality on the first Holter recording, the second Holter recording had major abnormalities in 9 (11%). Of the 72 patients without a major abnormality on the first 2 Holter recordings, only 3 patients (4.2%) had a major abnormality on the third Holter recording. Four factors were significantly associated with an increased likelihood of a major abnormality on 72 hours of monitoring: age >65 years, male gender, history of heart disease, and an initial nonsinus rhythm. These results suggest that 24 hours of Holter monitoring is not enough to identify all potentially important arrhythmias in patients with syncope. Monitoring may need to be extended to 48 hours if the first 24-hour Holter recording is normal.

Kapoor[74] from Pittsburgh, Pennsylvania, studied 433 patients with syncope to derive insights into the diagnostic evaluation and outcome of patients with this problem. This study shows that the etiology of syncope was not found in approximately 41% of patients. When a cause of syncope (Table 4-3) was determined, it was most frequently established on the basis of initial history, physical examination and an electrocardiogram. Furthermore, many of the other entities (e.g., AS, subclavian steal) were suggested by findings on the history and physical examinations that required directed diagnostic testing. Initial electrocardiogram was abnormal in 50% of patients but led to a cause of syncope infrequently. Prolonged electrocardiographic monitoring, which has assumed a central role in the evaluation of syncope, led to a specific cause in only 22% of patients. Other tests were less often helpful in assigning a cause of syncope. At 5 years, the mortality of 50.5% in patients with a cardiac cause of syncope was significantly higher than the 30% mortality in patients with a noncardiac cause or 24% in patients with an unknown

TABLE 4-3. *Causes of syncope. Reproduced with permission from Kapoor, et al.*[74]

	N
Noncardiac cause	
Vasodepressor syncope	35
Situational syncope	36
Drug-induced syncope	9
Orthostatic hypotension	43
Transient ischemic attacks	8
Subclavian steal syndrome	2
Seizure disorder	7
Trigeminal neuralgia	1
Conversion reaction	3
Total	144
Cardiac cause	
Ventricular tachycardia	49
Sick-sinus syndrome	15
Bradycardia	4
Supraventricular tachycardia	8
Complete heart block	6
Mobitz II atrioventricular block	2
Pacemaker malfunction	3
Carotid-sinus syncope	5
Aortic stenosis	8
Myocardial infarction	5
Dissecting aortic aneurysm	1
Pulmonary embolus	2
Pulmonary hypertension	2
Total	110
Unknown cause	179

TABLE 4-4. *Patient characteristics. Reproduced with permission from Kapoor, et al.*[74]

	Cardiac Cause (n = 110)	Non-Cardiac Cause (n = 144)	SUO (n = 179)	p value*
Mean age (yrs)	61	52	56	0.001
	%	%	%	
Men	54	38	35	0.001
Syncope witnessed	88	81	80	NS
Trauma with syncope	32	31	41	NS
Syncope last year	49	51	47	NS
Past history of:				
Hypertension	30	28	34	NS
Angina	30	17	12	0.0006
Ventricular arrhythmia	54	3	2	0.0001
Myocardial infarction	21	10	11	0.02
Congestive heart failure	25	8	8	0.0001
Diabetes	15	15	9	NS
Stroke	11	6	8	NS
Renal insufficiency (Cr > 2)	5	7	4	NS

Abbreviations: SUO = Syncope of unknown origin, Cr = Creatinine.
* p value refers to the comparison of differences between the 3 groups of causes of syncope.

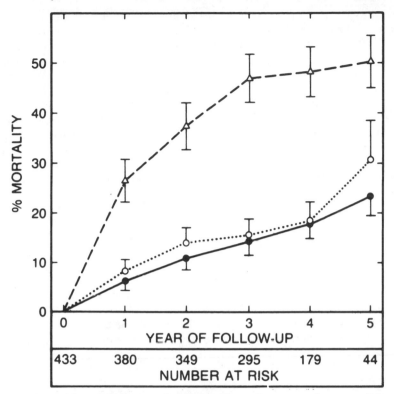

Fig. 4-4. Actuarial mortality rates of patients with cardiac cause of syncope (triangles), noncardiac cause of syncope (open circles), and syncope of unknown cause (solid circles). The mortality in patients with a cardiac cause of syncope was significantly higher than in patients with noncardiac cause (p <0.00001) or patients with syncope of unknown cause (p <0.00001). Reproduced with permission from Kapoor, et al.[74]

cause (Table 4-4; Figure 4-4). At 5 years, a mortality of 50.5% in patients with a cardiac cause of syncope was noted. There were 54 actual deaths in this group as compared to 11 expected deaths based on mortality data from Allegheny County, PA. At 5 years, a 33% incidence of sudden death was noted in patients with a cardiac cause of syncope, as compared with 5% in patients with a noncardiac cause and 8.5% in patients with a noncardiac cause and 8.5% in patients with an unknown cause. Mortality and sudden death remained significant for the first 3 years after which the survival curves were parallel. A cardiac cause of syncope was an independent predictor of sudden death and mortality. Recurrences were common but were not associated with an increased risk of mortality or sudden death. Major vascular events were also more frequent in patients with cardiac causes of syncope.

PACING AND PACEMAKERS

Bedotto and associates[75] in Dallas, Texas, and Tucson, Arizona, determined whether the asynchronous LV contraction-relaxation sequence that occurs during RV pacing alters LV relaxation. Measurements of both the maximal rate of decline of LV pressure and the time constant of LV relaxation were obtained during atrial and AV pacing in 25 patients referred for diagnostic cardiac catheterization. Heart rate was maintained at 10 to 15 beats above the sinus rate at rest, and relaxation was assessed during atrial pacing, AV pacing, and finally repeat atrial pacing. Patients were classified into 2 groups: group 1 had 10 patients with normal LV systolic function at rest and an EF >0.55 and without prior AMI and group 2 included 15 patients with a depressed LVEF or akinesia of one or more LV segments on the contrast ventriculogram. Heart rate, peak LV systolic pressure, end-systolic pressure and end-diastolic pressure remained constant during atrial, AV pacing and repeat atrial pacing in all patients. In group 1 patients, the decrease in peak negative dP/dt and the increase in the time constant of LV relaxation during AV pacing were not significantly different when compared with values during atrial pacing. In group 2 patients, peak negative dP/dt decreased during AV pacing as compared to atrial pacing and the time constant of LV relaxation increased. Maximal rate of rise of LV pressure also decreased during LV pacing in patients in groups 1 and 2. Thus, these data suggest that asynchronous contraction-relaxation occurs during RV pacing and alters LV relaxation in patients with abnormal LV systolic function.

Morgan and associates[76] from Croydon, UK, analyzed the clinical assessment and the investigations required in 150 patients with various electrophysiologic disorders and provided an algorithm to assist decision of pacemaker implantation and what type of pacemaker to implant (Figure 4-5).

CARDIOVERTERS/DEFIBRILLATORS

The automatic implantable cardioverter/defibrillator (AICD) has been shown to decrease the mortality of patients who have survived cardiac arrest due to VT or VF and are at high risk for recurrence. Kupperman and co-authors[77] in Washington, D.C., performed a cost-effectiveness analysis of this seemingly expensive new technology with data obtained from the 1984 Medicare data base, the medical literature, Medicare carriers, individual pharmacies and hospitals, and expert opinion. Analyzing combinations of principal and secondary discharge diagnoses across 18 diagnosis-related groups, they estimated the cost of hospitalization for a comparison group of patients. Hospitalization costs for the defibrillator group were obtained from reported empirical data. Rehospitalization rates and other health care use estimates were solicited from an expert panel of physicians, and mortality rates for both groups were obtained from the literature. Using a decision-analytic model, the investigators estimated that the net cost effectiveness of the defibrillator, when used in the high risk patient, is approximately $17,100 per life year saved, with sensitivity analyses suggesting that the true value lies between $15,000 and $25,000. It was also estimated that this was well within the range that is currently accepted by the US medical care system for other life saving interventions. The investigators also estimated the cost effectiveness of the defibrillator in a 1991 scenario to be $7,400 per life year saved, when the device would have greater longevity, and would be programmable, and would not require a thoracotomy. Sensitivity analyses suggest that the true value lies between a value that is cost saving (less expensive than pharmacologic therapy) and $19,600 per life year saved.

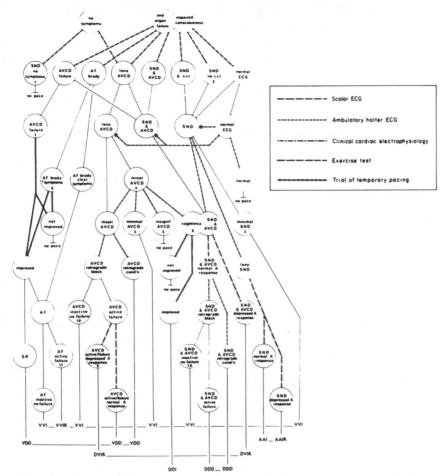

Fig. 4-5. Algorithm for pacemaker mode selection. Abbreviations: SND: Sinus node disease; AVCD: atrioventricular conduction disease; AF: atrial fibrillation; SR: sinus rhythm; svt: supreventricular tachyarrhythmias; ECG: electrocardiogram; A: atrial; VVIR, AAIR, DVIR: rate-responsive VVI, AAI, DVI pacing. Notes: 1: Asymptomatic sinus node disease does not require pacing. 2: Sinus node disease requires Holter monitoring only to demonstrate svt. 3: Minimal SND or AVCD: minimally apparent SND or AVCD with very infrequent manifestation. 4: Minor AVCD: low-grade AVCD: first-degree or type 1 second-degree heart block, bundle branch block or hemiblock. 5: Insignificant AVCD: AV nodal conduction delay or prolonged refractory period with doubtful or no symptoms. 6: Vagotonia: carotid sinus syncope or malignant vaso-vagal syndrome, where electrophysiology fails to demonstrate significant disease. 7: Failure: usually heart failure but also cerebral, renal or peripheral hypoperfusion. 8: Atrial fibrillation and bradycardia with doubtful symptoms. 9: AVCD with depressed evoked atrial response to exercise does not require atrial sensing. 10: Sedentary lifestyle, old age etc. in absence of failure does not require dual chamber pacing. 11: Active lifestyle or failure requires rate-responsive VVI pacemakers. Reproduced with permission from Morgan, et al.[76]

Multiple defibrillations by the AICD have been reported to result in localized epicardial damage. No data exist, however, regarding whether this damage can be detected in the clinical setting or whether it interferes with the detection of true myocardial infarction. Avitall and colleagues[78] in Milwaukee, Wisconsin, prospectively studied 49 patients who received defibrillations by patch electrodes. The investigators attempted to document the presence of myocardial injury with the following 3 commonly used modalities for the detection of AMI: serial electrocardiographic changes, serial creatine phosphokinase and CPK-MB release, and technetium 99 m pyrophosphate scanning. Fifteen patients received defibrillations by AICD patches at the time of generator replacement. Nine patients received defibrillations at the time of new AICD lead placement. No patient had detectable myocardial injury. Ten patients had defibrillations by the AICD patches at the time of CABG. One patient in this group developed AMI in the inferior wall after CABG. Fifteen patients were evaluated for spontaneous AICD discharges. Thirteen had a maximum of 5 consecutive shocks, and cumulative energy delivered was not greater than 330 J. No patient had detectable injury. Two patients had creatine phosphokinase-MB release of 15% and 8% respectively, and one of these patients had a positive pyrophosphate scan. These 2 patients received 12 and 17 rapid and consecutive AICD discharges. Twenty-one patients developed nonspecific ST-T segment changes that normalized within 48–72 hours after AICD discharges. Investigators concluded that 1) defibrillation efficacy testing limited to 85J does not cause detectable myocardial injury; 2) spontaneous discharges of the AICD with a maximum cumulative energy of 330J does not result in detectable myocardial injury when the rate of discharge for five rapid shocks is less than one shock per minute; 3) rapid consecutive (more than 12 at less than 1 minute apart) AICD discharges can result in a positive scan and creatine phosphokinase-MB release; 4) the appearance of new Q waves or persistent T wave changes, together with significant release of creatine phosphokinase enzymes is probably because of myocardial infarction caused by vascular occlusion; and 5) transient ST-T segment changes are common after AICD discharges.

Fogoros and associates[79] in Pittsburgh, Pennsylvania evaluated the ability of the AICD to prolong overall survival in patients with significantly depressed cardiac function. One hundred and nineteen patients who had an AICD placed were evaluated. Forty patients had LVEFs <30% (Group A) and 79 had LVEFs ≥30% (Group B). Cumulative survival was compared with the projected survival if the AICD had not been used with the assumption that the first appropriate shock would have resulted in death without the defibrillator. Among patients in group A, the 3 year cumulative survival rate was 67 ± 12% versus a projected survival rate of 6 ± 15%. Among patients in group B, the 3 year cumulative survival rate was 96 ± 3% as compared to a projected survival rate of 46 ± 8%. Cumulative and projected survival rates for patients in group A were significantly worse than those in patients in group B. These data demonstrate that the AICD significantly prolongs overall survival, even in patients with poor cardiac function.

The Defibrillator Working Group of the Food and Drug Administration in an article authored by Cummins and associates[80] from several medical centers reviewed data from the Medical Device Reporting System and a recent 5-state survey, as well as information presented at 2 Food and Drug Administration-sponsored conferences. These data include 156 reports of defibrillator problems to the Emergency Care Research Institute Problem Reporting Network, 495 reports of device problems to the Medical Device Reporting System, 676 reports of "defibrillator failure" in the 5-state survey, 594 inspections of in-service defibrillators, and site visits to 212 emergency care facilities. The Defibrillator Working Group concluded that the frequency of defibrillator failures during clinical use may be unacceptably high. While some failures are attributable to component malfunctions, evidence suggests that errors in operator use and errors in defibrillator care and maintenance account for a high proportion of defibrillator failures. Inadequate initial training and cursory continuing education increases the chances of operator errors at the moment when correct operation is needed most. Failure of operators to perform daily equipment checks leads to poor familiarity with the equipment and failure to identify component failures or damaged devices. Many defibrillators and batteries are kept in service beyond an expected useful life, given their level of clinical use. In smaller hospitals and emergency medical services systems periodic maintenance responsibilities are not always appropriately delegated between qualified engineering personnel and defibrillator operators, and some systems completely lack services from clinical engineers. The objectives of the Defibrillator Working Group are to make personnel who use defibrillators more aware of the potential for errors in operator performance and in periodic maintenance and to recommend improvements in training, maintenance, and defibrillator design. This article presents the initial observations and recommendations of the working group.

References

1. Sanfilippo AJ, Abascal VM, Sheehan M, Oertel LB, Harrigan P, Hughes RA, Weyman AE: Atrial Enlargement as a Consequence of Atrial Fibrillation A prospective Echocardiographic Study. Circulation 1990 (September);82:792–797.
2. Koskinen P, Kupari M, Leinonen H: Role of alcohol in recurrences of atrial fibrillation in persons 65 years of age. Am J Cardiol 1990 (Oct 15);66:954–958.
3. Petersen P, Kastrup J, Helweg-Larsen S, Boysen G, Godtfredsen J: Risk factors for thromboembolic complications in chronic atrial fibrillation: The Copenhagen AFASAK Study. Arch Intern Med 1990 (April);150:819–821.
4. Cabin HS, Clubb KS, Hall C, Perlmutter RA, Feinstein AR: Risk for systemic embolization of atrial fibrillation without mitral stenosis. Am J Cardiol 1990 (May 1);65:1112–1116.
5. Feinberg WM, Seeger JF, Carmody RF, Anderson DC, Hart RG, Pearce LA: Epidemiologic features of asymptomatic cerebral infarction in patients with nonvalvular atrial fibrillation. Arch Intern Med 1990 (Nov);150:2340–2344.
6. Rawles JM, Metcalfe MJ, Jennings K: Time of occurrence, duration, and ventricular rate of paroxysmal atrial fibrillation: The effect of digoxin. Br Heart J 1990 (Apr);63:225–227.
7. Coplen SE, Antman EM, Berlin JA, Hewitt P, Chalmers TC: Efficacy and Safety of Quinidine Therapy for Maintenance of Sinus Rhythm After Cardioversion A Meta-Analysis of Randomized Control Trials. Circulation 1990 (October);82:1106–1116.
8. Juul-Moller S, Edvardsson N, Rehnqvist-Ahlberg: Sotalol Versus Quinidine for the Maintenance of Sinus Rhythm After Direct Current Conversion of Atrial Fibrillation. Circulation 1990 (December);82:1932–1939.
9. Antman EM, Beamer AD, Cantillon C, McGowan N, Friedman PL. Therapy of refractory symptomatic atrial fibrillation and atrial flutter: A staged care approach with new antiarrhythmic drugs. J Am Coll Cardiol 1990 (March);15:698–707.
10. Wong CK, Lau CP, Leung WH, Cheng CH: Usefulness of labetalol in chronic atrial fibrillation. Am J Cardiol 1990 (Nov 15);66:1212–1215.
11. Wipf JE, Lipsky BA: Atrial fibrillation: Thromboembolic risk and indications for anticoagulation. Arch Intern Med 1990 (Aug);150:1598–1603.
12. The Boston Area Anticoagulation Trial for Atrial Fibrillation Investigators: The effect of low-dose warfarin on the risk of stroke in patients with nonrheumatic atrial fibrillation. N Engl J Med 1990 (Nov 29);323:1505–1511.
13. Paul T, Guccione P, Garson A Jr: Relation of syncope in young patients with Wolff-Parkinson-White Syndrome to rapid ventricular response during atrial fibrillation. Am J Cardiol 1990 (Feb 1);65:318–321.

14. Beckman KJ, Gallastegui JL, Bauman JL, Hariman RJ. The predictive value of electro-physiologic studies in untreated patients with Wolff-Parkinson-White syndrome. J Am Coll Cardiol 1990 (March);15:640–7.

15. Perry JC and Garson A: Supraventricular Tachycardia Due to Wolff-Parkinson-White Syndrome in Children: Early Disappearance and Late Recurrence. J Am Coll Cardiol 1990 (November);16:1215–1220.

16. Perry JC, Gluffre RM, Garson AJ, Jr.: Clues to the Electrocardiographic Diagnosis of Subtle Wolff-Parkinson-White Syndrome in Children. J Pediatr 1990 (December); 117:871–875.

17. Kupari M, Koskinen P, Leinonen H: Double-peaking circadian variation in the occur-rence of sustained supraventricular tachyarrhythmias. Am Heart J 1990 (December);120:1364–1369.

18. Haines DE, DiMarco JP. Sustained intraatrial reentrant tachycardia: Clinical, electro-cardiographic and electrophysiologic characteristics and long-term follow-up. J Am Coll Cardiol 1990 (May);15:1345–54.

19. Rankin AC, Oldroyd KG, Chong E, Dow JW, Rae AP, Cobbe EM: Adenosine or adenosine triphosphate for supraventricular tachycardias? Comparative double-blind random-ized study in patients with spontaneous or inducible arrhythmias. Am Heart J 1990 (February);119:316–323.

20. Sharma AD, Klein GJ, Yee R: Intravenous adenosine triphosphate during wide QRS complex tachycardia: Safety, therapeutic efficacy, and diagnostic utility. Am J Med 1990 (April);88:337–343.

21. DiMarco JP, Miles W, Akhtar M, Milstein S, Sharma AD, Platia E, McGovern B, Scheinman MM, Govier WC, The Adenosine for PSVT Study Group: Adenosine for paroxysmal supraventricular tachycardia; Dose ranging and comparison with verapamil: As-sessment in placebo-controlled, multicenter trials. An Intern Med 1990 (July 15);113:104–110.

22. Mostow ND, Vrobel TR, Noon D, Rakita L: Rapid control of refractory atrial tachyar-rhythmias with high-dose oral amiodarone. Am Heart J 1990 (December);120:1356–1363.

23. Cox JL, Ferguson B Jr, Lindsay BD, Cain ME: Perinodal cryosurgery for atrioventricular node reentry tachycardia in 23 patients. J Thorac Cardiovasc Surg 1990 (Mar);99:440–450.

24. Noh CI, Gillette PC, Case CL, Zeigler VL: Clinical and electrophysiological characteristics of ventricular tachycardia in children with normal hearts. Am Heart J 1990 (Decem-ber);120:1326–1333.

25. Paul T, Marchal C, Garson A Jr: Ventricular couplets in the young: Prognosis related to underlying substrate. Am Heart J 1990 (March);119:577–582.

26. Ahern DK, Gorkin L, Anderson JL, Tierney C, Hallstrom A, Ewart C, Capone RJ, Schron E, Kornfeld D, Herd JA, Richardson DW, Follick MJ, CAPS Investigators: Biobehavioral variables and mortality or cardiac arrest in the cardiac arrhythmia pilot study (CAPS). Am J Cardiol 1990 (July 1);66:59–62.

27. Lindsay BD, Ambos HD, Schechtman KB, Arthur RM, Cain ME. Noninvasive detection of patients with ischemic and nonischemic heart disease prone to ventricular fi-brillation. J Am Coll Cardiol 1990 (December);16:1656–64.

28. Stern S, Banai S, Keren A, Tzivoni D: Ventricular ectopic activity during myocardial ischemic episodes in ambulatory patients. Am J Cardiol 1990 (Feb 15);65:412–416.

29. Sheps DS, Herbst MC, Hinderliter AL, Adams KF, Ekelund LG, O'Neil JJ, Goldstein GM, Bromberg PA, Dalton JL, Ballenger MN, Davis SM, Koch GG: Production of arrhythmias by elevated carboxyhemoglobin in patients with coronary artery disease. An Intern Med 1990 (Sept 1);113:343–351.

30. Marieb MA, Beller GA, Gibson RS, Lerman BB, Kaul S: Clinical relevance of exercise-induced ventricular arrhythmias in suspected coronary artery disease. Am J Cardiol 1990 (July 15);66:172–178.

31. Yli-Mayry S, Huikuri HV, Korhonen UR, Airaksinen KEJ, Ikaheimo MJ, Linnaluoto MK, Takkunen JT: Prevalence and prognostic significance of exercise-induced ventricular arrhythmias after coronary artery bypass grafting. Am J Cardiol 1990 (Dec 15);66:1451–1454.

32. Chelsky LB, Cutler JE, Griffith K, Kron J, McClelland JH, McAnulty JH: Caffeine and ventricular arrhythmias: An electrophysiological approach. JAMA 1990 (Nov 7);264:2236–2240.

33. Manolis AS, Estes NAM III: Value of programmed ventricular stimulation in the evaluation and management of patients with nonsustained ventricular tachycardia associated with coronary artery disease. Am J Cardiol 1990 (Jan 15);65:201–205.

34. Kowey PR, Waxman HL, Greenspon A, Greenberg R, Poll D, Kutalek S, Gessman L, Muenz L, Philadelphia Arrhythmia Group: Value of electrophysiologic testing in patients with previous myocardial infarction and nonsustained ventricular tachycardia. Am J Cardiol 1990 (Mar 1);65:594–598.

35. Hammill SC, Trusty JM, Wood DL, Bailey KR, Vatterott PJ, Osborn MJ, Holmes DR Jr, Gersh BJ: Influence of ventricular function and presence or absence of coronary artery disease on results of electrophysiologic testing for asymptomatic nonsustained ventricular tachycardia. Am J Cardiol 1990 (Mar 15);65:722–728.

36. Wilber DJ, Olshansky B, Moran JF, Scanlon PJ: Electrophysiological Testing and Nonsustained Ventricular Tachycardia Use and Limitations in Patients with Coronary Artery Disease and Impaired Ventricular Function. Circulation 1990 (August);82:350–358.

37. Silka MJ, Kron J, Cutler JE, McAnulty JH: Analysis of programmed stimulation methods in the evaluation of ventricular arrhythmias in patients 20 years old and younger. Am J Cardiol 1990 (Oct 1);66:826–830.

38. Morganroth J, Bigger JT Jr, Anderson JL: Treatment of ventricular arrhythmias by United States cardiologists: A survey before the cardiac arrhythmia suppression trial results were available. Am J Cardiol 1990 (Jan 1);65:40–48.

39. Salerno DM, Gillingham KJ, Berry DA, Hodges M: A comparison of antiarrhythmic drugs for the suppression of ventricular ectopic depolarizations: A meta-analysis. Am Heart J 1990 (August);120:340–353.

40. Griffith MJ, Linker NJ, Garratt CJ, Ward DE, Camm AJ: Relative efficacy and safety of intravenous drugs for termination of sustained ventricular tachycardia. Lancet 1990 (Sept 15);336:670–673.

41. Task Force of the Working Group on Arrhythmias of the European Society of Cardiology: CAST and beyond implications of the Cardiac Arrythmia Suppression Trial. Eur Heart J 1990 (Mar);11:194–199.

42. Herre JM, Titus C, Oeff M, Eldar M, Franz MR, Griffin JC, Scheinman MM: Inefficacy and proarrhythmic effects of flecainide and encainide for sustained ventricular tachycardia and ventricular fibrillation. An Intern Med 1990 (Nov);113:671–676.

43. Aronow WS, Mercando AD, Epstein S, Kronzon I: Effect of quinidine or procainamide versus no antiarrhythmic drug on sudden cardiac death, total cardiac death, and total death in elderly patients with heart disease and complex ventricular arrhythmias. Am J Cardiol 1990 (Aug 15);66:423–428.

44. Pratt CM, Francis MJ, Seals AA, Zoghbi W, Young JB: Antiarrhythmic and hemodynamic evaluation of indecainide and procainamide in nonsustained ventricular tachycardia. Am J Cardiol 1990 (July 1);66:68–74.

45. Friehling TD, Lipshutz H, Marinchak RA, Stohler JL, Kowey PR: Effectiveness of propranolol added to a type I antiarrhythmic agent for sustained ventricular tachycardia secondary to coronary artery disease. Am J Cardiol 1990 (June 1);65:1328–1333.

46. Trippel DL and Gillette PC: Atenolol in Children with Ventricular Arrhythmias. Am Heart J 1990 (June);119:1312–1316.

47. Kerin NZ, Aragon E, Marinescu G, Faitel K, Frumin H, Rubenfire M: Long-term efficacy and side effects in patients with chronic drug-resistant potentially lethal ventricular arrhythmias. Arch Intern Med 1990 (Feb);150:381–384.

48. Funck-Brentano C, Kroemer HK, Lee JT, Roden DM: Propafenone. N Engl J Med 1990 (Feb 22);322:518–525.

49. Shen EN: Propafenone: A promising new antiarrhythmic agent. Chest 1990 (Aug);98:434–441.

50. Myers M, Peter T, Weiss D, Nalos PC, Gang ES, Oseran DS, Mandel WJ: Benefit and risks of long-term amiodarone therapy for sustained ventricular tachycardia/fibrillation: Minimum of three-year follow-up in 145 patients. Am Heart J 1990 (January);119:8–14.

51. Mooss AN, Mohiuddin SM, Hee TT, Esterbrooks DJ, Hilleman DE, Rovang KS, Sketch MH: Efficacy and tolerance of high-dose intravenous amiodarone for recurrent, refractory ventricular tachycardia. Am J Cardiol 1990 (Mar 1);65:609–614.

52. Guccione P, Paul T, Garson A Jr.: Long-Term Follow-up of Amiodarone Therapy in the Young: Continued Efficacy, Unimpaired Growth, Moderate Side Effects. J Am Coll Cardiol 1990 (April);15:1118–24.

53. Dusman RE, Stanton MS, Miles WM, Klein LS, Zipes DP, Fineberg NS, Heger J: Clinical Features of Amiodarone-Induced Pulmonary Toxicity. Circulation 1990 (July);82:51–59.

54. Svenson RH, Littmann L, Gallagher JJ, Selle JG, Zimmern SH, Fedor JM, Colavita PG. Termination of ventricular tachycardia with epicardial laser photocoagulation: A clinical comparison with patients undergoing successful endocardial photocoagulation alone. J Am Coll Cardiol 1990 (January);15:163–70.

55. Landymore RW, Gardner MA, McIntyre AJ, Barker RA. Surgical intervention for drug-resistant ventricular tachycardia. J Am Coll Cardiol 1990 (July);16:37–41.

56. Bourke JP, Hilton CJ, McComb JM, Cowan JC, Tansuphaswadikul S, Kertes PJ, Campbell RWF. Surgery for control of recurrent life-threatening ventricular tachyarrhythmias within 2 months of myocardial infarction. J Am Coll Cardiol 1990 (July);16:42–8.

57. Roberts D, Landolfo K, Light RB, Dobson K: Early predictors of mortality for hospitalized patients suffering cardiopulmonary arrest. Chest 1990 (Feb);97:413–419.

58. Moosvi AR, Goldstein S, Medendorp SV, Landis JR, Wolfe RA, Leighton R, Ritter G, Vasu CM, Acheson A: Effect of empiric antiarrhythmic therapy in resuscitated out-of-hospital cardiac arrest victims with coronary artery disease. Am J Cardiol 1990 (May 15);65:1192–1197.

59. Poole JE, Mathisen TL, Kudenchuk PJ, McAnulty JH, Swerdlow CD, Bardy GH, Greene HL. Long-term outcome in patients who survive out of hospital ventricular fibrillation and undergo electrophysiologic studies: Evaluation by electrophysiologic subgroups. J Am Coll Cardiol 1990 (September);16:657–65.

60. Weaver WD, Fahrenbruch CE, Johnson DD, Hallstrom AP, Cobb LA, Copass MK: Effect of Epinephrine and Lidocaine Therapy on Outcome After Cardiac Arrest Due to Ventricular Fibrillation: Circulation 1990 (December);82:2027–2034.

61. Sager PT, Choudhar R, Leon C, Rahimtoola SH, Bhandari AK: The long-term prognosis of patients with out-of-hospital cardiac arrest but no inducible ventricular tachycardia. Am Heart J 1990 (December);120:1334–1342.

62. Paradis NA, Martin GB, Rivers EP, Goetting MG, Appleton TJ, Feingold M, Nowak RM: Coronary perfusion pressure and the return of spontaneous circulation in human cardiopulmonary resuscitation. JAMA 1990 (Feb 23);263:1106–1113.

63. Longstreth WT Jr, Cobb LA, Fahrenbruch CE, Copass MK: Does age affect outcomes of out-of-hospital cardiopulmonary resuscitation? JAMA 1990 (Oct 24);264:2109–2110.

64. Gillum RF: Geographic variation in sudden coronary death. Am Heart J 1990 (February);119:380–389.

65. Tresch DD, Thakur RK, Hoffman RG, Aufderheide TP, Brooks HL: Comparison of outcome of paramedic-witnessed cardiac arrest in patients younger and older than 70 years. Am J Cardiol 1990 (Feb 15);65:453–457.

66. Dolack GL, Callahan DB, Bardy GH, Greene HL: Signal-averaged electrocardiographic late potentials in resuscitated survivors of out-of-hospital ventricular fibrillation. Am J Cardiol 1990 (May 1);65:1102–1104.

67. Corrado D, Thiene G, Nava A, Rossi L, Pennelli N: Sudden death in young competitive athletes: Clinicopathologic correlations in 22 cases. Am J Med 1990 (Nov);89:588–596.

68. Antecol DH, Roberts WC: Sudden death behind the wheel from natural disease in drivers of four-wheeled motorized vehicles. Am J Cardiol 1990 (Dec 1);66:1329–1335.

69. Kelly P, Ruskin JN, Vlahakes GJ, Buckley MJ, Freeman CS, Garan H. Surgical coronary revascularization in survivors of prehospital cardiac arrest: Its effect on inducible ventricular arrhythmias and long-term survival. J Am Coll Cardiol 1990 (February);15:267–73.

70. Santini M, Alexidou G, Ansalone G, Cacciatore G, Cini R, Turitto G: Relation of prognosis in sick sinus syndrome to age, conduction defects and modes of permanent cardiac pacing. Am J Cardiol 1990 (Mar 15);65:729–735.

71. Weintraub RG, Gow RM, Wilkinson JL: The Congenital Long QT Syndromes in Childhood. J Am Coll Cardiol 1990 (September);16:674–80.

72. Manolis AS, Linzer M, Salem D, Estes NAM III: Syncope: Current diagnostic evaluation and management. An Intern Med 1990 (June 1);112:850–863.
73. Bass EB, Curtiss EI, Arena VC, Hanusa BH, Cecchetti A, Karpf M, Kapoor WN: The duration of Holter monitoring in patients with syncope: Is 24 hours enough? Arch Intern Med 1990 (May);150:1073–1078.
74. Kapoor WN: Evaluation and outcome of patients with syncope. Medicine 1990 69:160–175.
75. Bedotto JB, Grayburn PA, Black WH, Raya TE, McBride W, Hsia HH, Eichhorn EJ. Alterations in left ventricular relaxation during atrioventricular pacing in humans. J Am Coll Cardiol 1990 (March);15:658–64.
76. Morgan JM, Joseph SP, Bahri AK, Ramdial J, Crowther A: Choosing the pacemaker; a rational approach to the use of modern pacemaker technology. Eur Heart J 1990 (Aug);11:753–764.
77. Kupperman M, Luce BR, McGovern B, Podrid PJ, Bigger Jr T, Ruskin JN: An analysis of the cost effectiveness of the implantable defibrillator. Circulation 1990 (Jan);81:91–100.
78. Avitall B, Port S, Gal R, McKinnie J, Tchou P, Jazayeri M, Troup P, Akhtar M: Automatic Implantable Cardioverter/Defibrillator Discharges and Acute Myocardial Injury. Circulation 1990 (May);81:1482–1487.
79. Fogoros RN, Elson JJ, Bonnet CA, Fiedler SB, Burkholder JA. Efficacy of the automatic implantable cardioverter-defibrillator in prolonging survival in patients with severe underlying cardiac disease. J Am Coll Cardiol 1990 (August);16:381–6.
80. Cummins RO, Chesemore K, White RD, Defibrillator Working Group: Defibrillator failures: Causes of problems and recommendations for improvement. JAMA 1990 (Aug 22/29);264:1019–1025.

Systemic Hypertension

Measuring blood pressure in the elderly

Sykes and associates[1] from Cardiff, UK, compared the interobserver and intraobserver variability of BP measurements in geriatric patients in AF and in sinus rhythm. Fifty elderly patients in sinus rhythm were compared to 50 in AF. Interobserver variability was significantly greater in the patients with AF for both systolic and diastolic BP. Intraobserver variability was significantly greater in the AF group for diastolic BP but the difference was not significant for systolic BP. These differences were not related to the pulse rate, age, or level of BP. Thus, these findings suggest that in the presence of AF physicians' interpretations of Korotkoff sounds are less uniform, a finding which may have important clinical implications.

Self determination of blood pressure

In Tecumseh, Michigan, Mejia and associates[2] from Ann Arbor, Michigan, obtained BP self-determination data in 608 healthy adults (327 men, 281 women; average age 33 ± 4 years) representing a wide range of educational backgrounds. The average (± SD) home BP (average 13 readings >1 week) was 121/75 ± 10/9 for men and 111/70 ± 11/8 mm Hg for women. One hundred thirty-three subjects remeasured their home BP 1 year later and a strong correlation between the 2 readings was obtained. Large-scale BP self-determination is feasible. Based on the BP distribution in Tecumseh, the upper limit of normalcy for home BP is 142/92 mm Hg for men and 131/85 mm Hg for women.

Ambulatory blood pressure monitoring

In a highly select group of patients with stable systemic hypertension, Prisant and Carr[3] from Augusta, Georgia, assessed the strength of association between various BP measurements (24 hour average automated ambulatory BP, 4 hour automated ambulatory morning average BP, multiple office visit average BP, and a single office visit average BP) and various echocardiographic indices of hypertensive cardiac target organ damage (LA diameter, LV end diastolic diameter, posterior LV wall thickness, combined wall thickness, relative wall thickness, LV mass and mass index, and combined wall thickness/LV diastolic diameter ratio). These data demonstrated that a single 24 hour average diastolic BP by automatic noninvasive ambulatory monitoring was a significantly better predictor of echocardiographic posterior wall thickness, combined wall thickness or relative wall thickness than the multiple office or single office average diastolic BP. Also there were highly significant correlations between both 24 hour average systolic and diastolic BP and these echocardiographic parameters (in descending order of correlation coefficient): combined wall thickness, posterior wall thickness, combined wall thickness/LV diastolic diameter, left ventricular mass index, relative wall thickness, and LV mass. LV end diastolic dimension did not linearly correlate with any systolic or diastolic BP measurement. Left atrial dimension demonstrated only a significant association with 24 hour average diastolic BP. Single office average BP did not linearly correlate with any echocardiographic parameter. Multiple office and 4 hour morning average automated ambulatory BP yielded correlation coefficients that were intermediate to the 24 hour and single office average BP. Multiple office average BP correlations with echocardiographic parameters tended to be higher than the morning BP correlations. However, only the correlation coefficients of posterior wall thickness, combined wall thickness, relative wall thickness and the combined wall thickness/LV diastolic diameter ratio were significantly higher between 24 hour average diastolic BP than multiple office average diastolic BP. Therefore, these data indicate the superiority of ambulatory BP monitoring over multiple casual office BP in predicting LV wall thickness and mass.

It has been suggested that ambulatory BP monitoring is superior to casual cuff methods in predicting cardiovascular events, but lack of reference data from a normal population seriously limits this method's clinical applicability. Broadhurst and colleagues[4] from Harrow, UK, performed 24-hour intra-arterial ambulatory BP monitoring in 50 normal volunteers (cuff BP <140/90 mm Hg) whose ages ranged from 18 to 74 years. There were 30 men and 20 women in the study, but there was no significant difference between the sexes with respect to age, cuff BP, or body mass index. A diurnal variation in BP was observed, qualitatively similar to that seen in hypertensive individuals, including a prewaking BP rise. Mean daytime intra-arterial pressures differed little between the sexes (124/74 mm Hg for women and 127/76 mm Hg for men), but was lower at night in women than in men (96/52 vs 102/59 mm Hg, respectively). Based on this group of individuals, the upper limit of normal daytime BP in both men and women is 150/90 mm Hg and the upper limit of mean nighttime BP is 130/80 mm Hg for men and 115/65 mm Hg for women. The lower nighttime pressures in women compared with their male counterparts with similar daytime pressures may explain why women appear to tolerate similar levels of BP better than men.

The National High Blood Pressure Education Program Coordinating Committee[5] reviewed the literature on ambulatory BP monitoring and addressed the current state of ambulatory BP monitoring methods, normal BP profiles, the clinical and research uses of ambulatory BP monitoring, cost considerations, and recommendations for use of ambulatory

BP monitoring in selected circumstances. Current ambulatory BP monitoring devices use either auscultatory or oscillometric methods to determine BP. A rigorous comparison of these methods is needed to determine whether 1 method is more reliable. A nonbiased assessment of all available equipment is necessary. Normative data provided by ambulatory BP monitoring research are needed for populations by age, race, gender, body habitus, and conditions, such as pregnancy. While ambulatory BP monitoring is not cost-effective for all hypertensive patients, it can assist in the evaluation of such problems as target organ complications, syncope, episodic hypertension, and autonomic dysfunction.

Blood pressure measuring artifacts

To determine the relative importance of factors known to cause therapy resistant systemic hypertension and to derive an efficient approach to the evaluation of the problem, Mejia and associates[6] from Ann Arbor, Michigan, studied 15 patients referred for management of refractory hypertension with a seated diastolic BP greater than 95 mm Hg while taking a standard dose of *hydrochlorothiazide*, *propranolol*, and *hydralazine* or its equivalent for at least 4 weeks. Seven patients (Group 1) had normal, resting mean intra-arterial BP (mean pressure <107 mm Hg) and 8 had elevated pressure (Group 2). Patients in Group 1 had minimal or no target organ involvement whereas those in Group 2 had higher minimum vascular resistance by forearm plethysmography and greater ventricular septal wall thickness. Factors contributing to resistant hypertension, particularly in Group 1, were "office hypertension" (clinical systolic BP at least 20 mm Hg higher than home systolic BP), pseudohypertension (cuff diastolic BP at least 15 mm Hg higher than simultaneously determined intra-arterial pressure), and "cuff-inflation hypertension" (intra-arterial diastolic BP rise of at least 15 mm Hg during cuff inflation). The authors recommended home BP monitoring and echocardiography as initial steps in the evaluation of patients with resistant hypertension. Intra-arterial BP measurement is particularly helpful in patients with resistant hypertension who do not have office hypertension yet have normal ventricular septal thickness on echocardiography.

Circadian blood pressure changes

Verdecchia and co-workers[7] in Perugia, Italy, investigated the effects of cicadian BP changes on the echocardiographic parameters of LV hypertrophy in 235 consecutive subjects (137 unselected untreated patients with essential hypertension and 98 healthy normotensive subjects) who underwent 24-hour noninvasive ambulatory BP monitoring and cross-sectional and M-mode echocardiography. In the hypertensive group, LV mass index correlated with nighttime systolic and diastolic BP more closely than with daytime systolic and diastolic or with casual systolic and diastolic BP. Hypertensive patients were divided into 2 groups by presence (group 1) and absence (group 2) of a reduction of both systolic and diastolic BP during the night by an average of >10% of the daytime pressure. Casual BP, ambulatory daytime systolic and diastolic BP, sex, body surface area, duration of hypertension, prevalence of diabetes, quantity of sleep during monitoring, funduscopic changes, and serum creatinine did not differ between the 2 groups. LV mass index, after adjustment for the age, the sex, the height, and the daytime BP differences between the 2 groups was 82 g/m^2 in normotensive group, 83 g/m^2 in the hypertensive patients of group 1 and 98 g/m² in the hypertensive patients of group 2. The other echocardiographic parameters of LV anatomy differed between the groups as did LV mass index. A statistically significant inverse correlation was found between LV mass index and percentage of nocturnal reduction of daytime ambulatory systolic and diastolic BP. These findings suggest that in unselected hypertensive patients, an ambulatory BP decline from day to night is associated with a lower LV muscle mass. In these patients, a nocturnal reduction of systolic and diastolic BP by >10% of daytime values could delay or prevent the development of cardiac LV hypertrophy.

Blacks vs whites

Previous biochemical assessment of sympathetic nervous system activity including plasma catecholamines, plasma renin activity, and plasma dopamine beta-hydroxylase levels has suggested racial differences in the contribution of the sympathetic nervous system to the pathogenesis or maintenance of hypertension. Palmer and co-investigators[8] in San Diego, California, performed physiological and pharmacological studies in white and black subjects with essential hypertension and their age-matched normotensive counterparts to assess autonomic and sympathetic nervous system function. One hundred one men (47 white hypertensive, 17 black hypertensive, 22 white normotensive, and 15 black normotensive subjects) were evaluated for baroreceptor reflex sensitivity to low-pressure (amyl nitrite inhalation) and high pressure (phenylephrine infusion) stimuli; cold pressor test, heart rate and blood pressure responses; and BP response to phentolamine alpha-adrenergic blockade. Hypertensive subjects exhibited an increase in resting heart rate, a decrease in baroreceptor reflex sensitivity, and an exaggerated decline in mean arterial BP in response to phentolamine. These abnormalities were present to a comparable degree in black and white hypertensive subjects. Cold pressor testing revealed greater increases in heart rate in blacks as compared with whites; however, this racial difference was present regardless of BP status, occurring in black normotensive and black hypertensive subjects to comparable degree. Cold pressor test blood pressure increments were similar in the 4 groups. The investigators concluded that both white hypertensive and black hypertensive subjects demonstrate similar abnormalities in autonomic and sympathetic nervous system function including blunting of baroreceptor reflex sensitivity and an increased alpha-adrenergic receptor participation in BP maintenance. The results do not suggest major racial differences in autonomic pathogenetic mechanisms in hypertension.

After exclusion of persons on BP medication or with prevalent cardiovascular disease, Ekelund and colleagues[9] in Chapel Hill, North Carolina studied 83 blacks and 2,548 white men and 113 black and 1,519 white women 20–69 years old from the Lipid Research Clinics population sample who had performed a standardized treadmill exercise test. Resting systolic and diastolic BPs were similar in black and white men, but the diastolic BP was significantly higher in black than in white women (81 vs 77 mm). Body weight was higher in black than in white women, and reported physical activity was higher in black than in white men. The proportion of smokers were somewhat higher in blacks than in whites. During treadmill exercise test with a modified Bruce protocol, mean systolic BP at stage 2 was 174 mm in black men and 166 mm in white men, but the stage 2 BP did not differ between black and white women. Even after adjustments were made for levels of baseline characteristics (age, weight, resting systolic BP, smoking, LDL-cholesterol, physical activity, and alcohol intake), black men responded with a 7-mm higher systolic BP during exercise than white men. Another new finding was a highly significant positive association between stage 2 systolic BP and LDL-cholesterol in men. The findings suggest a higher systemic vascular resistance during exercise in the selected sample of black men, which is consistent with a high incidence of hypertension in black men.

Multiple risk factor intervention trial

The Multiple Risk Factor Intervention Trial or MRFIT in Minneapolis, Minnesota, is a randomized primary prevention trial that tested the effect of a multifactor intervention program on CAD mortality in 12,866 high-risk men aged 35–57 years.[10] Men were randomly assigned to either a special intervention program, which consisted of dietary advice for lowering blood cholesterol levels, counseling aimed at cessation for cigarette smokers, and stepped-care treatment for hypertension for those with elevated BP, or to their usual sources of health care within the community. Among the 12,866 randomized men, 8,012 were hypertensive at baseline. For this subgroup, mortality rates with 10.5 years of follow-up were lower for the special intervention than for the usual care group by 15% for CAD and 11% for all causes. These results reflected more favorable outcomes for special intervention compared with usual care hypertensive men during the 3.8 post-trial years than during the preceding 6–8 years. During the post-trial years, death rates were lower for special intervention than for usual care by 26% for CAD and 23% for all causes. For those with diastolic BP ≥100 mm Hg, this post-trial trend was a continuation of a trend during the trial; therefore, with 10.5 years of follow-up, death rates were markedly lower for special intervention than for usual care by 36% for CAD and 50% for all causes. Similarly, for those without baseline resting electrocardiographic abnormalities, the favorable post-trial outcome for the special intervention group was a continuation of a trend during the trial. In contrast, for those with baseline diastolic BP of 90–99 mm Hg and for those with baseline resting electrocardiographic abnormalities, the variable post-trial mortality findings for the special intervention group were a reversal of unfavorable trends recorded during the trial. Two factors appear to have contributed to this more favorable mortality trend for the special intervention group: 1) a change in the diuretic treatment protocol for special intervention men about 5 years after randomization, which involved replacement of hydrochlorothiazide with chlorthalidone at a daily maximum dose of 50 mg; and 2) a favorable effect of intervention on nonfatal cardiovascular events during the trial years. In addition, delay until the full impact of beneficial effects on mortality end-points from smoking cessation and cholesterol lowering could have contributed. These 10.5-year mortality data support the inference that multifactor intervention program such as that used in the MRFIT has long-term beneficial effects for persons with hypertension.

Relation to stroke and coronary artery disease

MacMahon and associates[11] from multiple medical centers in several countries investigated the associations of diastolic BP with stroke and with CAD in 9 major prospective observational studies: total 420,000 individuals, 843 strokes, and 4,856 CAD events, 6–25 (mean 10) years of follow-up. The combined results demonstrate positive, continuous, and apparently independent associations, with no significant heterogeneity of effect among different studies. Within the range of diastolic BP studied (about 70–110 mm Hg), there was no evidence of any "threshhold" below which lower levels of diastolic BP were not associated with lower risks of stroke and of CAD. Previous analyses have described the uncorrected associations of diastolic BP measured just at "baseline" with subsequent disease rates. But, because of the diluting effects of random fluctuations in diastolic BP, these substantially underestimate the true associations of the usual diastolic BP (i.e., an individual's long-term average diastolic BP) with disease. After correction for this "regression dilution" bias, prolonged differences in usual diastolic BP of 5, 7.5, and 10 mm Hg were respectively associated with at least 34%, 46%, and 56% less stroke and at least 21%, 29%, and 37% less CAD. These associations are about 60% greater than in previous uncorrected analyses. (This regression dilution bias is quite general, so analogous corrections to the relations of cholesterol to CAD or of various other risk factors to CAD or to other diseases would likewise increase their estimated strengths.) The diastolic BP results suggest that most individuals, whether conventionally "hypertensive" or "normotensive," a lower BP should eventually confer a lower risk of vascular disease.

There are 14 unconfounded randomized trials of antihypertensive drugs (chiefly diuretics or beta-blockers): total 37,000 individuals, mean treatment duration 5 years, mean diastolic BP difference 5 mm Hg (Figure 5-1). In prospective observational studies, a long-term difference of 5–6 mm Hg in usual diastolic BP is associated with about 35–40% less stroke and 20–25% less CAD (Figure 5-2). For those dying in the trials, the diastolic BP difference had persisted only 2–3 years, yet an overview showed that vascular mortality was significantly reduced; non-vascular mortality appeared unchanged. Stroke was reduced by 42%, suggesting that virtually all the epidemiologically expected stroke reduction appears rapidly. CAD was reduced by 14%, suggesting that just over half the epidemiologically expected CAD reduction appears rapidly. Although this significant CAD reduction could well be worthwhile, its size remains indefinite for most circumstances (though beta-blockers after AMI are of substantial benefit). At present, a sufficiently high risk of stroke (perhaps because of age, BP, or history of cerebrovascular disease) may be the clearest indication for antihypertensive treatment.[12]

Silent myocardial ischemia

Electrocardiographic evidence of silent ischemia occurs commonly in patients with systemic hypertension, but its relationship to LV hypertrophy, large-vessel CAD, and neurohumoral factors remains unclear. Accordingly, Yurenev and associates[13] from Moscow, USSR, Los Angeles, California, and New York, New York, validated the results of echocardiographic methods used to measure LV mass by comparison with necropsy measurements in 30 patients; and then examined the relations in 46 men with essential hypertension among ST segment depression during ambulatory monitoring, exercise stress and transesophageal pacing (n = 38) to LV mass, catheterization evidence of CAD (n = 25), and neurohumoral factors (plasma catecholamines and platelet aggregability). Echocardiographic measurements of LV mass were closely correlated with necropsy values. During ambulatory monitoring from 1 to 17 episodes ≥1 mm ST depression occurred in 26 of 46 (65%) patients with hyper-

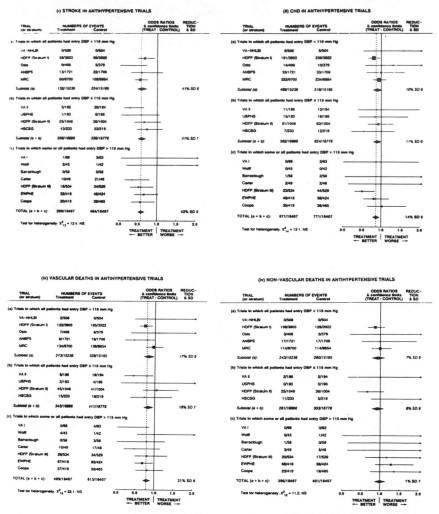

Fig. 5-1. Effects on (i) stroke, (ii) coronary heart disease, (iii) vascular death, and (iv) non-vascular death in the unconfounded randomised trials of antihypertensive drug treatment. Reproduced with permission from Collins, et al.[12]

tension; ischemia was also provoked by exercise or pacing stress in most but not all of these patients (65% and 80%, respectively). Neither ST depression nor the occurrence of additional episodes of symptomatic angina was related to the presence of coronary obstruction at catheterization; patients with and without ST depression did not differ in age, BP, and LV mass. No systemic differences between patients with and without CAD or ST depression were noted in catecholamine levels or platelet aggregability, but the subset in whom ischemia developed at a lower heart rate BP product during pacing stress than during exercise stress had significantly lower norepinephrine levels at rest and during pacing stress. Thus, asymptomatic ST depression occurs commonly during normal activity and induced stress in patients with systemic hypertension but is not consistently related to the presence of large-vessel CAD, LV hypertrophy, or neurohumoral abnormalities.

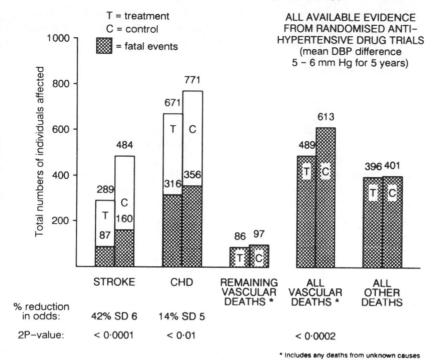

Fig. 5-2. Crudely summated results of the unconfounded randomised trials of antihypertensive drug therapy. All were evenly randomised: total 37,000 individuals, mean DBP at entry 99 mm Hg, mean DBP difference during follow-up 5–6 mm Hg, mean time from entry to vascular event 2–3 yr. Reproduced with permission from Collins, et al.[12]

Relation to job strain

To determine whether job strain (defined as high psychological demands and low decision latitude on the job) is associated with increased workplace diastolic BP and the LV mass index, Schnall and associates[14] from New York, Stoneybrook, and Bronx, New York, conducted a case-controlled study at 7 urban work sites of 215 employed men aged 30 to 60 years without evidence of CAD. After comprehensive BP screening of male employees (N = 2556) at the work site, 87 cases of hypertension and a random sample of 128 controls were studied. In a multiple logistic regression model, job strain was significantly related to hypertension, with an estimated odds ratio of 3.1, after adjusting for age, race, body-mass index, type A behavior, alcohol intake, smoking, work site, 24-hour urine sodium excretion, education, and physical demand level of the job. Controlling for the above variables in subjects aged 30 to 40 years with job strain, the authors found that the echocardiographically determined LV mass index was, on average, 10.8 g/m² greater than in subjects without job strain. The authors concluded that job strain may be a risk factor for both hypertension and structural changes of the heart in working men.

Obesity related

The hypothesis that obesity-related hypertension is relatively innocuous was explored by an examination of cardiovascular events over 34 years of follow-up when related to biennially measured weights and BP measurements using time-dependent covariate proportional hazards analysis in a study performed by Kannel and associates[15] from Boston, Massachusetts, and Bethesda, Maryland. The 5209 participants were also classified by age, cigarette smoking, and antihypertensive treatment at each of 4 baseline examinations with 8-year follow-up periods. Over the period of follow-up, there were 978 cardiovascular events in men and 836 in women. Risk of cardiovascular morbidity and mortality in general and of CAD in particular was as strongly related to hypertension at all levels of body mass index. This was also found to apply when adjustment was made for possible confounding by cigarette smoking. Age and smoking-adjusted absolute risks of cardiovascular events were found to be higher in hypertensive individuals with high than with low body mass indexes. Furthermore, the relative risk of cardiovascular disease did not vary significantly with body mass index. Thus hypertension is at least as dangerous in obese as in lean persons at all ages in either sex, providing no support for the hypothesis that hypertension in the obese is more benign. This is important, since obesity predisposes to hypertension and most who have hypertension are obese. This report examines the hypothesis for cardiovascular disease outcomes considered by previous reports and also the subcategories of cardiovascular disease such as myocardial infarction and stroke, and includes data on both men and women and on young and old.

Relation to fetal and placental size

Barker and associates[16] from South Hampton, UK, studied the effect of intrauterine growth and maternal physique on BP in adult life by following up infants born 50 years previously whose measurements at birth were recorded in detail. The study involved 449 men and women born in-hospital in 1935–1943 and still living in the same city 50 years later. Placental weight, birth weight, weight and BP at age 46–54 years were recorded. In both sexes systolic and diastolic BP were strongly related to placental weight and birth weight. Mean systolic BP rose by 15 mm Hg as placental weight increased from ≤1 lb. (0.45 kg) to >1.5 lb. and fell by 11 mm Hg as birth weight increased from ≤5.5 lb. to >7.5 lb. These relations were independent so that the highest BP occurred in people who had been small babies with large placentas. Higher body mass index and alcohol consumption also were associated with higher BP. These findings show for the first time that the intrauterine environment has an important effect on BP and the presence or absence of systemic hypertension in adults.

Alcohol consumption

Moore and associates[17] from Baltimore, Maryland, examined the relation between alcohol consumption and BP in the 1982 Maryland Hypertension Survey, a cross-sectional population-based household survey of BP control in adults residing in Maryland. In individuals <50 years old, a J-shaped dose-response association was found with abstainers and heavy alcohol consumers having significantly higher BP than moderate alcohol consumers (1 to 2 beverages per day) (Figure 5-3). In individuals 50 years and older, alcohol was associated with higher BP only at the highest levels of intake (>2 beverages per day). The prevalence of hypertension was similarly affected in each age group. This association between alcohol consumption and BP was independent of several vari-

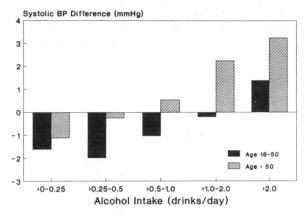

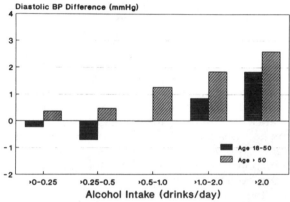

Fig. 5-3. The top half of this figure depicts the difference in mean systolic blood pressure (mm Hg) between successive level of alcohol intake compared to abstention for individuals of age 18 to 50, or age 50 and older. The differences are significant (P <.05) at >2.0 drinks/day in both younger and older age groups and for >0 to .25 drinks/day and >.25 to .5 drinks/day in younger individuals. The bottom half of this figure depicts the difference in mean diastolic blood pressure (mm Hg) between successive level of alcohol intake compared to abstention for individuals of age 18 to 50, or age 50 and older. The differences are significant (P <.05) at >1.0 to 2.0 drinks/day and >2.0 drinks/day in older individuals and for >2.0 drinks/day in younger individuals. Reproduced with permission from Moore, et al.[17]

ables that are associated with increased BP such as age, sex, race, smoking, education, Quetelet index, social participation, and physical activity. The population attributable risk for hypertension due to heavy alcohol consumption is 5 to 7% in those <50 years old and 6 to 8% in those >50 years old. These data suggest that alcohol consumption is a potentially important risk factor for elevations in BP and hypertension.

Witteman and associates[18] from Rotterdam, The Netherlands, and Boston, Massachusetts, studied the relation between alcohol consumption and the risk of development of systemic hypertension among 58,218 US female registered nurses aged 39 to 59 years who were free of diagnosed systemic hypertension and other major diseases. In 1980, all of these women completed an independently validated dietary questionnaire, which included use of alcoholic beverages. During 4 years of follow-up, 3,275 women reported an initial diagnosis of hypertension; validity of the self-report measure was demonstrated in a subsample. When compared to nondrinkers, women drinking 20 to 34 g of alcohol per day (about 2 or 3 drinks) had a significantly elevated relative risk of 1.4. For women consuming ≥35 g/day, the relative risk was 1.9. Adjustment for smoking and dietary variables did not alter these results. Independent significant associations were observed for the consumption of beer, wine and liquor. These prospective data suggest that alcohol intake of up to about 20 g/day does not increase the risk of hypertension among women, but beyond this level, the risk increases progressively.

Exaggerated blood pressure response to exercise

To determine whether normal, nonhypertensive subjects who have unusually large increases of systolic BP with exercise have LV hypertrophy, Gottdiener and associates[19] from Washington, D.C., and Baltimore, Maryland, studied 39 men aged 34 to 71 years (mean 45) including 25 participants in a health fitness screening program and another 14 normal men with atypical chest pain. Twenty-two subjects with a systolic BP during peak exercise of 210 mm Hg or greater were compared with 17 others with systolic BP less than 210 mm Hg during exercise. LV hypertrophy (LV mass index >134 g/m²) was found in 14 of 22 men with a systolic BP of ≥210 mm Hg but in only 1 person with a lower exercise BP. LV mass was linearly related with maximum exercise BP. Whereas LV hypertrophy was mild in about 50%, substantial LVH was present in the others. The presence of LV hypertrophy was not related to superior physical conditioning and was accompanied by increased LA size suggesting impaired LV filling. Thus, even in the absence of systemic hypertension, exaggerated BP responses during exercise testing suggest a possibility of 0.64 of LV hypertrophy, a finding associated with the cardiac "end-organ" manifestations of hypertension.

Left ventricular exercise dysfunction

To elucidate determinants of abnormal LV functional responses to exercise in hypertensive patients, Blake and associates[20] from New York, New York, studied 127 patients with uncomplicated systemic hypertension by rest and exercise radionuclide angiography and by echocardiography at rest. The 24 patients with subnormal LVEF at peak exercise (<54%) were similar in age and rest and exercise BP to the 103 with normal exercise EF, but were more obese and had greater LV mass and internal dimensions. The parallel increase in LV chamber size and mass (eccentric hypertrophy) in the group with exercise dysfunction was associated with higher resting end-systolic wall stress and abnormal increases of end-systolic LV volume from rest to peak exercise. Multivariate analysis revealed that exercise LV dysfunction was independently associated with higher LV mass, end-systolic wall stress, dietary sodium intake, and body mass index.

Target organ changes

The Tecumseh project investigates the evolution of systemic hypertension in a healthy population. Of 946 subjects aged 18–38 years, 124 had clinic BP readings >140/90 mm Hg (the mean for borderline hypertensive subjects was 130/94 mm Hg). Compared with normotensive subjects, borderline hypertensive subjects had higher home BP (mean 12/7 mm Hg higher) as determined by Julius and colleagues[21] from Ann Arbor, Michigan. The childhood and post-pubertal BP were elevated (6/4 mm

Hg higher than normal at age 6 years and 12/7 mm Hg higher than normal at age 21 years), and hypertensive target organ changes were detected. Borderline hypertensive subjects also had elevated minimal forearm resistance (0.22 U higher than normal), decreased stroke index (1.8 mL/m² lower than normal), and impaired ventricular diastolic relaxation (mitral Doppler peak early diastolic blood flow [E] to peak late diastolic blood flow [A] ratio 0.13 lower than normal). Borderline hypertensive subjects had significant abnormalities in other coronary risk factors (cholesterol levels were 0.39 mmol/L higher, triglyceride levels were 0.45 mmol/L higher, HDL levels were 0.08 mmol/L lower, insulin levels were 38 mmol/L higher, and 16.5% more of them were overweight). Borderline hypertension is neither transient nor innocuous.

Captopril test

Renovascular hypertension is potentially curable but of low prevalence. A previous retrospective study has demonstrated the use of a potentiated increase in plasma renin activity after captopril administration as a diagnostic test for renovascular hypertension. This test requires 2 blood samples for plasma renin activity determination and 3 inclusive criteria for a positive test result. Frederickson and associates[22] from Gainesville, Florida, and Atlanta, Georgia, applied this test prospectively to screen 100 hypertensive patients with renovascular hypertension. They evaluated 29 patients with renovascular hypertension; the remainder were diagnosed as having essential hypertension. In the patient population, a postcaptopril plasma renin activity of 5.7 ng of angiotensin/ml/hr (ngA1•mL^{-1}•h^{-1}) or greater had a 100% sensitivity and an 80% specificity for renovascular hypertension. An absolute increase in plasma renin activity with captopril of 4.7 ngA1•mL^{-1}•h^{-1} or greater had a lower sensitivity of 90% and a specificity of 87%, whereas a fractional increase in plasma renin activity after captopril of 150% or higher had the lowest sensitivity of 69% and a specificity of 86%. A subgroup analysis of 38 patients who were receiving diuretic therapy demonstrated that the test sensitivity was unchanged but the specificity was reduced. In conclusion, a single post-captopril plasma renin activity value of 5.7 ngA1•mL^{-1}•h^{-1} or greater is a simplified screening test for renovascular hypertension, with excellent sensitivity and acceptable specificity. This test is well tolerated, inexpensive, and easy to perform.

Patterns of left ventricular hypertrophy

In some patients with systemic hypertension it may be difficult to ascertain whether LV hypertrophy is a secondary end-organ consequence of long-term elevations in BP or a manifestation of a coexistent primary HC. To address this issue and better characterize LV hypertherapy in patients with systemic hypertension, Lewis and Maron[23] from Washington, D.C., and Bethesda, Maryland, used 2-dimensional echocardiography to define the patterns of LV hypertrophy in 102 patients with sustained systemic hypertension and marked degrees of LV wall thickness. Patients ranged in age from 31 to 88 years (mean 61) and were predominantly female (58%); all were black. By selection, each patient had a maximal LV wall thickness of >15 mm (range 16 to 29). Distribution of hypertrophy was judged to be symmetric (i.e., concentric) in most patients (67 of 102, 66%). However, a substantial proportion (35 patients, 34%) demonstrated nonuniform, asymmetric patterns of hypertrophy in which at least 1 segment of the LV wall was at least 1.5 times the thickness of any other. In these 35 patients, the distribution of hypertrophy was similar to that characteristic of the morphologic spectrum of HC, with thickening of portions of both the ventricular septum and free wall in 16 patients, anterior and posterior ventricular septum alone in 11 patients and segmental involvement of only the anterior ventricular septum in 8. Patients with asymmetric patterns of wall thickening did not differ from the patients with symmetric hypertrophy with regard to age, sex or clinical findings. Asymmetric LV hypertrophy appears to represent an important feature of the morphologic spectrum of severe hypertensive heart disease. Moreover, the diverse patterns of hypertrophy observed in hypertensive patients with marked LV wall thickening often cannot be distinguished definitively, on a morphologic basis alone, from those characteristic of HC.

Risk of left ventricular hypertrophy

LV hypertrophy has been repeatedly shown to be associated with a marked increase in mortality risk. Available data, however, do not provide evidence that the risk associated with the increase in cardiac muscle mass is independent of the severity of preexistent CAD. In a cohort of predominantly black patients with a high prevalence of systemic hypertension and LV hypertrophy, Cooper and associates[24] from Chicago, Illinois, estimated LV mass by echocardiography and found it to be a powerful prognostic factor independent of EF and CAD. After excluding patients with either a dilated LV cavity (diastolic internal diameter >5.8 cm) or asymmetric septal hypertrophy (septal: posterior wall ratio >1.5) LV mass/height remained significantly increased in decedents compared to survivors (116 ± 38 vs 131 ± 47 g/m), while the thickness of the ventricular septum and the posterior wall were even more highly predictive of a fatal outcome. After exclusion of patients with eccentric LV hypertrophy, differences in LV muscle mass in survivors and decedents were due entirely to increased thickness of the ventricular wall, and no differences in cavity dimensions of LVEF were noted. Stepwise regression analysis was used to demonstrate that measures of LV hypertrophy were the most important predictors of survival and eliminated the contribution of all other prognostic factors to the model except the number of stenotic vessels. The relative risk associated with a 100-g increase in mass was 2.1 while a 0.1-cm increase in posterior wall thickness was associated with approximately a 7-fold increase in the risk of dying. These findings suggest that hypertension is an important risk factor for cardiac death over and above its effect on accelerating the development of coronary atherosclerosis and that echocardiographically derived measures of LV hypertrophy can add significant discriminatory information over angiographic data.

Ventricular arrhythmias

Siegel and associates[25] from San Francisco, California, reported echocardiographic predictors of ventricular arrhythmias for the Hypertension Arrhythmia Reduction Trial. Men with mild hypertension were withdrawn from their diuretic therapy and repleted with 40 mEq/day of oral potassium and 20 mEq/day of oral magnesium for 1 month. M-mode echocardiography was performed on 123 men, mean age 62 years. Forty-eight men (39%) had echocardiographic evidence of LV hypertrophy defined as an LV mass index >134 g/m^2 and this finding was not related to the presence of LV hypertrophy on electrocardiogram or to age. Men who had echocardiographic LV hypertrophy were more likely than men without echocardiographic LV hypertrophy to have ≥30 VPCs/hr and the combination of frequent (≥30 VPCs/hr) or complex (ventricular couplets, multiform extrasystoles or episodes or VT) ventricular arrhythmia. Similar associations between echocardiographic LV hypertrophy and ventricular arrhythmias were observed on 24-hour tracings obtained on entry to the study (before electrolyte repletion) in the 96 men who were taking diuretics at this time. The combination of a frequent or complex arrhythmia was also more common in men aged 60 to 70 compared to men aged 35 to 59. These findings suggest that ventricular arrhythmias occur more commonly in older hypertensive men and in hypertensive men with echocardiographic LV hypertrophy.

Ventricular arrhythmias occur with increased frequency in patients with systemic hypertension with LV hypertrophy. The relations, however, between ventricular arrhythmias and coexistent CAD, LV dysfunction, and LV fibrosis have not been examined in patients with systemic hypertension and LV hypertrophy. McLenachan and Dargie[26] of Glasgow, UK, performed coronary arteriography on 15 hypertensive patients with LV hypertrophy and nonsustained VT (≥3 consecutive ventricular complexes) of whom 9 were free of coronary ventricular narrowings >50% in diameter. To identify other possible correlates of LV arrhythmias, 28 patients with LV hypertrophy, comprising 17 with VT and 11 without ventricular arrhythmias, underwent quantitative assessment of LV function (angiographic EF), LV mass by echocardiography, and LV fibrosis by endomyocardial biopsy. EF was not significantly different between the 2 groups (15 ± 8% vs 62 ± 2%). LV mass was significantly greater (442 ± 28 g vs 339 ± 34 g), and percentage fibrosis significantly higher (19 ± 4% vs 3 ± 1%) in those patients with VT. Thus, ventricular arrhythmias in hypertensive patients with LV hypertrophy cannot be entirely attributed to coexistent CAD nor to LV dysfunction but are related to the degree of LV hypertrophy and subendocardial fibrosis.

Diastolic filling abnormalities

Hypertension and aging are both associated with changes of LV diastolic filling and increased LV mass. To determine whether diastolic filling abnormalities are present in hypertension independent of aging and significant hypertrophy, Szlachcic and associates[27] from San Francisco, California, studied 19 hypertensive patients following a period of 4 weeks when they were not receiving therapy and 18 normotensive subjects matched for sex, age, and LV mass. All subjects had normal systolic function and EF as assessed by radionuclide angiography. Measured were peak velocity of early filling, late filling, and their ratio by Doppler echocardiography. Filling indices were abnormal in hypertensive patients, but none of the filling indices were significantly correlated with LV mass. Early filling was inversely related to age and diastolic BP in normotensive individuals, but these correlations were not significant in hypertensive patients. Early filling was not significantly correlated to LV mass or wall thickness. In contrast, late filling was influenced by septal wall thickness and BP in both groups. The early to late filling ratio correlated inversely with age in both normal individuals and hypertensive patients. These findings indicate that diastolic filling abnormalities in hypertension are not solely caused by either LV hypertrophy or by aging and therefore must be in part related to the hemodynamic load or altered myocardial or chamber properties.

Predicting salt sensitivity

The overall prevalence of salt sensitivity was studied by Dimsdale and associates[28] from San Diego, California, in 75 men stratified by diagnosis (hypertensive vs normotensive) and race (black vs white). All were studied in a crossover design employing a 200 mEq and 10 mEq Na/day. High salt led to a decrease in diastolic pressure for all groups. For systolic pressure, there was no salt effect on BP across the whole group; however amongst the hypertensives, particularly the black hypertensives, high salt led to increases in systolic pressure. Obese patients were more likely to increase their systolic pressure in response to salt loading. The patients whose pressure increased on high salt were those who manifested less of a decrease in plasma levels of norepinephrine and renin in response to salt loading. Systolic salt sensitivity was predicted with high statistical power by a multiple regression equation employing: race; diagnosis; the change in renin and norepinephrine levels with diet; and the change in BP sensitivity to infused norepinephrine across the 2 diets. In view of the findings of increased norepinephrine, renin and diastolic pressure on low salt and in view of the particular physiological and epidemiological setting associated with systolic salt sensitivity, one wonders about the advisability of across-the-board recommendations of low salt diets for all hypertensive patients.

Abnormal endothelium-dependent vascular relaxation

Endothelium regulates vascular tone by influencing the contractile activity of vascular smooth muscle. This regulatory effect of the endothelium on blood vessels has been shown to be impaired in atherosclerotic arteries in humans and in non-human animals with hypertension. To determine whether patients with essential hypertension have an endothelium-dependent abnormality in vascular relaxation, Panza and associates[29] from Bethesda, Maryland, studied the response of the forearm vasculature to acetylcholine (an endothelium-dependent vasodilator) and sodium nitroprusside (a direct dilator of smooth muscle) in 18 hypertensive patients (mean age 51 ± 10 years; 10 men and 8 women) 2 weeks after the withdrawal of antihypertensive medicines and in 18 normal controls (mean age 50 ± 9 years; 9 men and 9 women). The drugs were infused at increasing concentrations into the brachial artery, and the response in forearm blood flow was measured by strain-gauge plethysmography. The basal forearm blood flow was similar in the patients and controls (mean ± SD, 3.4 ± 1.3 and 3.7 ± 0.8 ml per minute per 100 ml of forearm tissue, respectively). The responses of blood flow and vascular resistance to acetylcholine were significantly reduced in the hypertensive patients; maximal forearm flow was 9 ± 5 ml per minute per 100 ml in the patients and 20 ± 8 ml per minute per 100 ml in the controls. There were no significant differences between groups in the responses of blood flow and vascular resistance to sodium nitroprusside. Because the vasodilator effect of acetylcholine might also be due to presynaptic inhibition of the release of norepinephrine by adrenergic nerve terminals, the effect of acetylcholine was assessed during phentolamine-induced a-adrenergic blockade. Under these conditions, it was also evident that the responses to acetylcholine were significantly blunted in the hypertensive patients. Endothelium-mediated vasodilation is impaired in patients with essential hypertension. This defect may play an important part in the functional abnormalities of resistance vessels that are observed in hypertensive patients.

TREATMENT

Weight reduction

Schotte and Stunkard[30] from Houston, Texas, and Philadelphia, Pennsylvania, assessed the effects of weight reduction on BP in 301 persons ≥20% above their ideal body weights by the 1959 Metropolitan Life Insurance standards. Weight reduction was achieved by behavior modification, medication, or their combination and was associated with significant reductions in systolic and diastolic BP. The weight reduction method was less important than the amount of weight lost in determining reductions in BP. The greatest reductions in weight and BP occurred during the first half of weight loss, suggesting that even brief treatment (i.e., 8 to 10 weeks) may benefit obese, hypertensive patients (Figure 5-4). Despite repeated measurements, 36 patients who failed to lose weight showed no decrease in BP. Although BP rose during follow-up in patients who regained weight, it remained below baseline levels. These findings provide further support for weight reduction in the control of hypertension.

Diet of decreased calories ± decreased sodium ± increased potassium

The Hypertension Prevention Trial Research Group, directed by Albert Oberman from Birmingham, Alabama,[31] randomly assigned 841 healthy men and women aged 25 to 49 years with diastolic BP of 78–89 mm Hg to a controlled treatment group (no dietary counseling) or to one of four dietary counseling treatment groups (reduced calories, reduced sodium, reduced sodium and calories, or reduced sodium and increased potassium). Participants were followed for a 3-year period to assess the effect of dietary changes on BP. After 6 months, counseling had resulted in a net (of control) mean overnight urinary sodium reduction of 13%, a potassium increase of 8%, and a decrease in mean body weight of 7%. At 3 years, the sodium and weight reductions were 10% and 4%, respectively; the potassium change was nil. All 4 dietary counseling treatment groups had lower mean BP than the control group. The largest net reduction in BP occurred in the calorie group: diastolic BP was 2.8 mm Hg and 1.8 mm Hg and systolic BP, 5.1 mm Hg and 2.4 mm Hg at 6 months and 3 years, respectively. All 4 dietary counseling treatment groups experienced fewer hypertensive events; significantly fewer occurred in the sodium groups. The beneficial effects on BP achieved in this trial have implications for the prevention of cardiovascular disease through dietary reduction of calories and sodium.

Eicosapentaenoic and docosahexaenoic acids

Studies of whether polyunsaturated fatty acids in fish oil—in particular, eicosapentaenoic and docosahexaenoic acids—lower BP have varied in design and results. Bonaa and associates[32] from Tromso, Norway,

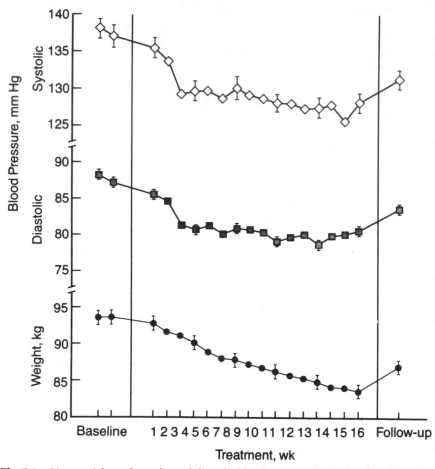

Fig. 5-4. Mean weight and systolic and diastolic blood pressure during baseline (2 weeks), treatment (16 weeks), and follow-up in 265 weight losers. Reproduced with permission from Shotte, et al.[30]

conducted a population based, randomized, 10-week dietary supplementation trial in which the effects of 6 grams/day of 85% eicosapentaenoic and docosahexaenoic acids were compared with those of 6 grams/day of corn oil in 156 men and women with previously untreated, stable, mild essential hypertension. The mean systolic BP fell by 4.6 mm Hg, and diastolic BP by 3.0 mm Hg in the group receiving fish oil; there was no significant change in the group receiving corn oil. The differences between the groups remained significant for both systolic (6.4 mm Hg) and diastolic (2.8 mm Hg) pressure after control for anthropometric, lifestyle, and dietary variables. The decreases in BP were larger as concentrations of plasma phospholipid n-3 fatty acids increased. Dietary supplementation with fish oil did not change mean BP in the subjects who ate fish 3 or more times a week as part of their usual diet, or in those who had a base-line concentration of plasma phospholipid n-3 fatty acids above 175.1 mg per liter. The authors concluded that eicosapentaenoic and docosahexaenoic acids reduces BP in essential hypertension, depending on increases in plasma phospholipid n-3 fatty acids.

Aerobic exercise

To determine the antihypertensive efficacy of aerobic exercise training in mild essential hypertension, Martin and co-workers[33] in San Diego, California, conducted a prospective randomized controlled trial comparing an aerobic exercise regimen to a placebo exercise regimen, with a crossover replication of the aerobic regimen in the placebo exercise group. Twenty-seven men with untreated diastolic BP of 90–104 mm were randomized to 2 exercise regimens. Ten patients completed the aerobic regimen. Nine patients completed the control regimen, 7 of whom subsequently entered and completed the aerobic regimen. The aerobic regimen consisted of walking, jogging, stationary bicycling, or any combination of these activities for 30 minutes, 4 times a week, at 65–80% maximal heart rate. The control regimen consisted of slow calisthenics and stretching for the same duration and frequency but maintaining <60% maximal heart rate. The diastolic BP decreased 10 mm in the aerobic exercise group but increased 0.8 mm in the placebo control exercise group. Systolic BP decreased 6 mm in the aerobic group and increased 0.9 mm in the control group. Subsequently, 7 of the 9 controls entered a treatment crossover and completed the aerobic regimen with significant reductions in both diastolic and systolic BP. BP changes were not associated with any significant changes in weight, body fat, urinary electrolytes, or resting heart rate. This randomized controlled trial provides evidence for the independent BP lowering effect of aerobic exercise in unmedicated mildly hypertensive men.

In diabetes mellitus

Hypertension occurs with twice the frequency in the diabetic population compared with the general nondiabetic population. Christlieb[34] from Boston, Massachusetts, reviewed various therapeutic options for treatment of systemic hypertension in diabetics with an eye on the effect of diabetes on the treatment itself and the potential for adverse effects from selective antihypertensive agents in the diabetic patients (Table 5-1, Figure 5-5). A rational approach to antihypertensive therapy in diabetics with or without concurrent diabetic complications incorporates a "stepped" approach to therapy that includes alternative step 1 agents (e.g., angiotensinconverting enzyme inhibitors and calcium channel blockers) rather than traditional agents (e.g., diuretics and β-blockers). Evolving evidence with angiotensin-converting enzyme inhibitors reveals that they do not exacerbate complications of diabetes mellitus and also may arrest or slow the progression of diabetic nephropathy. Treatment algorithms for a stepped approach to the management of the hypertensive diabetic patient are proposed.

Daily dose frequency of patient compliance

Eisen and associates[35] from St. Louis, Missouri, determined the relation between described daily dose frequency and patient medication compliance. The medication compliance of 105 patients receiving antihypertensive medications was monitored by analyzing data obtained from special pill containers that electronically record the date and time of medication removal, inaccurate compliance estimates derived using the simple pill count method were thereby avoided. Compliance was defined

TABLE 5-1. *Possible adverse and beneficial effects of antihypertensive drugs used in patients with diabetes mellitus.* Reproduced with permission from Christlieb, et al.*[34]

Drug Class	Possible Adverse Effects and Precautions	Possible Benefits
Adrenergic antagonists		
Cardioselective β-blockers	Obscure hypoglycemic symptoms; impotence, hypertriglyceridemia, ↓ HDL cholesterol, heart failure, renal excretion (except metoprolol), same as noncardioselective in high doses	Effective in coronary heart disease
Noncardioselective β-blockers	Same as cardioselective, plus delayed recovery from hypoglycemia, deterioration of glucose control (NIDDM), hyperosmolar coma, hypertension if hypoglycemic, aggravated peripheral vascular disease, ↑ potassium (hypoaldosteronism)	Effective in coronary heart disease
Combined α- and β-blockers	Same as noncardioselective blockers	...
Peripheral adrenergic inhibitors	Orthostatic hypotension, impotence, sodium retention	...
Central adrenergic inhibitors	Same as peripheral inhibitors	...
α₁-Adrenergic inhibitors	Orthostatic hypotension, sodium retention	Rarely cause impotence, no adverse effects on glucose or lipids
Angiotensin converting enzyme inhibitors	Severe hyperkalemia (hypoaldosteronism); further compromise of renal function in renal failure	Rarely cause impotence, no effect on glucose or lipids, minimize adverse metabolic effects of diuretics, rarely cause orthostatic hypotension, ↓ albuminuria, may ↓ rate of renal deterioration
Calcium channel blockers	Orthostatic hypotension (occasionally), glucose intolerance (?)	Rarely cause impotence, no adverse effects on lipids
Direct vasodilators	Aggravate coronary disease, sodium retention	Rarely cause orthostatic hypertension, rarely cause impotence, no effect on glucose or lipids
Diuretics		
Thiazide	↑ glucose (NIDDM), impotence, orthostatic hypotension, hypercholesterolemia, ineffective in renal failure, may accelerate renal failure	Minimize sodium retention when used with sodium-retaining drugs
Loop	Same as thiazides (except regarding renal failure)	Effective in renal failure, impotence unusual
Potassium-sparing	Severe hyperkalemia (renal failure and hypoaldosteronism), impotence	...

*HDL indicates high-density lipoprotein; NIDDM, non-insulin-dependent diabetes mellitus.

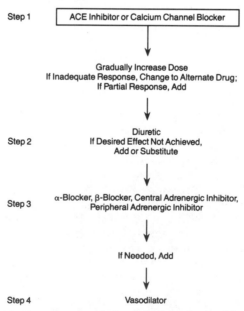

Step 1 — ACE Inhibitor or Calcium Channel Blocker

Gradually Increase Dose
If Inadequate Response, Change to Alternate Drug;
If Partial Response, Add

Step 2 — Diuretic
If Desired Effect Not Achieved,
Add or Substitute

Step 3 — α-Blocker, β-Blocker, Central Adrenergic Inhibitor,
Peripheral Adrenergic Inhibitor

If Needed, Add

Step 4 — Vasodilator

Fig. 5-5. Proposed treatment approach for diabetic patients with essential or isolated systolic hypertension. ACE indicates angiotensin converting enzyme. Reproduced with permission from Christlieb, et al.[34]

as the percent of days during which the prescribed number of doses were removed. Compliance improved from 59% on a 3-time daily regimen to 84% on a once-daily regimen. Thus, compliance improves dramatically as prescribed dose frequency decreases. Probably the single most important action that health care providers can take to improve compliance is to select medications that permit the lowest daily prescribed dose frequency.

Thiazide therapy and hip fracture

Thiazide diuretic agents lower the urinary excretion of calcium. Their use has been associated with increased bone density, but their role in preventing hip fracture has not been established. LaCroix and associates[36] from multiple medical centers prospectively studied the effect of thiazide diuretic agents on the incidence of hip fracture among 9518 men and women 65 years of age or older residing in 3 communities. At base line, 24 to 20% of the subjects were thiazide users. In the subsequent 4 years, 242 subjects had hip fractures. The incidence rates of hip fracture were lower among thiazide users than nonusers in each community; the Mantel-Haenszel relative risk of hip fracture, adjusted for community and age, was 0.63. The protective effect of the use of thiazides was independent of sex, age, impaired mobility, body-mass index, and current and former smoking status; the multivariate adjusted relative risk of hip fracture was 0.68. Furthermore, the protective effect was specific to thiazide diuretic agents, since there was no association between the use of antihypertensive medications other than thiazides and the risk of hip fracture. These prospective data suggest that in older men and women the use of thiazide diuretic agents is associated with a reduction of approximately one third in the risk of hip fracture.

Of hypertensive crisis

A review article on the treatment of hypertensive crisis appeared in the October 25, 1990, issue of the New England Journal of Medicine[37] (Tables 5-2, 5-3, and 5-4).

TABLE 5-2. *Types of hypertensive emergency and treatment recommendations. Reproduced with permission from Calhoun, et al.*[37]

Type of Hypertensive Emergency	Recommended Treatment	Drugs to Avoid
Hypertensive encephalopathy	Sodium nitroprusside, labetalol, diazoxide	β-Antagonists, methyldopa, clonidine
Cerebral infarction	No treatment, sodium nitroprusside, labetalol	β-Antagonists, methyldopa, clonidine
Intracerebral hemorrhage, subarachnoid hemorrhage	No treatment, sodium nitroprusside, labetalol	β-Antagonists, methyldopa, clonidine
Myocardial ischemia, myocardial infarction	Nitroglycerin, labetalol, calcium antagonists, sodium nitroprusside	Hydralazine, diazoxide, minoxidil
Acute pulmonary edema	Sodium nitroprusside and loop diuretic, nitroglycerin and loop diuretic	Hydralazine, diazoxide, β-antagonists, labetalol
Aortic dissection	Sodium nitroprusside and β-antagonist, trimethaphan and β-antagonist, labetalol	Hydralazine, diazoxide, minoxidil
Eclampsia	Hydralazine, diazoxide, labetalol, calcium antagonists, sodium nitroprusside*	Trimethaphan, diuretics, β-antagonists
Acute renal insufficiency	Sodium nitroprusside, labetalol, calcium antagonists	β-Antagonists, trimethaphan
Grade III or grade IV Keith–Wagener funduscopic changes†	Sodium nitroprusside, labetalol, calcium antagonists	β-Antagonists, clonidine, methyldopa
Microangiopathic hemolytic anemia	Sodium nitroprusside, labetalol, calcium antagonists	β-Antagonists

*Because of the potential risk to the fetus, reserve for patients with eclampsia that is refractory to treatment with other agents.

†Grade III changes include exudates and hemorrhage, and grade IV changes papilledema.

TABLE 5-3. *Parenteral medications used in the treatment of hypertensive emergencies. Reproduced with permission from Calhoun, et al.*[37]

Drug	Administration*	Onset	Duration of Action	Dosage	Adverse Effects and Comments
Sodium nitroprusside	IV infusion	Immediate	2–3 min	0.5–10 μg/kg/min (initial dose, 0.25 μg/kg/min for eclampsia and renal insufficiency)	Hypotension, nausea, vomiting, apprehension. Risk of thiocyanate and cyanide toxicity is increased in renal and hepatic insufficiency, respectively; levels should be monitored. Must shield from light.
Diazoxide	IV bolus	1–5 min	6–12 hr	50–100 mg every 5–10 min, up to 600 mg	Hypotension, tachycardia, nausea, vomiting, fluid retention, hyperglycemia. May exacerbate myocardial ischemia, heart failure, or aortic dissection. May require concomitant use of a β-antagonist.
	IV infusion			10–30 mg/min	
Labetalol	IV bolus	5–10 min	3–6 hr	20–80 mg every 5–10 min, up to 300 mg	Hypotension, heart block, heart failure, bronchospasm, nausea, vomiting, scalp tingling, paradoxical pressor response. May not be effective in patients receiving α- or β-antagonists.
	IV infusion			0.5–2 mg/min	
Nitroglycerin	IV infusion	1–2 min	3–5 min	5–100 μg/min	Headache, nausea, vomiting. Tolerance may develop with prolonged use.
Phentolamine	IV bolus	1–2 min	3–10 min	5–10 mg every 5–15 min	Hypotension, tachycardia, headache, angina, paradoxical pressor response.
Trimethaphan	IV infusion	1–5 min	10 min	0.5–5 mg/min	Hypotension, urinary retention, ileus, respiratory arrest, mydriasis, cycloplegia, dry mouth. More effective if patient's head is elevated.
Hydralazine (for treatment of eclampsia)	IV bolus	10–20 min	3–6 hr	5–10 mg every 20 min (if no effect after 20 mg, try another agent)	Hypotension, fetal distress, tachycardia, headache, nausea, vomiting, local thrombophlebitis; infusion site should be changed after 12 hr.
Nicardipine†	IV infusion	1–5 min	3–6 hr	5 mg/hr, increased by 1–2.5 mg/hr every 15 min, up to 15 mg/hr	Hypotension, headache, tachycardia, nausea, vomiting.

*IV denotes intravenous.

†Not yet approved by the Food and Drug Administration for this use.

TABLE 5-4. *Oral medications used in the treatment of urgent hypertensive crisis. Reproduced with permission from Calhoun, et al.*[37]

Drug	Administration	Onset	Duration of Action	Dosage*	Adverse Effects and Comments
Nifedipine	Sublingual	5–10 min	3–6 hr	10–20 mg (sublingual and buccal'doses can be repeated at intervals of 5–15 min)	Headache, tachycardia, hypotension, flushing, dizziness.
	Buccal	5–10 min			
	Oral	15–20 min			
Clonidine	Oral	30–60 min	8–12 hr	0.1–0.2 mg, then 0.05–0.1 mg every hour, up to 0.7 mg	Sedation, dry mouth. Should be avoided in patients with second-degree or third-degree heart block, bradycardia, or sick sinus syndrome. Overdose should be treated with tolazoline.

*The initial dose of either agent should be lower (nifedipine, 10 mg; clonidine, 0.05 mg) in elderly patients, patients who have recently been treated with other antihypertensive agents, patients with a history of cerebrovascular or coronary disease, and patients with volume depletion.

Costs of antihypertensive therapy

To evaluate the comparative efficacy and cost-effectiveness of various anti-hypertensive medicines in persons aged 35–64 years with diastolic BP of ≥95 mm Hg and no known CAD, Edelson and associates[38] from Boston, Massachusetts, used the Coronary Heart Disease Policy Model, which is a computer simulation of overall mortality as well as the mortality, morbidity, and cost of CAD in the U.S. population. From the pooled publications, the authors estimated the anti-hypertensive and total cholesterol effects of various anti-hypertensive regimens. For 20 years of simulated therapy from 1990 through 2010, the cost per year of life saved was projected to be $10,900 for *propranolol* hydrochloride; $16,400 for *hydrochlorothiazide;* $31,600 for *nifedipine;* $61,900 for *prazosin* hydrochloride; and $72,100 for *captopril.* Doubling the cholesterol effects of the agents under study did not significantly change their effectiveness because, in general, lowering diastolic BP by 1 mm Hg was equivalent to lowering the cholesterol level by 6%. Although any projection requires multiple estimates, each of which may be open to debate, propranolol appears to be the preferred initial option under most of a variety of alternative assumptions.

Hydrochlorothiazide

Kochar and associates[39] from Milwaukee, Wisconsin, studied the effects of reduction in dose of hydrochlorothiazide from 50 to 25 mg/d, and its discontinuation for up to 22 months in 36 well-controlled patients with systemic hypertension. Hydrochlorothiazide was discontinued if the diastolic BP remained less than or equal to 94 mm Hg after a 6-month period on the lower dose of hydrochlorothiazide. No other changes were made in medications or diet. Sitting systolic BP rose from 135 ± 15 mm Hg to 140 ± 14 mm Hg on reduction of the hydrochlorothiazide dose and rose still further to 145 ± 20 mm Hg on discontinuation. Even greater increases in standing BP were observed. There were no significant effects on the diastolic BP with reduction of dose or discontinuation of hydrochlorothiazide. A significant decrease in the serum uric acid and a rise in serum potassium occurred. There were no changes in serum glucose or lipids on reduction in the dose of hydrochlorothiazide; whereas, with discontinuation, the serum lipids and hemoglobin A,C fell significantly. These results suggest that the benefits of a reduced dose of hydrochlorothiazide may not be as great as considered heretofore.

Effects on blood lipids of withdrawing hydrochlorothiazide or atenolol

Middeke and associates[40] from Munich, Federal Republic of Germany, assessed BP and serum lipoprotein concentrations in 40 men with essential hypertension at the end of a long-term, controlled intervention study (HAPPHY) after 5.2 ± 1.4 years of treatment with *hydrochlorothiazide* (n = 23) or *atenolol* (n = 17) and after a wash-out period. After withdrawal from antihypertensive medication, the BP of patients treated with diuretics or beta blockers rose from 142/93 and 145/91 to 159/106 and 165/104 mm Hg, respectively. At the same time, LDL cholesterol decreased by 17 and 12 mg/dl, respectively, in the diuretic and beta blocker groups (Table 5-5). In addition, total cholesterol decreased by 16 mg/dl in the diuretic group, whereas HDL cholesterol increased by 8 mg/dl and triglycerides decreased by 27 mg/dl in the beta blocker group at the end of the wash-out period as compared to the final phase of the HAPPHY study. The data indicate the persistence of lipid changes during long-term treatment with hydrochlorothiazide and atenolol. For the first time, it was clearly demonstrated that the well-known unfavorable effects

TABLE 5-5. *Characteristics of hypertensive men during therapy and after a wash-out period. Reproduced with permission from Middeke, et al.*[40]

Characteristics	HAPPHY trial (5.2±1.4 yrs)		Wash-out period (4.6±1.5 wks)	
	Diuretic	Beta blocker	Diuretic	Beta blocker
N	23	17	23	17
Blood pressure, systolic/diastolic (mm Hg)	145/91±16/6	142/93*±14/6	165/104±17/7	159/106*±16/7
Heart rate (beats/min)	79±6	69±5	75±9	74±7‡
Weight (kg)	83.2±9.3	84.9±9.0	83.9±9.0	84.1±8.9
Cholesterol (mg/dl)	247±39	240±52	231±35‡	233±36
LDL chol (mg/dl)	167±35	162±44	150±43‡	150±35‡
HDL chol (mg/dl)	46±17	37±7	45±17	45±11†
Triglycerides (mg/dl)	176±106	196±97	182±106	169±93‡

*p<0.001, †p<0.01, ‡p<0.05 compared to the HAPPHY trial.
Chol=cholesterol, LDL=low density lipoprotein, HDL=high density lipoprotein.
The diuretic used was hydrochlorothiazide; the beta-blocker was atenolol.

of diuretics and beta blockers on lipid metabolism are reversible after cessation of long-term therapy of several years' duration.

Risk of discontinuing beta-blocker therapy on coronary risk

Psaty and associates[41] from Seattle, Washington, conducted a population-based, case-control study of risk factors for the first events of CAD in patients with high BP. All subjects had hypertension treated with medication. The 248 cases presented with new CAD from 1982 through 1984, and the 737 controls were a probability sample of health maintenance organization patients free of CAD. The health maintenance organization's computerized pharmacy database identified recent stoppers—patients who did not fill their prescriptions regularly enough to be at least 80% compliant. After adjustment for potential confounding factors, subjects who had recently stopped using β-blockers had a transient fourfold increase in the relative risk of CAD. The association was specific to β-blockers but not diuretics. A withdrawal syndrome immediately following the cessation of β-blocker use may be an acute precipitant of angina and AMI in hypertensive patients who have no prior history of CAD.

Supplemental potassium chloride

Clinical and epidemiologic studies suggest that the intake of potassium chloride lowers BP. To investigate whether supplemental potassium chloride (96 mmol of microcrystalline potassium chloride a day) reduced the need for antihypertensive medicine in hypertensive men on a restricted-sodium diet, Grimm and associates[42] from Minneapolis, Minnesota, and Miami, Florida, conducted a randomized, placebo-controlled, double-blind clinical trial. A total of 287 men 45 to 68 years of age, 142 given potassium chloride and 145 given placebo, were followed for an average of 2.2 years after the withdrawal of their antihypertensive medication. Men in both groups received instructions on following a low-sodium diet. Overnight urinary sodium excretion fell from 63 mmol/8 hours at base line to an average of 45 mmol/8 hours during follow-up. Participants given supplemental potassium chloride had significantly higher serum potassium levels and urinary potassium excretion (averaging 4.5 mmol/L and 42.5 mmol/8 hours, respectively) during follow-up than participants given placebo (4.2 mmol/L and 20 mmol/8 hours). Seventy-nine participants in each group required reinstitution of antihypertensive medication according to strict indications defined by the protocol. No significant differences in systolic or diastolic BP were observed between the 2 groups. During follow-up, systolic and diastolic BP averaged 131 and 83 mm Hg, respectively, for participants given supplemental potassium, and 133 and 83 mm Hg for participants given placebo. The authors concluded that supplemental potassium chloride does not reduce the need for antihypertensive medication in hypertensive men on a restricted-sodium diet.

Atenolol vs acebutolol

Neutel and associates[43] from Long Beach and Irvine, California, and Birmingham, Alabama, used whole-day automated ambulatory BP monitoring to assess the duration of the antihypertensive actions of the β-blockers atenolol (50 to 100 mg; n = 20) and acebutolol (400 to 800 mg;

n = 19) each given once daily at 9 A.M. When compared with its pre-treatment 24-hour average, atenolol decreased diastolic BP by 10 ± 2 mm Hg and systolic BP by 12 ± 2 mm Hg. Acebutolol decreased the 24-hour diastolic BP by 11 ± 1 mm Hg and systolic BP by 13 ± 2 mm Hg. More specifically, a comparison of the 2 drugs during the final 6 hours (3 A.M. to 9 A.M.) of the dosing interval showed that the mean decrease in diastolic BP of 10 ± 1.5 mm Hg with acebutolol was greater than the decrease of 6.2 ± 1.3 mm Hg with atenolol. Moreover, this final 6-hour effect of atenolol was less than that observed during the first 18 hours of the day. The late effects of acebutolol did not change significantly from its early effects. The 2 agents also differed in their trough (final 2-hour decrease in diastolic BP) and peak (maximum 2-hour decrease in diastolic BP) effects: for atenolol the peak-to-trough difference was 7.8 ± 3.1 mm Hg, whereas for acebutolol it was 3.8 ± 4.2 mm Hg. This study confirms the efficacy of atenolol and acebutolol. Moreover, acebutolol given once daily maintains its antihypertensive effects throughout the entire 24-hour period, including the important early to mid-morning hours.

Atenolol vs captopril vs verapamil

Saunders and associates[44] from multiple medical centers compared in a double-blind, positively controlled, forced dose titration study the efficacy and safety of atenolol, captopril, and verapamil sustained release as single agents in the treatment of black patients with mild to moderate systemic hypertension (diastolic BP, 95 to 114 mm Hg). A total of 394 patients were randomized to 1 of the 3 therapies. Mean BP during a 2- to 4-week placebo treatment period (baseline) ranged from 100 to 101 mm Hg diastolic and 152 to 153 mm Hg systolic for the 3 groups. Of the patients, 355 (of whom 345 had assessable data) completed the first treatment period, which consisted of therapy with either 50 mg/d of atenolol, 25 mg every 12 hours of captopril, or 240 mg/d of verapamil sustained release. During the second 4-week treatment period, which 319 patients completed (307 assessable), half of the patients had their antihypertensive medication increased and the other half continued the same dose. Goal BP was defined as a supine diastolic BP of <90 mm Hg or a 10-mm Hg or greater drop in supine diastolic BP from pretreatment levels. Atenolol, captopril, and verapamil sustained release therapy was associated with goal BP achievement during the first treatment period 55%, 44%, and 65% of the time, respectively, and during the second treatment period 60%, 57%, and 73% of the time. Side effects were minimal and comparable for all 3 drugs.

Croog and associates[45] from multiple medical centers conducted a randomized, double-blind trial among 306 black men and women with mild to moderate hypertension to determine effects of atenolol, captopril, and verapamil sustained release on measures of quality of life. Patients were randomly assigned to a stable or forced-dose titration sequence. After an 8-week treatment period, the rate of withdrawal from treatment because of adverse effects was low and did not differ by drug treatment group or titration level. Patients taking verapamil SR showed a significantly greater reduction in mean BP than patients treated with atenolol or captopril. Along with absence of worsening on any quality of life total scale scores examined over the treatment period, the authors found either improvement or no change in the total scale scores for all 3 treatment groups. Among both male and female patients, comparisons between drug treatment groups showed no differences in degree of change on the total scale scores. In comparisons within each treatment group, improvement in scores of male patients after 8 weeks appeared among those taking atenolol in general well-being and physical symptoms reduction; among male patients taking captopril in general well-being, physical symptoms, and sexual performance; and among male patients receiving verapamil SR in scores in irritability, sleep, and the Digit Span test. Improvement in scores among female patients taking atenolol was found in scores on general well-being, physical symptoms, and sleep; among women taking captopril on general well-being, physical symptoms, and irritability; and among women taking verapamil SR on general well-being. Patients in all treatment groups improved on measures of visuomotor functioning. The research shows that with the 3 newer generation antihypertensive medications studied, BP control was achieved during the treatment period without negative effects on some measures.

LV mass sometimes decreases during treatment of systemic hypertension, but this response is inconsistent and its effects on LV function are unknown. In a 6-month randomized trial, Schulman and associates[46] from Baltimore, Maryland, studied the ability of verapamil and atenolol to reduce LV mass in 42 patients over 60 years of age with systemic hypertension and the effects of this reduction in mass on cardiac function. The mean BP ($\pm$ SE) decreased in both the group that received verapamil (from $171 \pm 3/93 \pm 2$ mm Hg to $143 \pm 3/79 \pm 2$ mm Hg) and the group that received atenolol (from $180 \pm 5/99 \pm 2$ mm Hg to $148 \pm 3/83 \pm 1$ mm Hg), but the atenolol-treated patients more frequently required the addition of chlorthalidone to achieve BP reduction. Verapamil resulted in a reduction in the LV mass index from 104 ± 5 g/m^2 of body-surface area to 85 ± 5 g/m^2. Atenolol did not produce a reduction in the LV mass index (109 ± 9 g/m^2 before treatment vs 112 ± 10 g/m^2 after treatment). Two weeks after the withdrawal of antihypertensive therapy, BP returned to pretreatment values. Nevertheless, in patients whose LV mass had decreased, 2 measures of diastolic filling, the peak diastolic filling rate of the LV and the ratio of the peak filling rate to the peak ejection rate, were significantly higher than before treatment (2.32 ± 0.2 vs 3.32 ± 0.4 and 0.61 ± 0.03 to 0.85 ± 0.05, respectively). Diastolic filling was unchanged in the group that had no reduction in LV mass. Cardiac output and the EF at rest and during mild exercise were unchanged in both groups as compared with baseline values. The authors concluded that LV mass can be reduced in elderly patients with hypertension and mild ventricular hypertrophy who receive antihypertensive therapy. Reduction occurs more frequently with verapamil than with atenolol therapy, increases diastolic filling, and does not impair systolic function.

Labetalol

Giles and associates[47] from New Orleans, Louisiana, Long Beach, California, Rockford, Illinois, and Washington, D.C., evaluated antihypertensive therapy with labetalol in a prospective, randomized, multiple center, double-blind study of 133 patients >60 years of age with isolated systolic hypertension (standing systolic BP $\geq$160 mm Hg; diastolic BP <95 mm Hg). Following a placebo-washout period, patients received either labetalol (n = 70) or placebo (n = 63), which was titrated as necessary from 100 to 400 mg twice a day over a 6-week period. Once the BP was controlled (standing systolic BP <160 mm Hg, and $\geq$10 mm Hg decrease from baseline) or the maximum dosage had been given, patients continued receiving the same regimen until the end of the titration period and throughout a 4-week maintenance period. BP was controlled in 57 (81%) of 70 of the labetalol-treated patients (86% receiving ≤200 mg twice a day) compared with 34 (54%) of 63 of the placebo-treated patients. Throughout the active treatment periods, BP was significantly lower in patients treated with labetalol compared with those taking placebo; mean standing systolic BP decreased 26 mm Hg in the labetalol group vs 9 mm Hg in the placebo group. Side effects were generally mild, and the dropout rates due to adverse experiences were similar between treatment groups (14% in the labetalol group vs 10% in the placebo group). In summary, labetalol can effectively lower systolic BP in the elderly without causing adverse orthostatic changes.

Clark and associates[48] from Rockville, Maryland, and Washington, D.C., reviewed reports of 11 patients (3 fatal) in the U.S.A. in which hepato-cellular damage was associated with labetalol therapy for systemic hypertension. The temporal circumstances strongly implicate labetalol; the conditions of 9 patients improved after cessation of labetalol therapy, and 1 patient had a recurrence after therapy was restarted. Follow-up with each reporting physician failed to provide historic or laboratory evidence for other viral, toxic, or drug-induced causes of hepatocellular damage, and the case series did not show the demographic and historic risk factors that would be expected if non-A, non-B hepatitis were the cause. Reports of microscopic liver examinations were available in the 5 cases in which they were done. The reported histologic changes were consistent with hepatocellular necrosis in 4 instances and chronic active hepatitis in one. The clinical presentation of the cases was most compatible with the mechanism of metabolic idiosyncrasy, but other pathogenetic explanations could not be entirely excluded.

Diltiazem

Lund-Johansen and Omvik[49] from Bergen, Norway, studied the effects of long-term treatment with diltiazem on blood pressure, central hemodynamics and exercise endurance in 16 men (mean age 52 years) with essential hypertension. Intra-arterial pressure and heart rate were monitored continuously. Cardiac output was measured by Cardiogreen at rest (supine and sitting) and during 50 W, 100 W and 150 W bicycle exercise. Hemodynamic measurements were repeated after continuous bicycling at 150 W for 20 min or until exhaustion. After 1 year on diltiazem (mean daily dose 278 mg) intra-arterial pressure was reduced in all situations (at rest sitting from 183/108 mm Hg to 157/92 mm Hg (14%) due to reduction in total peripheral resistance. HR was reduced at rest (7%) and during exercise (10%). Stroke volume tended to increase while CO was unchanged. Exercise time at constant workload increased by 25%. After a peak level, intra-arterial pressure fell by 3% to 5% due to a decrease in total peripheral resistance both before and during diltiazem treatment. Stroke volume and CO remained unchanged during endurance exercise while HR showed a small increase. Thus, there was no reduction in the overall cardiac pump function after long-term diltiazem treatment, and blood flow during exercise was maintained.

Diltiazem ± hydrochlorothiazide

Burris and associates[50] from 5 USA medical centers assessed in a multicenter, factorial-design trial the safety and additive antihypertensive efficacy of a slow-release (SR) formulation of diltiazem hydrochloride given alone or in combination with hydrochlorothiazide for treatment of mild to moderate systemic hypertension (supine diastolic BP 95–110 mm Hg). After 4–6 weeks placebo run-in period, 297 qualifying patients were randomized to receive placebo, 1 of 4 doses of diltiazem SR monotherapy, 1 of 3 doses of hydrochlorothiazide monotherapy, or 1 of 12 possible combinations of diltiazem SR and hydrochlorothiazide for 6 weeks. A dose-related reduction in BP was demonstrated for each drug as monotherapy and for the 2 drugs in combination. Absolute BP of patients who received combination therapy were lower by an overall mean of 3 mm Hg diastolic and 8 mm Hg systolic vs diltiazem SR used alone and 3.5 mm Hg diastolic and 4 mm Hg systolic vs hydrochlorothiazide used alone. At the largest doses used, 50% of patients achieved goal BP while taking hydrochlorothiazide, 57% while taking diltiazem SR, and 75% while taking combination therapy. Combination therapy was well tolerated. This trial clearly demonstrates that diltiazem SR and hydrochlorothiazide have additive antihypertensive effects.

Nifedipine

To assess the changes in sodium excretion and sodium balance after withdrawal of nifedipine used for a long time, Pevahouse and associates[51] from London, UK, performed a single-blind, placebo-controlled study of 8 patients with mild to moderate uncomplicated essential hypertension who had been taking nifedipine 20 mg twice daily for at least 6 weeks. The patients received fixed sodium and potassium intakes and were withdrawn from nifedipine and replaced with matching placebo for 1 week. Urinary sodium excretion and cumulative sodium balance, body weight, plasma atrial natriuretic peptide concentrations, plasma renin activity and aldosterone concentrations and BP were measured. During nifedipine withdrawal there was a significant reduction in urinary sodium excretion (day 1: -63 mmol/24 h) and each patient retained a mean of 146 mmol sodium over the week of replacement with placebo. Body weight and plasma atrial natriuretic peptide concentrations increased during the placebo period and seemed to be associated with the amount of sodium retained. Systolic BP rose from 157 to 165 mm Hg when nifedipine was replaced with matching placebo, and the rise seemed to be related to the amount of sodium that was retained. Nifedipine causes a long term reduction in sodium balance in patients with essential hypertension. This long term effect may contribute to the mechanism whereby nifedipine lowers BP.

Verapamil vs nifedipine

The effect of different calcium antagonists on LV function during exercise and on exercise performance in patients with hypertension is not clear. Fifteen patients with essential hypertension (diastolic BP 95 to 110 mm Hg) were enrolled in a placebo-controlled, single-blinded crossover study comparing nifedipine with verapamil for rest/exercise heart rate and BP, exercise performance, and rest/exercise LV function in a study carried out by Ashmore and associates[52] from Denver, Colorado. Each drug was titrated to achieve resting diastolic pressures <90 mm Hg. All patients underwent maximal exercise testing and rest/exercise gated radionuclide ventriculography at the end of 3-week placebo, nifedipine, and verapamil treatment periods. Both calcium antagonists significantly reduced BP at rest and during exercise compared with placebo.

Neither calcium antagonist altered resting heart rate; however, both verapamil and nifedipine significantly reduced heart rate at maximal exercise. Verapamil but not nifedipine impaired LV peak emptying rate and LV peak filling rate during exercise but not at rest. Neither verapamil nor nifedipine, however, significantly altered rest or exercise global LVEF compared with placebo. There was a trend, however, for impairment in the LVEF response to exercise in the verapamil treatment group. Exercise capacity was not significantly altered by either calcium antagonist compared with placebo. Thus, verapamil but not nifedipine impairs LV function during exercise in hypertensive patients.

Isradipine

Lacourciere and associates[53] from Montreal, Canada, compared the antihypertensive efficacy of sustained released isradipine administered once daily to the immediate-release formulation administered twice daily as assessed by ambulatory BP monitoring in a double-blind randomized crossover study of 76 mild-to-moderate hypertensive patients. Conventional BP and heart rate parameters were evaluated after a 4-week placebo period and patients qualified for entry if sitting diastolic BP was between 95 and 114 mm Hg. Ambulatory BP monitoring was measured at baseline and after active treatment with both formulations. The 2 regimens induced a significant and almost identical reduction in the mean 24-hour BP without affecting heart rate. Isradipine was more effective in patients whose clinical hypertension was confirmed by ambulatory BP monitoring than in patients who remained normotensive by ambulatory BP monitoring criteria. The isradipine-treated ambulatory hypertensive group experienced significantly greater decreases in BP during 24-hour, work, awake and sleep periods than did the ambulatory normotensive group. These data suggest that sustained-release isradipine has a sustained antihypertensive effect throughout 24 hours comparable to that of isradipine given twice daily and may improve compliance with long-term treatment. In addition, the results confirm the usefulness of ambulatory BP monitoring in determining truly hypertensive patients likely to respond to drug administration.

Lacidipine

Heber and associates[54] from Middlesex, UK, examined the efficacy of the new once daily dihydropyridine calcium antagonist, lacidipine, in reducing ambulatory intraarterial BP in 12 untreated hypertensive patients. The intraarterial recording was commenced 24 hours before the first 4-mg dose and was continued for a further 24 hours thereafter. After dose titration and chronic therapy, a second 24-hour ambulatory BP recording was made. There was a steady onset of drug action, maximal at 2 hours, but with a reflex tachycardia after the first dose. Chronic administration reduced BP throughout the 24-hour period, without tachycardia. Mean daytime reduction in BP was 20 mm Hg systolic and 12 mm Hg diastolic. Mean nighttime reduction was 8-mm Hg systolic and 6-mm Hg diastolic. There was no postural decrease in BP on 60° head-up tilting and hypotensive action was maintained during isometric exercise (reduction at peak of 23/18 mm Hg) and throughout dynamic exercise (reduction at peak of 23/14 mm Hg). Lacidipine is an effective once-daily antihypertensive agent, with good control of stress response.

Nitrendipine vs metoprolol vs mepindolol vs enalapril

In a randomized 6-month study of 201 patients, Schrader and associates[55] from Göttingen, West Germany, compared the antihypertensive efficacy of the calcium antagonist nitrendipine, and β_1-selective blocker metoprolol, mepindolol, the β-blocker with intrinsic activity and the angiotensin-converting enzyme inhibitor enalapril as monitored by 24-hour ambulatory BP measurements. The study was designed so that a comparable decrease in casual BP values was obtained with all 4 drugs. If normotension was not achieved with monotherapy, a diuretic also was administered. Pretreatment casual BP and mean 24-hour ambulatory BP values did not differ between the 4 groups. Normotension as assessed by casual BP measurements was observed in all 4 groups after 6 months of therapy, there being no significant differences between the groups. Significantly more diuretics were required in the mepindolol (n = 14) and in the enalapril (n = 20) groups compared to the nitrendipine (n = 5) and metoprolol (n = 7) groups. Despite comparable casual BP control, the 4 groups differed significantly in their mean 24-hour measurements. The greatest systolic and diastolic BP decreases were seen in the metoprolol group. Metoprolol was also the most effective drug in decreasing the frequency of systolic pressure peaks >180 mm Hg. Both β-blockers and enalapril significantly decreased the morning BP increase compared to the values before treatment, while nitrendipine did not. These data show that casual BP measurement is not a good predictor of 24-hour BP in patients taking hypertensive therapy. Despite an equal degree of "office" BP control, different antihypertensive regimens do not confer the same degree of "nonoffice" BP control.

Captopril

Successful long-term treatment of systemic hypertension must include consideration of individual patients' lifestyles interfaced with the potential for adverse drug events. In a postmarketing surveillance study, Schoenberger and associates[56] from Chicago, Illinois, evaluated 30,515 patients who received captopril monotherapy evaluated by 7,792 physicians. Mean systolic and diastolic BP were reduced 17 and 11 mm Hg, respectively. Mean diastolic BP was reduced 10% for patients with mild hypertension; larger mean reductions were noted for patients with moderate (16.5%) and severe (21.5%) hypertension. Captopril therapy was equally effective in all races (white, Hispanic, and black patients), age groups, and in isolated instances of systolic hypertension. Only 4.9% of patients reporting an adverse event required discontinuation of therapy. Headache (1.8%) and dizziness (1.6%) were the most frequently reported adverse events. Quality-of-life measures improved.

Lisinopril vs hydrochlorothiazide

To investigate whether sodium restriction might replace thiazides in promoting BP reduction with lisinopril Omvik and Lund-Johansen[57] from Bergen, Norway, compared the long-term hemodynamic effect of lisinopril plus sodium restriction versus lisinopril plus hydrochlorothiazide at rest and during dynamic exercise in 2 groups of patients with essential hypertension. Mean pretreatment intraarterial BP at rest sitting was 177/107 mm Hg. The patients were randomly allocated to lisinopril combined with either low salt diet (low salt group, n = 13) or hydrochlorothiazide (diuretic group, n = 12). After 1 year of treatment the mean dose of lisinopril was 25 mg in both groups. In the low salt group sodium excretion was reduced from 188 to 129 mmol/24 hours. Total peripheral resistance was reduced in both groups: at rest 14 and 7% and during exercise 8 and 5% in the low salt and the diuretic groups, respectively. Overall cardiac output was reduced in the diuretic group but remained unchanged in the low salt group. Thus, lisinopril—either in combination with a diuretic or sodium restriction—induces marked reduction in BP due to decreases in peripheral vascular resistance both at rest and during exercise. Lisinopril plus low salt diet reduces the risk of unwanted metabolic effects and leads to more complete hemodynamic normalization than lisinopril plus a diuretic and should be preferred when this leads to satisfactory BP control.

References

1. Sykes D, Dewar R, Mohanaruban K, Donovan K, Nicklason F, Thomas DM, Fisher D: Measuring blood pressure in the elderly: Does atrial fibrillation increase observer variability? Br Med J 1990 (Jan 20);300:162–163.
2. Mejia AD, Julius S, Jones KA, Schork NJ, Kneisley J: The Tecumseh blood pressure study: Normative data on blood pressure self-determination. Arch Intern Med 1990 (June);150:1209–1213.
3. Prisant LM, Carr AA, Wilson B, Converse S: Ambulatory blood pressure monitoring and echocardiographic left ventricular wall thickness and mass. Am J Hypertens 1990 (Feb);3:81–89.
4. Broadhurst P, Brigden G, Dasgupta P, Lahiri A, Raftery EB: Ambulatory intra-arterial blood pressure in normal subjects. Am Heart J 1990 (July);120:160–166.
5. National High Blood Pressure Education Program Coordinating Committee: National High Blood Pressure Education Program Working Group report on ambulatory blood pressure monitoring. Arch Intern Med 1990 (Nov);150:2270–2280.
6. Mejia AD, Egan BM, Schork NJ, Zweifler AJ: Artefacts in measurement of blood pressure and lack of target organ involvement in the assessment of patients with treatment-resistant hypertension. An Intern Med 1990 (Feb 15);112:270–277.
7. Verdecchia P, Schillaci G, Guerrieri M, Gatteschi C, Benemio G, Boldrini F, Porcellati C: Circadian blood pressure changes and left ventricular hypertrophy in essential hypertension. Circulation 1990 (February);81:528–536.
8. Parmer R, Cervenka J, Stone R, O'Connor: Autonomic Function in Hypertension Are There Racial Differences? Circulation 1990 (April);81:1305–1311.
9. Ekelund L, Suchindran, Karon J, McMahon R, Tyroler H: Black-White Differences in Exercise Blood Pressure The Lipid Research Clinics Program Prevalence Study. Circulation 1990 (May);81:1568–1574.
10. Multiple Risk Factor Intervention Trial Research Group: Mortality After 10½ Years for Hypertensive Participants in the Multiple Risk Factor Intervention Trial. Circulation 1990 (November);82:1616–1628.
11. MacMahon S, Peto R, Cutler J, Collins R, Sorlie P, Neaton J, Abbott R, Godwin J, Dyer A, Stamler J: Blood pressure, stroke, and coronary heart disease: Part 1, prolonged differences in blood pressure: prospective observational studies corrected for the regression dilution bias. Lancet 1990 (Mar 31);335:765–774.
12. Collins R, Peto R, MacMahon S, Hebert P, Fiebach NH, Eberlein KA, Godwin J, Qizilbash N, Taylor JO, Hennekens CH: Blood pressure, stroke, and coronary heart disease. Lancet 1990 (April 7);335:827–838.

13. Yurenev AP: DeQuattro V, Devereux RB: Hypertensive heart disease: Relationship of silent ischemia to coronary artery disease and left ventricular hypertrophy. Am Heart J 1990 (October);120:928–933.

14. Schnall PL, Pieper C, Schwartz JE, Karasek RA, Schlussel Y, Devereux RB, Ganau A, Alderman M, Warren K, Pickering TG: The relationship between 'job strain,' workplace diastolic blood pressure, and left ventricular mass index: Results of a case-controlled study. JAMA 1990 (April 11);263:1929–1935.

15. Kannel WB, Zhang T, Garrison RJ: Is obesity-related hypertension less of a cardiovascular risk? The Framingham Study. Am Heart J 1990 (November);120:1195–1201.

16. Barker DJP, Bull AR, Osmond C, Simmonds SJ: Fetal and placental size and risk of hypertension in adult life. Br Med J 1990 (Aug 4);301:259–262.

17. Moore RD, Levine DM, Southard J, Entwisle G, Shapiro S: Alcohol consumption and blood pressure in the 1982 Maryland hypertension survey. Am J Hypertens 1990 (Jan);3:1–7.

18. Witteman JCM, Willett WC, Stampfer MJ, Colditz GA, Kok FJ, Sacks FM, Speizer FE, Rosner B, Hennekens CH: Relation of moderate alcohol consumption and risk of systemic hypertension in women. Am J Cardiol 1990 (Mar 1);65:633–637.

19. Gottdiener JS, Brown J, Zoltick J, Fletcher RD: Left ventricular hypertrophy in men with normal blood pressure: Relation to exaggerated blood pressure response to exercise. An of Intern Med 1990 (Feb);112:161–166.

20. Blake J, Devereux RB, Borer JS, Szulc M, Pappas TW, Laragh JH: Relation of obesity, high sodium intake, and eccentric left ventricular hypertrophy to left ventricular exercise dysfunction in essential hypertension. Am J Med 1990 (May);88:477–485.

21. Julius S, Jamerson K, Mejia A, Krause L, Schork N, Jones K: The association of borderline hypertension with target organ changes and higher coronary risk: Tecumseh blood pressure study. JAMA 1990 (July 18);264:354–358.

22. Frederickson ED, Wilcox CS, Bucci M, Loon NR, Peterson JC, Brown NL, Thompson RD, Smith TB, Wingo CS: A prospective evaluation of a simplified captopril test for the detection of renovascular hypertension. Arch Intern Med 1990 (Mar);150:569–572.

23. Lewis JF, Maron BJ: Diversity of patterns of hypertrophy in patients with systemic hypertension and marked left ventricular wall thickening. Am J Cardiol 1990 (Apr 1);65:874–881.

24. Cooper RS, Simmons BE, Castaner A, Santhanam V, Ghali J, Mar M: Left ventricular hypertrophy is associated with worse survival independent of ventricular function and number of coronary arteries severely narrowed. Am J Cardiol 1990 (Feb 15);65:441–445.

25. Siegel D, Cheitlin MD, Black DM, Seeley D, Hearst N, Hulley SB: Risk of ventricular arrhythmias in hypertensive men with left ventricular hypertrophy. Am J Cardiol 1990 (Mar 15);65:742–747.

26. McLenachan JM, Dargie HJ: Ventricular arrhythmias in hypertensive left ventricular hypertrophy: Relationship to coronary artery disease, left ventricular dysfunction, and myocardial fibrosis. Am J Hpertens 1990 (Oct);3:735–740.

27. Szlachcic J, Tubau JF, O'Kelly B, Massie BM: Correlates of diastolic filling abnormalities in hypertension: A Doppler echocardiographic study. Am Heart J 1990 (August);120:386–391.

28. Dimsdale JE, Ziegler M, Mills P, Berry C: Prediction of salt sensitivity. Am J Hypertens 1990 (June);3:429–435.

29. Panza JA, Quyyumi AA, Brush JE Jr, Epstein SE: Abnormal endothelium-dependent vascular relaxation in patients with essential hypertension. N Eng J Med 1990 (July 5);323:22–7.

30. Schotte DE, Stunkard AJ: The effects of weight reduction on blood pressure in 301 obese patients. Arch Intern Med 1990 (Aug);150:1701–1704.

31. Hypertension Prevention Trial Research Group: The hypertension prevention trial: Three-year effects of dietary changes on blood pressure. Arch Intern Med 1990 (Jan);150:153–162.

32. Bonaa KH, Bjerve KS, Straume B, Gram IT, Thelle D: Effect of eicosapentaenoic and docosahexaenoic acids on blood pressure in hypertension: A population-based intervention trial from the Tromso Study. N Eng J Med 1990 (Mar 22);322:795–801.

33. Martin J, Dubbert P, Cushman W: Controlled Trial of Aerobic Exercise in Hypertension. Circulation 1990 (May);81:1560–1567.

34. Christlieb AR: Treatment selection considerations for the hypertensive diabetic patient. Arch Intern Med 1990 (June);150:1167–1174.

35. Eisen SA, Miller DK, Woodward RS, Spitznagel E, Przybeck TR: The effect of prescribed daily dose frequency on patient medication compliance. Arch Intern Med 1990 (Sept);150:1881–1884.

36. Lacroix AZ, Wienpahl J, White LR, Wallace RB, Scherr PA, George LK, Cornoni-Huntley J, Ostfeld AM: Thiazide diuretic agents and the incidence of hip fracture. N Engl J Med 1990 (Feb 1);322:286–290.

37. Calhoun DA, Oparil S: Treatment of hypertensive crisis. NEJM 1990 (Oct 25);323:1177–1183.

38. Edelson JT, Weinstein MC, Tosteson ANA, Williams L, Lee TH, Goldman L: Long-term cost-effectiveness of various initial monotherapies for mild to moderate hypertension. JAMA 1990 (Jan 19);263:407–413.

39. Kochar MS, Landry KM, Ristow SM: Effects of reduction in dose and discontinuation of hydrochlorothiazide in patients with controlled essential hypertension. Arch Intern Med 1990 (May);150:1009–1011.

40. Middeke M, Richter WO, Schwandt P, Beck B, Holzgreve H: Normalization of lipid metabolism after withdrawal from antihypertensive long-term therapy with beta blockers and diuretics. Arteriosclerosis 1990 (Jan/Feb);10:145–147.

41. Psaty BM, Koepsell TD, Wagner EH, Logerfo JP, Inui TS: The relative risk of incident coronary heart disease associated with recently stopping the use of β-blockers. JAMA 1990 (Mar 23/30);263:1653–1657.

42. Grimm RH, Neaton JD, Elmer PJ, Svendsen KH, Levin J, Segal M, Holland L, Witte LJ, Clearman DR, Kofron P, Labounty RK, Crow R, Prineas RJ: The influence of oral potassium chloride on blood pressure in hypertensive men on a low-sodium diet. N Engl J Med 1990 (Mar 1);322:569–574.

43. Neutel JM, Schnaper H, Cheung DG, Graettinger WF, Weber WA: Antihypertensive effects of β-blockers administered once daily: 24-hour measurements. Am Heart J 1990 (July);120:166–171.

44. Saunders E, Weir MR, Kong W, Hollifield J, Gray J, Vertes V, Sowers JR, Zemel MB, Curry C, Schoenberger J, Wright JT, Kirkendall W, Conradi EC, Jenkins P, McLean B, Massie B, Berenson G, Flamenbaum W: A comparison of the efficacy and safety of a β-blocker; a calcium channel blocker; and a converting enzyme inhibitor in hypertensive blacks. Arch Intern Med 1990 (Aug);150:1707–1713.

45. Croog SH, Kong W, Levine S, Weir MR, Baume RM, Saunders E: Black Hypertension Quality of Life Multicenter Trial Group. Arch Intern Med 1990 (Aug);150:1733–1741.

46. Schulman SP, Weiss JL, Becker LC, Gottlieb SO, Woodruff KM, Weisfeldt ML, Gerstenblith G: The effects of antihypertensive therapy on left ventricular mass in elderly patients. N Engl J Med 1990 (May 10);322:1350–1356.

47. Giles TD, Weber M, Bartels DW, Silberman HM, Gilderman LP, Burris JF: Treatment of isolated systolic hypertension with labetalol in the elderly. Arch Intern Med 1990 (May);150:974–976.

48. Clark JA, Zimmerman HJ, Tanner LA: Labetalol hepatotoxicity. An Intern Med 1990 (Aug 1);113:210–213.

49. Lund-Johansen P, Omvik P: Effect of long-term diltiazem treatment on central hemo-dynamics and exercise endurance in essential hypertension. Eur Heart J 1990 (June);11:543–551.

50. Burris JF, Weir MR, Oparil S, Weber M, Cady WJ, Stewart WH: An assessment of diltiazem and hydrochlorothiazide in hypertension: Application of factorial trial design to a multicenter clinical trial of combination therapy. JAMA 1990 (Mar 16);263:1507–1512.

51. Pevahouse JB, Markandu ND, Cappuccio FP, Buckley MG, Sagnella GA, MacGregor GA: Long term reduction in sodium balance: Possible additional mechanism whereby nifedipine lowers blood pressure. Br Med J 1990 (Sept 22);301:580–584.

52. Ashmore RC, Corkadel LK, Green CL, Horwitz LD: Verapamil but not nifedipine impairs left ventricular function during exercise in hypertensive patients. Am Heart J 1990 (March);119:636–641.

53. Lacourciere Y, Poirier L, Dion D, Provencher P: Antihypertensive effect of isradipine administered once or twice daily on ambulatory blood pressure. Am J Cardiol 1990 (Feb 15);65:467–472.

54. Heber ME, Broadhurst PA, Brigden GS, Raftery EB: Effectiveness of the once-daily calcium antagonist, lacidipine, in controlling 24-hour ambulatory blood pressure. Am J Cardiol 1990 (Nov 15);66:1228–1232.

55. Schrader J, Schoel G, Buhr-Schinner, Kandt M, Warneke G, Armstrong VW, Scheler F: Comparison of the antihypertensive efficiency of nitrendipine, metoprolol, mepindolol and enalapril using ambulatory 24-hour blood pressure monitoring. Am J Cardiol 1990 (Oct 15);66:967–972.

56. Schoenberger JA, Testa M, Ross AD, Brennan WK, Bannon JA: Efficacy, safety, and quality-of-life assessment of captopril antihypertensive therapy in clinical practice. Arch Intern Med 1990 (Feb);150:301–306.

57. Omvik and Lund-Johansen: Comparison of long-term hemodynamic effects at rest and during exercise of lisinopril plus sodium restriction versus hydrochlorothiazide in essential hypertension. Am J Cardiol 1990 (Feb 1);65:331–338.

Valvular Heart Disease

Cystic medial necrosis without the Marfan syndrome

Marsalese and associates[1] in Cleveland, Ohio, performed a retrospective analysis to determine the surgical outcome and long-term follow-up of 93 patients with cystic medial necrosis of the aorta diagnosed at the Cleveland Clinic between July 1963 and December 1987. Among these patients, 72% were men with a mean age of 55 (range 26 to 77). Patients who met diagnostic criteria for the Marfan syndrome were excluded. Sixty-eight percent of the patients had a diastolic murmur and chest roentgenogram revealed a dilated ascending aorta in 58% and cardiomegaly in 63%. Cardiac catheterization in 76 patients demonstrated aortic root dilatation in 78%, AR in 72%, aortic dissection in 32%, and CAD in 32%. Ninety patients underwent surgery, including composite graft repair with reimplantation of the coronary arteries in 34%. Follow-up data obtained on 90 (97%) of the 93 patients at a mean of 29 months (range 0 to 137) indicated that 34 of the 90 patients died at a mean age of 60 years and 94% of the known causes of death were related to the cardiovascular system. Included among the causes of death were 65% resulting from aortic dissections, rupture, or sudden death (Figures 6-1 and 6-2). Ninety-six percent of survivors were in New York Heart Association functional class I or II. Estimated survivals at 1, 3, and 5 years were 72.2%, 63.5% and 57.4%, respectively. Actuarial survivals in patients who underwent composite graft reconstructions were 84% at 5 years. The presence of a diastolic murmur at initial presentation was associated with a poor prognosis. These data indicate that patients with cystic medial necrosis of the aorta without other features of the Marfan syndrome have an increased risk of cardiovascular abnormalities, including dissecting aortic aneurysms and AR. Moreover, because these patients lack the external stigmata of the Marfan syndrome and clinically identifiable markers for

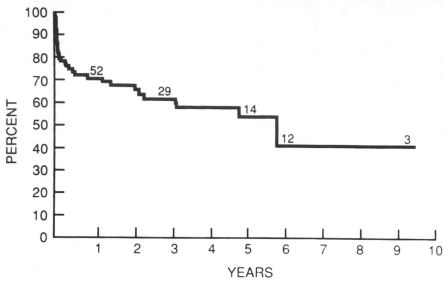

Fig. 6-1. Overall survival of 90 of the 93 patients. Estimated survival at 1, 3 and 5 years is 72.2%, 63.3% and 57.4%, respectively. The number of patients remaining at risk for each follow-up interval is noted. Reproduced with permission from Marsalese, et al.[1]

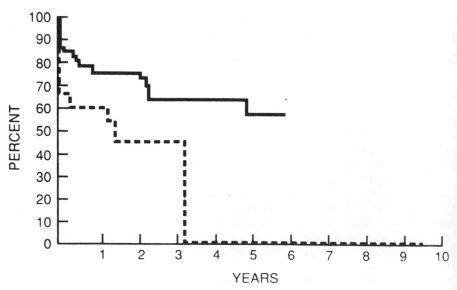

Fig. 6-2. Survival in patients who had a diastolic murmur (dashed line) versus those who did not (solid line). The presence of a diastolic murmur on initial cardiac examination was associated with a poor prognosis (p = 0.03). Reproduced with permission from Marsalese, et al.[1]

aortic root disease, they are often seen at older ages and with more advanced disease.

Systemic lupus erythematosis

Khamashta and associates[2] from 3 medical centers carried out a prospective echocardiographic study on 132 consecutive patients with systemic lupus erythematosis (SLE). The prevalence of valvular lesions was 22% compared with 3% in a control group of 68 healthy volunteers: 50 SLE patients had antibodies against phospholipids. The prevalence of valvular vegetations (8/50 [16%]) and of MR (19/50 [38%]) was significantly higher among the SLE patients with antiphospholipids than among those without (1% vs 12%). During follow-up of the patients with valvular lesions, hemodynamically significant clinical valve disease developed in 6 but surgery was required in only 1; 9 had cerebrovascular occlusions; and 7 died, although no death was due directly to the cardiac involvement. Thus, valvular heart disease, particularly affecting the mitral valve, is common in patients with SLE, and the presence of antibodies against phospholipids is associated with a higher prevalence of valvular abnormalities.

Carcinoid heart disease

Lundin and associates[3] from Uppsala, Sweden, performed transthoracic and transoesophageal echocardiography and Doppler investigations in 31 consecutive patients with malignant mid-gut carcinoid tumors. The transoesophageal images allowed measurement of the thickness of the atrioventricular valve leaflets and the superficial wall layers on the cavity side of both atria. The mean thickness of the anterior tricuspid leaflet was significantly greater than that of the mitral valve—a difference not seen in a control group of age-matched patients without carcinoid tumors and with normal cardiac ultrasound findings. In addition, the edges of the tricuspid leaflets were thickened giving them a clubbed appearance. TR was detected transoesophageally in 71% of the patients with carcinoid compared with 57% by transthoracic investigation. The inner layer of the RA wall in the carcinoid patients was significantly thicker than that of the left atrium and that of both atria in the controls. Patients with other signs of the carcinoid heart disease had significantly thicker mean RA luminal wall layer than those with less or no signs of right sided heart disease. Thus, transoesophageal cardiac ultrasound investigation improves the diagnostic accuracy and often shows the structural changes typical of carcinoid heart disease.

Lundin and associates[4] from Uppsala, Sweden, described results of tricuspid and pulmonic valve replacement in 4 patients with progressive right-sided CHF from carcinoid heart disease. The tricuspid and pulmonic valve replacement operations resulted in dramatic improvement in 3 of the 4 patients and these patients are still free of symptoms of cardiac dysfunction 10, 12, and 38 months postoperatively (Figure 6-3). One patient died 5 days postoperatively. The authors also reviewed previous reports of replacement of the tricuspid and/or mitral valve in patients with carcinoid heart disease.

MITRAL VALVE PROLAPSE

Auscultatory observations

Mitral systolic clicks and murmurs together with associated symptoms constitute a major reason for cardiologic referral. Although echocardiography and Doppler study enables characterization of the mitral valve apparatus and quantification of MR, its use has resulted in an over-

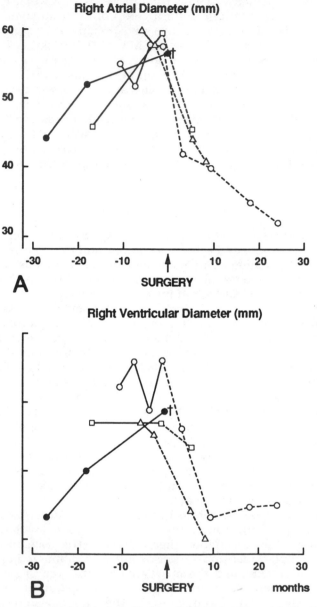

Fig. 6-3. Mean right atrial (A) and maximal medial-lateral right ventricular (B) diameters by two-dimensional echocardiography before and after valve replacement operations in four patients with severe carcinoid heart disease. Reproduced with permission from Lundin, et al.[3,4]

emphasis of the technical diagnosis of MVP and an under-evaluation of diagnosis based on physical examination. To determine the clinical significance of an auscultatory classification of mitral systolic clicks with or without precordial systolic murmurs, Tofler and Tofler[5] from Boston, Massachusetts, reviewed 291 patients with these signs. Based on initial auscultatory findings, patients were divided into: (1) single or multiple apical systolic clicks with no murmur (n = 99); (2) single or multiple apical systolic clicks and a late systolic murmur (n = 129); and (3) single or multiple apical clicks and an apical pansystolic murmur or murmur beginning in the first half of systole (n = 63). The average duration of patient follow-up was 8 years (range 1 to 30). The prognosis was excellent for patients from all 3 classes. Two cardiac-related deaths occurred: 1 each from classes 1 and 2. Mitral valve surgery was performed in 3 class 2 patients (2%) and in 2 class 3 patients (3%). No patient developed endocarditis during follow-up. Palpitations, with varying anxiety overlay, constituted a major indication for cardiologic referral in all 3 classes. Auscultatory findings were valuable to the physician for explanation and relief of patient anxiety. For patient management, use of an auscultatory classification may be preferable to the technically generated term "mitral valve prolapse."

Echocardiographic observations

To assess the serial phonocardiographic and echocardiographic changes in patients with MVP, You-Bing and associates[6] from Tokyo, Japan, reviewed phonocardiograms and echocardiograms retrospectively in 116 patients (48 men and 68 women, mean age 27 years) who had been determined to have MVP and were reexamined 1 to 14 years (mean 4.3) later by phonocardiography and echocardiography between 1971 and 1988. Follow-up phonocardiograms showed periods when 5 of 18 patients with silent MVP developed mid- or late systolic clicks. Of 57 patients with mid- or late systolic clicks, 15 had silent MVP, 6 developed a late systolic murmur with or without systolic clicks and 1 developed a pansystolic murmur. Two of 9 patients with an isolated late systolic murmur developed a pansystolic murmur. M-mode echocardiograms showed that left atrial and LV dimensions at end-diastole and end-systole increased in patients with systolic murmur (33 ± 10 vs 35 ± 11, 46 ± 6 vs 50 ± 7 and 29 ± 4 vs 31 ± 5 mm, respectively) and no statistically significant changes in any of these dimensions were found in patients without a systolic murmur. The degree of MVP evaluated by the anteroposterior mitral leaflet angle on the 2-dimensional echocardiogram was more severe in patients with a systolic murmur than in patients without systolic murmur (157 ± 12 vs $131 \pm 16°$). The degree of prolapse did not change during the follow-up periods. The number of patients with mitral regurgitation detected by pulsed Doppler echocardiography increased from 21 of 72 (29%) to 31 of 72 (43%). The present study suggests that the systolic murmur confirmed by phonocardiography should be taken into consideration in evaluating severity and in assessing prognosis of MVP.

Few data exist regarding the relation of valvular anatomy and coaptation to the presence of MR in patients with MVP. Grayburn and associates[7] from Lexington, Kentucky, assessed the ability of 2-dimensional echocardiographic features of mitral valve morphology to predict the presence, direction, and magnitude of MR as assessed by color Doppler flow imaging. MR was present in 21 of 46 patients with MVP on 2-dimensional echocardiography. Echocardiograms were specifically evaluated for leaflet apposition, leaflet morphology, and mitral anular diameter. Color flow images were analyzed for presence of MR, direction of the regurgitant jet, and area encompassing the largest jet visible in any view. Abnormal mitral leaflet coaptation on 2-dimensional echocardiography was strongly associated with the presence of MR, being present in 15 of 21 patients as compared with 5 of 25 patients without MR. Similarly, mitral leaflet thickness and MR were closely associated with the latter being present in 9 of 30 patients with normal and 12 of 16 patients with excessive leaflet thickness. MR jet direction tended to be anterior to central with posterior leaflet prolapse and posterior or central with anterior leaflet prolapse. Maximal jet area of MR tended to be larger in patients with compared with those without mitral anular dilatation (5.4 ± 2.3 vs 2.1 ± 1.9 cm²), and in those with abnormal rather than normal leaflet thickness (4.5 ± 2.7 vs 2.0 ± 1.6 cm²). Thus the presence, direction, and size of MR jets in MVP are related to structural abnormality of the mitral apparatus on echocardiography.

MITRAL REGURGITATION

Pai and co-workers[8] evaluated a new Doppler-derived index of the rate of LV pressure rise (DP/DT) for the prognostic stratification of patients with MR. The index is derived from the continuous wave Doppler mitral regurgitation signal by dividing magnitude of LV-LA pressure gradient rise (delta-p) between 1 and 3 m/sec of the MR velocity signal by the time take (delta-t) for this change. The investigators studied the LV (delta-p/delta-t) and other echocardiographic indexes of LV function before and after mitral valve surgery in 25 patients with chronic, severe MR in the absence of significant CAD. There was a good correlation between post-operative EF and the derived LV (delta-p/delta-t). The other echocardiographic parameters that correlated with postoperative EF were LV end-systolic dimension, end-systolic volume, end-diastolic dimension, end-diastolic volume, preoperative EF, end-systolic wall stress, and end-systolic wall stress normalized for end-systolic volume index. With multiple regression, the LV (delta-p/delta-t) and LV end-systolic dimension were shown to be independent predictors of postoperative EF. The investigators concluded that the Doppler-derived index of LV (delta-p/delta-t) and end-systolic dimension are afterload-independent predictors of post-operative EF in patients with chronic, severe MR.

MITRAL STENOSIS

Mitral area comparison

Mitral valve area determined by the Gorlin formula in patients with combined MS and MR underestimates the true orifice size. Recent data suggest Doppler ultrasound and 2-dimensional echocardiography more accurately estimate the mitral valve area in patients with mixed mitral valvular disease. This study by Fredman and associates[9] from St. Louis, Missouri, assessed the accuracy of an alternate method, the hemodynamic pressure half-time method, for mitral valve area determination in such patients. In 22 patients, 28 separate mitral valve areas were calculated by the hemodynamic pressure half-time method, the Gorlin formula, and the Gorlin formula corrected for MR, and were compared with results calculated by the Doppler pressure half-time method. Six patients were studied both before and after balloon mitral valvuloplasty. In addition, mitral valve areas calculated by all 4 methods were compared with results obtained by planimetry in 15 patients with technically optimal echocardiograms. The mitral valve areas determined by hemodynamic pressure half-time correlated closely with the valve areas determined by Doppler, whereas mitral valve areas determined by the Gorlin formula (both without and with correlation for MR) did not correlate as well with the Doppler-estimated valve areas. Correlation between the Doppler-derived mitral valve areas and the planimetered valve areas was also good, as was that between the mitral valve areas calculated by hemodynamic pressure half-time and those calculated by planimetry. The mitral valve areas calculated by the Gorlin formula, even with correction for MR, did not correlate well with the planimetered valve areas. These comparisons indicate that in patients with combined MS and MR, the hemodynamic pressure half-time method is more accurate than the Gorlin formula and should be considered for hemodynamic assessment of mitral valve orifice area in patients with mixed mitral valve disease.

Percutaneous mitral commissurotomy

A fine review of percutaneous balloon valvuloplasty was provided by Nishimura and associates[10] from Minneapolis, Minnesota, and it appeared in the *Mayo Clinic Proceedings*, February 1990.

To compare the single rubber-nylon balloon and double polyethylene balloon techniques, 94 patients with rheumatic MS underwent percutaneous transseptal balloon mitral valvuloplasty between November 1985 and September 1988 in a study reported by Chen and associates[11] from Guangzhou, China, and Washington, D.C. The single balloon technique was used in 73 patients and the double balloon technique was used in 21. The 2 groups were similar in age, weight, severity of the lesion, and cardiac functional status. The mean mitral valve diastolic gradient decreased from 18 ± 6.5 to 2.9 ± 3.1 mm Hg, 19 ± 7 to 6 ± 3 mm Hg, and 18 ± 6 to 3 ± 4 mm Hg in the single balloon group, double balloon group, and the entire series, respectively. The final mitral diastolic gradient in the single balloon group was lower than in the double balloon group. Complications in the single balloon group were lower than in the double balloon group. Additional advantages of single over double balloon technique were easier maneuverability and higher success rate. The initial and long-term follow-up results confirmed the earlier impressions that percutaneous transseptal balloon mitral valvuloplasty is an effective and safe nonsurgical method of treatment for rheumatic MS, and the single rubber-nylon balloon technique is at least as effective as, if not superior to, the double polyethylene balloon technique.

Ruiz and associates[12] from Los Angeles, California, successfully performed percutaneous double balloon valvotomy for severe rheumatic MS in 281 of 285 consecutive patients. The changes evoked were a decrease of the mean transvalvular gradient from 16 ± 7 to 5 ± 3 mm Hg, an increase in cardiac output from 3.8 ± 1.0 L/min to 5.4 ± 1.5 L/min and an increase in mitral valve area from 0.86 ± 0.24 cm^2 to 2.41 ± 0.54 cm^2. The mean PA pressure decreased from 37 ± 13 mm Hg to 27 ± 12 mm Hg and the pulmonary vascular resistance decreased from 307 ± 181 to 238 ± 122 dynes/s/cm^{-5}. Symptomatic improvement occurred in 272 of the 285 (95%) patients. There were 3 procedure-related deaths (1%). Post-dilatation MR was not significant in most patients. Therefore, this procedure can be performed at a low risk with effective results and a fast recovery.

Herrmann and associates[13] in Philadelphia, Pennsylvania, evaluated initial results, complications, and early follow-up of 74 patients undergoing percutaneous balloon mitral valvuloplasty in 7 hospitals participating in a multicenter study. Seventy-four patients with a mean age of 53 years had 75 valvuloplasty procedures over a 2.5 year period. Eighty-nine percent of the attempted procedures were completed and resulted in an increase in mean mitral valve area from 1.0 ± 0.04 to 2.0 ± 0.1 cm^2; the valve area increased $\geq 50\%$ of the baseline valve area in 73% of patients. Procedure related deaths, cardiac tamponade, systemic embolism, and emergent surgery were required in 2.7%, 6.7%, 2.7%, and 6.7% of patients, respectively. At a mean follow-up period of 15 months, the condition of most patients had improved and 89% of 55 patients treated with only valvuloplasty were in New York Heart Association functional class I or II.

Casale and associates[14] in Boston, Massachusetts, followed 150 patients who had percutaneous mitral balloon valvuloplasty, including 124 women and 26 men with a mean age of 53 ± 1 years. A left-to-right shunt through the created atrial communication was present in 28 patients (19%) after valvuloplasty. The pulmonary to systemic flow ratio was $\geq 2:1$ in 4 patients and $<2:1$ in 24. Univariate predictors of left-to-right shunting after valvuloplasty included older age, lower cardiac output before mitral valvuloplasty, higher New York Heart Association functional class before valvuloplasty, presence of mitral valve calcification under fluoroscopy, and higher echocardiographic score. Multiple stepwise logistic regression analysis identified the presence of mitral valve calcium and lower cardiac output as independent predictors of a left-to-right shunt through the atrial communication after balloon valvuloplasty. Follow-up (10 ± 1 months) of patients with an ASD after valvuloplasty showed that 1) 6 patients died; 2) an ASD was demonstrated in 3 of 6 patients who underwent MVR at 6 ± 0.8 months after valvuloplasty; and 3) 13 patients were in functional class I, 2 patients were in functional class II, and 1 patient was in class III at 13 ± 1 months after valvuloplasty. A persistent ASD was demonstrated by oximetry in only 5 of 13 patients who underwent elective right sided heart catheterization at 11 ± 1 months after mitral valvuloplasty. Doppler color flow echocardiography demonstrated a left-to-right shunt in only 1 of the remaining 3 patients who did not undergo cardiac catheterization. Therefore, 13 (59%) of 22 patients who had a left-to-right shunt after mitral balloon valvuloplasty were demonstrated to have no evidence of a left-to-right shunt through a created atrial communication at follow-up study.

Abascal and co-workers[15] in Boston, Massachusetts, studied 130 patients undergoing percutaneous balloon mitral valvotomy. The relation between valvular morphology according to a previously described echo- ocardiographic scoring system and hemodynamic outcome expressed as qualitative ("good" and suboptimal) and as absolute change in valve area was analyzed. The relative importance of the individual components of this echocardiographic score (valvular thickening, mobility, calcium, and subvalvular disease) to the change in valve area after valvotomy was also examined. Mean transmitral pressure gradient decreased from 16 to 6 mm Hg, and mitral valve area increased from 0.9 to 1.8 cm^2. Results in individual patients were variable. Eighty-four percent of patients with an echocardiographic score of ≤ 8 had a good outcome, whereas 58% of patients with an echocardiographic score of 8 or more had a suboptimal result. The echocardiographic score correlated negatively with the absolute increase in mitral valve area after valvotomy, but there was substantial scatter in the data. Of the 4 components of the total echocardiographic score, valvular thickening correlated best with the absolute change in valve area. Multiple regression analysis selected valvular thickening as the only morphological predictor of the change in valve area, followed by a larger effective balloon dilating area and sinus rhythm. The equation derived from this multivariate analysis was used to predict the absolute change in valve area after valvotomy.

To estimate the incidence of residual atrial septal perforation following percutaneous transvenous mitral commissurotomy with the Inoue balloon catheter and to examine the factors contributing to atrial septal perforation, Ishikura and associates[16] from Osaka, Japan, studied 46 patients with MS undergoing percutaneous transvenous mitral commissurotomy. Residual atrial septal perforation was evaluated by Doppler color flow imaging 1 day after percutaneous transvenous mitral commissurotomy, and was detected in 7 out of 46 patients (15%). Examined were the relations between the development of atrial septal perforation and age of the patient, the LA dimension before percutaneous transvenous mitral commissurotomy, the mean pressure difference between left and right atrium after percutaneous transvenous mitral commissurotomy, and duration of the procedure from atrial septal puncture by the Brockenbrough method to balloon inflation. There was a good correlation between the development of residual atrial septal perforation and the duration of the procedure. There was no correlation between the development of atrial septal perforation and other factors. In the follow-up study, atrial septal perforation disappeared in 4 patients within 3 months. Atrial septal perforation persisted in 2 patients for 1 year after percutaneous transvenous mitral commissurotomy. The shunt in these 2 patients was clinically insignificant. These data suggest that residual atrial septal perforation may depend on the duration of the procedure, and that most cases of atrial septal perforation disappear within 1 year after percutaneous transvenous mitral commissurotomy.

Acute mitral obstruction may lead to an increase in atrial natriuretic peptide (ANP) due to increased LA pressure and a large increase in arginine vasopressin due to simultaneous arterial and ventricular baroreceptor unloading. Lewin and colleagues[17] from Milwaukee, Wisconsin, measured ANP and arginine vasopressin concentrations after transseptal puncture and during percutaneous retrograde mitral balloon valvuloplasty in 11 patients (mean age 57 ± 12 years; 9 women) with MS and CHF. Atrial septal puncture per se resulted in a significant increase in ANP and arginine vasopressin without a significant change in aortic pressure. Subsequent percutaneous retrograde mitral balloon valvuloplasty led to a further increase in ANP, a transient decrease in aortic pressure from 89 ± 7 to 45 ± 4 mm Hg, and a 5-fold increase in arginine vasopressin. ANP and arginine vasopressin were no longer different from baseline values after the procedure. This study suggests that transseptal puncture and acute mitral obstruction are major stimuli to ANP release and that combined unloading of arterial and LV mechanoreceptors is a very potent vasopressinergic stimulus.

AORTIC VALVE STENOSIS

Outcome in asymptomatic patients

Pellikka and associates[18] in Rochester, Minnesota, studied the natural history of asymptomatic, hemodynamically significant, valvular AS in adults. Among 471 patients with AS identified by Doppler echocardiography as evidenced peak systolic flow velocity ≥ 4 m/s from January 1984 through August 1987, 143 were asymptomatic and had isolated valvular AS. Thirty patients underwent AVR within 3 months (group 1); the remaining 113 patients did not have an intervention within 3 months (group 2). Follow-up information was available for all patients; the mean duration of follow-up was 20 months. Three cardiac events occurred in the 30 group 1 patients after operation, including 2 deaths and 1 reoperation. Among the 113 group 2 patients, 3 had cardiac death apparently the result of AS, and all 3 had developed symptoms ≥3 months before death. The actuarial probability of remaining free of symptoms of angina, dyspnea or syncope for group 2 was 86% at 1 year and 62% at 5 years. For this group, the 1 and 2 year probabilities of remaining free of cardiac events, including AVR or cardiac death were 93% and 74%, respectively. Among the clinical and echocardiographic variables, only Doppler flow velocity and EF were independent predictors of subsequent cardiac events. Among the 44 patients (group 1 and 2) with a flow velocity ≥4.5 m/s, the relative risk of having a cardiac event was 4.9. Patients with asymptomatic, hemodynamically significant AS are at increased risk for cardiac events within 2 years. However, during the time they are asymptomatic, the risk of sudden death is small. The asymptomatic patient may be treated medically but requires careful follow-up evaluation for the development of symptoms at which time AVR is indicated.

Brachioradial delay

During the assessment of patients with severe or symptomatic AS, Leach and McBrien[19] from London, UK, observed a detectable delay between the brachial and radial pulses. This delay was not present in normal subjects. The timed delay of 53.5 ms in severe AS was significantly longer than that in normal volunteers (22.6 ms) or in patients with low cardiac output. This increased delay was clinically detectable before the occurrence of LV failure and often before the onset of symptoms.

Progression

Roger and associates[20] from Rochester, Minnesota, examined progression of AS as assessed by Doppler echocardiography in 112 consecutive adult patients with AS. All underwent 3 examinations during a mean 25-month period (range 7 to 54). At the time of entry into the study, mean values for initial peak aortic velocity and EF were 2.9 ± 0.7 m/sec and 63 ± 10%, respectively; 52% of the patients were symptomatic. At the third examination the percentage of symptomatic patients increased to 65%, and the aortic peak velocity increased to 3.3 ± 0.8 m/sec. Age, sex, and EF were not predictors of progression. Documented CAD (in 57 patients) did not affect progression, and neither did the aortic peak velocity at the time of entry into the study. Thirty-eight patients reported an increase in symptoms from the first to third examination, and their rate of progression was significantly different from that of the rest of the population: 0.33 ± 0.50 m/sec/yr compared to 0.18 ± 0.26 m/sec/yr.

Percutaneous valvulotomy

To evaluate the serial changes in LV performance after percutaneous aortic balloon valvuloplasty, 15 patients, mean age 75 ± 18 years, and in New York Heart Association class III, were studied by Harpole and associates[21] from Durham, North Carolina, with first-pass radionuclide angiocardiography immediately before, then 5 minutes, 2 hours, 4 hours, 6 hours, and 3 days after valvuloplasty. No change was observed in heart rate, aortic root systolic pressure, Fick, or radionuclide angiocardiography cardiac output, amount of AR measured either angiographically or with the regurgitant fraction determination immediately after valvuloplasty. Significant changes were observed in the peak-to-peak aortic valve gradient (63 to 35 mm Hg), mean aortic valve gradient (54 to 33 mm Hg), aortic valve area (0.6 to 0.9 cm²), and meridional wall stress (79 to 50 10³ dynes/cm²) immediately following valvuloplasty. In addition, LV end-diastolic volume decreased from 186 to 153 ml, end-systolic volume decreased from 114 to 86 ml, micromanometric LV end-diastolic pressure decreased from 20 to 14 mm Hg, and LVEF increased from 39 to 45%. Peak positive LV dP/dt and end-systolic pressure-volume ratio did not change after valvuloplasty. The serial radionuclide angiocardiographic data revealed that LVEF gradually increased (45 to 52%) and end-systolic volume decreased (86 to 69 ml) during the first 6 hours after valvuloplasty, while heart rate, BP, and end-diastolic volume did not change. The improved systolic performance persisted at 3 days and appeared to be due to reduced LV outflow obstruction and to recovery from balloon-induced LV dysfunction.

Rodriguez and associates[22] from Houston, Texas, described the short- and long-term outcome of 44 consecutive percutaneous balloon aortic valvuloplasty procedures performed in 42 elderly patients (age 78 ± 7 years) with AS. The initial success rate was 95%, with the peak aortic valve pressure gradient declining from a mean of 82 ± 32 to 44 ± 23 mm Hg and aortic valve area increasing from a mean of 0.59 ± 0.15 to 0.83 ± 0.40 cm². One procedure-related death occurred and an additional 3 patients died ≤30 days after balloon aortic valvuloplasty. These patients all had New York Heart Association class IV CHF symptoms prior to the procedure and their mean LVEF (28 ± 7%) was lower than that of hospital survivors (52 ± 13%). At the time of hospital discharge after valvuloplasty, 76% of patients were asymptomatic or markedly improved (New York Heart Association class I or II). After a mean follow-up of 16 months (range 2 to 26 months), however, 10 patients had died and 15 had undergone AVR for recurrence of New York Heart Association class III or IV symptoms. The adjusted 1- and 2-year survivals were 0.68 and 0.62, respectively, and adjusted 2-year event-free survival was 0.25. Proportional hazard regression analysis indicated that LVEF <40% was the only variable affecting survival and was a possible indicator of event-free survival. Patients with LVEF <40% had a 2-year survival of 0.36 compared with 0.80 for those with LVEF ≥40% and 2-year event-free survival was 0 vs 0.34, respectively. This study showed that balloon aortic valvuloplasty is not an effective long-term alternative for management of AS in patients with depressed LV function.

Davidson and associates[23] from Durham, North Carolina, performed a second balloon aortic valvuloplasty in 17 of 138 patients having balloon aortic valvuloplasty. The second procedure was done on average of 9 months (range 1–24 months) after the first attempt. The ages of the 17 patients ranged from 63 to 86 years (mean 76). The procedure was done in patients who were considered to be at high risk for AVR. The outcome for the 17 patients having repeat aortic valvuloplasty was dismal. Eight patients had cardiac death within a mean of 2 months of the repeat aortic valvuloplasty. Two patients had AVR 1 to 11 months after the repeat procedure. Thus, 10 patients died or had AVR within a mean of 2.5 months after repeat valvuloplasty. When compared with the initial procedure, the use of larger balloons during repeat valvuloplasty provided no additional improvement in aortic valve area or other variables measuring ventricular performance.

Effect of aortic valve replacement on degree of mitral regurgitation

Tunick and associates[24] from New York, New York, determined the severity of MR by color Doppler echocardiography in 44 adult patients with severe asymptomatic AS before and after isolated AVR. Preoperative MR was absent in 17, mild in 14, moderate in 11, and severe in 2 patients. Three to 388 (mean 58) days after surgery, 14 patients continued to have no MR. In the other 30 patients, MR decreased in 18 (60%), remained unchanged in 8 (27%) and increased in only 4 (13%). Furthermore, in 13 patients with significant (moderate or severe) MR, the severity decreased in 12 (92%). Thus, the severity of MR often decreases after AVR for AS.

AORTIC VALVE REGURGITATION

Vasodilator therapy

Dumesnil and associates[25] from Quebec, Canada, studied the long-term effects of hydralazine retrospectively in asymptomatic patients with significant AR followed annually for up to 4 years (mean 3.1 ± 7 years). Of the 19 patients, 12 were not receiving vasodilators and 7 were receiving hydralazine, 40 to 200 mg daily. In the patients not receiving vasodilators, LV diastolic and systolic dimensions increased progressively in all patients by an average of 8% and 13%, respectively, after 3 years. In the patients receiving hydralazine, LV dimensions increased by 9% and 5% in the year or more before hydralazine use and decreased by 7% and 7%, respectively, during the first year after using hydralazine. The reduction was observed in all patients during the first year, but an increase was detected in 3 patients followed up beyond that period. The results suggest that the progression of LV dilatation in asymptomatic patients with aortic regurgitation can be delayed by long-term therapy with vasodilators. Pending further confirmation, such therapy may possibly influence the natural history of the disease and delay the timing of operation.

Scognamiglio and associates[26] in Padua, Italy, evaluated the effect of 12 months of therapy with nifedipine on LV performance in 72 asymptomatic patients with severe AR. At 12 months of therapy, patients receiving nifedipine had a significant reduction in LV end-diastolic volume index and mass as measured by 2-dimensional echocardiography (Figure 6-4). They also had a reduced LV mean wall stress and an increase in LVEF from 60 ± 6% to 72 ± 8% (Figure 6-5). These data indicate that long-term unloading therapy with nifedipine may reverse LV dilatation and sustain improved LV function in asymptomatic patients with hemodynamically important AR.

Timing of aortic valve replacement

Out of 160 prospectively followed patients with AR, the clinical courses of 53 patients with pure, severe, and chronic AR and without CAD who were selected for surgery on the basis of predefined criteria are reported

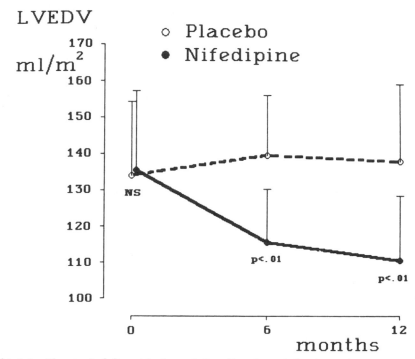

Fig. 6-4. Changes in left ventricular end-diastolic volume index (LVEDV) over time in 72 study patients. Measurements obtained at 6 and 12 months were compared with baseline measurements from the same patients. Left ventricular end-diastolic volume index did not change in the placebo-treated group, but decreased significantly in patients treated with nifedipine. Reproduced with permission from Scognamiglio, et al.[26]

by Tornos and associates[27] from Barcelona, Spain. Surgical criteria were either unequivocal symptoms or documentation of impaired LV dysfunction (defined as angiographic EF <50% plus an end-systolic volume index >60 ml/m²). According to preoperative status, patients were divided as follows: 11 asymptomatic patients (group A), 30 patients with moderate (classes II to III) symptoms (group B), and 12 patients with dyspnea at rest and pulmonary edema when first seen (group C). Surgical mortality was 1 patient (from group C). Late death occurred in 4 patients (1 from group B, 3 from group C). At the end of follow-up (minimum 1 year, mean 3.6 years) 41 patients were in functional class I, 4 patients in class II, and 1 patient in class III. All patients except 1 in functional classes II and III belonged to group C. Before surgery, patients from groups A and B had similar ventricular dimensions and EFs, whereas patients from group C had larger end-systolic diameters and volumes and lower EFs. End-diastolic and end-systolic diameters decreased significantly at 1 and 2 years after surgery. Patients from group C continued to have dilated hearts as did those patients from groups A and B who had preoperative end-systolic diameters >55 mm. Radionuclide EF increased in most patients with preoperative values <50%, except in those with preoperative values <30%. These results suggest that in asymptomatic patients, surgery can be delayed at least until the present criteria for LV dysfunction are reached. Although the postoperative outcome of patients with preoperative severe CHF was not as good as that of other patients, symptomatic improvement is likely to occur even in cases of severely impaired LV function.

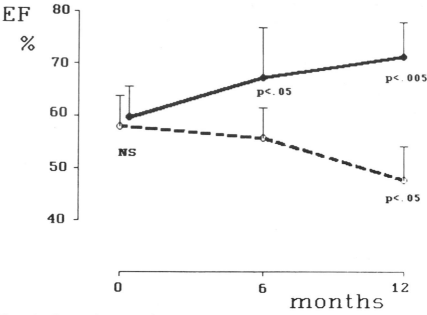

Fig. 6-5. Changes in ejection fraction (EF) over time in the two study groups. Ejection fraction decreased slightly in the placebo-treated group (open circles) but increased in the nifedipine-treated group (solid circles). Reproduced with permission from Scognamiglio, et al.[26]

TRICUSPID VALVE REGURGITATION

Minagoe and associates[28] from Los Angeles, California, defined the significance of laminar systolic regurgitant flow in TR, by performing pulsed-wave and continuous-wave Doppler, and 2-dimensional and M-mode echocardiography in 68 patients with TR, including 5 patients with tricuspid valvectomy. The pattern of TR flow (laminar versus turbulent), TR severity (the distance that the regurgitant flow extended into the right atrium, the peak flow velocity of TR, the presence or absence and the amount of systolic tricuspid cusp separation, and the dimension of the right ventricle and the inferior vena cava, were assessed. A laminar pattern of TR flow in systole was obtained in 21 patients, 5 of whom had undergone tricuspid valvectomy. Fourteen of 21 had visible tricuspid cusp separation in systole; of the 7 who had no visible tricuspid cusp separation during systole, 5 had undergone tricuspid valvectomy. All 47 patients with a turbulent pattern of TR flow had no visible systolic tricuspid cusp separation. Severe TR was present in 14 of 21 (67%) patients with laminar TR flow and in 4 of 47 (9%) patients with turbulent TR flow. The peak flow velocity of TR in patients with laminar TR flow (2.0 ± 0.7 m/sec) was lower than in those with turbulent TR flow (3.1 ± 0.7 m/sec). The dimension of the right ventricle and inferior vena cava were larger in patients with laminar TR flow (38 ± 9.4 mm and 27 ± 7.1 mm, respectively) than in those with turbulent TR flow (25 ± 9.55 mm and 19 ± 4.2 mm, respectively). The distance of systolic tricuspid cusp separation (tricuspid anulus in patients with tricuspid valvectomy) ranged from 3 to 40 mm and was inversely correlated with the peak flow velocity of TR in 19 patients with laminar TR flow. It was concluded that laminar TR flow is strongly suggestive of the presence of severe TR.

Treatment for TR in patients who have MVR remains controversial partly because of the lack of a convenient method for measuring reflux. Wong and associates[29] from Los Angeles, California, and Saitama, Japan, assessed Doppler measurement of TR in selecting patients for surgical or nonsurgical management and in evaluating the results. Thirty-three patients who had mitral valve surgery had 3 ultrasound examinations: before operation, before discharge from hospital, and 2 years after operation. Seventeen patients were assigned to tricuspid annuloplasty and 16 to no procedure. Assignment was based on visual grading of regurgitant velocity maps and intraoperative grading by direct palpation. Before operation patients in the annuloplasty group had larger mean jet velocity areas, RA size, and diastolic transvalvular velocities than had the nonsurgical group. The overlap of data precluded the definition of thresholds for separating the patients into either of 2 regimens. Early after operation the patients with annuloplasty had decreased regurgitant indexes similar to the preoperative levels of patients who had no procedure; the latter preoperative levels had not changed. Late after operation both groups had stabilization or trends toward less regurgitation, and continued decreases in tricuspid diastolic flow velocities. Thus, Doppler ultrasonography played a complementary role in selecting patients for annuloplasty or nonsurgical management and a major role in the longitudinal evaluation of treatment.

DOUBLE VALVE REGURGITATION

LV and RV performance characteristics in operative candidates with combined AR and MR have not been defined. Niles and associates[30] from New York, New York, determined radionuclide cineangiographic EF and echocardiographic and hemodynamic variables in 8 symptomatic patients undergoing double-valve replacement for pure, severe MR and AR. In order to gain insight into the basis for the poor postoperative survival in patients with this intrinsically biventricular disease, the authors compared these results with those of 29 symptomatic patients with isolated AR and with 18 symptomatic patients with isolated MR, all also undergoing valve replacement. Before operation, patients with AR/MR had significantly lower LVEF than patients with MR (rest, 40 ± 9% vs 52 ± 10%; exercise, 35 ± 12% vs 54 ± 12%) and tended to have lower LVEF than patients with AR alone (rest, 40 ± 9% vs 45 ± 12%, difference not significant; exercise, 35 ± 12% vs 39 ± 11%, difference not significant); RVEF was lower in AR/MR than in AR, and tended to be lower than in MR (difference not significant). At average postoperative follow-up of 72 to 76 months (survivors in each group), symptomatic patients with AR/MR had significantly poor survival than symptomatic patients with isolated MR and were more likely to have persistent symptoms than patients with AR. These findings suggest that symptomatic patients with AR/MR have poorer LV and RV performance than similarly symptomatic operative candidates with AR or MR alone. These findings are paralleled by poorer operative outcome, in terms of survival and symptom persistence, in the AR/MR group.

Isometric exercise produces well-defined hemodynamic changes in normal and diseased states. The effect of isometrics on the degree of valvular regurgitation recorded by color Doppler flow imaging had not been reported until Spain and associates[31] from Lexington, Kentucky, used color Doppler flow imaging to evaluate changes in valvular regurgitation in 34 patients, mean age 53 ± 16 years. Data were collected for 43 regurgitant lesions including 20 cases of AR and 23 cases of MR. Isometrics produced a significant increase in heart rate (71 to 83 beats/min) and BP (132/64 to 153/70 mm Hg) in all patients. Regurgitant jet area by color Doppler flow imaging increased significantly in both AR (4.5 to 6.2 cm^2) and MR (6.2 to 8.2 cm^2). Patients taking concurrent vasodilator or angiotensin-converting enzyme inhibitor therapy had similar responses to those not receiving long-term therapy. Thus, color Doppler flow imaging detects an increase in aortic and mitral regurgitant jet area induced by isometric exertion. The change in color Doppler flow imaging jet area with handgrip demonstrates the influence of loading conditions on the size of a regurgitant jet area, and suggests that isometric exertion may increase the magnitude of MR and AR.

INFECTIVE ENDOCARDITIS

Echocardiographic findings

Taams and associates[32] from Rotterdam, The Netherlands, studied 33 consecutive patients with clinically suspected infective endocarditis by both precordial cross-sectional echocardiography and transoesophageal echocardiography. The diagnostic value of both techniques was assessed. The data were compared with findings at operation in 25 patients. In 21 patients with native valve endocarditis precordial echocardiography showed evidence of vegetations in 6 patients and suggested their presence in 9. Transoesophageal echocardiography identified vegetations in 18 patients. Complications were seen in 4 patients at precordial echocardiography and in 9 patients at transoesophageal echocardiography. Precordial echocardiography did not show vegetations in any of the 12 patients with prosthetic valve endocarditis whereas transoesophageal echocardiography showed vegetations in four. Complications were seen in 4 patients at precordial echocardiography and in 10 at transoesophageal echocardiography. Echocardiographic findings were confirmed at operation in all 25 operated patients. In 2 patients both echocardiographic techniques had missed the perforation of the cusps of the aortic valve that was seen at operation, but this had no effect on patient management. Transoesophageal echocardiography is the best diagnostic approach when infective endocarditis is suspected in patients with either native or prosthetic valves.

Jaffe and associates[33] in Seattle, Washington, used the echocardiograms and clinical records of 70 patients with infective endocarditis evaluated between 1983 and 1988 to determine the role of 2-dimensional and Doppler echocardiography in diagnosis and in identifying risk factors for morbidity and mortality. A blinded observer reviewed the echocardiograms for the presence and size of vegetations and the severity of the valvular regurgitation. Vegetations were identified in 54 (78%) of 69 technically satisfactory echocardiograms. In 38 patients whose hearts were examined at surgery or autopsy, all vegetations diagnosed by echocardiography were confirmed, but six additional vegetations were found.

Abnormal ($\geq 2+$) valvular regurgitation occurred in 88% of patients. No patient with $\leq 1+$ regurgitation (n = 8) died or required valve surgery for heart failure, but 3 of the 8 patients underwent surgery for mycotic aneurysms, recurrent embolism, or paravalvular abscesses. In patients without embolism before echocardiography, there was a trend toward a greater incidence of subsequent embolization in those with vegetations >10 mm in size (26% compared with 11% with vegetations ≤ 10 mm). By multivariate analysis, risk factors for in-hospital death (n = 7) were an infected prosthetic valve, systemic embolism and infection with S. aureus. Thus, if valvular regurgitation is $\leq 1+$, the risk in-hospital for death is low and progression to cardiac surgery for hemodynamic instability is not likely; 2) there is a trend toward a higher risk of embolization in patients with vegetations >10 mm in size; 3) early mortality appears to be related importantly to infected prosthetic valves, systemic embolism, and S. aureus infections; and 4) when a paravalvular abscess or prosthetic valve endocarditis is suspected, transthoracic echocardiographic findings may be equivocal and transesophageal echocardiography may be helpful.

Staphylococcal species as a cause

To determine the characteristics of infective endocarditis in a single hospital, Sanabria and associates[34] from Worcester, Massachusetts, reviewed all patients with that diagnosis at the University of Massachusetts Medical Center between 1981 and 1988. Of 113 patients with infective endocarditis, 56 (50%) had staphylococcal endocarditis. Despite aggressive medical and surgical therapy, in-hospital mortality was 25%. Forty-five (80%) of the 56 cases of staphylococcal endocarditis involved *Staphylococcus aureus* with a mortality of 28% vs 9% in the non-S aureus group. Mortality was higher in patients with CHF (35%), AV block (45%), AF (42%), and prosthetic valve endocarditis (50%). Seventy-six percent of the patients with CHF had surgery. Patients with CHF and S aureus infection had a mortality of 45%. Thirty-six patients (64%) were alive at late follow-up (mean, 29 months). Mortality was highest (23%) during the first 3 months following diagnosis of staphylococcal endocarditis. Staphylococcal endocarditis represents an increasingly large proportion of patients with infective endocarditis. Mortality rates remain high despite aggressive management.

Antibiotic prophylaxis

The Endocarditis Working Party of the British Society for Antimicrobial Chemotherapy published recommendations for the antibiotic prophylaxis of infective endocarditis.[35] The recommendations are published in Table 6-1.

Dajani and associates[36] summarized recommendations of a committee of the American Heart Association for prevention of bacterial endocarditis. These recommendations are an update of those made by the committee in 1984 and they incorporate new data and include opinions of national and international experts. The recommended standard prophylactic regimen for dental, oral or upper respiratory tract procedures in patients who are at risk are summarized in Table 6-2. Alternate prophylactic regimens for dental, oral, and upper respiratory tract procedures in patients at risk are summarized in Table 6-3, and regimens for genitourinary/gastrointestinal procedures in Table 6-4.

TABLE 6-1. *Recommendations for endocarditis prophylaxis. Reproduced with permission from Simmons, et al.*[35]

(1) *Dental Extractions, Scaling, or Peridontal Surgery Under local or no anaesthesia*	*Special risk patients who should be referred to hospital:* (i) Patients with prosthetic valves who are to have a general anaesthetic
(a) For patients not allergic to penicillin and not prescribed penicillin more than once in the previous month:	(ii) Patients who are to have a general anaesthetic *and* who are allergic to penicillin or have had a penicillin more than once in the previous month
Amoxycillin Adults: 3 g single oral dose taken under supervison 1 hour before dental procedure Children under 10: half adult dose Children under 5: quarter adult dose	(iii) Patients who have had a previous attack of endocarditis Recommendations for these patients are:
(b) For patients allergic to penicillin: *Erythromycin stearate* Adults: 1·5 g orally taken under supervision 1–2 hours before dental procedure plus 0·5 g 6 hours later Children under 10: half adult dose Children under 5: quarter adult dose	*(d)* For patients not allergic to penicillin and who have not had penicillin more than once in the previous month: Adults: 1 g amoxycillin intramuscularly in 2·5 ml 1% lignocaine hydrochloride *plus* 120 mg gentamicin intramuscularly just before induction: then 0·5 g amoxycillin orally 6 h later Children under 10: amoxycillin, half adult dose; gentamicin 2 mg/kg body weight
or *Clindamycin* Adults: 600 mg single oral dose taken under supervision 1 hour before dental procedure Children under 10: 6 mg/kg body weight single oral dose taken under supervision 1 hour before dental procedure	*(e)* For patients allergic to penicillin or who have had penicillin more than once in the previous month. Adults: vancomycin 1 g by slow intravenous infusion over 60 min followed by gentamicin 120 mg intravenously just before induction or 15 min before the surgical procedure Children under 10: vancomycin 20 mg/kg intravenously, gentamicin 2 mg/kg intravenously
Under general anaesthesia *(c)* For patients not allergic to penicillin and not given penicillin more than once in the previous month:	**(2)** *Surgery or Instrumentation of Upper Respiratory Tract* Recommended cover is as for 1(a) to 1(e), but any postoperative antibiotic may have to be given intramuscularly or intravenously if swallowing is painful.
Amoxycillin intramuscularly Adults: 1 g in 2·5 ml 1% lignocaine hydrochloride just before induction plus 0·5 by mouth 6 hours later Children under 10: half adult dose	**(3)** *Genitourinary Surgery or Instrumentation* For patients with sterile urine the suggested cover is directed against faecal streptococci and is as for 1(d) or 1(e) above. If the urine is infected prophylaxis should also cover the pathogens involved.
or *Amoxycillin orally* Adults 3 g oral dose 4 hours before anaesthesia followed by a further 3 g by mouth as soon as possible after operation Children under 10: half adult dose Children under 5: quarter adult dose	**(4)** *Obstetric and Gynaecological Procedures* Cover is suggested only for patients with prosthetic valves, and is as for 1(d) or 1(e) because of the risk from faecal streptococci
or *Amoxycillin and probenecid orally* Adults: amoxycillin 3 g together with probenecid 1 g orally 4 hours before operation	**(5)** *Gastrointestinal Procedures* Cover is suggested only for patients with prosthetic valves and is as for 1(d) or 1(e).

TABLE 6-2. *Recommended standard prophylactic regimen for dental, oral, or upper respiratory tract procedures in patients who are at risk.** *Reproduced with permission from Dajani, et al.*[36]

Drug	Dosing Regiment
	Standard Regimen
Amoxicillin	3.0 g orally 1 h before procedure; then 1.5 g 6 h after initial dose
	Amoxicillin/Penicillin-Allergic Patients
Erythromycin or	Erythromycin ethylsuccinate, 800 mg, or erythromycin stearate, 1.0 g, orally 2 h before procedure; then half the dose 6 h after initial dose
Clindamycin	300 mg orally 1 h before procedure and 150 mg 6 h after initial dose

*Includes those with prosthetic heart valves and other high-risk patients.
†Initial pediatric doses are as follows: amoxicillin, 50 mg/kg; erythromycin ethylsuccinate or erythromycin stearate, 20 mg/kg; and clindamycin, 10 mg/kg. Follow-up doses should be one half the initial dose. **Total pediatric dose should not exceed total adult dose.** The following weight ranges may also be used for the initial pediatric dose of amoxicillin: <15 kg, 750 mg; 15 to 30 kg, 1500 mg; and >30 kg, 3000 mg (full adult dose).

VALVE REPLACEMENT

Transesophageal echocardiography

Sheikh and associates[37] in Durham, North Carolina, used intraoperative transesophageal echocardiography during cardiac surgery in 154 consecutive patients who had a valve operation with pre- and postcar-

TABLE 6-3. *Alternate prophylactic regimens for dental, oral, or upper respiratory tract procedures in patients who are at risk. Reproduced with permission from Dajani, et al.*[36]

Drug	Dosing Regimen*
Patients Unable to Take Oral Medications	
Ampicillin	Intravenous or intramuscular administration of ampicillin, 2.0 g, 30 min before procedure; then intravenous or intramuscular administration of ampicillin, 1.0 g, or oral administration of amoxicillin, 1.5 g, 6 h after initial dose
Ampicillin/Amoxicillin/Penicillin-Allergic Patients Unable to Take Oral Medications	
Clindamycin	Intravenous administration of 300 mg 30 min before procedure and an intravenous or oral administration of 150 mg 6 h after initial dose
Patients Considered High Risk and Not Candidates for Standard Regimen	
Ampicillin, gentamicin, and amoxicillin	Intravenous or intramuscular administration of ampicillin, 2.0 g, plus gentamicin, 1.5 mg/kg (not to exceed 80 mg), 30 min before procedure; followed by amoxicillin, 1.5 g, orally 6 h after initial dose; alternatively, the parenteral regimen may be repeated 8 h after initial dose
Ampicillin/Amoxicillin/Penicillin-Allergic Patients Considered High Risk	
Vancomycin	Intravenous administration of 1.0 g over 1 h, starting 1 h before procedure; no repeated dose necessary

*Initial pediatric doses are as follows: ampicillin, 50 mg/kg; clindamycin, 10 mg/kg; gentamicin, 2.0 mg/kg; and vancomycin, 20 mg/kg. Follow-up doses should be one half the initial dose. **Total pediatric dose should not exceed total adult dose.** No initial dose is recommended in this table for amoxicillin (25 mg/kg is the follow-up dose).

TABLE 6-4. *Regimens for genitourinary/gastrointestinal procedures. Reproduced with permission from Dajani, et al.*[36]

Drug	Dosage Regimen*
Standard Regimen	
Ampicillin, gentamicin, and amoxicillin	Intravenous or intramuscular administration of ampicillin, 2.0 g, plus gentamicin, 1.5 mg/kg (not to exceed 80 mg), 30 min before procedure; followed by amoxicillin, 1.5 g, orally 6 h after initial dose; alternatively, the parenteral regimen may be repeated once 8 h after initial dose
Ampicillin/Amoxicillin/Penicillin-Allergic Patient Regimen	
Vancomycin and gentamicin	Intravenous administration of vancomycin, 1.0 g, over 1 h plus intravenous or intramuscular administration of gentamicin, 1.5 mg/kg (not to exceed 80 mg), 1 h before procedure; may be repeated once 8 h after initial dose
Alternate Low-Risk Patient Regimen	
Amoxicillin	3.0 g orally 1 h before procedure; then 1.5 g 6 h after initial dose

*Initial pediatric doses are as follows: ampicillin, 50 mg/kg; amoxicillin, 50 mg/kg; gentamicin, 2.0 mg/kg; and vancomycin, 20 mg/kg. Follow-up doses should be half the initial dose. **Total pediatric dose should not exceed total adult dose.**

diopulmonary bypass. Prebypass imaging yielded unsuspected findings that either assisted or changed the planned operation in 29 (19%) of 154 patients. Imaging immediately after valve replacement revealed unsatisfactory operative results that necessitated immediate further surgery in 10 (6%) of 154 patients. Post valve replacement LV dysfunction prompting administration of inotropic agents was identified in 13 patients (8%). Transesophageal echocardiography proved most useful when both 2-dimensional and Doppler color flow imaging were employed in patients undergoing a MVR, where surgical decisions based on echocardiographic results were made in 26 (41%) of 64 cases. Postbypass echocardiographic findings identified patients at risk for an adverse postoperative outcome.

Among 123 patients whose postbypass valve function was judged to be satisfactory, 18 (15%) had a major postoperative complication and 6 (5%) died. In 7 patients with moderate residual valve dysfunction, 6 (86%) had a postoperative complication and 3 (43%) died (p <0.05). Among 131 patients with preserved postbypass LV function, 12 (9%) had a major complication and 7 (5%) died, whereas among 23 patients with reduced ventricular function, 17 (73%) had a postoperative complication and 6 (26%) died. These data include that intraoperative transesophageal echocardiography is useful in developing a surgical plan, assessing immediate operative results, and identifying patients with unsatisfactory results who may be at increased risk for postoperative complications.

Mitral valve repair vs replacement

Obarski and associates[38] from Cleveland, Ohio, reviewed 335 consecutive patients who had isolated mitral valve operations for MR and no significant CAD. The patients were reviewed for the presence of a perioperative AMI. Of 224 patients undergoing mitral valve repair, 12 (5.4%) had electrocardiographic and cardiac enzyme evidence of perioperative AMI. Of 111 patients undergoing MVR none had perioperative AMI develop as determined by electrocardiographic and enzyme criteria. All 12 infarctions after valve repair involved the inferior wall by electrocardiographic or echocardiographic criteria. Although no patient had significant clinical difficulty in recovery, 7 of the 12 patients were left with Q waves upon hospital discharge. The etiology of the AMI is believed to be air emboli introduced at the time of testing valve competence during LV insufflation under pressure. Changes in surgical technique may reduce or eliminate this complication.

Isolated mitral valve replacement

To determine how survival and clinical status were related to LV size and systolic function after MVR, Crawford and colleagues[39] from Albuquerque, New Mexico, evaluated 104 patients (48 MR, 33 MS, and 23 MS/MR) with isolated MVR before and after surgery. Preoperative hemodynamic abnormalities by cardiac catheterization were improved 6 months after surgery in all 3 patient groups. The patients with MR had reductions in LV end-diastolic volume index (117 to 89 ml/m, and EF (0.56 to 0.45); however the ratio of forward stroke volume to end-diastolic volume increased (0.32 to 0.245) because of the elimination of regurgitant volume. Survival analysis revealed that mortality was significantly higher in MS or MS/MR patients with postoperative end-diastolic volume index >101 ml/m and in MR patients with postoperative EF ≤0.50. Also, most patients with MR or MS/MR and postoperative end-diastolic volume index >101 ml/m and EF ≤0.50 were in New York Heart Association class III or IV. Multivariate logistic regression analysis in the patients with MR revealed that the strongest predictor of postoperative EF was preoperative EF. Preoperative mean PA pressure ≤20 mm was a significant determinant of postoperative end-diastolic volume increased index less than or equal to 101 ml/m in patients with MR. The most significant predictor of persistent LV enlargement in patients with MR or MS/MR was a large endsystolic volume index before operation. Therefore, these investigators concluded that surgery should be considered in MR and MS/MR patients before EF decreases to <0.50, end-diastolic volume index is >50 ml/m, or PA hypertension develops.

Hennein and associates[40] from Bethesda, Maryland, studied 69 patients with isolated MR who underwent MVR before and 6 months after operation by treadmill exercise testing, cardiac catheterization, echocardiography, and radionuclide angiography. Nine patients underwent MVR with preservation of the entire mitral apparatus and 5 with preservation of the posterior leaflet and attached chordae. The remaining 55 patients had MVR with complete excision of the native valve. Preoperatively, there were no differences among groups in age, gender, exercise capacity, cardiac index, rest or exercise EF, fractional shortening, or pulmonary artery pressures. There were 4 perioperative deaths (7%) and 8 late deaths among the 55 patients with chordal resection but no early or late deaths of patients whose chordae were preserved. In patients in whom the chordae were excised, exercise capacity, LV systolic dimensions, and cardiac index did not improve after MVR, and LV function deteriorated, as evidenced by a reduction of both the resting and exercise EF (from 46% ± 13% to 31% ± 13%, and from 49% ± 12% to 37% ± 14%, respectively) and fractional shortening (from 34% ± 10% to 26% ± 14%). In contrast, exercise capacity improved after MVR in patients in whom the entire apparatus was spared (by 4 ± 3 minutes), LV systolic dimensions decreased (from 44 ± 8 to 36 ± 9 mm), and LV function was maintained or improved, as evidenced by preservation of the resting EF (preoperative, 50% ± 14%; postoperative, 54% ± 11%), exercise EF (46% ± 16% versus 52% ± 9%), fractional shortening (from 31% ± 9% to 18% ± 9%), and an increase in the cardiac index (from 2.0 ± 0.3 to 2.7 ± 0.5 L/min/m²). No statistically significant differences between posterior chordal resection only and preservation of the entire apparatus were found. These data demonstrate that postoperative survival, exercise capacity, and LV function are better in patients who undergo MVR with chordal preservation than in patients in whom the chordae are excised.

Recent studies have suggested that excision of the mitral valve apparatus during MVR impairs LV performance. Functional measurements in humans have been difficult to obtain in a load-independent fashion. To investigate this concept, Harpole and associates[41] from Durham, North Carolina, studied 12 patients, mean age 65 ± 8 years and mean New York Heart Association functional class 3.3 ± 0.7, with 4+/4+ MR (n = 8) or MS (valve area, 1.2 ± 0.2 cm²) (n = 4) who underwent prosthetic valve replacement using crystalloid cardioplegia. No patient required therapeutic inotropic support, every patient had at least the anterior mitral leaflet excised, and paced heart rate was maintained constant throughout. LV volume was measured with radionuclide angiocardiography, LV pressure with a 3F micromanometer, and LV wall volume with 2-dimensional transesophageal echocardiography. LV preload was varied over a mean end-diastolic pressure range of 9 to 20 mm Hg and an end-diastolic volume range of 134 to 170 m to generate 4 to 5 steady-state pressure-volume loops before and 10 minutes after cardiopulmonary bypass. LV performance was estimated with the stroke work/end-diastolic volume relation. After bypass, no significant change was noted in wall volume for patients with MR or MS (175 ± 68 to 189 ± 63 mL/m² and 130 ± 22 to 127 ± 19 mL/m², respectively). The stroke work/end-diastolic volume relations were highly linear before and after bypass. These data suggest that partial excision of the mitral apparatus does not significantly impair LV performance during the early period after routine valve replacement.

Isolated aortic valve replacement

To evaluate the effect of LV dysfunction on Doppler-derived trans-prosthetic hemodynamic indexes in patients with normally functioning St. Jude medical prostheses in the aortic valve position, Ren and associates[42] from Philadelphia, Pennsylvania, studied 74 consecutive patients. LVEF was assessed by using Simpson's biplane rule. The 34 patients with normal EF (≥0.51) (group A) generally had the highest values of peak (31 ± 13 mm Hg) and mean (16 ± 6 mm Hg) gradients, whereas 19 patients with moderate to severe reduction of EF (≤0.31) (group C) had the lowest values (17 ± 6 and 9 ± 3 mm Hg, respectively). Significant decreases for acceleration and corrected (for heart rate) velocity time integral in group C were noted compared to group A, and group B (21 patients with mild to moderately reduced EF [0.50 to 0.32]). A significant inverse correlation for Doppler-derived peak and mean gradients and corrected velocity time integral was demonstrated with increasing aortic valve prosthetic sizes from 19 to 29 mm in group A patients but less so in group B or C. Thus, in addition to valve size, LV function should be considered an important factor in detecting prosthetic valvular flow characteristics and dysfunction. A normal derived velocity and gradient in patients with moderately to severely depressed LV function may not rule out significant valvular stenosis.

Dumesnil and associates[43] in Sainte-Foy, Quebec, Canada used Doppler echocardiographic evaluation of aortic valve prostheses to study the validity and usefulness of the Doppler valve gradient and area measurements in 31 patients with a mean age of 69 ± 10 years 20 ± 4 months after implantation of a given type of aortic bioprosthesis ranging in size from 19 to 29 mm. Valve area data obtained with both the standard and simplified continuity equations were compared with known in vitro prosthetic valve area measurements and an excellent correlation was obtained between the standard and simplified continuity equations and between in vivo and known in vitro prosthetic valve areas. Peak gradients ranged from 11 to 75 mm Hg and mean gradient from 8 to 44 mm Hg. The relations were improved by indexing valve area by body surface area. The best correlations were obtained between indexed valve area and a quadratic function of the gradient. This study has helped validate the use of either the standard or the simplified continuity equation for the noninvasive Doppler echocardiographic assessment of intrinsic aortic bioprosthesis function. Peak and mean valve gradient data are less useful because they depend on cardiac output.

Taniguchi and colleagues[44] in Osaka, Japan, evaluated LV ejection performance, wall stress, and contractile state in 35 patients with chronic AR. Cineangiography and pressure measurements were obtained before and a mean of 26 months after AVR, and data were compared with those from 30 normal control subjects. The relation between quantitative changes in wall stress and changes in EF after surgery was determined. Preoperatively, end-systolic stress was elevated in patients with AR and EF was depressed. End-systolic stress decreased postoperatively and EF increased. The magnitude of increase in EF correlated significantly and negatively with the quantitative change in end-systolic stress after surgery. Contractile function, as assessed by the ejection phase index-end-systolic stress relation, did not significantly change; 23 of 35 patients preoperatively and 18 of 35 patients postoperatively had values that clearly fell below the 95% confidence limit of the EF-end-systolic stress relation for controls. Moreover, persistent postoperative LV hypertrophy was significantly associated with persistent contractile dysfunction. Thus, late improvement in LV ejection performance after AVR can be attributed to the reduction in end-systolic stress. Contractile function itself was not improved by surgery.

Kurnik and associates[45] from Camden, New Jersey, measured LV mass and function using ultrafast computed tomography, and correlated it with clinical status in 17 patients with AS and/or AR undergoing AVR or balloon valvuloplasty. Wall mass was 159 ± 38 gm/m² initially, decreased 25% to 116 ± 29 gm/m² at 4 months, and decreased a total of 34% to 105 ± 33 gm/m² at 8 months after valve repair. By 8 months not only was the mean wall mass within the normal range, but only 3 patients retained abnormal hypertrophy. EF increased 8%. Clinical function improved in all patients, with only 3 patients remaining outside of New York Heart Association functional class I at 8 months. Regression of ventricular mass into the normal range correlated with attainment of class I functional status, despite a lack of increase of EF.

Hoffman and Burckhardt[46] from Basel, Switzerland, screened 100 patients aged 24 to 78 years prospectively a mean of 71 months after AVR for the presence of LV hypertrophy on the electrocardiogram and for repetitive VPCs (≥2 couplets/24 hr) during 24-hour Holter monitoring. During the subsequent 41-month follow-up (range 10 to 50 months), the yearly cardiac mortality rate was 1% in patients with LV hypertrophy, 3% in patients with VPCs, and 9% in patients with LV hypertrophy plus VPCs but only 0.6% when none of these factors was present. The patient groups did not differ with regard to age, time elapsed since operation, underlying valve lesions, and CAD. Both LV hypertrophy and VPCs occurred more frequently in patients with LV dysfunction. Thus, after AVR cardiac mortality is markedly increased in patients with LV hypertrophy and repetitive VPCs, since they are noninvasive markers of LV dysfunction.

Late follow-up of porcine bioprosthesis

Jones and associates[47] from Atlanta, Georgia, reported experiences in 440 patients having isolated MVR, 522 patients having isolated AVR, and in 88 patients having MVR plus AVR between 1974 and 1981. Patients with associated surgical procedures were excluded. Mean follow-up was 8.3 years. At 10 years, there was no difference in patient survival between those having AVR and those having MVR. Reoperations were performed on 192 patients. Endocarditis was the reason for reoperation in 3.7% of patients who had MVR and 10.6% of those who had AVR. Structural valve degeneration was the reason for reoperation in 90% of MVR patients and 79% of AVR patients. Hospital mortality among patients having valve reoperations was 5%. At 10 years, the freedom from valve reoperation for all causes and from structural valve degeneration was significantly better for the AVR group than the MVR group (74% ± 3% vs 61% ± 4%; and 79% ± 3% vs 63% ± 4%, respectively). For patients in their 60s, the 10-year freedom from reoperation was 92% ± 2% for AVR and 80% ± 6% for MVR. At 10 years, freedom from cardiac-related death and valve reoperation was best for MVR and AVR patients in their 60s. Patients 70 years old or older rarely had reoperation but died before valve failure occurred. The 10-year freedom from all major valve-related events (cardiac-related death, reoperation, thromboembolism, endocarditis, and anticoagulant-related bleeding) was practically the same for both MVR and AVR patients (48% ± 3%, respectively). Patients in their 70s have an extremely low rate of reoperation but a high rate of cardiac-related death and do not outlive the prostheses.

The Carpentier-Edwards standard porcine bioprosthesis was implanted in 1190 patients (1201 operations, 1303 bioprosthesis) between January, 1975 and June, 1986 and the results of these valve operations were reported by Jamieson and associates[48] from Vancouver, Canada. The mean age of patients was 57 years (range 8 to 85 years). The early mortality was 8% (AVR 5%, MVR 9%, and MVR 15%). Late mortality was 4% per patient-year (AVR 4%, MVR 4%, and MVR 4%). The total cumulative follow-up period was 6737 years. Thromboembolism was 2% per patient-year (fatal 0.4% per patient-year) (minor 0.6%, major 0.9%); antithromboembolic therapy-related hemorrhage was 0.5% (fatal 0.1%); prosthetic valve endocarditis was 0.6% (fatal 0.2%); nonstructural dysfunction was 0.5% (fatal 0.2%); and structural valve deterioration and/or primary tissue failure was 1.5% per patient-year (fatal, 0.2% per patient-year). Thromboembolism and structural valve deterioration were the significant complications, structural valve deterioration occurring primarily between the 6th and 10th year of evaluation. The overall patient survival was 65% for AVR and 55% for MVR at 10 years. The patients were classified as 93% New York Heart Association functional classes III and IV preoperatively and 92% classes I and II postoperatively. Freedom at 10 years from thromboembolism was 84% for AVR and 77% for MVR; structural valve deterioration was 79% for AVR and 72% for MVR; reoperation was 74% for AVR and 67% for MVR. Freedom from all valve-related complications at 10 years was 59% for AVR and 47% for MVR; valve-related mortality was 90% for AVR and 83% for MVR; mortality and reoperation was 59% for AVR and 47% for MVR; mortality and residual morbidity (treatment failure) was 87% for AVR and 75% for MVR; mortality, residual morbidity, and reoperation were 66% for AVR and 55% for MVR.

Flow characteristics of bioprostheses

Rashtian and associates[49] from Los Angeles and Loma Linda, California, and Atlanta, Georgia, reviewed the in vivo and in vitro fluid dynamic performance of 3 bioprosthetic heart valves, Hancock porcine valves (standard models 242 aortic and 342 mitral and modified orifice model 250 aortic), Carpentier-Edwards porcine valves (models 2625 aortic and 6625 mitral), and the Ionescu-Shiley pericardial valve. These valves were chosen because of their past or present popularity in clinical use and because of the variation in fluid dynamic performance reported by different investigators. The flow parameters reported include in vivo and in vitro mean pressure drop, cardiac output or cardiac index, regurgitant volume, effective orifice area, and performance index. These data provide a framework for differentiation of normal and abnormal bioprosthetic valve function.

St. Jude medical prosthesis

Nair and associates[50] from Omaha, Nebraska, reported their 10-year experience with 165 patients (100 men and 65 women, mean age 58 ± 13 years) who underwent valve replacement with a St. Jude medical prosthesis. Of the 165 patients, 147 were treated with warfarin. A prothrombin time 1.3 to 1.8 times control (range 15 to 20 seconds) was maintained in 134 patients with single valve and 1.8 to 2 times control (range 20 to 25 seconds) in 13 patients with double valve prostheses. The

10-year actuarial event-free incidence from thromboembolic and hemorrhagic complications was 84 and 95%, respectively. Of the 8 patients receiving antiplatelet therapy alone, 4 had thromboembolic events. Of the 10 patients on neither warfarin nor antiplatelet therapy, 3 had thromboembolic events. The 10-year actuarial event-free incidence from valve failure was 95%. The 10-year actuarial patient survival was 55%. Thus, the St. Jude valve is a safe and reliable prosthesis with acceptable overall long-term performance in patients given a modest anticoagulation regimen. Patients who receive St. Jude prosthetic valves without anticoagulants have a high incidence of thromboembolic events despite therapy with antiplatelet agents.

Left atrial dimensions and systemic emboli afterwards

Burchfiel and associates[51] in Denver, Colorado; Asheville, North Carolina; Hines, Illinois; San Antonio, Texas; and Los Angeles, California, evaluated the relationship between LA dimension measured by M-mode echocardiography and systemic embolization after valve replacement in 397 patients with a prosthetic valve enrolled in the Department of Veterans Affairs Cooperative Study on Valvular Heart Disease. Baseline clinical characteristics included several measures of LA dilatation that were compared in 31 patients who developed systemic embolism and 366 who did not during a 5-year follow-up. The incidence of systemic embolism was >3 times higher after MVR than after AVR (4.4 and 1.3 per 100 patient-years, respectively). This difference persisted after adjustment for other factors. Univariate analysis indicated a 3-fold higher incidence of systemic embolism in patients with a LA dimension ≥4 cm compared with that in patients with a LA dimension ≤4 cm. When the effect of valve location was taken into account, LA dimensions were not associated with an increased risk for systemic embolism. In multivariate analysis, AF, age, EF and location of the prosthetic valve were significantly associated with embolism. Thus, LA dimension is not independently related to the development of systemic embolism in patients undergoing valve replacement.

Anticoagulation

Saour and associates[52] from Riyadh, Saudi Arabia, and Bedford Park, Australia, compared the efficacy and complications of anticoagulation with warfarin in 258 patients with prosthetic cardiac valves treated with regimens of "moderate intensity" (prothrombin-time ratio, 1.5; international normalized ratio, 2.65) or "high intensity" (prothrombin-time ratio, 2.5; international normalized ratio, 9) in a prospective randomized study. The 2 patient groups were followed up for 421 patient-years and 436 patient-years, respectively. Eleven patients were lost to follow-up. Thromboembolism occurred with similar frequency in the 2 groups, but there was a total of 6.2 bleeding episodes per 100 patient-years in the moderate-intensity group and 12.1 episodes in the high-intensity group. There were 5.2 episodes of minor bleeding per 100 patient-years in the moderate-intensity group and 10.1 episodes in the high-intensity group. Major bleeding also was more common in the high-intensity group (2.1 episodes per 100 patient-years—including the only 2 fatal hemorrhages—as compared with 0.95 episode in the moderate-intensity group. The authors concluded that a moderate anticoagulant effect (prothrombin-time ratio, about 1.5) in patients with a mechanical prosthesis offers protection equivalent to that of more intensive therapy, but at a significantly lower risk.

Hospitalizations for patients with prosthetic heart valves undergoing non-cardiac surgery are frequently prolonged for intravenous heparin therapy to decrease the incidence of thromboembolism while patients are not taking oral anticoagulant agents. Because the rate of thromboembolic events is low and the period of increased risk is short, the cost of preventing these rare events can be great (Table 6-5). Eckman and associates[53] from Boston, Massachusetts, performed cost-effectiveness analyses addressing these issues. The authors calculated the marginal cost per additional quality-adjusted year of life gained per thromboembolic event averted and per death averted. The authors concluded that the marginal cost of prolonging hospitalization to administer heparin is prohibitively high compared with most contemporary therapies, except when the patient has the most thrombogenic of valves.

References

1. Marsalese DL, Moodie DS, Lytle BW, Cosgrove DM, Ratliff NB, Goormastic M, Kovacs A: Cystic medial necrosis of the aorta in patients without Marfan's syndrome: Surgical outcome and long-term follow-up. J Am Coll Cardiol 1990 (July);16:68–73.
2. Khamashta MA, Cervera R, Asherson RA, Font J, Gil A, Coltart DJ, Vazquez JJ, Pare C, Ingelmo M, Oliver J, Hughes GRV: Association of antibodies against phospholipids with heart valve disease in systemic lupus erythematosis. Lancet 1990 (June 30);335:1541–1544.
3. Lundin L, Landelius J, Andren B, Oberg K: Transoesophageal echocardiography improves the diagnostic value of cardiac ultrasound in patients with carcinoid heart disease. Br Heart J 1990 (Sept);64:190–194.
4. Lundin L, Hansson HE, Landelius J, Oberg K: Surgical treatment of carcinoid heart disease. J Thorac Cardiovasc Surg 1990 (Oct);100:552–561.
5. Tofler OB, Tofler GH: Use of auscultation to follow patients with mitral systolic clicks and murmurs. Am J Cardiol 1990 (Dec 1);66:1355–1358.

TABLE 6-5. *Thromboembolic complications of valvular prostheses. Reproduced with permission from Eckman, et al.*[53]

| Valve Position | Valve Type | Incidence of Thromboemboli per 100 Patient-Years | | | |
| | | Emboli in Patients Receiving Anticoagulant Therapy | | Valve Thrombosis | |
		Fatal	Nonfatal	Anticoagulant Therapy	No Anticoagulant Therapy
Aortic	Ball	0.61	2.75	0.03	1.32
	Bjork-Shiley	0.65	1.64	0.33	3.14
	Lillehei-Kaster	0.11	2.30	0.48	3.40
	St Jude	0.00	0.70	0.00	1.64
Mitral	Ball	1.11	7.59	0.55	...
	Bjork-Shiley	0.80	3.69	0.70	5.74*
	Lillehei-Kaster	1.04	3.27	2.26	10.40
	St Jude	0.00	3.60	0.00	1.64

*Sutton and colleagues reported this rate in patients treated with dipyridamole. While we could not find any adequate series describing the rate of thrombosis for Bjork-Shiley valves in the mitral position in patients not receiving anticoagulant therapy, Sutton et al reiterated Bjork's contention that the frequency of thromboembolism in patients treated with dipyridamole was the same as that in patients receiving no treatment at all.

6. You-Bing D, Takenaka K, Sakamoto T, Hada Y, Suzuki J, Shiota T, Amano W, Igarashi T, Amano K, Takahashi H, Sugimoto T: Follow-up in mitral valve prolapse by phonocardiography, M-mode and two-dimensional echocardiography and Doppler echocardiography. Am J Cardiol 1990 (Feb 1);65:349–354.

7. Grayburn PA, Berk MR, Spain MG, Harrison MR, Smith MD, DeMaria AN: Relation of echocardiographic morphology of the mitral apparatus to mitral regurgitation in mitral valve prolapse: Assessment by Doppler color flow imaging. Am Heart J 1990 (May);119:1095–1102.

8. Pai RG, Bansal RC, Shah PM: Doppler-Derived Rate of Left Ventricular Pressure Rise Its Correlation with the Postoperative Left Ventricular Function in Mitral Regurgitation. Circulation 1990 (August);82:514–520.

9. Fredman CS, Pearson AC, Labovitz AJ, Kern MJ: Comparison of hemodynamic pressure half-time method and Gorlin formula with Doppler and echocardiographic determinations of mitral valve area in patients with combined mitral stenosis and regurgitation. Am Heart J 1990 (January);119:121–129.

10. Nishimura RA, Holmes DR Jr, Reeder GS: Percutaneous balloon valvuloplasty. Mayo Clin Proc 1990 (Feb);65:198–220.

11. Chen CR, Huang ZD, Lo ZX, Cheng TO: Comparison of single rubber-nylon balloon and double polyethylene balloon valvuloplasty in 94 patients with rheumatic mitral stenosis. Am Heart J 1990 (January);119:102–111.

12. Ruiz CE, Allen JW, Lau FYK: Percutaneous double balloon valvotomy for severe rheumatic mitral stenosis. Am J Cardiol 1990 (Feb 15);65:473–477.

13. Herrmann HC, Kleaveland JP, Hill JA, Cowley MJ, Margolis JR, Nocero MA, Zalewski A, Pepine CJ, for the M-Heart Group: The M-heart percutaneous balloon mitral valvuloplasty registry: Initial results and early follow-up. J Am Coll Cardiol 1990 (May);15:1221–6.

14. Casale P, Block PC, O'Shea JP, Palacios IF. Atrial septal defect after percutaneous mitral balloon valvuloplasty: Immediate results and follow-up. J Am Coll Cardiol 1990 (May);15:1300–4.

15. Abascal VM, Wilkins GT, O'Shea JP, Choong CY, Palacios IF, Thomas JD, Rosas Emma, Newell JB, Block PC, Weyman AE: Prediction of Successful Outcome in 130 Patients Undergoing Percutaneous Balloon Mitral Valvotomy. Circulation 1990 (August);82:448–456.

16. Ishikura F, Nagata S, Yasuda S, Yamashita N, Miyatake K: Residual atrial septal perforation after percutaneous transvenous mitral commissurotomy with Inoue balloon catheter. Am Heart J 1990 (October);120:873–881.

17. Lewis R, Raff H, Findling JW, Dorros G: Stimulation of atrial natriuretic peptide and vasopressin during retrograde mitral valvuloplasty. Am Heart J 1990 (December);120:1305–1310.

18. Pellikka PA, Nishimura RA, Bailey KR, Tajik AJ: The national history of adults with asymptomatic, hemodynamically significant aortic stenosis. J Am Coll Cardiol 1990 (April);15:1012–7.

19. Leach RM, McBrien DJ: Brachioradial delay: A new clinical indicator of the severity of aortic stenosis. Lancet 1990 (May 19);335:1199–1201.

20. Roger VL, Tajik AJ, Bailey KR, Oh JK, Taylor CL, Seward JB: Progression of aortic stenosis in adults: New appraisal using Doppler echocardiography. Am Heart J 1990 (February);119:331–338.

21. Harpole DH, Davidson C, Skelton T, Jones RH, Bashore TM: Serial evaluation of ventricular function after percutaneous aortic balloon valvuloplasty. Am Heart J 1990 (January);119:130–135.

22. Rodriguez AR, Kleiman NS, Minor ST, Zoghbi WA, West MS, DeFelice CA, Samuels DA, Cashion R, Pickett JD, Lewis JM, Raizner AE: Factors influencing the outcome of balloon aortic valvuloplasty in the elderly. Am Heart J 1990 (August);120:373–380.

23. Davidson CJ, Harrison JK, Leithe ME, Kisslo KB, Bashore TM: Left ventricular performance and clinical outcome after repeat balloon aortic valvuloplasty. An Intern Med 1990 (Aug 1);113:250–252.

24. Tunick PA, Gindea A, Kronzoni: Effect of aortic valve replacement for aortic stenosis on severity of mitral regurgitation. Am J Cardiol 1990 (May 15);65:1219–1221.

25. Dumesnil JG, Tran K, Dagenais GR: Beneficial long-term effects of hydralazine in aortic regurgitation. Arch Intern Med 1990 (April);150:757–760.

26. Scognamiglio R, Fasoli G, Ponchia A, Dalla-Volta S: Long-term nifedipine unloading therapy in asymptomatic patients with chronic severe aortic regurgitation. J Am Coll Cardiol 1990 (August);16:424–9.

27. Tornos MP, Permanyer-Miralda G, Evangelista A, Worner F, Candell J, Garcia-del-Castillo H, Soler-Soler J: Clinical evaluation of a prospective protocol for the timing of surgery in chronic aortic regurgitation. Am Heart J 1990 (September);120:649–657.

28. Minagoe S, Rahimtoola SH, Chandraratna PAN: Significance of laminar systolic regurgitant flow in patients with tricusoid regurgitation: A combined pulsed-wave, continuous-wave Doppler and two-dimensional echocardiographic study. Am Heart J 1990 (March);119:627–635.

29. Wong M, Matsumura M, Kutsuzawa S, Omoto R: The valve of Doppler echocardiography in the treatment of tricuspid regurgitation in patients with mitral valve replacement: Perioperative and two-year postoperative findings. Thorac Cardiovasc Surg 1990 (June);99:1003–1010.

30. Niles N, Borer JS, Kamen M, Hochreiter C, Devereux RB, Kligfield P, Bucek J, Boccanfuso R: Preoperative left and right ventricular performance in combined aortic and mitral regurgitation and comparison with isolated aortic or mitral regurgitation. Am J Cardiol 1990 (June 1);65:1372–1378.

31. Spain MG, Smith MD, Kwan OL, Demaria AN: Effect of isometric exercise on mitral and aortic regurgitation as assessed by color Doppler flow imaging. Am J Cardiol 1990 (Jan 1);65:78–83.

32. Taams MA, Gussenhoeven EJ, Bos E, De Jaegere P, Roelandt JRTC, Sutherland GR, Bom N: Enhanced morphological diagnosis in infective endocarditis by transoesophageal echocardiography. Br Heart J 1990 (Feb);63:109–113.

33. Jaffe WM, Morgan DE, Pearlman AS, Otto CM: Infective endocarditis, 1983–1988: Echocardiographic findings and factors influencing morbidity and mortality. J Am Coll Cardiol 1990 (May);15:1227–33.

34. Sanabria TJ, Alpert JS, Goldberg R, Pape LA, Cheeseman SH: Increasing frequency of staphylococcal infective endocarditis: Experience at a university hospital, 1981 through 1988. Arch Intern Med 1990 (June);150:1305–1309.

35. British Society for Antimicrobial Chemotherapy: Antibiotic prophylaxis of infective endocarditis. Lancet 1990 (Jan 13);335:88–91.

36. Dajami AS, Bisno AL, Chung KJ, Durack DT, Freed M, Gerber MA, Karchmer AW, Millard HD, Rahimtoola S, Shulman ST, Watanakunakorn C, Taubert KA: Prevention of bacterial endocarditis: Recommendations by the American Heart Association. JAMA 1990 (Dec 12);264:2919–2922.

37. Sheikh KH, DeBruijn NP, Rankin JS, Clements FM, Stanley T, Wolfe WG, Kisslo J: The utility of transesophageal echocardiography and Doppler color flow imaging in patients undergoing cardiac valve surgery. J Am Coll Cardiol 1990 (February);15:363–72.

38. Obarski TP, Loop FD, Cosgrove DM, Lytle BW, Stewart WJ: Frequency of acute myocardial infarction in valve repairs versus valve replacement for pure mitral regurgitation. Am J Cardiol 1990 (Apr 1);65:887–890.

39. Crawford M, Souchek J, Oprian C, Miller D, Rahimtoola S, Giacomini J, Sethi G, Hammermeister K: Determinants of Survival and Left Ventricular Performance After Mitral Valve Replacement. Circulation 1990 (April);81:1173–1181.

40. Hennein HA, Swain JA, McIntosh CL, Bonow RO, Stone CD, Clark RE: Comparative assessment of chordal preservation versus chordal resection during mitral valve replacement. J Thorac Cardiovasc Surg 1990 (May);99:828–837.

41. Harpole DH Jr, Rankin JS, Wolfe WG, Clements FM, Vanstrigt P, Young WG, Jones RH: Effects of standard mitral valve replacement on left ventricular function. Ann Thorac Surg 1990 (June);49:866–874.

42. Ren JF, Chandrasekaran K, Mintz GS, Ross J, Pennock RS, Frankl WS: Effect of depressed left ventricular function on hemodynamics of normal St. Jude medical prosthesis in the aortic valve position. Am J Cardiol 1990 (Apr 15);65:1004–1009.

43. Dumesnil JG, Honos GN, Lemieux M, Beauchemin RT: Validation and applications of indexed aortic prosthetic valve areas calculated by Doppler echocardiography. J Am Coll Cardiol 1990 (September);16:637–43.

44. Taniguchi K, Nakano S, Kawashima Y, Sakai K, Kawamoto T, Sakaki S, Kobayashi J, Morimoto S, Matsuda H: Left Ventricular Ejection Performance, Wall Stress, and

Contractile State in Aortic Regurgitation Before and After Aortic Valve Replacement. Circulation 1990 (September);82:797–807.

45. Kurnik PB, Innerfield M, Wachspress JD, Eldredge WJ, Waxman HL: Left ventricular mass regression after aortic valve replacement measured by ultrafast computed tomography. Am Heart J 1990 (October);120:919–927.

46. Hoffmann A, Burckhardt D: Patients at risk for cardiac death late after aortic valve replacement. Am Heart J 1990 (November);120:1142–1147.

47. Jones EL, Weintraub WS, Craver JM, Guyton RA, Cohen CL, Corrigan VE, Hatcher CR Jr: Ten-year experience with the porcine bioprosthetic valve: Interrelationship of valve survival and patient survival in 1,050 valve replacements. Ann Thorac Surg 1990 (Mar);49:370–384.

48. Jamieson WRE, Allen P, Miyagishima RT, Gerein AN, Munro AI, Burr LH, Tyers GFO: The Carpentier-Edwards standard porcine bioprosthesis: A first-generation tissue valve with excellent long-term clinical performance. J Thorac Cardiovasc Surg 1990 (Mar);99:543–561.

49. Rashtain MY, Stevenson DM, Allen DT, Yoganathan AP, Harrison EC, Edmiston WA, Rahimtoola SH: Flow characteristics of bioprosthetic heart valves. Chest 1990 (Aug);98:365–375.

50. Nair CK, Mohiuddin SM, Hilleman DE, Schultz R, Bailey RT, Cook CT, Dketch MH: Ten-year results with the St. Jude medical prosthesis. Am J Cardiol 1990 (Jan 15);65:217–225.

51. Burchfiel CM, Hammermeister KE, Krause-Steinrauf H, Sethi GK, Henderson WG, Crawford MH, Wong M, and participants in the Department of Veterans Affairs Cooperative Study on valvular heart disease: Left atrial dimension and risk of systemic embolism in patients with a prosthetic heart valve. J Am Coll Cardiol 1990 (January);15:32–41.

52. Saour JN, Sieck JO, Mamo LAR, Gallus AS: Trail of different intensities of anticoagulation in patients with prosthetic heart valves. N Engl J Med 1990 (Feb 15);322:428–432.

53. Eckman MH, Beshansky JR, Durand-Zaleski I, Levine HJ, Pauker SG: Anticoagulation for noncardiac procedures in patients with prosthetic heart valves: Does low risk mean high cost? JAMA 1990 (Mar 16);263:1513–1521.

Myocardial Heart Disease

IDIOPATHIC DILATED CARDIOMYOPATHY

In children

Chen and associates[1] from St. Louis, Missouri, studied the clinical profile of 23 children with idiopathic dilated cardiomyopathy to detect any factors that might be predictive for their survival. There were 12 survivors; 8 survived 1 year, and 5 survived 5 years. Age at onset, gender, cardiothoracic ratio on chest radiograph, pattern of infarction, ST changes or arrhythmia, and LV end diastolic pressure were nonpredictive of outcome. Low shortening fraction (12% in nonsurvivors vs 21% in survivors), familial cardiomyopathy and endocardial fibroelastosis did indicate a poor prognosis. These authors show strikingly different findings than those presented by Griffin and associates (see *Cardiology, 1989*, page 371; J Am Coll Cardiol 1988; 11:139-144). Those authors showed that all children who presented at <2 years of age with congestive cardiomyopathy died during the follow-up. There remain some children in the present series, as well as in most pediatric follow-up studies, who do much better than initially predicted from data at presentation. The failure to improve in terms of LV shortening fraction over a 2–3 month period and particularly failure to achieve a shortening fraction of 15% or greater during this time period appears to be almost uniformly associated with poor outcome. Thus, this measurement might be useful in terms of follow-up and consideration for transplant in these patients.

Familial type

To evaluate the occurrence of familial cases of dilated cardiomyopathy, Mestroni and associates[2] from Trieste, Italy, studied 165 consecutive patients. Diagnosis of myocardial disease was based on clinical, hemodynamic, bioptic, postmortem or a combination of these criteria. Twelve patients (7% of cases) showed evidence of myocardial disease in 1 relative; 27 patients with myocardial disease were detected in the 12 families, but a suspected history of myocardial involvement was present in a further 16 cases. In 6 families proband and relatives were affected by dilated cardiomyopathy (total 14 cases); in 1 of these families the disease began with an AV block. In 4 families the relatives showed the presence of myocarditis at the endo-myocardial biopsy. In 2 families the relatives presented a RV cardiomyopathy. The mode of inheritance was autosomal dominant in 7 families, recessive in 4; X-linked pattern may be hypothesized in 1. Nine patients died under the age of 45 years: 2 of sudden death, 6 of chronic CHF and 1 of cerebral embolism. Familial transmission is not rare. Different modes of genetic transmission (autosomal dominant, recessive and X-linked) and different forms of myocardial disease suggest that familial cardiomyopathy may be a multifactorial disease.

Mildly dilated type

Prognosis in classically described dilated congestive cardiomyopathy has been reported to be related to ventricular size. Mildly dilated idiopathic dilated cardiomyopathy has been defined as end-stage CHF of unknown etiology (New York Heart Association class IV, LVEF <30%), occurring with neither typical hemodynamic signs of restrictive myopathy nor significant ventricular dilatation (<15% above normal range). Keren and colleagues[3] from Stanford, California, reviewed the follow-up of 12 nontransplant patients with mildly dilated congestive cardiomyopathy. In the first 4 months after diagnosis, 2 patients improved and are living, and 2 showed cardiac dilation and clinical deterioration and died. Six of the remaining 8 with persistent mildly dilated cardiomyopathy died without change in ventricular size before death, despite medical therapy over 12 months. Eight comparable transplanted patients with persistent mildly dilated congestive cardiomyopathy demonstrated improved total survival by life table analysis. A family history of congestive cardiomyopathy was found in 9 of 16 patients with persistent mildly dilated congestive cardiomyopathy. Nontransplant patients were older but other findings were similar in the 2 groups. Endomyocardial biopsies available in 14 of 16 patients showed little or no myofibrillar loss in spite of severe hemodynamic impairment. The degree of myofibrillar loss did not correlate with hemodynamic parameters but showed good correlation with LV size, that is, 5 of 6 patients with no myofibrillar loss had normal ventricular size, whereas all 8 patients with mild myofibrillar loss had mild cardiomegaly. This experience suggests a somewhat variable but negative prognosis after prospective diagnosis of mildly dilated congestive cardiomyopathy, with poor survival in patients with persistence of the original diagnostic features during follow-up. Thus, irrespective of heart size or myofibrillar preservation on biopsy, heart transplantation should be strongly considered in mildly dilated congestive cardiomyopathy if signs of severe cardiac dysfunction persist despite therapy.

Endothelium-dependent coronary microvasculature dilatation

Dilator reserve of the coronary microvasculature is diminished in patients with dilated cardiomyopathy. Although increased extravascular compressive forces, tachycardia, and increased myocardial mass can explain some impairment, recent evidence suggests the possibility of intrinsic microvascular disease. Treasure and colleagues[4] in Boston, Massachusetts, tested out the hypothesis that impairment of endothelium-dependent dilation of the microvasculature could be a contributing mechanism. Investigators infused the endothelium-dependent dilator acetylcholine and the smooth muscle vasodilator adenosine into the left anterior descending coronary artery in 8 patients with dilated cardiomyopathy (mean ejection fraction, 28%) and 7 controls (atypical chest pain). Small vessel resistance was assessed by measuring coronary blood flow at constant arterial pressure with a Doppler velocity catheter. Vascular colon control patients increased coronary blood flow, whereas coronary blood flow did not significantly change in the cardiomyopathy patients. With adenosine, control patients increased coronary blood flow 422% and cardiomyopathy patients increased coronary blood flow 268%. An index of the proportion of coronary flow reserve attributable to endothelium-dependent vasodilation was obtained by standardizing each patient's acetylcholine dose response to maximal adenosine flow response. In 7 control patients receiving both acetylcholine and adenosine, 56% of the maximal adenosine flow response was attained with the endothelium-dependent vasodilator acetylcholine, whereas in 7 cardiomyopathy patients receiving both acetylcholine and adenosine, only 23% of the maximal adenosine response was attained. Thus endothelium-dependent vasodilator function is impaired in the coronary microvasculature of patients with dilated cardiomyopathy.

Polymerase chain reaction gene amplification

Recent molecular studies have suggested that viral myocarditis frequently underlies human congestive cardiomyopathy; however, only moderately sensitive and specific techniques were used. Polymerase chain reaction gene amplification is a sensitive, specific technique ideally suited for the diagnosis of viral disease in small tissue samples where low copy numbers of the viral genome may be present. Using Polymerase chain reaction and high stringency condition, Jin and co-investigators[5] in Toronto, Canada, screened biopsies taken from 48 patients with clinically suspected myocarditis or dilated cardiomyopathy. Five patients demonstrated positive enteroviral signals by Polymerase chain reaction; 2 of them had myocarditis by pathology, were as the other 3 had changes consistent with cardiomyopathy. Four other patients had myocarditis diagnosed by pathology from 3 to 12 months earlier, but were now negative by both Polymerase chain reaction and pathology. Both pathology and Polymerase chain reaction were negative for active myocarditis in all other patients. Ventricular samples taken from LV myectomy in 4 additional patients with HC, normal human ventricle samples, and uninfected monkey kidney cells were also negative by Polymerase chain reaction. This study supports a link between viral infection and dilated cardiomyopathy in some patients.

G_{ia} protein

In myocardial membranes from heart with dilated cardiomyopathy, Bohm and co-investigators[6] in Munich, Germany observed a 37% increase of the G_{ia} protein as measured by ^{32}P-ADP-ribosylation of a $===$ 40kDa pertussis toxin substrate. Immunoblotting techniques also showed increased amounts of G_{ia} in dilated cardiomyopathy. In hearts with ischemic cardiomyopathy, G_{ia} was not altered compared with nonfailing myocardium. Basal and Gpp (NP)p-stimulated adenylate cyclase activity was reduced in dilated cardiomyopathy but not in ischemic cardiomy-opathy. The number of beta-adrenoceptors was similiarly reduced both in dilated and ischemic cardiomyopathy compared with nonfailing myo-cardium. Alterations of m-cholinoceptors or A_1-adenosine receptors did not occur. Consistently, "indirect" negative inotropic effects of the m-cholinoceptor agonist carbachol and the A_1-adenosine receptor agonist R-PIA were not different in ischemic, dilated nonfailing myocardium. In ischemic and dilated cardiomyopathy, there was a marked reduction of the positive inotropic responses to isoprenaline and milrinone. There was a further reduction in dilated cardiomyopathy compared with is-chemic. These investigators concluded that the increase of G_{ia} is accom-panied by a reduction of basal and guanine-nucleotide-stimulated adenylate cyclase activity. Alterations of m-cholinoceptors and A_1-adenosine receptors do not appear to be involved. The further decrease of the positive inotropic effects of isoprenaline and milrinone in dilated cardiomyopathy provides evidence that the increase of G_{ia} is functionally relevant in dilated but not ischemic cardiomyopathy and hence might contribute to the reduced effects of endogenous catecholamines and exogenous cAMP-dependent positive inotropic agents in the former but not the latter condition.

Cardiac autoantibodies

Caforio and associates[7] in London, UK and Pisa, Italy, determined whether organ specific cardiac autoantibodies are present in patients with dilated cardiomyopathy using indirect immunofluorescence on hu-man heart and skeletal muscles to test sera from 200 normal subjects and 65 patients with dilated cardiomyopathy and 41 patients with chronic CHF due to AMI and 208 with other cardiac diseases. Three immunoflu-orescence patterns were found: diffuse cytoplasmic on cardiac tissue only; fine striational on cardiac; and skeletal muscle and broad striations on both cardiac and skeletal muscle. Cardiac specificity of the cyto-plasmic patterns was confirmed by absorption studies with homogenates of human atrium, skeletal muscle and rat liver. Organ-specific cardiac antibodies were more frequent in patients with dilated cardiomyopathies (17 of 65) than in those with other cardiac diseases (2 of 208), patients with CHF (0 of 41), or in normal subjects (7 of 200). Organ-specific cardiac antibodies were more common in patients with dilated cardiomyopathies and in those with fewer symptoms. Cross-reactive antibodies were de-tected in a similar proportion of patients with dilated cardiomyopathies (11%), other cardiac diseases (7%), heart failure (2%), and normal subjects (5.5%). Therefore, the presence of organ-specific cardiac antibodies pro-vides a serologic marker of cardiac autoimmunity in some patients with dilated cardiomyopathies.

Percutaneous fiberoptic angioscopy

Uchida and associates[8] from Tokyo and Funabashi, Japan, examined LV endocardial changes by percutaneous fiberoptic angioscopy in 13 patients with dilated cardiomyopathy and in 4 patients with acute my-ocarditis. Angioscope-guided endomyocardial biopsy was also performed in 6 patients with dilated cardiomyopathy and in 2 with acute myocar-ditis. A balloon-tipped guiding catheter (9F) was introduced through the right femoral artery into the left ventricle; the balloon was inflated, and a 1.6 or 4.3F fiberscope was introduced through the catheter into the ventricle so as to locate the fiberscope tip at the tip of the catheter shaft. The balloon was then pushed against the desired portion of the ventricle and warmed saline was infused to observe the luminal changes. In contrast to the patients without organic heart disease whose LV luminal surface was brown in color, the luminal surface was white or light yellow in 4, light brown in 1, bluish-white in 1, with white and brown portions distributed in a mosaic pattern in 4, and it was reddish brown in the remaining 1 patient with dilated cardiomyopathy. Mural thrombi were observed in 2 of the patients. The luminal surface was light brown in 1, reddish brown in 1, rose in 1, and red in 1 patients with acute myocarditis. Thrombi and scattered bleeding were observed in 2 and 1 of these patients, respectively. The changes in luminal coloration in patients with dilated cardiomyopathy and acute myocarditis had no obvious relation to LV volume and EF. Angioscope-guided biopsy revealed that the white and light yellow portions were due to endocardial fibrosis, that the endocardia of brown portions were not fibrotic, and that the myocardium in the red portions contained mononuclear cells, indicating inflammation. These results indicate that the angioscopic features of the LV luminal surface were not uniform in patients with dilated cardiomyopathy or in those with acute myocarditis, and that angioscopy can be used as a guiding tool for endomyocardial biopsy.

Dobutamine ± amrinone

Nine consecutive patients having severe idiopathic dilated cardiomyopathy were studied by Sundram and colleagues[9] from Chicago, Illinois, for their response in ventricular function, coronary sinus blood flow and myocardial oxygen consumption, lactate extraction and efficiency following incremental doses of dobutamine, followed by the combination of dobutamine and the phosphodiesterase inhibitor amrinone. Results, presented as baseline and the response to the peak dose (15 μg/kg/min) of dobutamine and to the combination of dobutamine and amrinone (each at 15 μg/kg/min) (differences compared with baseline) were: PA wedge pressure decreased from 28 ± 7 to 26 ± 8 and to 20 ± 6 mm Hg; cardiac index rose from 1.47 ± 0.44 to 2.89 ± 1.1 and to 3.64 ± 1.05 L/min/m²; myocardial oxygen consumption remained invariant (18 ± 8, 17 ± 5, and 19 ± 5 ml/min) despite progressive increments in minute work from 2.96 ± 1.1 to 6.98 ± 3.9 and to 9.38 ± 4.3 kg-m/min; myocardial lactate extraction rose from 21 ± 10% to 30 ± 15% and to 35 ± 10% with the addition of amrinone. No patient had net lactate efflux into the coronary sinus, and myocardial efficiency improved from 9.5 ± 5% to 22 ± 13% and to 28 ± 18%. Thus, in idiopathic dilated cardiomyopathy, dobutamine and the combination of dobutamine and amrinone have additive beneficial effects on ventricular performance without an adverse elevation in myocardial oxygen consumption or lactate production, resulting in improved efficiency, suggesting the presence of significant metabolic reserve within the failing myocardium.

Labetalol

Leung and associates[10] from Hong Kong, administered labetalol, a combined alpha- and beta-blocking agent, to 12 patients (mean age 55 years) with idiopathic dilated cardiomyopathy to examine its effects on symptomatology and exercise performance. Studies were performed before treatment, after 8 weeks of placebo, and after 8 weeks of labetalol therapy in a randomized, crossover, double-blind design. The mean dose of labetalol for the group was 275 ± 29 mg. Compared to treatment with placebo, the maximum duration of symptom-limited exercise was significantly prolonged with labetalol (580 ± 72 seconds to 683 ± 71 seconds). Both the resting and peak exercise heart rate and systolic BP were significantly reduced. Ascending aortic blood blow velocity was also measured by continuous-wave Doppler technique during exercise. Compared to placebo, treatment with labetalol conferred no significant change in cardiac output at rest but significantly improved cardiac output at maximum exercise (14 ± 3%). Doppler-derived peak aortic flow velocity, acceleration, and flow velocity integral were also significantly improved at maximum exercise. Systemic vascular resistance, as derived from mean BP/cardiac output, was reduced by 12 ± 3% and 16 ± 3% at rest and at maximum exercise, respectively. New York Heart Association functional class was improved (3.2 ± 0.2 to 2.2 ± 0.3). No major side effects from labetalol were encountered. Thus labetalol improves symptomatology, exercise capacity, and exercise hemodynamics and reduces systemic vascular resistance in patients with idiopathic dilated cardiomyopathy.

Bucindolol

Bucindolol is a potent nonselective β-blocking agent with vasodilatory properties. Gilbert and associates[11] from Salt Lake City, Utah, evaluated the effects of long-term bucindolol therapy in the treatment of CHF from idiopathic dilated cardiomyopathy. Patients were eligible for enrollment if they had symptomatic CHF, idiopathic dilated cardiomyopathy, and LVEF <0.40. All patients received an initial test dose of 12.5 mg bucindolol orally every 12 hours for 2 or 3 doses. Patients tolerating the test dose were randomly assigned (double-blind) to receive bucindolol or placebo in a 3:2 ratio. Study medication was begun at a dose of 12.5 mg orally every 12 hours and gradually increased over a 1-month period until either a maximum tolerated dose or a target dose of 100 mg every 12 hours was reached. Study medication was then continued for an additional 2 months. A total of 24 patients were enrolled into the study. Twenty-three patients tolerated bucindolol test challenge; 14 were randomized to receive bucindolol, and 9 were randomly assigned to receive placebo. The placebo group (age 56 ± 2 years) was significantly older than the bucindolol group (46 ± 3 years), but by all other clinical and hemodynamic parameters the 2 groups were comparable. Twenty-two of 23 patients completed the study. Patients treated with bucindolol had significant improvements in clinical heart failure symptoms and in resting hemodynamic function, including an increase of LVEF (0.26 ± 0.02 to 0.35 ± 0.09), cardiac index (2.2 ± 0.1 to 2.5 ± 0.4 L/minute/m²), and LV stroke work index (25 ± 3 to 35 ± 7 g•m/m²) and a decrease in PA wedge pressure (17 ± 3 to 10 ± 5 mm Hg) and heart rate (86 ± 3 to 75 ± 9 beats/minute). Patients treated with bucindolol also had a significant increase in exercise LVEF (0.26 ± 0.03 to 0.32 ± 0.14) and reduction in questionnaire-measured symptoms and New York Heart Association functional class. Total treadmill exercise duration and maximal oxygen consumption with exercise did not change. No changes in rest or exercise parameters were observed in the placebo-treated group. Central venous plasma norepinephrine concentration decreased significantly in the bucindolol-treated group (423 ± 79 to 212 ± 101 pg/mL), but was unchanged in the placebo-treated group. Bucindolol is well tolerated in patients with idiopathic dilated cardiomyopathy and CHF, and therapy for 3 months is associated with improved resting cardiac function, improved CHF symptoms, and a reduction in venous norepinephrine concentration.

Dual-chamber pacing

The beneficial effects of physiologic dual-chamber (DDD) pacing in the treatment of end-stage idiopathic dilated cardiomyopathy were evaluated by Hochleitner and associates[12] from Vienna, Austria, in 16 patients in whom conventional drug therapy had failed. Candidates for cardiac transplantation as well as patients not accepted for transplantation participated. During DDD pacing at an atrioventricular delay of 100 ms, LVEF increased from 16 ± 8 to 26 ± 9% accompanied by a striking improvement in clinical symptoms, such as severe dyspnea at rest and pulmonary edema. The New York Heart Association class decreased from 3.6 ± 0.4 to 2.1 ± 0.5. The decrease in cardiothoracic ratio from 0.60 ± 0.06 to 0.56 ± 0.05 coincided with a decrease in LA and RV echocardiographic dimensions, indicating a decrease in preload. Systolic BP increased from 108 ± 29 to 126 ± 21 mm Hg and diastolic BP from 67 ± 15 to 80 ± 11 mm Hg. Normalization of heart rate was achieved. No major complications developed as a consequence of DDD pacing. All patients could be discharged from the hospital within 3 weeks after pacemaker implantation and return to a relatively normal life. Within 1 year after onset of DDD pacing only 4 of the patients died (from either sudden death or stroke). DDD pacing could represent an alternative approach to the management of chronic heart failure due to dilated cardiomyopathy, especially for heart transplant candidates and patients who are not accepted for cardiac transplantation, but no longer respond to drug therapy.

MYOCARDITIS

In peripartum period

Midei and colleagues[13] in Baltimore, Maryland, examined the clinical and pathological features of 18 consecutive patients with peripartum cardiomyopathy at The Johns Hopkins Hospital in an attempt to define the incidence of myocarditis and to determine its response to immunosuppressive agents. Fourteen of the 18 patients showed evidence of myocarditis. Of these, 10 were treated with immunosuppressive therapy. Nine of the 10 treated patients with myocarditis had subjective and objective improvement. Follow-up endomyocardial biopsies in these patients showed resolution or substantial improvement in myocarditis. Four patients with myocarditis not treated with immunosuppressive also improved. All patients improving spontaneously presented with CHF within 1 month of delivery and improved traumatically within days of presentation. Four of the 18 patients showed no evidence of myocarditis. Of these, two improved, and two deteriorated (both requiring cardiac transplantation). None of these 4 patients were treated with immunosuppressive therapy. The investigators concluded that in patients with peripartum cardiomyopathy, 1) the etiology remains unclear although myocarditis was present in 78% of those with this condition, 2) resolution of myocarditis is associated with significant improvement in LV function,

3) myocarditis may resolve spontaneously without detectable loss of cardiac function, and 4) immunosuppressive therapy in patients with myocarditis and persistent LV dysfunction may improve LV function and prognosis.

Indication for repeat biopsy

Dec and associates[14] in Boston, Massachusetts used repeated endomyocardial biopsy in 28 patients with dilated cardiomyopathy of ≤12 months' duration and symptomatic CHF or life-threatening ventricular arrhythmias to determine whether a second biopsy would detect myocarditis identified as "borderline myocarditis" on the initial biopsy. Myocarditis was strongly suspected clinically in all cases, yet was unconfirmed on initial RV biopsy. Seventeen patients underwent both RV and LV biopsies, 7 patients had a repeat RV biopsy and 4 patients underwent LV biopsy alone. The interval between the initial and repeat biopsies averaged 31 ± 6 days. Myocarditis was identified on repeat biopsy in 4 of 6 patients whose initial biopsies revealed "borderline" myocarditis, i.e., interstitial inflammation, but no evidence of myocyte necrosis compared with none of the 22 patients whose initial biopsies showed either myocyte hypertrophy, interstitial fibrosis, or both. Thus, repeated endomyocardial biopsy may identify myocarditis and potentially modify the treatment of patients with dilated cardiomyopathy and nondiagnostic initial endomyocardial histologic features. RV biopsies should be repeated in patients whose initial biopsy demonstrate "borderline" myocarditis.

Antibodies to human MHC antigens

Herskowitz and associates[15] in Baltimore, Maryland, and Atlanta, Georgia, studied 13 patients with active myocarditis and 8 control patients with other well defined cardiac diagnoses with a sensitive radioimmunoassay developed to be utilized with monoclonal antibodies to human MHC class I and class II antigens in order to quantitate the expression of both of these antigens within each biopsy. This approach was used because autoimmunity and viral disease are commonly associated with increased expression of major histocompatibility complex (MHC) antigens on target tissue. Abnormal MHC class I and II antigen expression was present in 11 of 13 myocarditis specimens and 1 of 8 controls (specificity 88% and sensitivity 85%). Active myocarditis samples had approximately a 10-fold increase in MHC class I and II expression. Immunoperoxidase staining localized abnormal MHC expression primarily within microvascular endothelium and along myocyte surfaces in 11 of 13 cases. This study is the first to demonstrate an increase in major histocompatibility complex antigen expression within the myocardium of patients with active myocarditis. This approach may prove useful in identifying myocarditis.

Antimyosin antibody cardiac imaging

Dec and associates[16] in Boston, Massachusetts used RV endomyocardial biopsies and antimyosin antibody scintigraphy to detect the presence of myocardial necrosis in 82 patients with suspected myocarditis. Seventy-four patients had dilated cardiomyopathies of less than 1 year's duration and a mean LVEF of 0.30 ± 0.02. Eight patients had normal LVEFs. Symptoms at presentation included CHF in 92%, chest pain suggesting myocardial ischemia (6%), and life-threatening ventricular tach-yarrhythmias in 2%. All patients had planar and single photon emission computed tomographic cardiac imaging after injection of indium-111-labeled antimyosin antibody fragments and an RV biopsy within 48 hours of imaging. Antimyosin images were interpreted as either abnormal or normal and correlated with biopsy results. On the basis of the RV histologic examination, the sensitivity of the antimyosin imaging was 83%, specificity 53%, and predictive value of a normal scan 92%. Improvement in LV function occurred within 6 months of treatment in 54% of patients with an abnormal antimyosin scan compared with 18% of those with a normal scan. These data indicate that antimyosin antibody cardiac imaging may be useful for the initial evaluation of patients with dilated and non-dilated cardiomyopathy and clinically suspected myocarditis. A normal antimyosin antibody scan is associated with a very low rate of myocarditis on endomyocardial biopsy.

HYPERTROPHIC CARDIOMYOPATHY

Sudden death

Spirito and Maron[17] in Bethesda, Maryland, evaluated the association between the magnitude of LV hypertrophy and the risk of sudden unexpected death in 29 asymptomatic or mildly symptomatic patients with HC who subsequently died suddenly or had a cardiac arrest with documented VF. The findings were compared with those obtained in a control group of 95 patients of similar age and symptomatic state. Maximal LV wall thickness was significantly greater in patients with sudden death (26 ± 7 mm) than in the control individuals (21 ± 5 mm). LV wall thickness index, a quantitative expression of the overall extent of hypertrophy, was also greater in patients with sudden death (76 ± 20 mm) than in surviving control patients (62 ± 13 mm). Marked and diffuse hypertrophy with maximal wall thickness ≥30 mm or wall thickness ≥25 mm in ≥2 of the 4 segments into which the LV had been divided was 8 times more common in patients with sudden death (11 of 29) than in control patients (5 of 95) (Figure 7-1). The prevalence of mild and localized hypertrophy with maximal wall thickness ≤17 mm involving only one segment was similar in patients with sudden death and in control patients. Thus, asymptomatic or mildly symptomatic patients with hypertrophic cardiomyopathy who die suddenly have marked and diffuse LV hypertrophy. Sudden cardiac death is uncommon in asymptomatic or mildly symptomatic adult patients with HC and relatively mild LV hypertrophy.

In patients ≥65 years of age

Fay and colleagues[18] in Rochester, Minnesota, evaluated the prognosis of patients diagnosed as having HC in 95 patients aged ≥65 years. Seventy-five percent of patients were symptomatic as evidenced by presence of chest pain, dyspnea, or syncope. The mean ventricular septal wall thickness was 20 mm. The median duration of follow-up study was 4 years. Survival rates at 1 and 5 years were 95% and 76%, respectively, which were not significantly different from those of an age- and gender-matched control group. Among patients presenting with New York Heart Association functional class I or II dyspnea, only 18% progressed to class III or

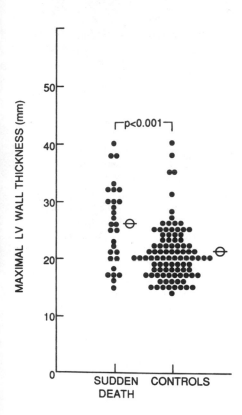

Fig. 7-1. Comparison of maximal left ventricular (LV) wall thickness in patients with sudden cardiac death and in surviving control patients. ⊖ = mean value. Reproduced with permission from Spirito et al.[17]

IV during the follow-up period. Patients presenting with class III dyspnea had a 1-year mortality of 36%, significantly higher than in control subjects. Among the echocardiographic variables, indexed LA size was the most strongly associated with reduced survival. These results suggest that the prognosis of older patients with HC is generally favorable.

Syncope

Nienaber and associates[19] in Hamburg, Federal Republic of Germany, evaluated 29 consecutive patients with symptomatic HC and a mean age of 45 ± 12 years who underwent complex invasive and noninvasive testing to identify a risk profile for syncope. Clinical, morphologic, electrophysiologic, and hemodynamic variables at rest and at a symptom-limited pacing rate were analyzed for a significant association with syncope. Logistic regression analysis identified 3 variables as independent predictors of syncope and HC: 1) age <30 years; 2) left ventricular end-diastolic volume index <60 ml/m²; and 3) non-sustained VT on 72 hours ambulatory electrocardiographic monitoring. Combined occurrence of all 3 variables had a sensitivity and specificity of 100% in identifying 8 patients with syncopal events. Thus, the risk for syncope in patients with HC is highest in young patients with a combination of low LV filling volume and episodes of nonsustained VT.

Atrial fibrillation

Robinson and associates[20] in London, UK, evaluated the clinical outcome of 52 consecutive patients with HC who developed paroxysmal (<1 week) or established (≥1 week) AF between 1960 and 1985. Follow-up study until death or the time of the report ranged from 6 months to 24 years (median 11 years) from diagnosis and from 6 months to 22 years (median 7 years) from the onset of AF. AF was present in 6 patients at the time of diagnosis, whereas it developed subsequently in 46. The acute onset of arrhythmias was associated with a change in symptoms in 41 (89%) of the patients. After initial treatment of acute AF, sinus rhythm was restored in 29 (63%) of the 46 patients; 43 (93%) of the 46 returned to their original symptom class. Stepwise logistic regression revealed that shorter duration of arrhythmias and amiodarone therapy were the most powerful predictors of return to sinus rhythm. Sinus rhythm was maintained during a median follow-up period of 5.5 years in 22 of the 29 patients in whom it was restored after initial therapy. During follow-up, 25 of the 52 patients were treated with conventional therapy alone and 7 with amiodarone alone. Amiodarone therapy was associated with better maintenance of sinus rhythm, fewer alterations in drug therapy, fewer embolic events, and fewer attempted direct current cardioversions. The remaining 20 patients initially received conventional therapy, but were not well controlled and they were converted to amiodarone (median 200 mg/day) after which there were fewer alterations in drug therapy and fewer direct current cardioversions during a similar follow-up period. There were 19 disease-associated deaths. Estimated probability of surviving 5, 10, 15 and 20 years HC was recognized clinically was 0.86, 0.71, 0.65 and 0.50 and was similar in a concurrent group of 122 patients with HC who remained in sinus rhythm (Figure 7-2).

Abnormal Q waves

Lemery and associates[21] in London, UK, evaluated potential causes of abnormal Q waves in patients with HC. Myocardial wall thickness was

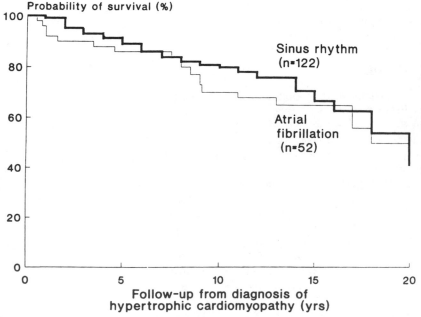

Fig. 7-2. Probability of survival for 52 patients with hypertrophic cardiomyopathy and atrial fibrillation and 122 concurrent patients with hypertrophic cardiomyopathy who remained in sinus rhythm. The difference is not significant. Reproduced with permission from Robinson, et al.[20]

evaluated by 2-dimensional echocardiography at 8 LV and 10 RV sites in 67 patients with HC and a mean age of 40 years. The findings were analyzed in relationship to the presence of abnormal Q waves on the 12 lead electrocardiogram. Nineteen (28%) of the 67 patients had abnormal Q waves. RV hypertrophy was significantly more common in patients without abnormal Q waves (25 or 52% of 48 patients as compared to 2 [11%] of 19 patients, respectively). With univariate analysis, six measurements were significantly associated with abnormal Q waves. However, with multivariate analysis, only the ratios of upper anterior septal to mean right ventricular wall thickness and upper posterior wall thickness were significantly related to the presence of abnormal Q waves and predicted Q wave location with a sensitivity, specificity and predictive accuracy of 90%, 88%, and 89%, respectively. These data indicate that in patients with HC, the presence of abnormal Q waves on 12 lead electrocardiogram is primarily a function of the relation of RV wall thickness and upper anterior septal thickness.

Signal-averaged electrocardiogram

Cripps and associates[22] in London, UK, utilized high gain signal-averaged electrocardiograms in 64 patients with HC and 50 age and gender-matched control patients to determine the utility of signal-averaged electrocardiograms in predicting arrhythmia risk. An abnormal signal-averaged electrocardiogram was more common in patients than in control subjects, including 13 (20%) of 64 patients with HC and 2 (4%) of the 50 control subjects. There was an association between the presence of nonsustained VT on 48 hour electrocardiographic Holter monitoring and the presence of an abnormal signal averaged electrocardiogram: 8 (47%) of the 17 patients with nonsustained VT and 6 (86%) of 7 patients with more than 3 episodes of nonsustained VT per 24 hours had signal-averaged electrocardiogram abnormalities. There was no association between an abnormal signal-averaged electrocardiogram and a family history of premature sudden cardiac death, history of syncope, symptomatic status, maximal LV wall thickness, the presence of systolic anterior motion of the mitral valve or maximal rate of oxygen uptake on exercise. However, among 4 patients with a history of cardiac arrest, 3 had an abnormal signal-averaged electrocardiogram. The sensitivity for the signal-averaged electrocardiogram in detecting patients with electrical instability defined as a history of cardiac arrest or the presence of nonsustained VT or both was 50% and the specificity was 93% with a predictive accuracy of 77%. In the younger age group (<25 years of age), the only patients with an abnormal signal-averaged electrocardiogram were 2 of the 3 patients with a history of cardiac arrest. Thus, these data suggest that the signal-averaged electrocardiogram may be a useful means to evaluate patients with HC, especially in the prediction of sudden death in the young age group for whom no reliable prognostic marker presently exists.

With infective endocarditis

Alessandri and associates[23] from Rome, Italy, reported 7 patients with infective endocarditis associated with obstructive HC. In 3 patients the mitral valve was the site of vegetations and in 4 patients both mitral and aortic valves were involved. Five patients had typical systolic anterior motion of the anterior mitral leaflet. The infective endocarditis was confirmed anatomically in 3 of the 7 patients by operation (MVR). The 7 cases of infective endocarditis with HC were among the authors' 43 patients with HC evaluated for cardiac surgery in a 4-year period. The authors also found from review of previous publications 54 reported cases of infective endocarditis in patients with HC. In most of these cases, however, the infective endocarditis was not confirmed anatomically (at operation or at necropsy). The authors concluded that HC should be considered a risk factor for the development of infective endocarditis. The authors also recommended that all patients with HC should be given antibiotic treatment any time they undergo surgery and/or invasive diagnostic procedures to prevent potentially fatal septicemia.

Without increased myocardial mass

McKenna and associates[24] from London, UK, described 2 families in which individuals had wide-spread myocardial disarray at histologic examination but no cardiomegaly grossly. In one family the clinical presentation was that of sudden unexpected cardiac death in 4 family members: members of the other family presented with electrocardiographic repolarization changes and abnormalities of LV diastolic function. The finding of myocardial disarray, the characteristic histological abnormality of HC, in the absence of increased cardiac mass suggests a wider range of abnormality in HC than is currently recognized.

Coronary vasodilatory capacity

Koga and associates[25] from Kurume, Japan, performed split-dose thallium-dipyridamole myocardial scintigraphy in patients with nonobstructive HC who had angiographically normal coronary arteries. The dipyridamole-induced increases in thallium-201 uptake, calculated to evaluate coronary vasodilatory capacity, were significantly lower in 30 patients with HC than in 13 control subjects (177 ± 58 vs 281 ± 46%) and the reductions were observed in both the septal and lateral segments. The reductions of the septal segment in HC patients were significantly greater than those in 10 hypertensive patients with comparable degrees of septal hypertrophy. Of patients with HC, 16 had increases in thallium uptake well below the normal range. Compared with those having normal increases, these patients had significantly lower exercise duration (11 vs 15 minutes), with 33% having ST depression develop at a workload ≤80 watts. These data indicate that approximately one-half of patients with HC have impaired coronary vasodilatory capacity that could be an important pathophysiologic abnormality of HC resulting in the development of myocardial ischemia and the impairment of cardiac performance during exercise.

Operative results with pulmonary hypertension

Stone and associates[26] from Bethesda, Maryland, reported results of operations for HC in which the PA systolic pressure was <35 mm HG with or without associated MR. Since 1962, 49 patients underwent LV myotomy and myectomy with 98% follow-up. Mean follow-up was 7.9 years with a range of 0.8 to 18.4 years. Early hospital mortality rate was 12% (n = 6); 2 deaths from low cardiac output and 4 from arrhythmia. There were 43 (88%) hospital survivors and 18 late deaths. Actuarial survival rate after operation was 87% ± 5% (n = 31) at 5 years and 55% ± 8% (n = 9) at 10 years (Figure 7-3). Thirty-nine of 43 survivors (91%)

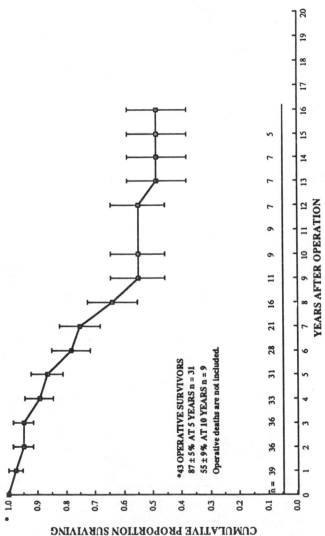

Fig. 7-3. Actuarial probability of survival after LV myotomy and myectomy for obstructive hypertrophic cardiomyopathy and pulmonary arterial hypertension. Operative mortality rate was 12%, n = 6, and was not included. Probability is expressed as the mean ± standard error of the mean. Reproduced with permission from Stone, et al.[26]

returned 9 ± 1 months postoperatively for follow-up evaluation including cardiac catheterization. Most (83%) were in New York Heart Association functional class I or II postoperatively. Cardiac catheterizations indicated a fall in PA systolic pressure from 62 ± 3 (range = 36 to 105) to 38 ± 2 (range = 21 to 65) mm Hg with no difference in RA pressure or cardiac output. PA wedge mean pressure decreased from 24 ± 1 to 16 ± 5 mm Hg and preoperative MR improved or was abolished in 85% of patients studied (n = 13). Rest and maximal provocable LV outflow tract gradients decreased from 81 ± 7 and 103 ± 5 to 14 ± 3 and 45 ± 8 mm Hg, respectively. Comparison of the above-mentioned patients, operated on since 1982, with a preoperatively matched group who underwent MVR in the same interval showed no statistically significant difference in mortality, morbidity, hemodynamic outcome, or functional outcome with a mean follow-up of 2 years (Tables 7-1 and 7-2). The authors concluded that a consistent, significant reduction (mean = 40%) in preoperative PA systolic pressure, clinical symptoms, and MR occurs with relief of outflow tract obstruction of LV myotomy and myectomy and that PA hypertension and MR are not indications for MVR in these patients.

ASSOCIATION WITH A CONDITION AFFECTING PRIMARILY NON-CARDIAC STRUCTURE(S)

Alcoholism

Systolic LV dysfunction is relatively common in asymptomatic alcoholics, but whether LV diastolic function is also altered is much less well-studied. Kupari and associates[27] from Helsinki, Finland, used M-mode and Doppler echocardiography to study LV size, mass, systolic function and diastolic filling in 32 alcoholics free of clinically detectable heart disease and in 15 healthy control subjects. LV mass index and posterior wall thickness were higher in alcoholics than in controls, but there was no statistically significant difference either in end-diastolic size or in systolic ventricular function. More abnormalities were found in the Doppler indexes of diastolic function, however. The alcoholics had a prolonged relaxation time (200 ± 6 vs 184 ± 5 ms [mean ± standard error],

TABLE 7-1. *Comparison of the results of LVMM versus MVR for obstructive hypertrophic cardiomyopathy with pulmonary hypertension. Reproduced with permission from Stone, et al.[26]*

	LVMM (n = 43)			MVR (n = 8)			
	Preop.	Postop.	p Value	Preop.	Postop.	p Value	Difference
PAS	62 ± 3	38 ± 2	p = 0.0001	58 ± 7	37 ± 6	p = 0.0056	p = NS
PAD	28 ± 1	17 ± 1	p = 0.0001	25 ± 5	18 ± 3	p = 0.042	p = NS
PAWP	24 ± 1	16 ± 5	p = 0.0001	21 ± 2	12 ± 2.1	p = 0.034	p = NS
RAP	9 ± 0.6	8 ± 0.7	p = NS	5 ± 2	7 ± 1	p = NS	p = NS
LVOTΔP							
Rest	81 ± 7	14 ± 3	p = 0.0001	108 ± 17	4 ± 2	p = 0.0085	p = NS
Max.	103 ± 5	45 ± 8	p = 0.0001	113 ± 11	16 ± 5	p = 0.0001	p = NS
LVEDP	25 ± 1	19 ± 1	p = 0.0068	18 ± 2	12 ± 3	p = 0.007	p = 0.004
ΔLVEDP		6 ± 0.3			6 ± 0.7		p = NS
CI	2.4 ± 0.1	2.2 ± 0.1	p = NS	2.5 ± 0.2	2.6 ± 0.3	p = NS	p = NS
MR (0-4+)	1.8 ± .2	0.6 ± 0.2	p = 0.0004	1.7 ± 0.4	0.6 ± 0.2	p = NS	p = NS
NYHA FC	3.3 ± 0.3	1.7 ± 0.1	p = 0.0001	3.1 ± 0.1	1.7 ± 0.2	p = 0.0002	p = NS

All data are from patients with paired preoperative and postoperative data available and are expressed as the mean value ± the standard error. PAS, Pulmonary artery systolic pressure; PAD, pulmonary arterial diastolic pressure; PAWP, mean pulmonary arterial wedge pressure; RAP, right atrial pressure; LVOTΔP, left ventricular outflow tract gradient; Max., left ventricular outflow tract gradient during maximal stimulation with isoproterenol; LVEDP, left ventricular end-diastolic pressure; ΔLVEDP, change in left ventricular end-diastolic pressure; CI, cardiac index; MR, angiographic degree of mitral regurgitation on a scale of one to four; NYHA FC, New York Heart Association functional class.

TABLE 7-2. *Operative mortality for all patients undergoing LVMM or MVR for hypertrophic cardiomyopathy versus those with pulmonary hypertension. Reproduced with permission from Stone, et al.[26]*

	No.	Age (yr)	PAS (mm Hg)	FC	OM (%)
LVMM (1960-1975)	83	41	36.7	3.3	7*
LVMM (1983-1987)	108	46	30.2	3.2	3*
MVR (1982-1987)	43	47	29.8	3.2	8.6
LVMM and PHTN (1962-1987)	49	49	62.4	3.4	12*
MVR and PHTN (1983-1987)	9	50	58.3	3.1	11

PAS, Pulmonary artery systolic pressure; FC, New York Heart Association functional class; OM, operative mortality (occurring within 30 days of operation or during the hospital stay); LVMM, left ventricular myotomy and myectomy; MVR, mitral valve replacement; PHTN, pulmonary hypertension (for this study defined solely as a pulmonary artery systolic pressure greater than 35 mm Hg); HCM, obstructive hypertrophic cardiomyopathy.

*There was a significant increase in mortality in patients with pulmonary hypertension who underwent LVMM; however, this was probably related to factors other than pulmonary hypertension. Patients with concomitant cardiac disease were excluded.

a decreased peak early diastolic velocity (52 ± 2 vs 60 ± 3 cm/s), a slower acceleration of the early flow (410 ± 18 vs 552 ± 43 cm/s²), and a higher atrial-to-early peak velocity ratio (0.74 ± 0.04 vs 0.60 ± 0.05). This pattern of changes suggests a primary abnormality in the relaxation of the LV. In multivariate analyses, the abnormalities in the Doppler indexes were independent of the duration of alcoholism, the quantity of the most recent ethanol exposure and the increased mass of the LV. Impaired early filling of the LV due to delayed relaxation is common in asymptomatic alcoholics and may in fact be the earliest functional sign of preclinical alcoholic cardiomyopathy.

Acromegaly

Chanson and associates[28] from Paris, France, and Basel, Switzerland, treated 7 patients with active acromegaly, 3 of whom had refractory CHF and the other 4 had no CHF, with octreotide, 100-500 μg subcutaneously 3 times daily. During octreotide therapy patients showed a rapid decrease in growth hormone and insulin like growth factor. Plasma volume returned to normal and heart rate decreased significantly. In the 4 patients without CHF, right-sided heart catheterization done before and after 3 months of octreotide therapy showed an 18% reduction in stroke volume and return to normal of the cardiac index. The 3 patients with CHF, evaluated before and after 40 days and up to 2 years of therapy, showed a dramatic clinical improvement that was associated with an increase of 24 to 51% in stroke volume. In these 3 patients the cardiac index remained in the normal range, filling pressures were markedly decreased, and PA wedge pressure returned to normal. Thus, octreotide therapy for patients with acromegaly may be highly beneficial even in those with advanced CHF.

Hypothyroidism

Polikar and associates[29] in San Diego, California studied cardiovascular sensitivity to catecholamines in 15 patients with hypothyroidism (mean age 45 ± 4 years), with a mean serum thyroxine index of 2.7 ± 0.5 µg/100 ml and mean thyroid stimulating hormone levels of 137 ± 48 µU/ml and compared their hemodynamic sensitivity to catecholamines to that of 8 control subjects. The studies were repeated in 10 patients with hypothyroidism 4 ± 0.5 months after thyroid replacement therapy when their T_4 indexes were 9.9 ± 2.1 µg/100 ml and TSH values were 3.5 ± 1.3 µU/ml. Basal, average, and maximal heart rates were measured using 24 hour ambulatory electrocardiographic monitoring and plasma levels of epinephrine and norepinephrine were determined before and after thyroid replacement. Heart rate increased less after bolus injection of 0.8, 1.6 and 3.2 µg of isoproterenol in the hypothyroid than in the euthyroid states. Control subjects had similar responses to patients receiving thyroid replacement. These data demonstrate that patients with hypothyroidism have a decreased cardiac chronotropic response to beta-adrenergic stimulation that may contribute to the decreased basal and maximal daily heart rates seen in patients with hypothyroidism.

Systemic lupus erythematosus

Crozier and associates[30] from Hong Kong assessed cardiac involvement by echocardiography in 50 patients with systemic lupus erythematosus (SLE). The LVEF was decreased in patients compared to control subjects (61 ± 9 vs 68 ± 7%), whereas ventricular septum (12 ± 3 vs 9 ± 1 mm), and posterior wall dimension (9 ± 2 vs 8 ± 1 mm), LV mass (186 ± 54 vs 130 ± 32 g) and mitral valve Doppler A:E ratio (0.8 ± 0.2 vs 0.7 ± 0.1) were increased. Pericardial effusion was detected in 27 patients and 5 control subjects, and valvular regurgitation was more frequent in the patients (aortic 2 vs 0; mitral 23 vs 5; tricuspid 34 vs 22 and pulmonary 28 vs 17). MR or AR was more common in patients with active SLE (60 vs 40%) but was not related to the duration of SLE or current dosage of prednisone. This study demonstrates that pericardial effusion, valvular regurgitation and myocardial abnormalities are frequently present in patients with SLE.

Subclinical myocardial involvement frequently occurs in patients with SLE. Leung and associates[31] from Hong Kong, assessed LV diastolic function in 58 patients (54 female and 4 male; mean age 32 ± 11 years) and in 40 sex-matched and age-matched healthy control individuals (37 female and 3 male; mean age 33 ± 9 years) by pulsed Doppler echocardiography. All subjects had no clinical evidence of overt myocardial disease or abnormal LV systolic function. Compared with the control group, patients with SLE had significantly prolonged isovolumic relaxation time (62 ± 12 vs 80 ± 14 msec), reduced peak early diastolic flow velocity (82 ± 18 vs 76 ± 16 cm/sec), increased peak late diastolic flow velocity (45 ± 7 vs 53 ± 8 cm/sec), reduced E/A ratio (1.81 ± 0.32 vs 1.46 ± 0.29), and lower deceleration rate of early diastolic flow velocity (489 ± 151 vs 361 ± 185 cm/sec². Subgroup analysis according to disease activity revealed that when compared to the inactive disease group, the active disease group had significantly longer isovolumic relaxation time (74 ± 21 msec vs 92 ± 18 msec), lower peak early diastolic flow velocity (78 ± 16 vs 70 ± 16 cm/sec), higher peak late diastolic flow velocity (51 ± 8 vs 57 ± 7 cm/sec), lower E/A ratio (1.56 ± 0.25 vs 1.26 ± 0.27), and lower early diastolic flow velocity (379 ± 169 cm/sec^2 vs 324 ± 172 cm/sec^2). In conclusion, an abnormal pattern of LV diastolic filling dynamics occurs in patients with SLE. These abnormalities may represent myocardial involvement in SLE and may be related to disease activity.

Nihoyannopoulos and co-workers[32] in London, UK, prospectively performed 2-dimensional echocardiographic studies in 93 patients with SLE to discover the incidence and spectrum of cardiac abnormalities and to relate these findings to the presence of high levels of anticardiolipin antibodies. Assessment of the intracardiac anatomy was also performed in an additional 12 patients who had increased anticardiolipin antibody levels but did not have lupus. Fifty patients with SLE had cardiac abnormalities, and 43 patients had normal hearts. Three categories of cardiac abnormalities were identified-valvular lesions, ranging from vegetations to valvular thickening, were found in 28%, pericardial effusion or thickening was found in 20%, and regional or global LV dysfunction was found in 5%. High levels of anticardiolipin antibodies were detected in 50 patients. Of those, only 11 had an entirely normal heart, whereas the remaining 39 had at least one cardiac abnormality. (For instance, valvular lesions in 20, pericardial effusion in 15, and myocardial dysfunction in 5 patients.) In patients with SLE the presence of abnormal intracardiac anatomy was strongly associated with increased levels of anticardiolipin antibodies. The overall sensitivity and specificity of high levels of anticardiolipin antibodies in the prediction of cardiac abnormalities was 78% and 74%. Eight of the 12 patients who had increased anticardiolipin antibodies but whose disease did not fulfill the American Rheumatism Association classification criteria for SLE had cardiac abnormalities similar to those in patients with SLE compared with only 4 who had normal hearts. High levels of anticardiolipin antibodies are strongly association with cardiac abnormalities, not only in SLE but also in other SLE-like syndromes.

Thalassemia major

The consequences of transfusional iron overload on left ventricular diastolic filling have never been investigated systematically in patients with thalassemia major. The pattern of LV filling was assessed by Spirito and co-workers[33] in Genoa, Italy, by Doppler echocardiography in 32 patients with thalassemia major who had not experienced symptoms of CHF and had normal LV systolic function. Data were compared with those obtained in 32 age-matched and sex-matched normal subjects. An abnormal Doppler pattern of LV filling with increased flow velocity at mitral valve opening followed by an abrupt and premature decrease of flow velocity in early diastole was identified in patients with thalassemia. Peak flow velocity in early diastole was increased in patients compared with controls, and rate of deceleration of flow velocity after the early diastolic peak and the ratio between the early and late peaks of flow velocity were also increased, whereas flow velocity deceleration time was reduced. This Doppler pattern of diastolic filling is usually described as "restrictive" and reflects a decrease in LV chamber compliance. A restrictive pattern of LV filling was also identified in the subgroup of 16 patients who had undergone optimal iron chelation therapy with deferoxamine.

Rate of deceleration of flow velocity after the early diastolic peak was increased, and flow velocity deceleration time was reduced in these 16 patients compared with controls. The results of this investigation demonstrated that LV filling is altered in patients with thalassemia major and that diastolic abnormalities developed in an early phase of cardiac involvement, when symptoms of CHF are absent and systolic function is normal. These findings also suggest that chelation therapy with deferoxamine does not completely protect patients with thalassemia from myocardial damage due to iron-related cardiac toxicity.

Facioscapulohumeral muscular dystrophy

Stevenson and associates[34] in Los Angeles, California, evaluated patients with facioscapulohumeral muscular dystrophy to determine the frequency of cardiac involvement. Facioscapulohumeral muscular dystrophy is an autosomal dominant neuromuscular disease with an incidence of 3 to 10 cases per million. The disease typically becomes clinically overt in late childhood or adolescence, it is slowly progressive but variable in expression, and it is characterized by facial and shoulder/arm weakness and atrophy (Figure 7-4). Previously, cardiac involvement had not been convincingly reported in patients with facioscapulohumeral muscular dystrophy. Thirty rigorously documented cases of facioscapulohumeral muscular dystrophy were studied. All patients had a 12-lead electrocardiogram, 22 had a 24 hour ambulatory electrocardiogram, 15 patients had 2-dimensional echocardiography/Doppler studies, and 10 patients had 12 intracardiac electrophysiologic investigations. LA, RA, or biatrial P wave abnormalities were identified in 60% of the surface electrocardiograms from these patients. Evidence of abnormal AV node or intranodal conduction was present on intracardiac electrophysiologic studies or surface electrocardiograms in 27% of patients. Atrial flutter or

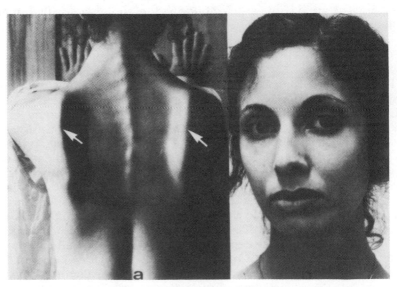

Fig. 7-4. Case 1. A 32 year old woman with facioscapulohumeral dystrophy. a, Winging of the scapulae (arrows) is exaggerated by pressing the extended arms against a resisting surface. b, Typical myopathic facies with dimpling at the corners of the mouth. Reproduced with permission from Stevenson, et al.[34]

AF was induced by single atrial extra stimuli in 10 of the 12 intracardiac electrophysiologic studies. Thus, this investigation provides evidence of cardiac involvement in patients with facioscapulohumeral muscular dystrophy. The cardiac involvement frequently takes the form of atrial rhythm disturbances which may be induced during electrophysiologic study and less frequent evidence of abnormal sinus node function and abnormal AV node or infranodal conduction.

Interleukin-2-based immunotherapy

Kragel and associates[35] from Bethesda, Maryland, described morphologic changes occurring in patients treated with interleukin-2 (IL-2), either alone or in combination with lymphokine-activated killer cells, tumor infiltrating lymphocytes, or other immunotherapeutic agents. They reviewed necropsy tissues from 19 patients with a variety of malignancies and the patients died after receiving IL-2-based immunotherapy. Death occurred at intervals ranging from less than 1 hour to 143 days following the last dose of therapy. All patients dying at or less than 43 days following cessation of therapy had lymphoid infiltrates of varying intensity in residual tumor. At necropsy, the major cause of death unrelated to the presence of metastatic tumor was bacterial sepsis. In addition, they found evidence of significant cardiac and pulmonary toxicity: 2 patients with AMI, 1 with and 1 without significant CAD, 2 cases of unexplained lymphocytic myocarditis, and 1 case of fatal pulmonary capillary plugging following an infusion of lymphokine-activated killer cells. Thus, not unlike other forms of therapy for cancer, IL-2-based immunotherapy does not appear to be without significant toxicity.

MISCELLANEOUS TOPICS

Arrhythmogenic right ventricular cardiomyopathy

Daliento and associates[36] from Padua, Italy, evaluated diagnostic sensitivity and specificity of cineangiography by multivariate logistic discriminant analysis in 32 patients with arrhythmogenic RV cardiomyopathy, 27 patients with biventricular dilated cardiomyopathy, 28 patients with ASD, and 18 normal subjects. In patients with arrhythmogenic RV cardiomyopathy and biventricular dilated cardiomyopathy, the diagnosis was confirmed by endo-myocardial biopsy. All RV values overlapped for the diagnosis of atrial septal defect and arrhythmogenic RV cardiomyopathy; overlapping extended to dilated cardiomyopathy for end-diastolic volume and infundibular dimensions. RVEF appeared reduced in all the disease; in particular, mean values in dilated cardiomyopathy and arrhythmogenic RV cardiomyopathy were 38 and 53%, respectively. LV quantitative studies showed a significant difference between dilated and arrhythmogenic RV cardiomyopathy, both in terms of pumping indexes (mean end-diastolic volumes 180 vs 91 ml/m^2 and mean EF 33 vs 60%), and indexes of contractility (stress/end-diastolic volume 3.7 vs 6.7). Multivariate analysis disclosed that transversally arranged hypertrophic trabeculae, separated by deep fissures, were associated with the highest probability of arrhythmogenic RV cardiomyopathy. Posterior subtricuspid and anterior infundibular wall bulgings were the only other independently significant variables. Coexistence of these signs was associated with 96% specificity and 87.5% sensitivity. Thus, arrhythmogenic RV cardiomyopathy presents quantitative volumetric and hemodynamic as well as qualitative features that clearly distinguish it from dilated cardiomyopathy and confirm its nosographic autonomy among the primary diseases of the myocardium.

Cardiac rhabdomyoma

Smythe and associates[37] from Toronto, Canada, report experience with rhabdomyoma diagnosed over a 20 year period. Diagnosis by angiography or echocardiography was accepted only if multiple tumors were present or if tuberous sclerosis was also diagnosed. Nine patients (3 diagnosed prenatally and the remaining 6 at age <8 months) were identified as having a total of 24 tumors. Measurements in 2 planes demonstrated at least some evidence of regression in 100%, with 20 of 24 having complete resolution. (Table 7-3) One patient required delayed surgery for excision of a subaortic ridge that appeared at the site of a resolved tumor. These authors show clearly the benign nature of most cardiac rhabdomyomas. Even tumors which appear to impinge on filling or emptying of the heart are tolerated amazingly well by many infants. Surgery should be reserved for patients with severe symptomatology. Cardiac arrhythmias which are difficult to treat will usually resolve over 6-18 months.

Noncompaction of ventricular myocardium

Chin and associates[38] from Los Angeles, California, studied isolated noncompaction of LV myocardium found as a rare disorder of endomyocardial morphogenesis characterized by numerous, excessively prominent ventricular trabeculations and deep intertrabecular recesses (Figure 7-5). This study comprised 8 patients, including 3 at necropsy. Ages ranged from 11 months to 22.5 years with a follow-up as long as 5 years. Gross morphological severity ranged from moderately abnormal ventricular trabeculations to profoundly abnormal, loosely compacted trabeculations. Echocardiographic images were diagnostic and corresponded to the morphological appearance at necropsy. The depth of the intertrabecular recesses was assessed by a quantitative echocardiographic ratio and was significantly greater than in normal control subjects. Clinical manifestations of the disorder included depressed LV systolic function in 5 patients, ventricular arrhythmias in 5, systemic embolization in 3, distinctive facial dysmorphism in 3, and familial recurrence in 4

TABLE 7-3. *Patient characteristics and tumor outcome. Reproduced with permission from Smythe, et al.[37]*

Case	Sex/Age	Presentation	Tumor Location				Follow-Up (regression)	Status (clinical)
			RA	RV	LV	IVS		
1	M/7 mo	Arrhythmia			1		1/1	Alive/TS
2	F/2 days	Arrhythmia				1	1/1	Alive/TS
3	M/3 mo	Murmur		1	1		2/2	Alive/TS
4	F/2 days	Murmur			1		1/1	Alive/TS
5	M/3 days	Murmur			1	1	1/2	Alive
6	F/prenat.	Screening U/S	1		2	2	4/5	Alive/TS
7	M/prenat.	Arrhythmia	1	2	2		5/5	Alive/TS
8	F/1 day	Murmur	2		2	1	4/5	Sub AS-Sx
9	F/prenat.	FHxTS			1	1	1/2	Alive/TS

Regression denotes complete resolution.
FH = family history; IVS = interventricular septum; LV = left ventricle; prenat. = prenatal; RA = right atrium; RV = right ventricle; Sub As-Sx = subaortic stenosis-surgical resection; TS = tuberous sclerosis; U/S = ultrasound.

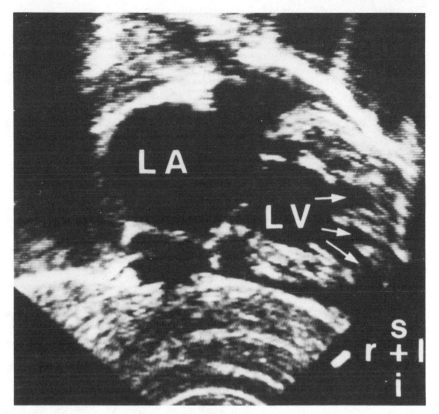

Fig. 7-5. Echocardiogram of patient 1. Subxiphoid long-axis view shows numerous prominent left ventricular trabeculations, increased depth of intertrabecular recesses (arrows), and apical thickening. LA, left atrium; LV, left ventricle; s, superior; i, inferior; r, right; l, left. Reproduced with permission from Chin, et al.[38]

patients. These authors present the largest series to date of this unusual abnormality which is believed to represent an arrest in endocardial morphogenesis.

References

1. Chen SU, Nouri SA, Balfour I, Jureidini S, Appleton RS: Clinical Profile of Congestive Cardiomyopathy in Children. J Am Coll Cardiol 1990 (January);15:189–93.

2. Mestroni L, Miani D, Di Lenarda A, Silvestri F, Bussani R, Gilippi G, Camerini F: Clinical and pathologic study of familial dilated cardiomyopathy. Am J Cardiol 1990 (June 15);65:1449–1453.

3. Keren A, Gottlieb S, Tzivoni D, Stern S, Yarom R, Billingham ME, Popp RL: Mildly dilated congestive cardiomyopathy: use of prospective diagnostic criteria and description of the clinical course without heart transplantation. Circulation 1990 (February);81;506–517.

4. Treasure CB, Vita JA, Cox DA, Fish, RD, Gordon JB, Mudge, GH, Colucci WS, St. John-Sutton MG, Selwyn AP, Alexander RW, Ganz P: Endothelium-dependent dilation of the coronary microvasculature is impaired in dilated cardiomyopathy. Circulation 1990 (March);81:772–779.

5. Jin O, Sole MJ, Butany JW, Chia WK, McLaughlin PR, Liu P, Liew CC: Detection of Enterovirus RNA in Myocardial Biopsies From Patients with Myocarditis and Car-

diomyopathy Using Gene Amplification by Polymerase Chain Reaction. Circulation 1990 (July);82:8–16.

6. Bohm M, Gierschik P, Jakobs KH, Pieske B, Schnabel P, Ungerer M, Erdmann E: Increase of G_{ia} In Human Hearts With Dilated but Not Ischemic Cardiomyopathy. Circulation 1990 (October);82:1249–1265.

7. Caforio ALP, Bonifacio E, Stewart JT, Neglia D, Parodi O, Bottazzo GF, McKenna WJ. Novel organ-specific circulating cardiac autoantibodies in dilated cardiomyopathy. J Am Coll Cardiol 1990 (June);15:1527–34.

8. Uchida Y, Nakamura F, Oshima T, Fujimori Y, Hirose J: Percutaneous fiberoptic angioscopy of the left ventricle in patients with dilated cardiomyopathy and acute myocarditis. Am Heart J 1990 (September);120:677–687.

9. Sundram P, Reddy HK, McElroy PA, Janicki JS, Weber KT: Myocardial energetics and efficiency in patients with idiopathic cardiomyopathy: Response to dobutamine and amrinone. Am Heart J 1990 (April);119:891–898.

10. Leung W-H, Lau C-P, Wong C-K, Cheng C-H, Tai Y-T, Lim S-P: Improvement in exercise performance and hemodynamics by labetalol in patients with idiopathic dilated cardiomyopathy. Am Heart J 1990 (April);119:884–890.

11. Gilbert EM, Anderson JL, Deitchman D, Yanowitz FG, O'Connell JB, Renlund DG, Bartholomew M, Mealey PC, Larrabee P, Bristow MR: Long-term B-blocker vasodilator therapy improves cardiac function in idiopathic dilated cardiomyopathy: A double-blind, randomized study of bucindolol versus placebo. Am J Med 1990 (Mar);88:223–229.

12. Hochleitner M, Hortnagl H, Ng CK, Hortnagl H, Gschnitzer F, Zechmann W: Usefulness of physiologic dual-chamber pacing in drug-resistant idiopathic dilated cardiomyopathy. Am J Cardiol 1990 (July 15);66:198–202.

13. Midei MG, DeMent SH, Feldman AM, Hutchins GM, Baughman KL: Peripartum myocarditis and cardiomyopathy. Circulation 1990 (March);81:922–928.

14. Dec GW, Fallon JT, Southern JF, Palacios I. "Borderline" myocarditis: An indication for repeat endomyocardial biopsy. J Am Coll Cardiol 1990 (February);15:283–9.

15. Herskowitz A, Ahmed-Ansari A, Neumann DA, Beschorner WE, Rose NR, Soule LM, Burek CL, Sell KW, Baughman KL. Induction of major histocompatibility complex antigens within the myocardium of patients with active myocarditis: A nonhistologic marker of myocarditis. J Am Coll Cardiol 1990 (March);15:624–32.

16. Dec GW, Palacios I, Yasuda T, Fallon JT, Khaw BA, Strauss HW, Haber E. Antimyosin antibody cardiac imaging: Its role in the diagnosis of myocarditis. J Am Coll Cardiol 1990 (July);16:97–104.

17. Spirito P, Maron BJ. Relation between extent of left ventricular hypertrophy and occurrence of sudden cardiac death in hypertrophic cardiomyopathy. J Am Coll Cardiol 1990 (June);15:1521–6.

18. Fay WP, Taliercio CP, Ilstrup DM, Tajik AJ, Gersh BJ. Natural history of hypertrophic cardiomyopathy in the elderly. J Am Coll Cardiol 1990 (October);16:821–6.

19. Nienaber CA, Hiller S, Spielmann RP, Geiger M, Kuck K. Syncope in hypertrophic cardiomyopathy: multivariate analysis of prognostic determinants. J Am Coll Cardiol 1990 (April);15:948–55.

20. Robinson K, Frenneaux MP, Stockins B, Karatasakis G, Poloniecki JD, McKenna WJ. Atrial fibrillation in hypertrophic cardiomyopathy: A longitudinal study. J Am Coll Cardiol 1990 (May);15:1279–85.

21. Lemery R, Kleinebenne A, Nihoyannopoulos P, Aber V, Alfonso F, McKenna WJ. Q waves in hypertrophic cardiomyopathy in relation to the distribution and severity of right and left ventricular hypertrophy. J Am Coll Cardiol 1990 (August);16:368–74.

22. Cripps TR, Counihan PJ, Frenneaux MP, Ward DE, Camm AJ, McKenna WJ. Signal-averaged electrocardiography in hypertrophic cardiomyopathy. J Am Coll Cardiol 1990 (April);15:956–61.

23. Alessandri N, Pannarale G, Del Monte F, Moretti F, Marino B, Reale A: Hypertrophic obstructive cardiomyopathy and infective endocarditis: A report of seven cases and a review of the literature. Eur H J 1990 (Nov);11:1041–1048.

24. McKenna WJ, Stewart JT, Nihoyannopoulos P, McGinty F, Davies MJ: Hypertrophic cardiomyopathy without hypertrophy: Two families with myocardial disarray in the absence of increased myocardial mass. Br Heart J 1990 (May);63:287–290.

25. Koga Y, Yamaguchi R, Ogata M, Kihara K, Toshima H: Decreased coronary vasodilatory capacity in hypertrophic cardiomyopathy determined by split-dose thallium-dipyridamole myocardial scintigraphy. Am J Cardiol 1990 (May 1);65:1134–1139.

26. Stone CD, Hennein HA, McIntosh CL, Quyyumi AA, Greenberg GJ, Clark RE: The results of operation in patients with hypertrophic cardiomyopathy and pulmonary hypertension. J Thorac Cardiovasc Surg 1990 (Sept);100:343–352.

27. Kupari M, Koskinen P, Suokas A, Ventila M: Left ventricular filling impairment in asymptomatic chronic alcoholics. Am J Cardiol 1990 (Dec 15);66:1473–1477.

28. Chanson P, Timsit J, Masquet C, Warner A, Guillausseau PJ, Birman P, Harris AG, Lubetzki J: Cardiovascular effects of the somatostatin analog octreotide in acromegaly. An Intern Med 1990 (Dec 15);113:921–925.

29. Polikar R, Kennedy B, Maisel A, Ziegler M, Smith J, Dittrich H, Nicod P. Decreased adrenergic sensitivity in patients with hypothyroidism. J Am Coll Cardiol 1990 (January);15:94–8.

30. Crozier IG, Li E, Milne MJ, Nicholls MG: Cardiac involvement in systemic lupus erythematosus detected by echocardiography. Am J Cardiol 1990 (May 1);65:1145–1148.

31. Leung W-H, Wong K-L, Lau C-P, Wong C-K, Cheng C-H, Tai Y-T: Doppler echocardiographic evaluation of left ventricular diastolic function in patients with systemic lupus erythematosus. Am Heart J 1990 (July);120:82-87.

32. Nihoyannopoulos P, Gomez PM, Joshi J, Loizou S, Walport MJ, Oakley CM: Cardiac Abnormalities in Systemic Lupus Erythematosus Association with Raised Anticardiolipin Antibodies. Circulation 1990 (August);82:369–375.

33. Spirito P, Gabriele L, Melevendi C, Vecchio C: Restrictive Diastolic Abnormalities Identified by Doppler Echocardiography in Patients with Thalassemia Major. Circulation 1990 (July);82:88–94.

34. Stevenson WG, Perloff JK, Weiss JN, Anderson TL. Facioscapulohumeral muscular dystrophy: Evidence for selective, genetic electrophysiologic cardiac involvement. J Am Coll Cardiol 1990 (February);15:292–9.

35. Kragel AH, Travis WD, Feinberg L, Pittaluga S, Striker LM, Roberts WC, Lotze MT, Yang JJ, Rosenberg SA: Pathologic findings associated with interleukin-2-based immunotherapy for cancer: A postmortem study of 19 patients. Hum Pathol 1990 (May);21:493–502.

36. Daliento L, Rizzoli G, Ghiene G, Nava A, Rinuncini M, Chioin R, Volta SD: Diagnostic accuracy of right ventriculography in arrhythmogenic right ventricular cardiomyopathy. Am J Cardiol 1990 (Sept 15);66:741–745.

37. Smythe JF, Dyck JD, Smallhorn JF, Freedom RM: Natural History of Cardiac Rhabdomyoma in Infancy and Childhood. Am J Cardiol 1990 (November);66:1247–1249.

38. Chin TK, Perloff JK, Williams RG, Kenneth J, Mohrmann R: Isolated Noncompaction of Left Ventricular Myocardium. A Study of Eight Cases. Circulation (August) 1990;82:507–513.

Congenital Heart Disease

Transesophageal Doppler echocardiography

Morimoto and associates[1] from Ube, Japan, used transesophageal echocardiography in 11 patients with secundum ASD, ages 15 to 55 years. The defect was clearly seen in all 11 patients with clear laminar shunt flow with two peaks in late systole and late diastole. The defect size measured by echocardiography correlated well with the surgical measurement in horizontal width and vertical length. In addition, significant high correlation was shown between shunt volume measured by echocardiography and by Fick's method. This modality can be extremely useful in patients whose standard echocardiographic imaging is suboptimal. It has also been useful for patients undergoing transcatheter closure of ASD.

Double-umbrella closure

Rome and associates[2] from Boston, Massachusetts, reported 40 patients catheterized for closure of ASD using 3 different devices. Patients weighed 8 kg or more which was a requirement for the transvenous access with the 11F delivery sheath. The new device was at least 1.6 times the diameter of the ASD. Closure was attempted in 34 patients with ASD size ranging from 3 to 22 mm with devices ranging from 17 to 33 mm. Initial device position immediately after release was correct in all patients. A cerebral embolus occurred in 1 elderly patient before device placement and the patient died 1 week later. Two instances of early device embolization occurred and devices were retrieved by catheter without complication. Follow-up of 31 patients discharged with devices in place for a 31 patient/year follow-up has yielded no complications. Adequate imaging in 19 patients 6.5 months after placement revealed no atrial shunt in 12; residual flow through separate, previously unrecognized defects in 2; and small residual leaks (<3 mm) around devices in 5 patients. The data represent continued improvement of the device for transcatheter closure of ASD. This has been a particularly useful device in patients with residual right-to-left atrial shunts which in some patients are left purposely after Fontan operation. This procedure, in all likelihood, will become a standard for treatment of small to moderate sized ASD.

Late follow-up after operative closure

ASD has been surgically correctable for >30 years. The long-term survival rates among patients treated in the early era of cardiac surgery are poorly documented, but such data are of critical importance to the future medical care, employability, and insurability of these patients. To determine the natural history of surgically corrected ASD, Murphy and associates[3] from Rochester, Minnesota, and Birmingham, Alabama, studies all 123 patients who underwent repair of an isolated ostium secundum or sinus venosus ASD at the Mayo Clinic between 1956 and 1960, 27 to 32 years before the procedure. The follow-up status of all patients was determined by written questionnaires and telephone interviews. Hospital records and death certificates were obtained if interim hospitalization or death had occurred. The overall 30-year actuarial survival rate among survivors of the perioperative period was 74%, as compared with 85% among controls matched for age and sex. The perioperative mortality was 3% (4 deaths). Actuarial 27-year survival rates among patients in the younger 2 quartiles according to age at operation (≤11 years and 12 to 24 years) were no different from rates among controls—97% and 93%, respectively. In the 2 older quartiles (25 to 41 years and >41 years), 27-year survival rates were significantly less—84% and 40%, respectively—than in controls (91 and 59%). Independent predictors of long-term survival according to multivariate analysis were age at operation and systolic pressure in the pulmonary trunk before operation (Figure 8-1). When repair was performed in older patients, late cardiac failure, stroke, and AF were significantly more frequent (Figure 8-2). Among patients with surgically repaired ASD, those operated on before the age of 25 have an excellent prognosis, but older patients require careful, regular supervision.

ATRIOVENTRICULAR CANAL

Clapp and associates[4] from Detroit, Michigan, reviewed experience over a 10 year period with patients with Down's syndrome and complete AV canal defect. Forty-five patients with Down's syndrome catheterized <1 year of age had a lower pulmonary blood flow and higher pulmonary vascular resistance than did 34 normal chromosome counterparts with similar diagnoses. When all ages were included 47% of children with Down's syndrome and 80% of normal children were considered operable. Of the 34 patients who did not have operation because of pulmonary vascular disease, 31 had Down's syndrome. In 10 of 81 children with Down's syndrome, fixed pulmonary vascular obstructive disease was diagnosed before the age of 1 year while this was found in none of 40 normal children. These authors provide reasonably good data indicating the early development of pulmonary vascular obstructive disease in children with Down's syndrome. The data are not as clean as one would

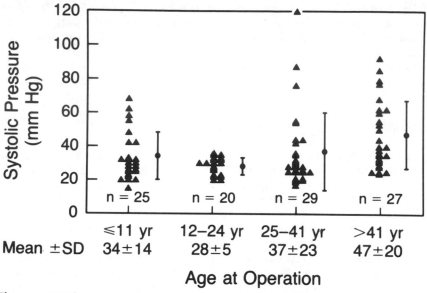

Fig. 8-1. Systolic pressure of main pulmonary artery before closure of atrial septal defect, according to age at operation (P = 0.0034 by Analysis of Variance). Reproduced with permission from Murphy, et al.[3]

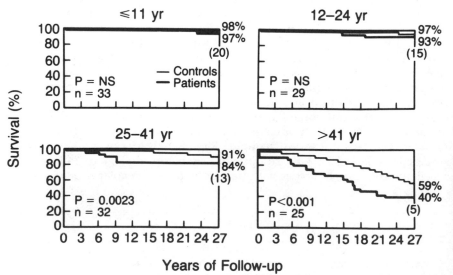

Fig. 8-2. Long-term survival of patients surviving the perioperative period, according to age at operation. Expected survival in an age- and sex-matched control population is also shown. P values for the comparison of observed with expected survival were calculated by the log-rank test; NS denotes not significant. Values in parentheses denote the numbers of patients alive at the end of the follow-up periods shown. Reproduced with permission from Murphy, et al.[3]

like because of the age differences between groups and the retrospective analysis. The question of upper airway obstruction and pulmonary disease contributing to pulmonary vascular disease in the Down syndrome child is difficult to sort out, although the authors believed that chronic airway problems were not a contributing factor in (most) patients. The recommendations for early catheterization and repair in patients with suspected pulmonary vascular resistance elevation are prudent.

VENTRICULAR SEPTAL DEFECT

Doppler color flow imaging for multiple defects

Chin and associates[5] from Philadelphia, Pennsylvania, used Doppler color flow imaging compared with axial contrast angiography in the preoperative detection of additional VSDs in the setting of a large known defect. One hundred seventy-nine infants with 2 ventricles and a large, nonrestrictive VSD underwent reparative surgery before 2 years of age. The reference standard for the presence of additional defects was intraoperative verification or subsequent identification at postoperative angiography or postoperative color Doppler exam or reoperation. Only 6 patients had additional VSDs confirmed at repair; an additional 5 had defects found postoperatively. The negative predictive value of Doppler color flow imaging and angiography was .95 and .97, respectively. The sensitivity was .27 (3 of 11) and .45 (5 of 11), respectively. These authors again show the difficulty of being absolutely sure about additional VSDs with color flow Doppler mapping before surgery in patients with a known large VSD. The authors represent an institution with considerable experience and expertise in this modality. Most institutions will continue to need to rely on angiography for detecting additional VSDs in this setting.

Late follow-up with aortic regurgitation

Rhodes and associates[6] from Boston, Massachusetts, followed 92 patients with VSD and audible AR with the median age of onset of AR of 5.3 years. The VSD was subcristal in 62 patients and subpulmonary in 21 and unknown in the remaining 9. The risk of developing AR was 2.5 times greater in those with subpulmonary VSD. The aortic valve was tricuspid in 90% and bicuspid in 10%. Prolapse was seen in 90% of those with subcristal VSD and in all of those with subpulmonary VSD. Pulmonary stenosis was seen in 46% of patients with gradients ranging from 10 to 55 mmHg. The prevalence of infective endocarditis was 15 episodes per 1,000 patient years. Among 20 patients followed medically for 297 patient years, 1 died and most have been stable, including 2 followed for >30 years. In the 72 patients operated on, there were 15 perioperative and 5 late deaths. Operations consisted of VSD closure alone in 7, VSD closure and valvuloplasty in 50 and VSD closure and aortic valve replacement in the other 15. Valvuloplasty was more effective in those operated on under age 10 compared to those older than 15 years. The durability of the valvuloplasty was 76% at 12 years and 51% at 18 years. These authors present excellent long-term followup on this important management problem.

Diazoxide for secondary pulmonary vascular disease

Rao[7] from Madison, Wisconsin, presented results of short- and long-term effects of diazoxide on the pulmonary vascular resistance in patients with pulmonary vascular obstructive disease secondary to delayed surgical correction of VSD. Six children, aged 4 to 10 years, who had closure of VSD and who on lung biopsy showed pulmonary vascular obstructive disease, received intravenous diazoxide (1, 2, 4, 5, and 6 mg/kg) after measurements of PA pressure, pulmonary flow index by thermodilution technique, and pulmonary vascular resistance were made. The PA pressure (51 ± 19 mm Hg vs 45 ± 16 mm Hg) and pulmonary vascular resistance (12 ± 2.7 units vs 8.9 ± 3.8 units) though decreased, did not attain statistical significance. The pulmonary flow index (3.2 ± 1.1 vs 3.4 ± 0.6 L/min/m²) did not change. After oral diazoxide (5 to 10 mg/kg/day) for 20 ± 3.4 months, the PA pressure (51 ± 19 mm Hg) and pulmonary vascular resistance (11 ± 5.8 units) did not decrease, but pulmonary flow index (4.4 ± 0.9 L/min/m²), though increased, did not attain significance. However, 1 of these children who had a fall in pulmonary vascular resistance from 8.5 to 4.5 units following intravenous diazoxide also had a lower resistance (3.9 units) after 20-months of oral diazoxide therapy and improved symptomatically. No complications other than hypertrichosis were encountered on long-term therapy. Based on this experience, it is suggested that oral diazoxide therapy may be used to improve pulmonary vascular obstructive disease if there is favorable response to intravenous diazoxide.

PULMONIC VALVE STENOSIS—BALLOON VALVULOPLASTY

Caspi and associates[8] from Toronto, Canada, evaluated management of neonatal critical PS with intact ventricular septum. Thirty-nine patients ages <3 months were treated initially by operation (n = 19) or with balloon valvuloplasty (n = 20). Surgical patients were younger (5 versus 18 days) and had a greater degree of hypoxia (PO₂ 55 vs 80 mmHg). RV hypoplasia was present in 10 of 19 surgical patients and 8 of 20 balloon patients. Balloon therapy was attempted in 20 patients at initial catheterization but was unsuccessful in 9 because of inability to catheterize the hypoplastic RV outflow tract. Patents with failed balloon therapy were subsequently operated on within 24 hours. The early operative mortality was 25% (7 of 28) and 1 death occurred after successful balloon valvotomy due to associated critical AS. The early postoperative gradient was 20 mmHg; post balloon gradient was 18. These authors conclude that balloon valvotomy yields good results in patients with critical PS with essentially normal sized RV whereas surgical valvotomy is required for patients with RV hypoplasia. Other centers have reported success with presumed hypoplastic right ventricles with balloon therapy. Unfortunately the precise quantification of RV size was lacking in this report as well as other reports and the determination of when RV hypoplasia is truly present is a bit nebulous.

Stanger and associates[9] from San Francisco, California, reported results of the Valvuloplasty Registry for Congenital Anomalies in 822 patients. Pre- and post-valvuloplasty gradients were available in 784 patients and showed a decrease from 71 to 28 mmHg. The site of residual obstructions could be ascertained in 196 patients in whom the total gradient decreased from 85 to 34 with 16 mmHg transvalvular and 18 mmHg infundibular. The procedure was less effective in reducing outflow gradients in patients with dysplastic valves with or without Noonan's syndrome. There were 5 major complications including 2 deaths (.2%), a cardiac perforation with tamponade (.1%) and 2 instances of tricuspid insufficiency (.2%). There were 11 minor complications including venous thrombosis in 5, vein tears in 2, respiratory arrest in 1, arrhythmia in 2, and pulmonary leaflet evulsion in 1. The prevalence of major and minor complications was inversely related to age. These authors show the expected good results in pulmonary valvuloplasty. Potential problems in infants indicate that the procedure should be undertaken only in centers where emergency is available and considerable continuing experience in treating critical heart disease in infancy is available.

Kan and associates[10] from Baltimore, Maryland, reported the results from the Valvuloplasty and Angioplasty Registry for Congenital Anomalies for 182 procedures in 156 patients ranging in age from 2 to 46 years for treatment of PA stenosis. Vessel dimension at the site of the stenosis increased from 4.5 to 6.8 mm with greater increases in diameter if the balloon was >3 times the original stenosis dimension. There was no significant benefit related to age or prior surgical intervention. The mean peak systolic pressure gradient was reduced from 49 to 37 mmHg and pressure proximal to the stenosis decreased from 69 to 63 mmHg. Complications occurred in 21 patients and included vessel rupture and deaths in 2, vessel perforation or rupture with survival in 3, cardiac arrest and death in 1, paradoxical embolism and death in 1 and low output and death in 1. These authors report only modest success in treatment of this condition. The risk of vessel rupture and death is significant with death or major rupture associated with 6 of 182 procedures. The procedure may be of significant benefit in selected patients with stenoses that are not amenable to surgical intervention.

Khan and associates[11] from Riyadh, Saudi Arabia, used follow-up cardiac catheterization studies to evaluate 105 patients who had undergone percutaneous balloon pulmonary valvuloplasty. Fifteen of those patients who had peak systolic pulmonary valve gradients ≥40 mm Hg at follow-up underwent repeat balloon valvuloplasty. For the initial balloon pulmonary valvuloplasty, the mean ratio of the balloon diameter to pulmonary valve anulus diameter was 0.98 ± 0.2; at repeat valvuloplasty the mean was 1.19 ± 0.12. The immediate post-repeat balloon valvuloplasty results showed a reduction in the peak systolic gradient from a mean of 70 ± 18 to 29 ± 19 mm Hg. This reduction in the gradient was maintained at a mean of 14 ± 5.0 mm Hg in 8 of the 10 patients who underwent further follow-up studies. It was concluded that successful repeat balloon pulmonary valvuloplasty with the use of larger sized balloons is feasible in patients who have restenosis after the initial percutaneous balloon valvuloplasty—including partial but not complete dysplasia of the pulmonary valve.

TETRALOGY OF FALLOT

Primary repair in infancy

Touati and associates[12] from Paris, France, reported primary repair of symptomatic TF in 100 consecutive infants ranging in age from .5 to 12 months. Twenty patients were ≤3 months and mean weight was 6.5 kg. Seventy patients received a transannular patch and 90% of patients ≤3 months had a transannular patch. The hospital mortality was 3% and there were no late deaths with a cumulative follow-up of 180 patient-years. Causes of death included hypoplastic pulmonary arteries in 2 and RV failure in 1. The most important factors influencing RV outflow tract reconstruction were the ratio between weight and pulmonary arterial outflow diameter and the ratio between body surface area and pulmonary arterial outflow diameter. The last 48 patients were operated on with no deaths during a time when myocardial protection with blood cardioplegia was instituted. No ventricular arrhythmias have been detected after repair with a mean follow-up of 22 months. These results lend further support to infant repair of TF in the hands of an experienced surgical group.

Late follow-up of repair before age 20

Horneffer and associates[13] from Baltimore, Maryland, reported 170 children aged 10 years or less who underwent total repair of TF between 1958 and 1978. Follow-up 10 to 28 years postoperatively on 90% of the 143 who survived the operation was performed with a mean follow-up of 18 years. All patients completed an extensive questionnaire and 59 returned for history and physical examination, electrocardiogram, exercise stress testing, pulmonary function testing and echocardiography. Late survival was excellent with only two of four known late deaths due to cardiac-related causes and with all 59 patients asymptomatic or showing only mild symptoms. Sinus rhythm was present in 90% and 1 patient had complete heart block. RV function was estimated to be normal by echocardiography in 78% and residual mild to moderate pulmonary stenosis was noted by Doppler study in 8 patients. Pulmonary regurgitation was present in 78% but in only 11 patients was it graded as moderate and in none was it severe. Stress testing documented the excellent functional status of most patients with 92% of predicted exercise time and 94% of maximum heart rate being attained. These data show excellent results late after TF repair in (most) patients. The echocardiogram is, however, not a very sensitive or specific method for assessing RV function and the authors may have underestimated this potential right sided heart dysfunction.

Ventricular arrhythmias postoperatively

Chandar and associates[14] from Miami, Florida, reported results of a multicenter retrospective study of 359 patients with postoperative TF repaired before 20 years of age who had electrophysiological study including programmed stimulation in the RV outflow or apex. The mean age at repair was 5 years with a mean follow-up of 7 years. Spontaneous VPCs on ambulatory monitoring was found in 48% and inducible VT on electrophysiologic stimulation was found in 17%. Both spontaneous VPCs and inducible VT were significantly related to delayed age at repair, longer follow-up interval, symptoms of syncope or presyncope, RV systolic pressure >60 mmHg, but not to RV diastolic pressure >80 mmHg. VPCs on ambulatory monitoring were more complex with increasing age at repair and follow-up duration. Induction of VT on electrophysiologic stimulation correlated with spontaneous VPCs including VT on 24 hour monitoring. While induced sustained monomorphic VT was related to all forms of spontaneous VPCs, induced nonsustained polymorphic VT was related to more complex forms of VPCs on monitoring. VT was not induced in asymptomatic patients who had normal 24 hour ambulatory monitoring and normal RV systolic pressure. Late sudden death occurred in 5 patients, most of whom had spontaneous VPCs on ambulatory monitoring and RV systolic pressure >80 mmHg but none had induced VT with a nonagressive electrophysiologic protocol. These data show that early repair of TF is associated with decreased prevalence of ventricular ectopic activity. Electrophysiological protocols have not been found useful in a broad range of TF patients but may provide further data in selected patients with significant ventricular ectopic activity on monitoring.

Vaksmann and associates[15] from Montreal, Canada, report follow-up on 224 consecutive patients operated on for TF who were followed from 1 to 28 years with a mean of 11. Mean age at surgery was 5.3 years (range 1 to 14). Postoperative RV systolic pressure was 60 mmHg in 19 of 213 patients. Fourteen patients (6%) had VPCs on surface electrocardiograms. Seventy-nine patients underwent treadmill exercise test and VPCs were induced in 22%. Twenty-four hour ambulatory monitoring in 92 patients demonstrated significant ventricular arrhythmias (≥grade 2 of the Lown classification) in 45%. The frequency of ventricular arrhythmias correlated with length of follow-up and duration of cardiopulmonary bypass. No correlation was found with age at surgery, postoperative RV systolic pressure and importance of conduction defects on electrocardiogram. There were no sudden or unexpected deaths during follow-up. This follow-up study suggests that treatment of asymptomatic ventricular rhythm disorders in postoperative may not be indicated. In contrast, patients with poor hemodynamic results and ventricular arrhythmias or those with complex arrhythmia with symptoms should be treated.

Late left ventricular dysfunction

Hausdorf and associates[16] from Hamburg, FRG, studied 32 patients after surgical correction of TF in childhood. The age of investigation was 19 ± 6 years and repair had been performed at the age of 8 ± 3 years. In 20 patients a one-stage operation was performed and in 12 patients a two-stage correction was performed. The control group consisted of 30 healthy volunteers, aged 18-30 years. The severity of preoperative hypoxemia was an important risk factor for late LV as dysfunction was LV end diastolic volume as a percentage of RV end diastolic volume. There was no influence on LV dysfunction of preoperative hypoxic spells, need for palliative shunt, or the age at surgical repair.

PULMONIC VALVE ATRESIA

Hawkins and associates[17] from Salt Lake City, Utah, studied the early and late results of treatment of 29 consecutive infants with pulmonary atresia and intact ventricular septum. Transventricular pulmonary valvotomy and central shunt were performed in 19 of 22 infants who had a patent infundibulum. Pulmonary valvotomy was performed in 3 of 22 infants with a patent infundibulum but 2 of these required subsequent shunts. Primary shunting was used to palliate 7 infants who had absent infundibular portions of the right ventricle and a very diminutive RV cavity. Tricuspid valve excision and atrial septectomy were also performed in 5 of these 7 infants to decompress large fistulous communications between the right ventricle and coronary arteries. Two early deaths occurred in infants with a very small right ventricle. Definitive operation has been accomplished in 16 patients with 13 having closure of residual interatrial communications and shunt ligations with no deaths. Fontan repair has been performed in 3 with 1 death. Actuarial survival for the entire group is 86% at 5 years. These authors present excellent results from dealing with this very difficult problem. Apparently they had no patients with coronary fistulous communication associated with coronary lesions. These patients probably have no real possibility for effective treatment other than cardiac transplantation. The use of tricuspid valve excision and atrial septectomy remains experimental until further data are obtained.

COMPLETE TRANSPOSITION OF THE GREAT ARTERIES

"Laid-back" aortogram for coronary anatomy

Mandell and associates[18] from Boston, Massachusetts, demonstrated a new angiographic project for evaluating coronary artery anatomy in infants with TGA. This view results in excellent demonstration of coronary anatomy (Figures 8-3, 8-4, and 8-5). These authors found superior detail to echocardiography in evaluating coronary anatomy in these infants. Intramural coronary arteries were suspected in 2 patients who were not

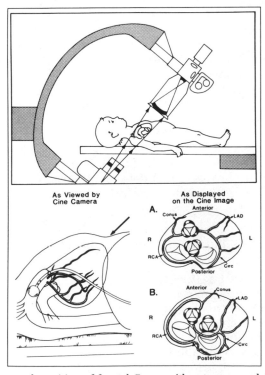

Fig. 8-3. Upper panel, position of frontal C-arm with extreme caudal angulation of the tube. The lateral tube, necessary for balloon positioning, is not shown. Lower left panel, view of heart and balloon position as "seen" by lateral image intensifier. Solid arrow in right upper corner shows "viewpoint" of frontal camera when it assumes its caudal view of heart and coronary arteries as displayed by frontal cine camera. An example of coronary course in front-to-back (A) and side-to-side (B) great arteries is shown. Circ = circumflex artery; LAD = left anterior descending artery; RCA = right coronary artery. Reproduced with permission from Mandell, et al.[18]

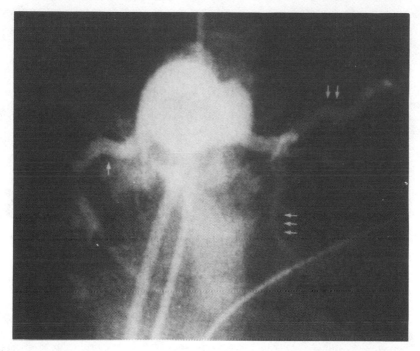

Fig. 8-4. Laid-back view in patient with most common anatomy found in transposition of great arteries. Great arteries are front-to-back and the right coronary artery (single arrow) arises from right posterior-facing sinus and gives off a conal branch, while the left coronary artery arises from left-posterior-facing sinus and gives rise to left anterior-descending (double arrow) and circumflex arteries (triple arrow). Reproduced with permission from Mandell, et al.[18]

suitable candidates for arterial switch repairs. These data should be studied by all cardiologists and surgeons who treat infants with TGA. The data are extremely useful in preparing for surgery and in quickly assessing the coronary anatomy at the operating table to confirm the suspected patterns seen on angiography.

Arterial switch operation

Wernovsky and associates[19] from Boston, Massachusetts, reviewed 30 of 290 patients who underwent arterial switch operation for TGA and had associated abnormalities of LV outflow tract or mitral valve or both. Abnormalities included isolated pulmonary valve stenosis in 9, dynamic subpulmonary stenosis in 5, fixed subpulmonary stenosis in 7, abnormal mitral chordal attachments in 2, or a combination in 7. There were 2 early deaths, 1 of which was due to MS and a subpulmonary (neo-aortic) membrane and 1 late death due to presumed coronary obstruction. Of 9 patients with pulmonary valve abnormalities, peak systolic ejection gradients preoperatively ranged from 0 to 50 mmHg, only 1 underwent valvotomy and at follow-up 5 to 30 months postoperativley the neo-aortic gradient was ≤15 mmHg in all patients and 3 of 9 had mild AR. No patients with dynamic subpulmonary obstruction had a surgical procedure performed on the LV outflow and none had obstruction after operation. Likewise no patient with anatomic subpulmonary obstruction due to accessory valve tissue or a subpulmonary membrane had a resid-

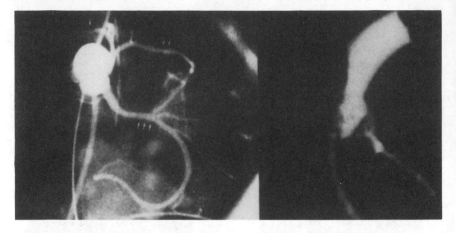

Fig. 8-5. Left, caudal view in a patient whose great arteries are more side-by-side in relation and whose coronary anatomy is atypical. From anterior-facing sinus, a coronary artery originates and gives rise to the left anterior descending artery (double arrow), which crosses anterior to the pulmonary artery, and a small right coronary artery (single arrow), the latter essentially supplying only the conus. From the posterior-facing sinus arises a very dominant circumflex artery (triple arrow), which courses behind the pulmonary artery and supplies the lateral, posterior and inferior walls of the left ventricle. This view clearly shows the large amount of myocardium supplied by this vessel, far in excess of that supplied by the left anterior descending artery, which arises separately from the anterior-facing sinus. Right, lateral view of the same showing ideal balloon position and occlusion of the aorta at time of injection. Reproduced with permission from Mandell, et al.[18]

ual gradient or abnormal atrioventricular valve function after arterial switch, combined with tissue or membrane resection. The only patients with significant residual LV outflow obstruction were 3 children with a combination of abnormalities that included obstruction due to posterior deviation of the infundibular septum. These authors have extended the arterial switch operation for TGA to patients with mild to moderate abnormalities of mitral valve or LV outflow tract. These patients must be screened carefully before operation but this form of therapy may be the most useful currently available for this group.

Mayer and associates[20] Boston, Massachusetts, studied the origins and distribution of coronary arteries in patients with TGA presenting for arterial switch operation. There were 314 patients who underwent surgery with the intent to perform an arterial switch operation with this operation actually performed in 290. There were 20 deaths with 12 deaths clearly related to problems with the coronary arteries. The arterial switch was aborted to a Senning operation in 24 patients primarily due to coronary anatomy. The authors found that all coronary patterns appear to be switchable but single right coronary artery and the inverted coronary artery pattern carried increased risk. Patients with intramural coronary arteries represent a difficult problem. These authors chose to do a Senning operation in 50% of patients when this abnormality was encountered. Alternative techniques for dealing with this unusual pattern are discussed. Cardiologists should strive for careful delineation of the coronary arterial pattern prior to surgery by both angiography and echocardiography. Despite these studies, exact patterns must be identified at the operating table and the presence or absence of an intramural coronary artery delineated before mobilization of the coronary ostium is performed.

Ventricular function postoperatively

Martin and associates[21] from London, UK, investigated RV and LV function in 21 patients after anatomical correction and 21 patients after atrial repair for TGA. Radionuclide angiography was used to measure RV and LV ejection fractions between 17 and 78 (mean 47) months after anatomical correction and between 3 and 187 (mean 67) months after intra-atrial repair. The mean age of the patient groups at the time of study was 52 and 84 months respectively. The RV ejection fraction ranged from 35 to 78% (mean 58%) in patients after anatomical repair and 27 to 68% (mean 51%) after intra-atrial repair. The LV ejection fraction ranged from 39 to 74% (mean 58%) after anatomical repair and from 35 to 74% (mean 58%) after intra-atrial repair (p = 0.86). The mean right and left ventricular ejection fractions of both groups were significantly lower than those of normal children. Individuals with systemic ventricular dysfunction were identified after both types of operations; symptomatic dysfunction occurred only after intra-atrial repair. These authors show abnormal resting systemic ventricular function in 38% of patients following intra-atrial repair of TGA, and a similar percentage of patients (29%) in the anatomical correction group. These authors also show 38% of patients after atrial repair and 32% of patients after anatomical repair had abnormal pulmonary ventricular ejection fraction. These data suggest that preoperative or perioperative myocardial damage occurred which resulted in biventricular dysfunction. Such patients obviously would not be amenable to subsequent anatomical repair after intra-atrial repair had been carried out as an initial operation.

CORRECTED TRANSPOSITION

Lundstrom and associates[22] from London, UK, reviewed data on 111 patients with congenitally corrected transposition and 2 separate ventricles managed over the 20 year period prior to 1988. The ages of survivors ranged from 1 to 58 years with a median of 20 years and all but 10 had additional anatomic abnormalities. Tricuspid valve abnormalities were more prevalent in patients symptomatic with heart failure (26 of 43) than those whose main problem was cyanosis (11 of 52). All dysplastic or Ebstein valves were at least moderately incompetent. Intracardiac repair was attempted in 51 patients with 11 early deaths. The risk factors for early death or poor result six months later related to poor preoperative symptomatic status, impaired systemic ventricular function, heart block, and younger age at surgery. Patients with more than mild preoperative TR did poorly if their valves were not replaced. Patients symptomatic from heart failure should be repaired early in the natural history of disease before the systemic ventricles dilate. By contrast, patients who predominantly cyanosed were more stable in early childhood and their surgical outcome was less compromised by poor preoperative symptomatic status. These data present excellent follow-up from a large number of patients with congenitally corrected transposition. Actuarial survival within the acyanotic group was <60% by 20 years of age.

DOUBLE INLET LEFT VENTRICLE

Nakazawa and associates[23] from Tokyo, Japan, studied ventricular volume characteristics in 10 patients with double-inlet LV before and after septation. Preoperative end diastolic volume was 291 ± 111% of normal and EF was .59 ± 0.7. Postoperatively end diastolic volume of the right sided ventricle was 82 ± 24% and the left sided ventricle was 153 ± 41%. EF of the RV was 77 ± 10 and LVEF was 49 ± 13%. On 2-dimensional echocardiography fractional change of the cross sectional area was .65 ± .16 for the RV and .23 ± .11 for the LV. Fractional shortening of the septum-to-ventricular free wall axis was .51 ± .17 in the RV and − .05 ± 0.9 in the LV right and left ventricle. Analysis of the curvature of the new septum revealed that the septum shifted to the right during systole in all patients in whom the systolic LV/RV pressure ratio was larger than 1. The septum shifted toward the LV during diastole in 8 patients in whom end diastolic pressure in the RV was higher than or equal to that in the LV, whereas it remained low in the right side in 2 patients with higher left sided pressure. The cardiac index of these 2 patients was 2.4 and 2.6 whereas it averaged 4.4 ± 1 in the other 8 patients. These data suggest that the single ventricle should be divided unevenly with the RV/LV end diastolic ratio being approximately 2:3. Additionally because the insertion of a noncontractile prosthesis as a part of the ventricular wall could compromise pump function of the LV, end diastolic volume must be larger than "normal" to maintain cardiac output. These authors present outstanding results in postoperative follow-up of septation in selected patients with double-inlet LV who have fairly large ventricular chambers. Their data suggest that most patients are considerably better off than those with the Fontan repair.

DOUBLE OUTLET RIGHT VENTRICLE

Shen and associates[24] from Rochester, Minnesota, analyzed results for repair of double outlet right ventricle (DORV) from 1965 to 1985. There were 118 operations with 23 deaths in the hospital and 6 patients lost to follow-up. The remaining 89 patients made up the study population and were 10 ± 8 years at the time of repair. Mean duration of follow-up was 82 months. There were 22 late deaths and 73% were sudden. Eight of the sudden deaths occurred within 1 year of operation. Multivariate analysis revealed the following significant risk factors for late sudden death: older age at operation, perioperative or postoperative ventricular tachyarrhythmias, and third degree AV block. Factors not associated with late sudden death included year of operation, sex, type and number of associated anomalies, preoperative functional class, previous palliative operations, surgical technique, perioperative or postoperative single VPC, and postoperative left or right BBB with or without fascicular block. These authors present an alarmingly high prevalence of sudden death in patients with repair of DORV. A previous report by Luber, et al (Circulation, 1983; 68 (Suppl II): II-144-II-147) showed a much lower mortality. The major differences between the studies were an earlier age at operation and early repeat operation for persistent hemodynamic abnormalities in the 1983 study. These data support early repair of DORV.

AORTIC VALVE STENOSIS

Operative valvotomy

Burch and associates[25] from London, UK, performed open valvotomy on 13 patients under the age of 1 year with critical AS with all patients surviving operation. There were 2 late deaths: 1 38 days after operation with an unrelated neurosurgical procedure and the other 2.5 years later after aortic valve replacement was performed. During this period 2 other infants presented with AS and 1 died before operation could be performed. The second patient had a hypoplastic left ventricle with a small mitral valve ring and was considered to be part of a different subgroup. Follow-up was from 7 months to 5 years and LV function in terms of percentage of systolic wall thickening was impaired in all age groups. In addition, peak diastolic thinning was abnormal in those children aged 3-5 years. The aortic gradient assessed by Doppler was <40 mmHg in 5 patients and between 40 and 70 mmHg in 7 patients. These authors presented excellent results for open valvotomy with critical AS. They excluded patients with hypoplastic left ventricle. These results need to be compared with similar patients undergoing balloon therapy. To date there has not been a similar group undergoing balloon therapy. Comparison studies continue to suffer because of the difficulty of matching patient groups in terms of pertinent risk factors for poor outcome.

Turley and associates[26] from San Francisco, California, Ann Arbor, Michigan, and Newark, New Jersey, reviewed data from 40 neonates, aged 1–30 days with isolated AS associated with PDA, coarctation of the aorta, or both, who underwent operative therapy. Perioperative conditions included CHF in 38 and MR in 16. LV-aortic gradients ranged from 15 to 130 mmHg (mean 67). There were 30 open valvotomies and 10 transventricular dilatations. The hospital survival rate was 88% with no significant difference between the methods of valvotomy. Although multiple methods of perfusion and valvotomy were used, the single unifying factor of cardiopulmonary bypass stabilization was present in all 40 patients. No significant difference in survival was noted between institutions, methods of cardiopulmonary bypass, cardiopulmonary bypass times, crossclamp times, or method of valvotomy. There have been 5 reoperations with 1 late death in a patient requiring MVR and an apical-aortic conduit. One sudden death occurred and autopsy revealed endocardial fibroelastosis. These authors presented excellent survival for this difficult group of patients. They operated on patients whose aortic annulus was ≥5 mm and excluded patients with borderline small left ventricles. The problem of determining when a patient is not a candidate for a valvotomy and should be considered for a Norwood procedure or transplantation still remains.

DeBoer and associates[27] from Bethesda, Maryland, presented follow-up data on 51 patients aged 1–18 years, having aortic valvotomy for congenital AS between 1956 and 1986. Average age at operation was 11.5 years with an operative mortality of 4%. The aortic gradient decreased from a preoperative value of 91 to 27 mmHg postoperatively. Current follow-up was 90% and averaged 17 years. Late cardiac mortality was 18% with actuarial survival of 94% at 10 and 15 years, 82% at 20 and 25 years and 71% at 28 years. Nineteen patients required reoperation at a mean of 18 years postoperatively with a reoperation-free survival of 98% at 10 years. The reoperation rate accelerated in the following decade to 3.3% per year. Ten patients without symptoms were evaluated by Doppler echocardiography and were found to have a mean gradient of 22 mmHg and 90% had mild to moderate AR. This study indicates the effectiveness of surgery for congenital AS in most patients for at least 10 years following initial operation. Progression of stenosis to require reoperation may be less rapid than previously estimated.

Balloon valvuloplasty

Rocchini and associates[28] from Ann Arbor, Michigan, and the Valvuloplasty and Angioplasty for Congenital Anomalies Registry reported data from 204 children and infants who underwent balloon valvuloplasty for aortic stenosis. The procedure was successful in 192 of 204 children reducing the peak ejection gradient from 77 to 30 mmHg. The same degree of gradient reduction was noted in both the 38 children under 1 year of age and the 166 over 1 year of age. Major life threatening complications occurred in 11 patients (5%). There were 5 deaths, all <1 year of age with 4 dying during the procedure and 1 within 2 days of the procedure. Arterial or aortic tears were responsible in 4 and 1 patient died with severe AR. Other major complications included life threatening arrhythmias in 3 patients, dislodgement of the balloon in the ascending aorta requiring emergency surgery in 1 patient, perforation of the mitral valve in 1 patient and perforation of the left ventricle in 1 patient. Development or increasing severity of AR occurred in 21 of 204 children. Significant bleeding requiring transfusion occurred in 5 of 204 and arterial thrombosis or damage associated with valvuloplasty procedure occurred in 25 of 204. Patients with permanent loss of the femoral arterial pulse occurred in 5 of these 25 children. Femoral artery patency was restored either with medical or surgical therapy in 80% of patients. These data indicate that percutaneous aortic balloon valvuloplasty does provide effective relief of AS in infants and children. There are significant risks for complications, including death, in this group and procedures should be carried out only by centers in which emergency surgery is available and where considerable experience in the treatment of critically ill infants is available.

Shaddy and associates[29] from Salt Lake City, Utah, performed balloon aortic valvuloplasty in 32 patients with congenital AS ranging in age from 2 days to 28 years. One balloon was used in 17 patients and 2 in 15 patients. Immediately after valvuloplasty, peak systolic pressure gradient decreased from 77 ± 27 to 23 ± 16 mmHg. At follow-up 19 months later, reduction in gradient averaged 40 ± 29%. There was echocardiographic evidence of significantly increased AR in 10 patients (31%) and aortic valve prolapse in 7 patients (22%). There was no correlation between the balloon/annulus ratio and the subsequent development of AR or prolapse. No patient who showed a significant increase in AR had a balloon/annulus ratio >100%. The degree of AR increased in approximately 33% of these patients but all tolerated this increase in AR well. Patients with unicommissural aortic valves appear to be at increased risk for significant AR following valvuloplasty.

SUBAORTIC STENOSIS

Douville and associates[30] from Charleston, South Carolina, reviewed records of 36 patients who underwent 39 operations for subaortic stenosis. Seventeen had associated anomalies. One perioperative death occurred in a patient with TF. The mean preoperative LV outflow tract systolic pressure gradient was 64 ± 5 mmHg and decreased to 9 ± 2 mmHg postoperatively. Reliable preoperative and postoperative information regarding aortic valve function was available for 27 patients. AR was found in 63% of those patients preoperatively. Postoperatively, AR increased in 3 patients and decreased in 4; none of these changes were major. Severity of preoperative AR increased significantly with age but did not correlate with LV outflow tract gradient. Reoperation was required in 3 patients and effectively relieved the residual obstruction.

Stewart and associates[31] from Nashville, Tennessee, reported 45 patients with fixed subaortic stenosis who underwent localized resection. Discrete membranous stenosis was present in 28 patients and tunnel stenosis in 13. Four patients had associated double outlet right ventricle. Mean age at operation ranged from 6 months to 21 years and averaged 7 years. Local resection of the fibrous tissue was performed in 26 patients and resection combined with myectomy in 18 patients. Aortoventriculoplasty by the modified Konno procedure was required in 3 patients. There were 3 perioperative deaths at initial operation and 2 deaths at the time of reoperation. Follow-up ranged from 1 month to 17 years with a mean follow-up of 47 months. Reoperation for recurrent obstruction was required in 27% and 3 patients have required a third operation. Mild to moderate AR was present in 17 patients. Successful removal of discrete fibrous subaortic stenosis is not infrequently followed by recurrent stenosis necessitating repeat operation with myectomy and in some patients aortoventriculoplasty. Recurrent stenosis necessitating reoperation can occur as long as 17 years after the initial procedure.

SUPRAVALVULAR AORTIC STENOSIS ± PULMONIC STENOSIS

Wren and associates[32] from Newcastle upon Tyne and London, UK, studied 35 patients with supravalvular AS or PA stenosis, or both, undergoing catheterization. Twenty-seven patients had supravalvular AS: 11 required surgery after the first study and 8 of 10 others having serial investigation showed an increase in pressure gradient. Angiographic data indicated the aortic pressure gradient increased related to failure of normal growth of the ascending aorta lumen. Nineteen patients had PA stenosis with RV pressure >33 mmHg. At restudy RV pressure had decreased in 9 of 11 patients. This decrease was associated with an increase in the systolic distensibility of the proximal PAs although there was no increase in the diastolic diameters. One patient had a rapid early increase in RV pressure and no PA growth and 2 patients showed multiple stenoses that became evident with time and produced persistent RV hypertension. Supravalvular AS is usually a progressive lesion whereas PA stenosis usually improves with time and only rarely limits prognosis.

AORTIC ISTHMIC COARCTATION

Balloon angioplasty

Hellenbrand and associates[33] from New Haven, Connecticut, reported results of balloon angioplasty in 200 patients with recoarctation of the aorta in a multicenter prospective study. The average age at the procedure was 7 years and systolic pressure in the ascending aorta decreased from 135 to 127 mmHg while descending aortic pressure rose from 93 to 114 mmHg. Peak systolic pressure difference decreased from 42 to 13 mmHg and the diameter of the recurrent coarctation site increased from 5 to 9 mmHg. After angioplasty residual pressure differences of <20 mmHg were found in 79% of patients. There were 5 deaths related to the procedure (2.5%). Two deaths were directly related to technical aspects of the procedure and 3 patients died because of the severity of the underlying disease. One additional patient had a stroke. Femoral artery complications occurred in 17 patients and 8 patients required surgical thrombectomy. These data indicate that recoarctation can frequently be relieved with balloon aortoplasty but that complications are not uncommon. There is still no clear indication as to the frequency or severity of aneurysm formation following this procedure.

Burrows and associates[34] from Toronto, Canada, reviewed 64 consecutive infants and children who underwent transfemoral balloon dilation of the aorta or aortic valve. Balloon angioplasty or balloon valvotomy was performed with 8F and 9F catheters without an arterial sheath. Patients ranged in age from 5 days to 15 years with a mean of 6 years. Acute iliofemoral complications occurred in 29/64 (45%) including thrombosis in 18 of 64, complete disruption in 5 of 64, incomplete disruption in 3 of 64 and arterial tear in 3 of 64. The arterial pathology was confirmed in 23 of 29 by one or a combination of surgical exploration and repair in 18 of 29, angiography in 6 of 29 and magnetic resonance imaging in 3 of 29. Complications were diagnosed by acute hypotension requiring transfusion in 3 and absent pedal pulses after procedure in 5. Of these 5, 3 developed bleeding during thrombolytic therapy and underwent surgical exploration and 2 were diagnosed by angiography after ineffective thrombolytic therapy. Reduced or absent pedal pulses at the time of discharge were present in 11 patients (17% of the entire group and 38% of the group with complications). A significant correlation was found between arterial complications and low patient weight. These authors show a high incidence of traumatic complications of transfemoral therapeutic procedures using large, high profile catheters. Patients weighing <20 kg were at increased risk for such complications and medical and surgical treatment was effective in only 62%. The introduction of low profile, 5F catheters introduced a 6F sheath in patients <10 kg and low profile 8F catheters in older children have been associated with no further arterial disruptions. Further data is needed with the use of these catheters to provide further data regarding risk-benefit ratio of procedures in individual patients.

Rao and associates[35] from Madison, Wisconsin, and Riyadh, Saudi Arabia, presented intermediate-term results of balloon angioplasty of native aortic coarctation in neonates and infants <1 year of age. During a 60-month-period that ended in January 1990, 19 infants ages 3 days to 12 months (median 2.5 months), underwent balloon angioplasty of native coarctation with resultant reduction in peak-to-peak systolic pressure gradient from 39 ± 12 mm Hg to 11 ± 7 mm Hg and increase in coarctation segment size from 2.2 ± 0.8 mm to 4.7 ± 1.0 mm. None required immediate surgical intervention. Thirteen of the 19 (68%) had severe associated cardiac defects. There was 1 death (5%) 2 days after balloon angioplasty, and it was related to associated cardiac defect. One infant was lost to follow-up. It was too soon to restudy 1 infant. The remaining 16 infants had clinical (36 ± 18 months) and catheterization (12 ± 4 months) follow-up data. The residual coarctation gradient (22 ± 15 mm Hg) and coarcted segment size (4.45 ± 1.6 mm) remain improved when compared with pre-balloon angioplasty values. Five of the 16 (31%) infants (4 were neonates at the time of balloon angioplasty) had evidence for recoarctation (defined as gradient >20 mm Hg) and underwent surgical resection (2) or repeat balloon angioplasty (3), all with success. None developed aneurysms. On the basis of this experience and the reported high morbidity and mortality rates after surgical repair in neonates and young infants, balloon angioplasty was recommended as the procedure of choice for relief of symptomatic native coarctation in the neonate and infant <1 year of age.

The purpose of this article by Rao and associates[36] from Madison, Wisconsin, and Riyadh, Saudi Arabia, was to present immediate and follow-up results of balloon angioplasty of aortic recoarctations following previous surgery in infants and children. During a 45-month period that ended in June 1989, 9 infants and children, ages 6 months to 7 years, underwent balloon angioplasty of recoarctation with resultant reduction in peak-to-peak systolic pressure gradient from 52 ± 20 mm Hg to 16 ± 8 mm Hg and increase in coarctation segment size from 3.4 ± 1.4 mm to 6.1 ± 1.6 mm. None required surgical intervention. There were no significant complications. Follow-up catheterization (16 ± 7 months) data in 6 children and follow-up clinical (17 ± 6 months) data in all children were available for review. Both the residual coarctation pressure gradient (6 ± 6 mm Hg) and coarctation segment size (8.2 ± 2.4 mm) remain improved when compared with pre-balloon angioplasty values and the pressure gradient fell further (p<0.01) when compared with that measured immediately after balloon angioplasty. None developed restenosis, although 1 child required surgical relief of severe narrowing of isthmus of the aortic arch. None developed aneurysms. On the basis of this experience and that reported previously and because of high morbidity and mortality rates associated with repeat surgery for postoperative recoarctation, balloon angioplasty was recommended as the procedure of choice for relief of postoperative recoarctation with significant hypertension.

Resection in infancy

Lacour-Gayet and associates[37] from Le Plessis Robinson, France, reported 66 consecutive neonates with coarctation and severe hypoplasia of the transverse arch who underwent repair by resection of the coarctation and reconstruction of the arch. Mean age at operation was 14 days and ranged from 2 to 30 days. The coarctation was isolated in 23%, associated with a VSD in 39%, and associated with complex anomalies in 38%, including 16 patients with TGA or double outlet right ventricle plus VSD, 2 with simple TGA, 2 with congenitally corrected TGA plus VSD and 5 with hypoplastic left ventricle. The surgical technique comprised a wide resection of the coarctation contiguous ductal tissue followed by reconstruction of the aortic arch by bringing the descending aorta into the concavity of the arch. The technique can relieve arch obstruction provided that the descending aorta is widely dissected to allow mobilization and the incision of the transverse arch is extended proximal to the ostium of the left carotid artery. The operation was performed through a left thoracotomy in 62 patients and through a sternotomy in 4 neonates who in addition, underwent a one stage repair of TGA plus VSD. The overall early mortality was 14% and there were 6 late deaths with an overall mortality of 23%. The mean follow-up was 21 months and ranged from 6 to 66 months. Actuarial survival at 5 years was 72% for the overall group, 87% for simple coarctation, 88% for coarctation and VSD and 52% for complex coarctation. The rate of recurrent coarctation was 13%, leading to 5 reoperations with no deaths. Freedom from reoperation was 90% at 5 years. These authors present excellent results for this difficult problem. There continues to be some quibbling about what is truly a hypoplastic arch and certainly what is truly a hypoplastic left ventricle. Their determination of a hypoplastic arch by comparing the diameter of the transverse arch or isthmus with the ascending aorta seems reasonable. Their diagnosis of hypoplastic left ventricle based on the aortic annulus diameter is not reasonable. The ventricle can be either small, normal or large in patients with the aortic annulus size used in their study to diagnose a small left ventricle.

Subclavian flap angioplasty

Van Son and associates[38] from Nijmegen, The Netherlands, studied Doppler spectral analysis of blood flow velocities in the left brachial artery at rest and during postocclusive reactive hyperemia in patients following subclavian flap angioplasty repair of coarctation of the aorta and compared results with patients with resection and end-to-end anastomosis and controls. There were 9 patients after subclavian flap surgery with a median age of 8 years, 14 patients after end-to-end anastomosis with a median age of 8 years, and 10 control subjects, median age 9.5 years. At rest there was a highly significant decrease of blood flow velocities to the left brachial arteries measured in all patients of the subclavian flap group compared with the other 2 groups. During reactive hyperemia a moderate capacity of augmentation of blood flow was observed in 5 patients of the subclavian flap group. This capacity was marginal in 2 patients with complaints of claudication in the left upper arm during strenuous exercise which could be related to the number of branches of the left subclavian artery ligated during operation. These authors bring interesting data to bear on the question of left arm blood flow problems following subclavian flap angioplasty in infancy. The data suggests that if possible the internal mammary artery, the thyro cervical trunk, and any additional branches of the left subclavian artery should be left undisturbed at the time of repair to avoid potential adverse sequelae for the hemodynamics of the affected arm.

Exercise-induced hypertension after repair

Kavey and associates[39] from Syracuse, New York, studied 10 patients with successful repair of coarctation defined as a resting arm/leg gradient of ≤18 mmHg. Mean age at repair was 5.5 years and age at study was 18 years. Patients had treadmill exercise before and after atenolol therapy. At baseline evaluation, systolic BP at termination of exercise ranged from 201 to 270 mmHg (mean 229 mmHg). Arm/leg gradients at exercise termination ranged from 30 to 143 mmHg (mean 84). Follow-up treadmill exercise after beta blockade revealed normal upper extremity systolic pressure at exercise termination in 9 of 10 patients. Maximal systolic BP at termination ranged from 163 to 223 mmHg (mean 196 mmHg) and was significantly different from pre-therapy value. Arm/leg pressure gradient at termination also decreased significantly to a mean of 51 mmHg. No patient had symptoms on atenolol and exercise endurance times were unchanged. These authors showed excellent short-term results for use of atenolol in significantly decreasing systolic hypertension post treadmill exercise. Whether or not these patients would be better off on long-term atenolol therapy as opposed to relief of their mild residual coarctation is unclear.

Left ventricular function after repair

Moskowitz and associates[40] from Richmond, Virginia, investigated whether LV structural or functional abnormalities persist in children on long-term follow-up after successful correction of coarctation of the aorta. Two-dimensional directed M-mode and Doppler echocardiographic examinations were performed on 11 such individuals and 22 age-matched controls. Digitized tracings were made from M-mode recordings of the LV and Doppler mitral valve inflow recordings to measure septal, posterior wall, and LV dimensions, LV mass, shortening fraction, peak shortening and lengthening velocities, diastolic filling time, peak E velocity, peak A velocity and velocity time integrals. Despite group similarities in age, body size, and systolic BP, greater fractional shortening, indexed peak shortening velocity, and greater LV mass index were seen in the coarctation group in the face of lower LV wall stress. LV mass index correlated with the resting arm-leg gradient, which ranged from −4 to +10 mm Hg. The coarctation group had decreased early filling with compensatory increased late diastolic filling. Diastolic filling abnormalities were prominent in the older coarctation individuals and were related to both systolic BP and LV mass index. Despite apparently successful repair of coarctation of the aorta, persistent alterations in both systolic and diastolic LV function and LV mass are present in children at long-term follow-up, which are related to the resting arm-leg gradient. It is suggested that these small measured arm-leg gradients represent persistent alterations in flow, which may result in LV hypertrophy and hyperkinesia.

AORTIC VALVE ATRESIA

Echocardiographic features

Chin and associates[41] from Philadelphia, Pennsylvania, studied anomalous attachment of the septum primum in patients with hypoplastic left heart syndrome using 2 dimensional echocardiography. Anomalous attachment was found in 37% of 129 patients with normally aligned great arteries and 34% of 29 patients with double outlet right ventricle and left AV valve underdevelopment. This anomaly was also found in 50% of 8 patients with single ventricle. The most reliable view to identify anomalous attachment was the subcostal left oblique-equivalent cut. The anomalies should be carefully studied by all physicians dealing with complex congenital heart disease. Resection of the atrial septum which is frequently needed at the time of palliation will be incomplete if this anomaly is not recognized.

Ludman and associates[42] from London, UK, compared cross sectional echocardiographic studies of 10 neonates with hypoplastic left heart syndrome and compared these with 15 neonates with other causes of RV overload in 15 normal controls. LV and RV cavity dimensions, the shape and size of the mitral valve annulus and aortic root were recorded as absolute values and corrected for body surface area. The diameter of the mitral valve annulus was the single most discriminative variable. There was considerable overlap of all of the calculated valves between neonates with hypoplastic left heart and those with other causes of RV overload. With RV overload the left ventricle is compressed posteriorly and can appear hypoplastic. Most infants with hypoplastic left heart have an apex which is formed solely by the right ventricle, however, and this is a distinctive feature which can be used as an aid in making this diagnosis. This distinction becomes extremely important in deciding about therapy in AS. There is obviously a lower limit of size to the left ventricle for which operative valvotomy or balloon valvotomy is futile and these patients should be submitted only for transplantation or Norwood procedure.

Results of first-stage palliation

Meliones and associates[43] from Ann Arbor, Michigan, reviewed the results of 57 infants who underwent first stage Norwood palliation for hypoplastic left heart syndrome. There were 21% long-term survivors with 31 infants dying within the first 30 days after surgery. Causes of early mortality included low output, sepsis, sudden death, and pulmonary vein atresia. Late deaths occurred in 14 infants due to sepsis, sudden death, and death at reoperation. Of the 31 patients who survived more than 24 hours, complications noted by echocardiography and catheterization were significant arch obstruction in 13%, branch PA stenosis in 23%, small ASD in 16%, inadequate shunt in 26%, neoaortic regurgitation in 13%, TR in 13%, ventricular dysfunction in 29%, thrombus in 6%, and superior vena cava obstruction in 3%. Of the 12 long-term survivors, 4 have had a successful Fontan procedure, 1 has had a transplant and 7 are waiting a second stage procedure. These authors present only 21% first stage survival in patients with hypoplastic left heart syndrome. The optimal management of these patients still is unclear. Infant transplantation remains a viable option but donor supply is limited. Most groups, including this outstanding unit, have been unable to duplicate the results which Dr. Norwood has reported.

MITRAL STENOSIS-BALLOON COMMISSUROTOMY

Spevak and associates[44] from Boston, Massachusetts, attempted balloon angioplasty in 9 children ages 0.1 to 10 years with congenital MS. All were symptomatic with severe CHF and failure to thrive. Effective reduction in mitral gradient was initially achieved in 7 patients. For the entire group mean valve gradient decreased from 15 ± 5 to 8 ± 7 mmHg and mean valve area increased from $1.1 \pm$ to 1.8 cm^2/m^2. More than mild MR developed in 2 patients but none required surgery for MR. Poor gradient relief followed dilation of valves with unbalanced chordal attachments, with restriction to the valve apparatus as in mitral arcade, and where the obstruction was not purely valvar as with a supramitral ring. Patients with true parachute mitral valves were excluded from the procedure. The reduction in the degree of MS was clinically effective in 5 cases and in 3 the gradient relief persisted for >3 months. This procedure should be considered in younger patients before MVR.

TRICUSPID VALVE ATRESIA

Banding of pulmonary trunk

Franklin and associates[45] from London, UK, studied the development of subaortic stenosis in 102 consecutive infants presenting with double inlet ventricle or tricuspid atresia with a dominant left ventricle and TGA. Obstruction of the aortic arch was present in 52 patients and in 28 patients subaortic stenosis was apparent at presentation. Of the remaining 74 patients, 19 received no palliative surgery and 55 underwent banding of the pulmonary trunk either with aortic arch repair in 22 or without repair in 33. Outcome was significantly worse in patients with associated aortic arch obstruction with either death or development or subaortic stenosis by 3 years of age in 22 of 33 with aortic arch obstruction and in 0 of 22 without arch obstruction. There was a lower ratio of VSD to ascending aorta diameter at presentation in those patients who developed subaortic stenosis after banding than in those who did not. Of the latter patients, 18 of 19 fulfilled criteria for a Fontan procedure at recatheterization. Thus the presence of aortic arch obstruction is associated with a rapid development of subaortic stenosis after banding and alternative initial surgery may be indicated. In the absence of such obstruction, banding the pulmonary trunk can be performed at reasonable risk provided the VSD is of adequate size. This procedure can satisfactorily prepare most patients for a later Fontan procedure. These authors present valuable data regarding use of pulmonary trunk banding in patients with single ventricle anatomy and TGA in whom the potential for subaortic obstruction is present. This clarification of the relatively small risk for developing subaortic stenosis in patients without aortic arch obstruction with pulmonary banding is a valuable bit of prognostic information.

Fontan operation

Gewillig and associates[46] from London, UK, and Nashville, Tennessee, determined LV dimensions and contractility by echocardiography in 33 patients with tricuspid atresia in 1985 and again in 1988. Eight patients remained palliated through the period and neither LV diameter nor a load independent index of contractility changed. Eleven patients underwent a Fontan operation and were reevaluated at least 6 months after surgery; LV dimensions decreased from 130 ± 15% to 114 ± 19% of predicted normal and the contractility index improved. Fourteen patients had undergone a Fontan operation before the initial study in 1985 and over the subsequent 3 year period LV dimensions did not change but the contractility index showed significant improvement. Eight additional patients were studied just before and after Fontan operations to examine the early effects of surgery. LV dimensions decreased from 130 ± 14% to 100 ± 13% of normal by 10 days with no further change at 2 months. An inappropriate degree of ventricular hypertrophy was observed only in the early postoperative period. These studies indicate that LV dimensions do decrease towards normal following the Fontan operation, as would be expected. The more marked changes occurred in the younger patients. In addition, the data here suggest that indices of contractility do improve after the Fontan operation. This study provides a more favorable impression of the Fontan operation than has been suggested by long-term follow-up data. Perhaps earlier age at operation and better myocardial protection in more recent patients may contribute to this change although the data to prove that point are not available to date.

Mair and associates[47] from Rochester, Minnesota, reported 176 patients with tricuspid atresia who had the Fontan procedure. Age at surgery ranged from 7 months to 42 years with 24% ≥16 years. Hospital mortality rate was 17% from 1973 through 1980 and 8% from 1981 through 1989. There have been 10 late cardiovascular deaths. Postoperative follow-up of 139 survivors for a mean of 5.5 years revealed 91% to be in excellent or good position and 9% in fair or poor condition. The latter patients had poor stamina and/or fluid retention with intermittent pleural effusions and ascites. Two factors that clearly influenced operative and late results are preoperative pulmonary arteriolar resistance and left ventricular diastolic function. A preoperative index devised by adding pulmonary arteriolar resistance to left ventricular end-diastolic pressure divided by Qp plus Qs may be helpful in selecting candidates most likely to survive and benefit. If this index is <4, then postoperative right atrial mean pressure will be 20 mmHg or less, a circumstance associated with 95% early and 89% overall survival rate. If this index is >4 breathing room air, the authors suggest repeating the measurement while breathing oxygen. These authors have added significantly to our understanding of the Fontan operation and the conditions under which this operation is useful. Difficult patients remain who have elevated ventricular end-diastolic pressures which might be due to volume loading and not to hypertrophy and fibrosis, which will not change following surgery. If the end-diastolic pressure is due to volume loading, then this should change following the Fontan procedure and must be as low as 12-14 mmHg for the Fontan repair to be successful.

CORONARY ARTERY ANOMALY

Associated anomalies

Tuzcu and associates[48] from Cleveland, Ohio, found that of 66,884 patients who underwent coronary arteriography between 1972 and 1982 at the Cleveland Clinic Foundation that 1,000 had coronary arterial anomalies. Of the 1,000, 101 had associated congenital anomalies: 29 had MVP, 18 had bicuspid aortic valve, 16 had tetralogy of Fallot, 11 had corrected transposition, 10 had a univentricular heart, 6 had coarctation of the aorta, 3 had VSD, and 8 had miscellaneous congenital heart disease. The most common coronary anomaly was ectopic origin of a coronary artery: 30 from the sinus of Valsalva, 12 from the ascending aorta, 11 from the pulmonary artery. Nineteen patients had no LM coronary artery. Thirteen patients had coronary artery fistulas and 21 had miscellaneous coronary anomalies.

Origin of left main from pulmonary trunk

Seguchi and associates[49] from Tokyo, Japan, evaluated post-operative myocardial perfusion and function using thallium-201 myocardial imaging and technetium-99m cardiac pool imaging in 5 patients with anomalous origin of the LM coronary artery from the pulmonary trunk. The patients underwent reimplantation of the left coronary artery at an age ranging from 10 months to 13 years. Postoperative electrocardiographic and radionuclide studies were performed both at rest and during stress 1 to 4 years after the operation. Electrocardiograms which were abnormal preoperatively returned to normal after surgery except that the T wave in lead a VL remained negative. Postoperatively, LVEF measured by technetium-99m cardiac pool imaging was normal in all patients. Postoperative thallium-201 myocardial imaging, however, showed a perfusion defect with incomplete redistribution at the high-lateral or antero-lateral segment in all patients after a stress test. These data suggest that although myocardial ischemic change decreases and global cardiac function improves after establishment of a dual coronary artery system, severe myocardial damage remains at the high-lateral or antero-lateral segment.

Coronary artery fistula

Sapin and associates[50] from Chapel Hill, North Carolina, described angiographic findings in 3 patients with a coronary artery fistula, i.e., an abnormal communication through which coronary artery blood is shunted into a cardiac chamber, great vessel, or other vascular structure without first passing through the myocardial capillary bed. Additionally, these authors reviewed numerous previous angiographic and case reports of coronary artery fistula reported by others.

THE FONTAN OPERATION

Results of "perfect" Fontan operation

Fontan and associates[51] from Bordeaux, France, and Birmingham, Alabama, performed a retrospective analysis to determine the early and long-term outcomes dictated by a "perfect" Fontan operation. Survival rate under optimal conditions was predicted to be 92%, 89%, 88%, 86%, 81%, and 73% at 1 month, 6 months, and 1, 5, 10, and 15 years, respectively, after the Fontan operation. The instantaneous risk of death at each moment after operation had an early rapidly declining phase of hazard that at about 6 months began to give way to a late hazard phase which was rising by about 6 years after the surgery. The functional capacity of patients was less the longer the period of follow-up and no risk factors other than older age at time of surgery were found for the late decline in survival or the decline in functional status. Although patients with a "perfect" Fontan operation, that is one associated with optimal age, less main chamber hypertrophy, larger pulmonary arteries, lower mean PA pressure, shorter ischemic time and direct RA to PA anastomosis show a slightly better present survival at the times indicated (Figure 8-6), there is still a late declining phase of survival and functional status. These data again indicate that the Fontan operation is a palliative rather than curative procedure.

For children <4 years of age

Bartmus and associates[52] from Rochester, Minnesota, reported on 54 children <4 years of age who had a modified Fontan operation between 1973 and 1987. Tricuspid atresia was present in 20, double inlet ventricle in 13, and other complex defects in 21. There were 14 early deaths and 6 late deaths. Multivariate analysis of survival for a larger group of 500 patients of all ages undergoing Fontan operation during the same time revealed the following factors to be associated with poor survival: absence of tricuspid atresia, asplenia, age <4 years, atrioventricular valve dysfunction, early calendar year of operation, and the presence of either 1 or more of the following: LVEF <60, mean PA pressure >15 mmHg, and pulmonary arteriolar resistance >4 Um². These authors show that in their hands age <4 years appears to be an independent risk factor for survival

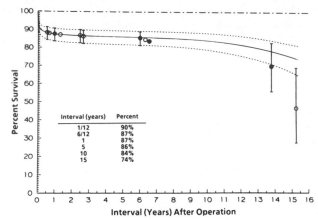

Fig. 8-6. Predicted survival (from secondary study design) after perfect Fontan operation. Depiction is as in Figure 1 (see text). Depiction is nomogram of specific solution of multivariate risk factor equation (see "Appendix 4"). For risk factor equation, values entered as multipliers of coefficients of variables for determining outcome were same as in "Appendix 2" except that ejection fraction was set to 0.6 and mean pulmonary artery pressure was not set because variable does not appear in model. Additionally, solid circles represent arrhythmic or sudden deaths occurring in patients in this analysis, and open circles represent deaths in other modes. Deaths are positioned in time along horizontal axis, and actuarially along vertical axis. In fact, actuarial estimate for death at 6.1 months was derived parametrically, and estimate for each succeeding individual death was then made in usual actuarial manner, beginning from death at 6.1 months. Reproduced with permission from Fontan, et al.[51]

after the modified Fontan operation. They did find, however, that patients who had no or only one adverse risk factors were not detectably different in mortality irrespective of age. The other important caveat of this study is that very few, if any, patients with small PA size or pulmonary arteriolar resistance >4 Um² were operated on and thus there was no true test of whether or not these factors might be independent risk factors of age. The debate continues about optimal use of the modified Fontan operation in children. The preservation of optimal ventricular function and treatment of patients before multiple shunts can distort PAs makes operation at 3-5 years of age seem optimal. Further studies by multiple groups in terms of minimizing operative mortality for this group will be extremely useful.

Univentricular atrioventricular connection

From April 1986 to September 1988, Kurosawa and associates[53] performed in 12 patients with double or common inlet LV and left anterior rudimentary RV, the septation procedure and in 17 patients with double or common inlet left or right ventricle, the Fontan operation. In the septation group 3 patients with pressure gradients between left ventricle and aorta underwent enlargement of the outlet foramen and all survived. One of the 12 patients had a common AV valve that was repaired by separating the valve by the procedure used for AV septal defect surgery. One patient had complete heart block before septation and another one after septation. One 17-year-old patient with the smallest LV (168% of normal) died in the hospital (mortality 8%). In the Fontan group 1 patient died in the hospital (6% hospital mortality) with high pulmonary resistance and 1 late death (6%) occurred in a patient who had complete heart block and high mean PA pressure. Because of outlet obstruction to the PA 2 patients had immediate takedown of the septation and substitution of the Fontan repair. Although RA pressure was almost equal in both groups after operation the cardiac index was significantly higher in the septation group than in the Fontan repair. These authors show outstanding results for septation in a group of patients with very complex univentricular anatomy. Their data indicate that septation for this type of anatomy is feasible and preferred in patients with ventricular end diastolic volume exceeding 170% of normal LV end diastolic volume. In addition, patients must have PS that is mild or can be relieved by surgery. These authors accept patients for Fontan if pulmonary resistance is <4 Um² and PA index >250 mm²/m² with morphological characteristics difficult for septation. They favor septation or Fontan under 10 years of age and would choose septation over Fontan in patients with characteristics favorable for either operation.

Lung biopsy with tricuspid-valve atresia or univentricular heart

Geggel and associates[54] from Boston, Massachusetts, reviewed lung biopsy data from 56 patients undergoing a modified Fontan procedure or recent palliative procedure with a diagnosis of tricuspid atresia (26) or other functional univentricular heart (30). PA structures were classified by both the Heath-Edwards and morphometric scales. Biopsy and autopsy grades were identical except for a minor difference in Heath-Edwards scale in 1 case. Elevated preoperative mean PA pressure >15 mmHg was associated with medial hypertrophy, although 6 patients with normal PA pressure had hypertrophy and 6 patients with mean PA pressure >15 mmHg did not have medial hypertrophy. Medial hypertrophy was a possible risk factor in patients with univentricular heart: patients with hypertrophy had a 9-fold greater risk of death. Controlling for confounding variables did not alter this result. Medial hypertrophy was not a risk factor for death in patients with tricuspid atresia: 4 patients had this finding and each survived while 4 patients without medial hypertrophy were operated and died. There was a trend toward a higher mean PA pressure gradient in patients with medial hypertrophy. These authors indicate that lung biopsy was not useful in patients with tricuspid atresia in terms of operability using the Fontan technique. It is of some potential value apparently in patients with univentricular anatomy other than tricuspid atresia.

Response to exercise afterwards

Rhodes and associates[55] from New York, New York, examined the effects of progressive and steady-state bicycle exercise performed by 11 patients with RA to RV Fontan anastomosis, 7 patients with RA-PA Fontan anastomosis, 13 patients after repair of TF and 34 control patients. All patients were clinically well and on no medications. The exercise function of the patients undergoing RA to RV and RA to PA Fontan procedures were similar. They achieved peak work loads 60% to 67% of control and peak oxygen consumption of 60% and 64% of control, respectively. Both groups displayed excessive ventilation, elevated dead space/tidal volume ratios, and depressed cardiac output during steady state exercise. In contrast, TF patients achieved peak work loads and oxygen consumptions 83% of control and maintained normal cardiac outputs and dead space/

tidal volume ratios during steady state exercise. These results indicate that the presence of a right ventricle within the pulmonary circulation of the Fontan patient does not result in improved exercise function. This may be due to the development of obstructive gradients across the right atrial-RV conduits during exercise or to the right ventricle's negative effect on LV compliance. In contrast to postoperative TF patients, the hypoplastic right ventricle in tricuspid atresia may not have sufficient myocardium to assume the active pumping function required by exercise.

Baffle fenestration and later transcatheter closure

Bridges and associates[56] from Boston, Massachusetts, created a baffle fenestration allowing right-to-left shunting to maintain cardiac output and limit RA pressure following Fontan operation in patients with excessive risk for standard treatment. Risk factors included PA pressure of 18 mmHg or end-diastolic pressure of 12 mmHg or more, valvular regurgitation, PA distortion, pulmonary vascular resistance of 2 units or more, ventricular outflow obstruction, and complex anatomy. There were 19 of 20 survivors with mean oxygen saturation 86%, mean RA pressure 15 mmHg, and mean duration of pleural effusion 6 days. Twelve of 19 survivors tolerated early test occlusion and had permanent transcatheter umbrella closure. Four patients failed early test occlusion with significant decrease in venous O_2 saturation and a rise in central venous pressure due to ventricular dysfunction, pulmonary distortion, and aortopulmonary collaterals. Three of 4 had successful late closure after correction of these abnormalities. These authors present outstanding early results for further enhancing the operability of patients with complex anatomy who would theoretically benefit from a Fontan procedure. Although the concept of leaving atrial defects in place following Fontan is not a new idea, the application of this technique to these patients and the use of transcatheter closure represents an extremely important advancement.

MISCELLANEOUS TOPICS

Transesophageal echocardiography

Stumper and associates[57] from Rotterdam, The Netherlands, performed transesophageal echocardiography with a single plane dedicated pediatric probe in 25 anesthetized children undergoing routine cardiac catheterization or surgery. The group ranged in age from 1 year to 15 years and weight from 6.5 to 52 kg. Studies were successful in all patients and no complications were encountered. Transesophageal echocardiography provided a more detailed evaluation of the morphology and of systemic and pulmonary venous return, the atria, interatrial baffles, AV valves and the LV outflow tract. Additional information over and above precordial echocardiography was obtained in 15 of 25 patients. Problem areas for transesophageal imaging were the apical ventricular septum, the RV outflow tract and the left PA. This technique will obviously add further "noninvasive" imaging information that can be extremely valuable in patients with poor echocardiographic windows. The decision as to when to use this modality will be one of the more important aspects of its use.

Sreeram and associates[58] from Rotterdam, The Netherlands, compared transthoracic and transesophageal echocardiography in 17 patients with major congenital abnormalities of the AV junction. The findings by either technique were correlated with cardiac catheterization in 12 patients and surgery in 5 patients. Ages ranged from 2 to 67 years with all but 3 patients 17 years of age or greater. In 2 of 6 patients with an absent AV connection as defined by transthoracic echocardiography, transesophageal imaging demonstrated an imperforate valve. In 11 of 11 patients with a discordant or criss-cross connection, assessment of AV valve and ventricular morphology was possible with transesophageal echocardiography but only in 3 of 11 by transthoracic studies. Anomalous pulmonary venous connection in 1 patient, ASD in 3 patients, and subpulmonary stenosis in 5 patients were better assessed by transesophageal imaging and atrial appendage morphology could be demonstrated in all. These transesophageal can be very useful in patients with complex anatomy. The esophageal studies are extremely helpful in patients beyond childhood in whom poor echo windows are common.

Doppler echocardiographic measurement of pulmonary artery pressure in the newborn

Musewe and associates[59] from Toronto, Canada, studied ductal flow velocities in 37 newborns: group 1 consisted of 16 with persistent PA hypertension, transient tachypnea in the newborn or other diagnoses; group 2 had respiratory distress syndrome. All patients were <48 hours of age, did not have congenital heart disease, weighed >1500 grams and had a gestational age ≥28 weeks. Clinical diagnosis of PA hypertension was based on sustained arterial oxygen tension ≤50 torr, in >90% oxygen in term newborns. Patients were excluded if PDA was not present on the first echocardiographic examination. Maximum TR Doppler velocity in 21 patients was used to estimate a PA pressure and compared with pressures derived from ductal flow velocities (Figure 8-7). There was a significant linear correlation between tricuspid regurgitant Doppler velocity and PA systolic pressure derived from ductal Doppler velocities in patients with unidirectional left-to-right or right-to-left shunting as well as those with bidirectional shunting. In those with bidirectional shunting duration of right-to-left shunting <60% of systole was found when PA pressure was systemic or less whereas duration ≥60% was associated with suprasystemic PA pressures. Serial changes in PA pressure reflected by changes in ductal Doppler velocities correlated with clinical status in persistent PA hypertension in the newborn. These authors show a new technique for evaluating PA pressure in patients with PDA. This method is more difficult than using the TR jet. It required a Doppler recording of ductal flow, a Doppler recording of ascending aorta for the timing of peak systole, and recording of central aortic blood pressure. Care must be taken not to confuse signals arising from flow in the adjacent left pulmonary artery with the right-to-left ductal shunt. Such distinctions can be difficult. Nevertheless this method can be useful in assessment of pulmonary arterial pressure in the newborn with a patent ductus.

Magnetic resonance imaging

Vick and associates[60] from Houston, Texas, reported 12 patients >8 years of age with complex congenital heart disease evaluated with magnetic resonance imaging (MRI) and with echocardiographic and angio-

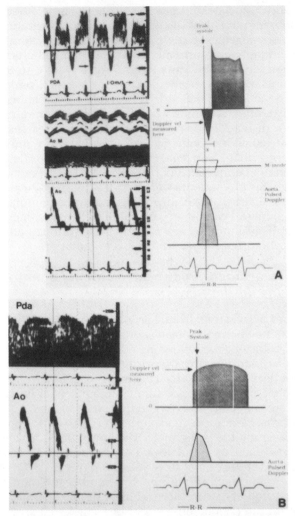

Fig. 8-7. Actual (left panels) and schematic (right panels) presentation of ductal shunting and the Doppler variables measured. A, Bidirectional ductal shunting. For ductal shunting, Doppler spectral display above the zero line is left to right whereas that below the zero line is right to left. Vertical dotted lines represent identical RR intervals for ductal and ascending aortic (Ao) Doppler and M-mode recordings. Peak systole is denoted by the vertical continuous line. Horizontal arrows indicate the point where ductal Doppler velocity (vel) corresponding to peak systole was measured. B, Pure left to right shunting. Format as in A; aortic M-mode recording is not included in this figure. Ao M = aortic valve M-mode recording; PDA = ductal Doppler display (pulsed in A, continuous wave in B); R-R = cardiac cycle duration; x = duration of right to left ductal shunt. Reproduced with permission from Musewe, et al.[59]

graphic techniques. The subpulmonary region, main PA, right and left PAs, and aorticopulmonary shunts were clearly visualized by MRI in all patients. Angiography defined the subpulmonary region and main PA in all patients, the right and left PAs along their length in 11 of 12 patients, and aorticopulmonary shunts in 7 of 8 patients. Except for the right PA, echocardiography defined the remaining structures in ≤50% of patients. Measurements of PA diameters by MRI correlated well with the angiographic measurements of both the left and right PAs. These data suggest that MRI might the preferable noninvasive parameter for assessment of PA anatomy in shunts in patients with complex congenital heart defects.

Complex ventricular anomalies are frequently associated with abnormalities of thoracic and abdominal situs, arterioventricular connection, and venous connection. The definition of all components of these anomalies is difficult to accomplish with imaging techniques. Kersting-Sommerhoff and colleagues[61] from San Francisco and Oakland, California, compared the effectiveness of electrocardiographic gated spin-echo MRI with cardiac angiography for the evaluation of all components of central cardiovascular anatomy in patients with the clinical diagnosis of single or common ventricle or complete AV septal (canal) defect. MRI studies and angiograms of 29 patients were evaluated independently. A sequential approach was used to define cardiac anatomy assessing 9 anatomic features in each patient. MRI provided 261 observations and angiography provided 209 observations. In the mutual 209 observations, only 17 discrepancies were found. Comparison of MRI and angiography in individual cases showed that MRI was as effective as angiography in the depiction of ventricular anomalies, including determination of morphology and evaluation of the size of the ventricles, the orientation of the ventricular septum relative to the AV valves, as well as the origins and spatial relations of the great arteries. MRI was more informative for the determination of thoracic and abdominal situs and systemic and pulmonary venoatrial connections, but was not as effective for the evaluation of semilunar valves. Thus, MRI provides complete evaluation of central cardiovascular anatomy and is effective in the anatomic assessment of most components of complex ventricular anomalies.

Angiographic demonstration of bifurcation of pulmonary trunk

Garcia-Medina and associates[62] from Minneapolis, Minnesota, demonstrated a new angiographic projection to delineate the origin of the right and left PAs. This technique is extremely important for patients with tetralogy of Fallot or pulmonary atresia, as well as patients with suspected isolated PA stenosis before and after repair. The report and the figures should be studied carefully by all angiographers of patients with congenital heart disease (Figure 8-8).

Polysplenia with normal heart

Debich and associates[63] from Pittsburgh, Pennsylvania, and London, UK, evaluated 10 cases of polysplenia without complex congenital heart disease. Left isomerism was present in only 4 patients and bilateral bilobed lungs present in 5. Biliary atresia was present in 8 of 10 and intestinal malrotation in 7 of 10. The status of the spleen is clearly an inaccurate marker of the presence of isomerism of the atrial appendage although one should obviously look for this abnormality when polysplenia is found.

The Marfan syndrome in infancy

Geva and associates[64] from Hanover, New Hampshire, and Boston, Massachusetts, reviewed the clinical, Doppler, echocardiographic, and pathologic findings in infantile Marfan syndrome in 9 infants. The age at diagnosis ranged from birth to 12 months with a mean of 2.7 months.

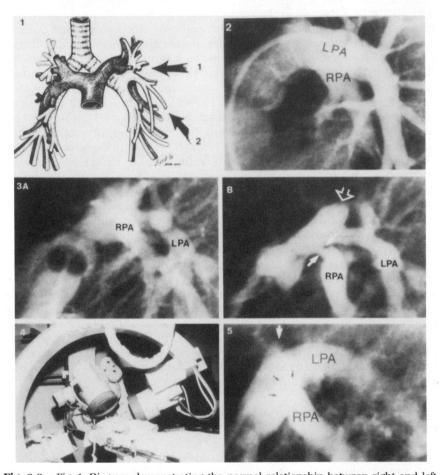

Fig. 8-8. Fig. 1. Diagram demonstrating the normal relationship between right and left pulmonary arteries with cranial angulation. The left pulmonary artery crosses over the left main stem bronchus, whereas the right pulmonary artery crosses in front of the right bronchus toward the right. The left pulmonary artery is therefore slightly higher in position than the right. Arrow 1 indicates left anterior oblique view without angulation, arrow 2 indicates left anterior oblique view with maximal caudal angulation. Fig 2. Steep left anterior oblique pulmonary arteriogram made without angulation as indicated by arrow 1 in Fig. 1. The true origin of right and left pulmonary arteries are superimposed. Fig. 3. (A) Steep left anterior oblique pulmonary arteriogram without tube angulation demonstrating superimposition of left and right pulmonary artery origins. (B) Same patient, same view with cardiac angulation demonstrating a normal left pulmonary artery, a severely stenotic right pulmonary origin (arrows) and a large ductus diverticulum of the pulmonary artery (open arrow). Fig. 4. Photograph demonstrating position of x-ray tubes for biplane demonstration of the pulmonary arteries. The AP tube is in shallow right anterior oblique position and angled maximally in cranial direction. The lateral tube is in steep left anterior oblique position and angled maximally in caudal direction. Fig. 5. Left anterior oblique pulmonary arteriogram with insufficient caudal angulation. Although the more distal right pulmonary artery is well demonstrated, the true origin (small black arrows) is still superimposed on the main pulmonary artery. Only the origin of the left pulmonary artery is well seen. There is a ductus diverticulum of the pulmonary artery (white arrows). Reproduced with permission from Garcia-Mendina, et al.[62]

Mitral valve prolapse was demonstrated in all with MR in 8. Tricuspid valve prolapse was present in 8, TR in 6. Marked aortic root dilatation was present in all and was progressive (Figure 8-9). Dilation of the pulmonary arterial root and PR was found in 3 of 7 infants. Severe heart failure associated with MR or TR was present in 7 of 9 patients and 4 infants died during the first year of life. Histologically the collagen and elastic fibers were severely disrupted, disarrayed and fragmented with increased interstitial ground substance. These data document that infantile Marfan syndrome is characterized by clinical and morphologic features that are distinctly different from the classic syndrome seen in adolescents and adults.

Enteral nutrition

Schwarz and associates[65] from Valhalla, New York, studied 19 infants with congenital heart disease and CHF using 3 feeding regimens: con-

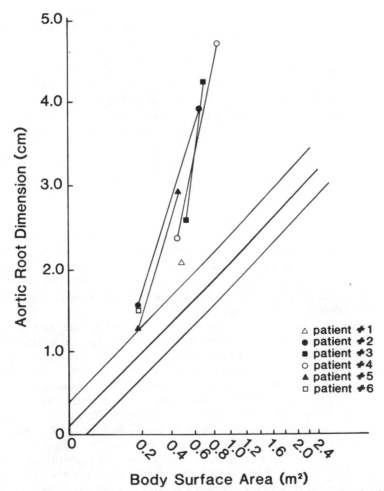

Fig. 8-9. Aortic root diameter in infantile Marfan syndrome. Two-dimensional echocardiographic aortic root dimension is plotted versus body surface area. The mean ± 2 standard deviations for aortic root dimension in normal infants and children (center) were reproduced with permission from Ichida et al. Reproduced with permission from Geva, et al.[64]

tinuous nasogastric alimentation, overnight nasogastric alimentation plus daytime oral feedings, and oral feedings. Infant formulas were supplemented to a caloric density of approximately 1 kcal/mL. During a 5 month study only infants with continuous nasogastric infusion achieved intakes >140 kcal/kg per day and serial anthropometric measurements demonstrated that only these infants had improved nutritional status when assessed by z scores for weight and length, as well as showing marked increases in midarm muscle circumference and subscapular skinfold thicknesses. These data provide important new data on the difficult problem of cardiac cachexia in infants with severe CHF. The marked superiority of the continuous nasogastric feeding regimen was apparent and no complications were encountered despite continuous infusion with a mean volume of 165 mL/kg/day.

Cavopulmonary shunt

Lamberti and associates[66] from San Diego, California, reported 17 patients who underwent a cavopulmonary shunt for single ventricle complex (4), hypoplastic right heart syndrome (10), and hypoplastic left ventricle (3). Age at primary operation ranged from 3.5 to 30 months with a median of 6 months. Seven cavopulmonary shunts were performed without cardiopulmonary bypass and 10 with bypass. All patients in the bypass group had additional procedures: takedown of modified Blalock-Taussig shunt (7), revision of RV outflow tract (4), reconstruction of pulmonary arteries (4), tricuspid valvuloplasty (1) and Damus procedure (1). There was 1 death and 1 patient required early revision. Follow-up from 1 to 53 months revealed a good to excellent result in 12 of 16 with a mean rise in oxygen saturation from 69 to 83%. Three patients died at 4 to 53 months with pulmonary vascular disease, pulmonary arteriovenous malformations, or pneumonia. There was one late failure converted to a standard Glenn shunt. The cavopulmonary shunt is an excellent palliative procedure when right atrium-PA connection must be deferred because of age, weight or anatomic considerations. These authors present excellent results with use of the bidirectional cavopulmonary anastomosis and demonstrate that the operation can be performed at 3.5 months with a good result. Of particular importance is a PA mean pressure of ≤20 mmHg with low pulmonary resistance, normal end diastolic pressure, and minimal systemic AV valvular regurgitation.

Bridges and associates[67] from Boston, Massachusetts, presented 38 patients considered to be at increased risk for Fontan repair who underwent bidirectional cavopulmonary anastomosis. Concurrent PA reconstruction was performed in 21 of the 38. Fontan risk factors included PA distortion, elevated PA resistance >2 Woods units and/or PA pressure >18 mmHg, AV valve regurgitation, systemic ventricular dysfunction, complex venous anatomy, and subaortic obstruction. There were no deaths early or late. Median arterial saturation increased from 79 to 84% and median hospital stay was 88 days. No patients had pleural effusions after 7 days. Inadequate relief of cyanosis occurred in 5 patients and 3 had venous collaterals and 2 had severe ventricular dysfunction. The latter 2 patients subsequently had strokes. One patient with persistent cyanosis required a systemic to pulmonary shunt. These authors present excellent results with use of the bidirectional cavopulmonary anastomosis. This procedure can be followed by the Fontan procedure if palliation is successful.

Kopf and associates[68] from New Haven, Connecticut, reported on follow-up of 91 patients who underwent a superior vena cava to pulmonary artery shunt at an age ranging from 2 days to 46 years with a mean of 7 years. Diagnoses were tricuspid atresia in 27, single ventricle in 22, TF in 14, TGA/VSD/PS in 9, simple TGA in 5, Ebstein's anomaly in 4, pulmonary atresia plus intact septum in 4 and other diagnoses in 6. Hospital mortality was 8% and there were 20 late deaths with actuarial survival of 84% at 10 and 66% at 20 years. Pulmonary arteriovenous fistula were found in 19 of 62 (31%) who had catheterization study. Therapeutic embolization with improvement in oxygen saturation was performed in 6 patients. The prevalence of arteriovenous fistula increases with time after shunt. There was no long-term shunt thrombosis or stricture formation and 50% of shunts were still functioning at 20 years. Palliation was limited because of decrease in blood flow to the contralateral pulmonary artery, collaterals between the inferior and superior vena cavae, and pulmonary arteriovenous fistula formation. Improvement in saturation was obtained in 8 otherwise inoperable patients by creation of a right axillary arteriovenous fistula up to 19 years after the shunt. Comparison of patients with and without a superior cava to pulmonary artery shunt before Fontan procedure revealed no difference in mortality but a higher prevalence of low cardiac output, pleural effusion, long intensive care unit stay and late death in patients without a prior shunt. These data provide useful information for physicians following patients with this shunt procedure. Currently the bidirectional cava-pulmonary shunt is favored and hopefully will not be associated with a high incidence of pulmonary arteriovenous fistulae late after operation.

Balloon valvuloplasty for branch pulmonary artery stenosis

Rothman and associates[69] from Boston, Massachusetts, reported 218 balloon angioplasty procedures in 135 patients with branch PA stenoses. Diagnoses include TF (49), TF/pulmonary atresia (64), isolated PA stenosis (58), and other lesions, including surgically induced PA stenosis (47). Mean age at dilation was 6.6 years and ranged from 1 month to 38 years. The mean diameter of the lesion increased from 3.8 ± 1.7 to 5.5 ± 2.1 mm. The overall success rate was 58%, assessed by an increase $\geq 50\%$ of predilation diameter, an increase $>20\%$ in flow to the affected lung or a decrease $>20\%$ in systolic RV to aortic pressure ratio. Success did not correlate with patient age. Mean balloon to artery ratio was higher in successful (4.2) than in failed (3.0) angioplasty procedures. There were 4 early deaths with 2 patients having PA rupture with angioplasty performed <1 month after PA surgery. An aneurysm occurred in 11 patients and transient pulmonary edema in 4 patients. At angiography a mean of 10 months after dilation, the mean post dilatation diameter of the 57 arteries was unchanged. However, 5 of 32 initially successfully dilated vessels had returned to predilation size as a result of restenosis. The most recent experience indicates a success rate of 60%, mortality rate of 1%, and a risk of aneurysm formation of 3%. These authors present excellent follow-up data in this difficult to treat condition. The natural history of the aneurysms is unknown but there have been no late ruptures or progressive dilation of these lesions to date.

Balloon angioplasty for obstructed Blalock-Taussig shunt

Six children with cyanotic congenital heart defect, aged 6 to 60 months, underwent percutaneous balloon angioplasty of a narrowed Blalock-

Taussig shunt to improve arterial oxygen saturation in a study carried out by Rao and colleagues[70] from Madison, Wisconsin. The indication for angioplasty was a cyanotic heart defect not amenable to total surgical correction, either because of the age and size of presentation or because of anatomic complexity, but at the same time requiring palliation of pulmonary oligemia. Following balloon angioplasty, there was an increase in arterial oxygen saturation from 71 ± 8% to 81 ± 6%. In 1 child with long segment narrowing, there was no significant improvement in oxygen saturation, and this child underwent an additional Blalock-Taussig shunt on the contralateral side. On follow-up 3 to 12 months after balloon angioplasty, the oxygen saturations remained improved (78 ± 10%) in the remaining 5 patients. In 2 children with either complete or almost complete blockage of the Blalock-Taussig shunt, it was not possible to advance any catheter across the shunt but was possible to advance a 2 or 3 mm balloon on a wire and dilate the shunt, followed by introduction of a catheter carrying a larger balloon for angioplasty. This procedure permitted obtaining PA pressure directly (this information was of obvious value in patient management) and resulted in an improvement in arterial oxygen saturation. It was concluded that 1) balloon angioplasty of narrowed Blalock-Taussig shunts is feasible, effective, and safe and 2) even completely occluded shunts can be cannulated and the balloon dilated with the newly available balloon-on-wire devices.

References

1. Morimoto K, Matsuzaki M, Tohma Y, Ono S, Tanaka N, Michishige H, Murata K, Anno Y, Kusukawa R: Diagnosis and Quantitative Evaluation of Secundum-Type Atrial Septal Defect by Transesophageal Doppler Echocardiography. Am J Cardiol (July) 1990;66:85–91.

2. Rome JJ, Keane JF, Perry SB, Spevak PH, Lock JE: Double-Umbrella Closure of Atrial Defects. Initial Clinical Applications. Circulation (September) 1990;82:751–758.

3. Murphy JG, Gersh BJ, McGoon MD, Mair DD, Porter CJ, Ilstrup DM, McGoon DC, Puga FJ, Kirklin JW, Danielson GK: Long-term outcome after surgical repair of isolated atrial septal defect: Follow-up at 27 to 32 years. N Engl J Med 1990 (Dec 13);323:1645–1650.

4. Clapp S, Perry BL, Farooki ZQ, Jackson WL, Karpawich PP, Hakimi M, Arciniegas E, Green EW, Pinsky WW: Down's Syndrome, Complete Atrioventricular Canal and Pulmonary Vascular Obstructive Disease. J Thorac Cardiovasc Surg (July) 1990;100:115–121.

5. Chin AJ, Alboliras ET, Barber G, Murphy JD, Helton G, Pigott JD, Norwood WI: Prospective Detection by Doppler Color Flow Imaging of Additional Defects in Infants with a Large Ventricular Septal Defect. J Am Coll Cardiol (June) 1990;15:1637–42.

6. Rhodes LA, Keane JF, Keane JP, Fellows KE, Jonas RA, Castaneda AR, Nadas AS: Long Follow-up (to 43 Years) of Ventricular Septal Defect with Audible Aortic Regurgitation. Am J Cardiol (August 1) 1990;66:340–345.

7. Rao PS: Long-term oral diazoxide therapy for pulmonary vascular obstructive disease associated with congenital heart defects. Am Heart J 1990 (June);119:1317–1321.

8. Caspi J, Coles JH, Benson LN, Freedom RM, Burrows PE, Smallhorn JF, Trusler GA, Williams WG: Management of Neonatal Critical Pulmonic Stenosis in the Balloon Valvotomy Era. Ann Thorac Surg (February) 1990;49:273–278.

9. Stanger P, Cassidy SC, Girod DA, Kan JS, Lababidi Z, Shapiro SR: Balloon Pulmonary Valvuloplasty and Angioplasty of Congenital Anomalies Registry. Am J Cardiol (March 15) 1990;65:775–783.

10. Kan JS, Marvin WJ, Bass JL, Muster AJ, Murphy J: Balloon Pulmonary Valvuloplasty and Angioplasty of Congenital Anomalies Registry. Am J Cardiol (March 15) 1990;65:798–801.

11. Ali Khan MA, Al-Yousef S, Moore JW, Sawyer W: Results of repeat percutaneous balloon valvuloplasty for pulmonary valvar restenosis. Am Heart J 1990 (October);120:878–881.

12. Touati GD, Vouhe PR, Amodeo A, Pouard P, Mauriat P, Leca F, Neveux JY, Castaneda R: Primary Repair of Tetralogy of Fallot in Infancy. J Thorac Cardiovasc Surg (March) 1990;99:396–403.

13. Horneffer PJ, Zahka KG, Rowe SA, Manolio TA, Gott VL, Reitz BA, Gardner TJ: Long-Term Results of Total Repair of Tetralogy of Fallot in Childhood. Ann Thorac Surg (August) 1990;50:179–185.

14. Chandar JS, Wolf GS, Garson A, Jr, Bell TJ, Beder SD, Bink-Boelkens M, Byrum CJ, Campbell RM, Deal, BJ, Dick M II, Flinn CJ, Gaum WE, Gillette PC, Hordof AJ, Kugler JD, Porter CJ, Walsh EP: Ventricular Arrhythmias in Postoperative Tetralogy of Fallot. Am J Cardiol (March) 1990;65:655–661.

15. Vaksmann G, Fournier A, Davignon A, Ducharme G, Houyel L, Fouron J-C: Frequency and Prognosis of Arrhythmias after Operative "Correction" of Tetralogy of Fallot. Am J Cardiol (August 1) 1990;66:346–349.

16. Hausdorf G, Hinrich C, Nienaber CA, Schark C, Keck EW: Left Ventricular Contractile State after Surgical Correction of Tetralogy of Fallot: Risk Factors for Late Left Ventricular Dysfunction. Pediatr Cardiol (April) 1990;11:61–68.

17. Hawkins JA, Thorne JK, Boucek MM, Orsmond GS, Ruttenberg HD, Veasy G, McGough EC: Early and Late Results in Pulmonary Atresia and Intact Ventricular Septum. J Thorac Cardiovasc Surg (October) 1990;100:492–497.

18. Mandell VS, Lock JE, Mayer JE, Parness IA, Kulik TJ: The "Laid-Back" Aortogram: An Improved Angiographic View for Demonstration of Coronary Arteries in Transposition of the Great Arteries. Am J Cardiol (June 1) 1990;65:1379–1383.

19. Wernovsky G, Jonas RA, Colan SD, Sanders SP, Wessel DL, Castaneda AR, Mayer JE: Results of the Arterial Switch Operation in Patients with Transposition of the Great Arteries and Abnormalities of the Mitral Valve or Left Ventricular Outflow Tract. J Am Coll Cardiol (November) 1990;16:1446–1454.

20. Mayer JE, Jr, Sanders SP, Jonas RA, Castaneda AR, Wernovsky G: Coronary Artery Pattern and Outcome of Arterial Switch Operation for Transposition of the Great Arteries. Circulation (suppl IV) (November) 1990;82:IV-139-IV-145.

21. Martin RP, Oureshi SA, Ettedgui JA, Baker EJ, O'Brien BJ, Deverall PB, Yates AK, Maisey MN, Radley-Smith R, Tynan M, Yacoub MH: An Evaluation of Right and Left Ventricular Function After Anatomical Correction and Intra-Atrial Repair Operations for Complete Transposition of the Great Arteries. Circulation (September) 1990;82:808–816.

22. Lundstrom U, Bull C, Wyse RKH, Somerville J: The Natural and "Unnatural" History of Congenitally Corrected Transposition. Am J Cardiol (May 15) 1990;65:1222–1229.

23. Hakazawa M, Aotsuka H, Imai Y, Kurosawa H, Fukuchi S, Satomi G, Takao A: Ventricular Volume Characteristics in Double-Inlet Left Ventricle Before and After Septation. Circulation (May) 1990;81:1537–1543.

24. Shen W-K, Holmes DR, Porter CJ, McGoon DW, Ilstrup DM: Sudden Death After Repair of Double-Outlet Right Ventricle. Circulation (January) 1990;81:128–136.

25. Burch N, Redington AN, Carvalho JS, Rusconi P, Shinebourne EA, Rigby ML, Paneth M, Lincoln C: Open Valvotomy for Critical Aortic Stenosis in Infancy. Br Heart J (January) 1990;63:37–40.

26. Turley K, Bove EL, Amato JJ, Iannettoni M, Yeh J, Cotroneo JV, Galdieri RJ: Neonatal Aortic Stenosis. J Thorac Cardiovasc Surg (April) 1990;99:679–84.

27. DeBoer DA, Robins RC, Maron BJ, McIntosh CL, Clark RE: Late Results of Aortic Valvotomy for Congenital Valvar Aortic Stenosis. Ann Thorac Surg (July) 1990;50:69–73.

28. Rocchini AP, Beekman RH, Shachar GB, Benson L, Schwartz D, Kan JS: Balloon Aortic Valvuloplasty: Results of the Valvuloplasty and Angioplasty of Congenital Anomalies Registry. Am J Cardiol (March 15) 1990;65:784–789.

29. Shaddy RE, Boucek MM, Sturtevant JE, Ruttenberg HD, Orsmond GS: Gradient Reduction, Aortic Valve Regurgitation and Prolapse After Balloon Aortic Valvuloplasty in 32

Consecutive Patients with Congenital Aortic Stenosis. J Am Coll Cardiol (August) 1990;16:451–456.

30. Douville EC, Sade RM, Crawford FA, Wiles HB: Subvalvar Aortic Stenosis: Timing of Operation. Ann Thorac Surg (July) 1990;50:29–34.

31. Stewart JR, Merrill WH, Hammon JW, Jr, Graham TP Jr, Bender JW Jr: Reappraisal of Localized Resection for Subvalvar Aortic Stenosis. Ann Thorac Surg (August) 1990;50:197–203.

32. Wren C, Oslizlok P, Bull C: Natural History of Supravalvular Aortic Stenosis and Pulmonary Artery Stenosis. J Am Coll Cardiol (June) 1990;15:1625–30.

33. Hellenbrand WE, Allen HD, Golinko RJ, Hagler DJ, Lutin W, Kan J: Balloon Angioplasty for Aortic Recoarctation: Results of Valvuloplasty and Angioplasty of Congenital Anomalies Registry. Am J Cardiol (March 15) 1990;65:793–797.

34. Burrows PE, Benson LN, Williams WG, Trusler GA, Coles J, Smallhorn JF, Freedom RM: Iliofemoral Arterial Complications of Balloon Angioplasty for Systemic Obstructions in Infants and Children. Circulation (November) 1990;82:1697–1704.

35. Rao PS, Thapar MK, Galal O, Wilson AD: Follow-up results of balloon angioplasty of native coarctation in neonates and infants. Am Heart J 1990 (December);120:1310–1314.

36. Rao PS, Wilson AD, Chopra PS: Immediate and follow-up results of balloon angioplasty of postoperative recoarctation in infants and children. Am Heart J 1990 (December);120:1315–1320.

37. Lacour-Gayet F, Bruniaux J, Seraff A, Chambran P, Blaysat G, Losay J, Petit J, Kachaner J, Planche C: Hypoplastic Transverse Arch and Coarctation in Neonates. J Thorac Cardiovasc Surg (December) 1990;100:808–816.

38. van Son JAM, van Asten WNJC, van Lier HJJ, Daniels O, Vincent JG, Skotnicki SH, Lacquet LK: Detrimental Sequelae on the Hemodynamics of the Upper Left Limb after Subclavian Flap Angioplasty in Infancy. Circulation (March) 1990;81:996–1004.

39. Kavey R-EW, Cotton JL, Blackman MS: Atenolol Therapy for Exercise-Induced Hypertension after Aortic Coarctation Repair. Am J Cardiol (November) 1990;66:1233–1236.

40. Moskowitz WB, Schieken RM, Mosteller M, Bossano R: Altered systolic and diastolic function in children after "successful" repair of coarctation of the aorta. Am Heart J 1990 (July);120:103–109.

41. Chin AJ, Weinberg PM, Barber G: Subcostal Two-Dimensional Echocardiographic Identification of Anomalous Attachment of Septum Primum in Patients with Left Atrioventricular Valve Underdevelopment. Am J Cardiol (March 1) 1990;15:678–81.

42. Ludman P, Foale R, Alexander N, Nihoyannopoulos P: Cross Sectional Echocardiographic Identification of Hypoplastic Left Heart Syndrome and Differentiation from other Causes of Right Ventricular Overload. Br Heart J (June) 1990;63:355–361.

43. Meliones JN, Snider AR, Bove EL, Rosenthal A, Rosen DA: Longitudinal results after First-Stage Palliation for Hypoplastic Left Heart Syndrome. Circulation (suppl IV) (November) 1990;82:IV-151–IV-156.

44. Spevak PJ, Bass JL, Ben-Sachar G, Hesslein P, Keane JF, Perry S, Pyles L, Lock JE: Balloon Angioplasty for Congenital Mitral Stenosis. Am J Cardiol (August 15) 1990;66:472–476.

45. Franklin RCG, Sullivan ID, Anderson RH, Shinebourne EA, Deanfield JE: Is Banding of the Pulmonary Trunk Obsolete for Infants with Tricuspid Atresia and Double Inlet Ventricle with a Discordant Ventriculoarterial Connection? Role of Aortic Arch Obstruction and Subaortic Stenosis. J Am Coll Cardiol (November) 1990;16:1455–1464.

46. Gewillig MH, Lundstrom UR, Deanfield JE, Bull C, Franklin RC, Graham TP, Wyse RK: Impact of Fontan Operation on Left Ventricular Size and Contractility in Tricuspid Atresia. Circulation (January) 1990;81:118–127.

47. Mair DD, Hagler DJ, Puga FJ, Schaff HV, Danielson GK: Fontan Operation in 176 Patients with Tricuspid Atresia. Results and a Proposed New Index for Patient Selection. Circulation (suppl IV) (November) 1990;82:IV-164–IV-169.

48. Tuzcu EM, Moodie DS, Chambers JL, Keyser P, Hobbs RE: Congenital heart diseases associated with coronary artery anomalies. Cleve Clin J Med 1990 (March/April) 57:147–152.

49. Seguchi M, Nakanishi T, Nakazawa M, Doi S, Momma K, Takao A, Imai Y, Kondoh C, Hiroe M: Myocardial perfusion after aortic implantation for anomalous origin of the left coronary artery from the pulmonary artery. Eur Heart J 1990 (Mar);11:213–218.

50. Sapin P, Frantz E, Jain A, Nichols TC, Dehmer GJ: Coronary artery fistula: An abnormality affecting all age groups. Medicine 1990;69:101–113.

51. Fontan F, Kirklin JW, Fernandez G, Costa F, Naftel DC, Tritto F, Blackstone EJ: Outcome after a "Perfect" Fontan Operation. Circulation (May) 1990;81:1520–1536.

52. Bartmus DA, Driscoll DJ, Offord KP, Humes RA, Mair DD, Schaff HV, Puga FJ, Danielson DK: The Modified Fontan Operation for Children Less than 4 years old. J Am Coll Cardiol (February) 1990;15:429–35.

53. Kurosawa H, Imai Y, Fukuchi S, Sawatari K, Koh Y, Nakazawa M, Takao A: Septation and Fontan Repair of Univentricular Atrioventricular Connection. J Thorac Cardiovasc Surg (February) 1990;99:314–319.

54. Gegel RL, Mayer JE, Fried R, Helgason H, Cook EF, Reid LM: Role of Lung Biopsy in Patients Undergoing a Modified Fontan Procedure. J Thorac Cardiovasc Surg (March) 1990;99:451–459.

55. Rhodes J, Garafano RP, Bowman FO, Grant GP, Bierman FZ, Gersony WM: Effect of Right Ventricular Anatomy on the Cardiopulmonary Response to Exercise. Implications for the Fontan Procedure. Circulation (June) 1990;81:1811–1817.

56. Bridges ND, Lock JE, Castancda AR: Baffle Fenestration with Subsequent Transcatheter Closure. Modification of the Fontan Operation for Patients with Increased Risk. Circulation (November) 1990;82:1681–1689.

57. Stumper OFW, Elzenga NJ, Hess J, Sutherland GR: Transesophageal Echocardiography in Children with Congenital Heart Disease: An Initial Experience. J Am Coll Cardiol (August) 1990;16:433–441.

58. Sreeram N, Stumper OFW, Kaulitz R, Hess J, Roelandt JRTC, Sutherland GR: Comparative Value of Transthoracic and Transesophageal Echocardiography in the Assessment of Congenital Abnormalities of the Atrioventricular Junction. Am J Coll Cardiol (November) 1990;16:1205–1214.

59. Musewe NN, Poppe D, Smallhorn JF, Hellman J, Whyte H, Smith B, Freedom RM: Doppler Echocardiographic Measurement of Pulmonary Artery Pressure from Ductal Doppler Velocities in the Newborn. J Am Coll Cardiol (February) 1990;15:446–456.

60. Vick III, GW, Rokey R, Huhta JC, Mulvagh SL, Johnston DL: Nuclear Magnetic Resonance Imaging of the Pulmonary Arteries, Subpulmonary Region, and Aorticopulmonary Shunts: A Comparative Study with Two Dimensional Echocardiography and Angiography. Am Heart J (May) 1990:1103–1110.

61. Kersting-Sommerhoff BA, Diethelm L, Stanger P, Dery R, Higashino SM, Higgins SS, Higgins CB: Evaluation of complex congenital ventricular anomalies with magnetic resonance imaging. Am Heart J 1990 (July);120:133–142.

62. Garcia-Medina V, Bass J, Braunlin E, Krabil KA, Pyles L, Castaneda-Zuniga WR, Hunter DW, Amplatz K: A Useful Projection for Demonstrating the Bifurcation of the Pulmonary Artery. Pediatr Cardiol (July) 1990;11:147–149.

63. Debich DE, Devine WA, Anderson RH: Polysplenia with Normally Structured Hearts. Am J Cardiol (May 15) 1990;65:1274–1275.

64. Geva T, Sanders SP, Diogenes MS, Rockenmacher S, VanPraagh R: Two-Dimensional and Doppler Echocardiographic and Pathologic Characteristics of the Infantile Marfan Syndrome. Am J Cardiol (May 15) 1990;65:1230–1237.

65. Schwarz SM, Gewitz MH, See CC, Berezin S, Glassman MS, Medow CM, Fish BC, Newman LJ: Enteral Nutrition in Infants with Congenital Heart Disease and Growth Failure. Pediatr (September) 1990;86:368–373.

66. Lamberti JJ, Spicer RL, Waldman JD, Grehl TM, Thomason D, George L, Kirkpatrick SE, Mathewson JW: The Bidirectional Cavopulmonary Shunt. J Thorac Cardiovasc Surg (July) 1990;100:22–30.

67. Bridges ND, Jonas RA, Mayer JE, Flanagan MF, Keane JF, Castaneda AR: Bidirectional Cavopulmonary Anastomosis as Interim Palliation for High-Risk Fontan Candidates. Circulation (suppl IV) (November) 1990;82:IV-170–IV-176.

68. Kopf GS, Laks H, Stansel HC, Hellenbrand WE, Kleinman CS, Talner NS: Thirty-year Follow-up of Superior Vena Cava-Pulmonary Artery (Glenn) Shunts. J Thorac Cardiovasc Surg (November) 1990;100:662–671.

69. Rothman A, Perry SB, Keane JF, Lock JE: Early Results and Follow-up of Balloon An-

gioplasty for Branch Pulmonary Artery Stenoses. J Am Coll Cardiol (April) 1990;15:1109–1117.

70. Rao PS, Levy JM, Chopra PS: Balloon angioplasty of stenosed Blalock-Taussig anastomosis: Role of balloon-on-a-wire in dilating occluded shunts. Am Heart J 1990 (November);120:1173–1178.

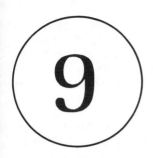

Congestive Heart Failure

Review

A superb symposium on CHF organized by Barry M. Massie and Milton Packer[1-10] appeared in *The American Journal of Cardiology*, August 15, 1990.

Hospitalization rates

Ghali and associates[11] from Chicago and Maywood, Illinois, and Atlanta, Georgia, examined hospital discharge data from a sample of short-stay US hospitals to obtain information regarding trends in the prevalence of CHF from 1973 through 1986. During this 14-year period, the number of discharges more than doubled and the age-adjusted rates increased from 53% to 88% among the 4 major sex-race groups. On average, non-white men had annual hospitalization rates 33% higher than white men while for women the corresponding nonwhite rates were 50% higher. Hospitalization rates during this period remained constant for persons younger than 55 years but rose sharply in those older than 55. The two factors accounting for the growing prevalence of CHF seem to be the increasing average age of the population and the longer survival of persons with chronic CHF. The roll of improved medical therapy during the period of the study remained uncertain.

Spontaneous improvement

Francis and associates[12] from Minneapolis, Minnesota, identified 11 patients with severe CHF (average EF 22 ± 4%) who developed spontaneous marked improvement over a period of follow-up lasting 4 ± 1 years. All 11 patients were initially symptomatic with exertional dyspnea and fatigue for a minimum of 3 months. They form a subset of a larger group of 97 patients with chronic CHF that the authors followed with sequential EF measurements. All 11 patients were treated with digitalis diuretics, and either converting-enzyme inhibitors or a combination of isosorbide dinitrate and hydralazine. Ten of the 11 patients had a history consistent with chronic alcoholism, and each reportedly abstained from alcohol during follow-up. During the follow-up period, the average EF improved in 11 patients from 22 ± 4% to 57 ± 10%. Late follow-up indicates an average EF of 53 ± 9% for the group. CHF resolved in each case. The authors concluded that selected patients with severe CHF can markedly improve their LV function in association with complete resolution of heart failure. This appears to be particularly evident in those patients with chronic alcoholism who subsequently abstain.

Basis of impaired exercise tolerance

Roubin and associates[13] in Sydney and Camperdown, Australia, evaluated hemodynamic and metabolic changes at rest and during exercise in 23 patients with chronic CHF and in 6 control subjects. Exercise was limited by leg fatigue in both groups and capacity was 40% lower in the patients with CHF. At rest, comparing patients with control subjects, heart rate, RA and pulmonary capillary wedge pressures were higher, cardiac output, stroke volume, work indexes, and EF were lower, mean arterial and RA pressure and systemic vascular resistance were similar during all phases of exercise in patients with CHF, pulmonary capillary wedge pressures and systemic vascular resistances were higher and pulmonary vascular resistance remained elevated compared with values in control subjects. Cardiac outputs were lower in the patients with CHF, but appeared to have the same physiologic distribution in both groups during exercise. Arterial-femoral venous oxygen content difference was higher in patients with CHF, but this increase did not compensate for a reduced blood flow. The maximal oxygen consumption was significantly reduced, femoral venous lactate and pH values were higher and femoral venous pH was similar in both groups at their respective levels of maximal exercise (Figure 9-1). LVEFs were lower in patients with CHF at rest and did not increase with exercise. Ventilation in relation to oxygen consumption was higher in patients with CHF than in control subjects. Therefore, in patients with CHF, exercise appears to be limited primarily by fatigue due to acidosis and reduced leg blood flow in exercising muscles.

Prognosis

In an attempt to identify which variables predict survival in advanced dilated cardiomyopathy, Keogh and associates[14] from Sydney, Australia, investigated 232 patients presenting for assessment for cardiac transplantation and followed for 10 ± 12 months (range 2 weeks to 5 years). Etiology of dilated cardiomyopathy included ischemic heart disease (33%), idiopathic (42%) and miscellaneous (25%). In each patient, 26 parameters were recorded. Whole group survival was 68% at 1 year, 56% at 2 years, 41% at 3 years and 25% at 4 years. On Cox multivariate regression analysis, 3 parameters predicted survival: New York Heart Association symptom class, PA wedge pressure and plasma atrial natriuretic factor level. On paired testing of actuarial survival curves, plasma noradrenaline also held predictive value, as did LVEF ≤20% on radionuclide ventriculography and presence of ≥4 beats of VT on Holter monitoring. Treatment with amiodarone did not appear to influence survival. Conventional deter-

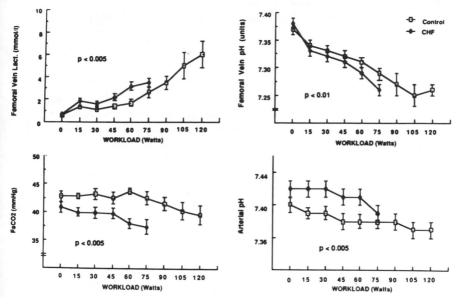

Fig. 9-1. Femoral venous lactate (Lact.), femoral venous pH, arterial carbon dioxide tension (PaCO2) and arterial pH at rest and during exercise in the control (□) and heart failure (CHF) (●) groups. Reproduced with permission from Roubin, et al.[13]

minants of prognosis in cardiomyopathy (symptom class, PA wedge pressure, nonsustained VT and EF) do not alone always adequately differentiate survival in this group of high risk patients. More attention to plasma noradrenaline and to atrial natriuretic factor levels may give important additional information in the context of assessment of patients for transplantation.

Kelly and associates[15] from San Diego, California, followed 133 patients with dilated heart failure, 80 with CAD and 53 with idiopathic dilated cardiomyopathy, for a mean of 29 months. Patients with CAD had a worse prognosis than those classified as having idiopathic cardiomyopathy. Features from history, physical examination, and diagnostic tests done when patients were referred were checked for univariate association with survival and were used in Cox model survival analysis to define risk groups. Neither the overall group nor either subgroup showed a relation between EF and survival. The best variables for predicting long-term mortality included underlying CAD, basal systolic BP <120 mm Hg, presence of congestion on chest radiogram, and age >64. Other variables did not improve risk prediction in the overall group. Among patients with CAD, BP, congestion, maximal heart rate on treadmill test, and the presence of left BBB on the initial electrocardiogram all contributed. Only systolic BP and the symptom score were related to survival in idiopathic cardiomyopathy.

C-reactive protein

Pye and associates[16] from Glasgow, UK, prospectively assessed in 37 patients with various degrees of CHF the serum concentration of C-reactive protein which was higher than normal in 26 (70%) patients. The concentration was directly related to the severity of the CHF and the state of decompensation. Thus, CHF is an additional cause of raised serum concentration of C-reactive protein, but the importance of this observation is not yet known.

Serum magnesium

Gottlieb and colleagues[17] in New York, New York and Baltimore, Maryland, evaluated the relation between serum magnesium concentration and clinical characteristics and long-term outcome of 199 patients with chronic CHF. The serum magnesium concentration was <1.6 mEq/L in 38 patients (19%), within the normal range in 134 patients (67%) and >2.1 mEq/L in 27 patients (14%). Patients with hypomagnesemia had more frequent VPCs and episodes of VT than did patients with normal serum magnesium concentrations. Even though the two groups of patients were similar with respect to severity of CHF and neurohormonal variables, patients with a low serum magnesium concentration had a poor prognosis during long-term follow-up with 45% and 71% surviving for 1 year, respectively. Patients with hypermagnesemia had more severe symptoms, greater neurohormonal activation and poorer renal function than did patients with a normal serum magnesium concentration, but they tended to have fewer ventricular arrhythmias. Hypermagnesemic patients had a poorer prognosis than patients with a normal magnesium concentration with 37% and 71% 1 year survivals, respectively. Thus, the measurement of serum magnesium concentration provides important clinical and prognostic information in patients with chronic CHF.

Late potentials

Middlekauff and associates[18] from Los Angeles, California, obtained signal-averaged electrocardiograms in 62 consecutive patients with advanced CHF undergoing evaluation for possible heart transplantation to determine if late potentials: 1) provide unique information compared to assessment of ventricular ectopic activity on ambulatory electrocardiogram, and 2) identify a subgroup of CHF patients with higher sudden death risk. Patients with a history of cardiac arrest or sustained VT were excluded. CHF was due to old myocardial infarction in 40 patients and idiopathic dilated cardiomyopathy in 22 patients. Late potentials were present in 16 of 40 (40%) patients with old infarction but in only 3 of 22 (14%) patients with nonischemic CHF. Twenty-four-hour ambulatory electrocardiograms were obtained in 34 patients (55%). Total ventricular ectopic activity and repetitive forms of ectopy were similar in patients with and without late potentials. Nine patients died suddenly, 9 had nonsudden death, 15 underwent heart transplantation and 29 were alive and well after a mean follow-up of 218 ± 154 days. At 1 year, the actuarial risk of death was 37% and of sudden death was 20%. Sudden death risk was 12% in patients with late potentials vs 21% in those without. Thus, the incidence of the arrhythmia substrate producing late potentials depends on the CHF etiology. The signal-averaged electrocardiogram and ambulatory electrocardiogram provide independent information for possible risk assessment in CHF. However, late potentials are poor predictors of sudden death risk when CHF is advanced, possibly due to the heterogeneity of causes of sudden death—VT being only 1 of many possible mechanisms.

Frequency of myocarditis as a cause

Vasiljevic and associates[19] from Belgrade, Zagreb, and Novi Sad, Yugoslavia, and London, UK, presented the combined experience of 3 Yugoslavian cardiovascular centers in the application of endomyocardial biopsy for the diagnosis of myocarditis in patients who present clinically with CHF. The study group comprised 107 patients (mean age 41 years; range 19 to 61 years). On the basis of patient history and diagnostic tests, the following clinical diagnoses were established: dilated cardiomyopathy (85), myocarditis (16), and alcohol-induced heart disease (6). Endomyocardial biopsy samples were taken from the left ventricle (95) or both ventricles (12) by use of a King's College bioptome, with a mean of 3.2 samples per patient. Histologic evidence of myocarditis was noted in 10 of 85 patients (12%) with a clinical diagnosis of dilated cardiomyopathy, in 2 of 6 patients (33%) with alcohol-induced heart disease, and in 12 of 16 patients (75%) with a clinical diagnosis of myocarditis. There was confirmation of the clinically suspected diagnosis in 63% of cases, a change of diagnosis based on histology in 15% of cases, and nonspecific findings in 22%. However, useful information was obtained in 78% of the cases, and there was a 22% incidence of histologically proven myocarditis for the entire group. These results indicate that endomyocardial biopsy is beneficial in determining the true incidence of myocarditis in patients with a clinical presentation of dilated cardiomyopathy.

Neuroendocrine investigations

To test the hypothesis that cardiac norepinephrine depletion related to CHF alters contractile responses to β-adrenergic agonists with a component of "indirect" action (acting by release of neuronal norepinephrine), Port and co-investigators[20] in Salt Lake City, Utah, examined the inotropic potential of several pharmacologically distinct β-agonists. Contractile responses to the nonselective β-agonist *isoproterenol*, the β2-selective agonist *zinterol*, and the direct- and indirect-acting agonists *dopamine* and *dopexamine* were compared in isolated RV trabeculae removed from failing, nonfailing innervated, and previously transplanted, and therefore, denervated nonfailing human hearts. In failing hearts, the contractile response isoproterenol was significantly lower (41%) than that in nonfailing innervated hearts. The responses to the mixed agonists dopamine and dopexamine were even more attenuated in failing hearts, to level 76–90% lower than those of nonfailing innervated hearts. In denervated, previously transplanted, nonfailing hearts, the contractile responses to the mixed agonists dopamine and dopexamine were 66–72% lower than those in the nonfailing innervated group, but the response to isoproterenol was not significantly different. The response to zinterol was not significantly heart failure, in vivo hemodynamic responses to dopexamine were compared with those of the direct-acting β-agonist dobutamine. Responses to dopexamine and dobutamine were measured before and after prolonged continuous infusions of each drug. The response to dopexamine, but not to dobutamine, diminished over time. The investigators conclude that a large component of the inotropic response to dopamine and dopexamine in human hearts is due to the ability of these agonists to promote the release of neuronal norepinephrine; when neuronal norepinephrine is depleted, indirect-acting agonists are less able to produce an inotropic response.

In the Studies of Left Ventricular Dysfunction (SOLVD), a multicenter study of patients with EF of ≤35%, Francis and co-investigators[21] in Bethesda, Maryland, compared baseline plasma norepinephrine, plasma renin activity, plasma atrial natriuretic factor, and plasma arginine vasopressin in 56 control subjects, 151 patients with dysfunction (no overt CHF), and 81 patients with overt CHF before randomization. Median values for plasma norepinephrine, plasma atrial natriuretic factor, plasma arginine vasopressin and plasma renin activity were significantly higher in patients with LV dysfunction than in normal control subjects (Figure 9-2). Neuroendocrine values were highest in patients with overt CHF. Plasma renin activity was normal in patients with LV dysfunction without CHF who were not receiving diuretics and was significantly increased in patients on diuretic therapy. The investigators concluded that neuroendocrine activation occurs in patients with LV dysfunction and no heart failure. Neuroendocrine activation is further increased as overt CHF ensues and diuretics are added to therapy.

Skeletal muscle findings

Recent studies in patients with long-term CHF have suggested that intrinsic abnormalities in skeletal muscle can contribute to the development of early lactic acidosis and fatigue during exercise. Sullivan and co-investigators[22] in Durham, North Carolina, provided an analysis of substate and enzyme content, fiber typing, and capillarization in skeletal muscle biopsy samples obtained at rest from the vastus lateralis in eleven patients with long-term CHF (LVEF 21%) and nine normal subjects. Patients demonstrated a reduced peak exercise oxygen consumption when

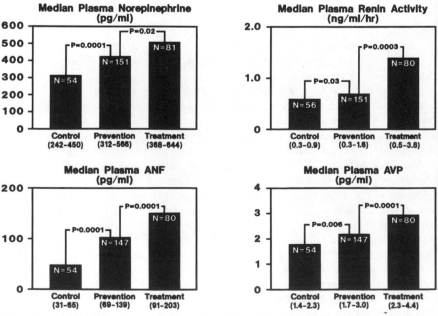

Fig. 9-2. Bar graphs of incremental and significant increase in plasma norepinephrine, plasma renin activity, plasma arginine vasopressin (AVP), and plasma atrial natriuretic factor (ANF) in control subjects, prevention patients, and treatment patients. Treatment values are higher than control values for each neurohormone. Median values and interquartile ranges 25% to 75%. Reproduced with permission from Francis, et al.[21]

compared with normals and had an accelerated rise in blood lactate levels during exercise. In mixed fiber skeletal muscle, total phosphorylase and glycolytic enzyme activities were not different in the 2 groups, whereas mitochondrial enzymes involved in terminal oxidation were decreased in patients as compared to normal subjects as indicated by reductions in succinate dehydrogenase and citrate synthetase. 3-Hydroxyacyl-CoA-dehydrogenase, an important enzyme mediating beta-oxidation of fatty acids, was also reduced in patients as compared with normals. There was no difference in high-energy phosphagens or lactate concentration of mixed muscle in the 2 groups, whereas glycogen content was decreased in patients. Patients demonstrated a reduced percentage of slow twitch type I fibers and had a high percentage of type IIb fast twitch fibers which were smaller than the type IIb fibers seen in normal subjects. In patients, the number of capillaries per fiber was decreased for type I and type IIa fibers but the ratio of capillaries to cross-sectional fiber area was not different for the two groups. These data demonstrate major alterations in skeletal muscle histology and biochemistry in patients with long-term CHF, including fiber atrophy, a decrease in percentage of composition of type I fibers, and an increase in type IIb fibers accompanied by a decrease in oxidative enzyme capacity. These skeletal muscle adaptations to the CHF state represent a potentially important mechanism underlying the very onset of anaerobic metabolism and fatigue seen in this disorder and might play a role in determining both day-to-day exercise tolerance and the response to therapeutic interventions in patients with long-term CHF.

Tumor necrosis factor

Although cachexia often accompanies advanced CHF, little is known about the causes of the cachectic state. To assess the potential role of tumor necrosis factor in the pathogenesis of cardiac cachexia, Levine and associates[23] from New York, New York, measured the serum levels of the factor in 33 patients with chronic CHF secondary to either CAD or idiopathic dilated cardiomyopathy and in 33 age-matched healthy subjects and in 9 patients with chronic renal failure. Mean (± SEM serum levels of tumor necrosis factor were higher in the patients with CHF (115 ± 25 U/ml) than in the healthy controls (9 ± 3 U/ml) (Figure 9-3). Nineteen of the patients with CHF had serum levels of tumor necrosis factor 39 U/ml (>2 SD above the mean value of the control group), whereas the remaining 14 patients had serum levels of tumor necrosis factor below this level. The patients with high levels of tumor necrosis factor were more cachectic than those with low levels (82 ± 3 vs 95 ± 6% of ideal body weight, respectively) and had more advanced CHF, as evidenced by their higher values for plasma renin activity (2.92 ± 0.53 vs 1.06 ± 0.53 ng/L/sec [10.5 ± 1.9 vs 3.8 ± 1.9 ng/ml/hr];) and lower serum sodium concentration (135 ± 1 vs 138 ± 1 mmol/L). The group with high levels of tumor necrosis factor also had lower hemoglobin levels (7.82 ± 0.2 vs 8.69 ± 0.4 mmol/L [12.6 ± 0.4 vs 14.0 ± 0.6 g/dl]) and higher values for blood urea nitrogen (19.5 ± 2.2 vs 12.5 ± 1.8 mmol/L) than the group with low levels of tumor necrosis factor. The high levels of tumor necrosis factor were not due solely to decreased renal clearance, however, since the levels in the patients with CHF were considerably higher than those in the 9 patients with chronic renal failure (115 ± 25 vs 45 ± 25 U/ml). These findings indicate that circulating levels of tumor necrosis factor are increased in cachectic patients with CHF and that this elevation is

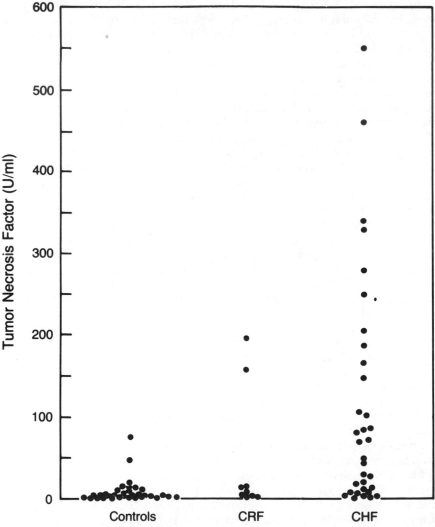

Fig. 9-3. Serum levels of tumor necrosis factor in 33 patients with chronic heart failure (CHF), 9 patients with chronic renal failure (CRF), and 33 healthy, age-matched controls. Reproduced with permission from Levine, et al.[23]

associated with the marked activation of the renin-angiotensin system seen in patients with end-stage cardiac disease.

Mountain sickness

Anand and associates[24] from Chandigarh, India, described a new type of mountain sickness in 21 men, mean age 22 ± 2 years, with severe CHF including severe peripheral edema and ascites after 11 ± 6 weeks at altitudes from 5800 to 6700 m. Investigation, within 3 days of transfer to 300 m, showed polycythemia, cardiomegaly with RV enlargement, and (in 17) pericardial effusion. The CHF resolved rapidly after transfer from high altitude.

TREATMENT

Physical training

Coats and associates[25] from Oxford, UK, treated 8 patients with chronic CHF secondary to CAD (mean age 63 years; LVEF 19 ± 8%) with 8 weeks of home-based bicycle exercise training and 8 weeks of activity restriction (rest) in a physician-blind, random-order, crossover trial. Training increased exercise duration from 14 ± 1 minute to 17 ± 1 minutes and peak oxygen consumption from 14 ± 1 ml/min^{-1}/kg^{-1} to 17 ± 1 ml/min^{-1}/kg^{-1}. Heart rates at submaximum workloads and rate-pressure products were significantly reduced by training, and there was also a significant improvement in patient-rated symptom scores. No adverse events occurred during the training phase. Thus home-based physical training programs are feasible even in severe chronic CHF and have a beneficial effect on exercise tolerance, peak oxygen consumption, and symptoms. The commonly held belief that rest is the mainstay of treatment of chronic CHF should no longer be accepted.

Digoxin

To appraise the effectiveness of digoxin for treatment of CHF in patients with sinus rhythm, Jaeschke and associates[26] from Hamilton, Canada, from review of publications on this subject, found 7 double-blind, randomized, controlled trials appraising the usefulness of digoxin in patients with CHF and sinus rhythm (Table 9-1). Analysis of these 7 studies disclosed the common odds ratio for CHF deterioration while receiving digoxin vs placebo was 0.28 with a 95% confidence interval. Predictors of digoxin benefit included presence of a third heart sound and the severity and duration of CHF. Data from these 7 trials of high methodologic quality suggest that 1 of 9 patients with CHF and sinus rhythm derive a clinically important benefit from digoxin.

TABLE 9-1. *Details of double-blind, randomized, controlled trials of digoxin therapy for patients with CHF and sinus rhythm. Reproduced with permission from Jaeschke, et al.[26]*

Reference (year)	Study Design	Sample Size	CHF Criteria	Interventions	Digoxin Dose in mg/day (and level)	Co-Intervention Allowed	Patients Excluded from the Analysis (%)	Excluded Patients Described
[25] (1989)	Parallel group	111*	Not stated	Digoxin vs milrinone vs both vs placebo	0.22 (mean 1.2 nmol/L, time not stated)	No (counted as treatment failure)	0	Not applicable
[22] (1988)	Parallel group	196*	Stated	Digoxin vs captopril vs placebo	0.125–0.375 (>0.9 nmol/L, 24-hour level)	Yes (increased diuretics)	0	Not applicable
[23] (1988)	Parallel group	213*	Not stated	Digoxin vs xamoterol vs placebo	0.25 (mean 1.12 nmol/L, time not stated)	No	0	Not applicable
[24] (1988)	Cross-over	28	Stated	Digoxin vs placebo	Mean 0.391 (1.75 nmol/L, 24-hour level)	No	8/28 (29)	Yes
[33] (1983)	Cross-over	22	Not stated	Digoxin vs placebo	"Regular" dose (mean 1.54 nmol/L, >6-hour level)	No	0	Not applicable
[32] (1982)	Cross-over	40	Stated	Digoxin vs placebo	Mean 0.24 (1.79 nmol/L, >6-hour level)	No	10/40 (25)	Yes
[34] (1982)	Cross-over	35	Stated	Digoxin vs placebo	Mean 0.435 (mean 1.46 nmol/L, 24-hour level)	No	10/35 (29)	Yes

vs = versus.
* For digoxin and placebo groups only.

Metalazone

Kiyingi and associates[27] from Sydney, Australia, treated 17 patients with New York Heart Association Class IV CHF refractory to conventional treatment with oral metolazone (1.25–10 mg daily), a potent quinazoline sulphonamide diuretic: 12 improved sufficiently to be discharged from the hospital with a mean weight loss of 8.3 kg, 1 of whom died at home 4 weeks later. The other 5 patients were treated with intravenous dobutamine for 72 hours: 2 responded (average weight loss 4.4 kg) and 2 responded to subsequent reintroduction of metolazone. Four of these 5 patients died, 2 in hospital of AMI. Overall, 15 patients with very severe refractory CHF improved sufficiently to be discharged from hospital. Treatment was associated with mild transient hypokalaemia in 7 patients, and hyponatremia and renal impairment in 1, for whom metolazone dosage had to be reduced. Failure to respond to the introduction of metolazone may indicate an especially poor prognosis.

Review of angiotensin-converting enzyme inhibitors

An excellent review of the usefulness of angiotensin converting enzyme inhibitors in patients with CHF was written by Prakash C. Deedwania[28] from Fresno, California, in the *Archives of Internal Medicine*, September 1990.

Captopril or enalapril

Osterziel and associates[29] from Heidelberg, West Germany, investigated the deranged autonomic control of heart rate in 34 patients with CHF (New York Heart Association functional class II to III) by examining the carotid sinus baroreflex. The carotid sinus baroreceptors were stimulated by graded suction. The slope of the regression line between increases in cycle length and the degree of neck suction was taken as an index of baroreflex sensitivity. The reflex response is mediated by a selective increase of vagal efferent activity. Baroreflex sensitivity therefore represents a measure of vagal reactivity. Using multiple regression analysis, baroreflex sensitivity correlated positively to stroke volume index and inversely to plasma renin activity and to age. In addition to digitalis and diuretics, angiotensin-converting enzyme inhibitors (captopril or enalapril) were given to 16 patients for a mean of 17 ± 3 days. The patients with hemodynamic improvement (group A) exhibited improved baroreflex sensitivity (1.4 ± 0.4 to 3.6 ± 1.2 msec/mm Hg). Baroreflex sensitivity remained unchanged in the patients without hemodynamic improvement (group B). The increase in reflex sensitivity did not correlate with hemodynamic alterations. Baroreflex sensitivity during angiotensin converting enzyme inhibition was only related to the baseline baroreflex sensitivity. In patients with CHF, reflex bradycardia decreases with age and with plasma renin activity and increases with stroke volume. Chronic therapy with angiotensin converting enzyme inhibitors enhances vagal reactivity in patients with hemodynamic improvement.

Enalapril

There is a varying hormonal activation in CHF. To be able to evaluate this activation and relate it to prognosis, Swedberg and co-workers[30] in Gothenburg, Sweden, took blood samples at baseline and after 6 weeks from 239 patients with severe CHF (all in New York Heart Association class IV) randomized to additional treatment with enalapril or placebo. In this study which has previously been reported, there was a significant reduction in mortality among patients treated with enalapril. The present data show in the placebo group a significant positive relation between mortality and levels of angiotensin II, aldosterone, noradrenaline, adrenaline, and atrial natriuretic factor. A similar relation was not observed among the patients treated with enalapril. Significant reductions in mortality in the groups of patients treated with enalapril were consistently found among patients with baseline hormone levels above median values. There were significant reductions in hormone levels from baseline to 6 weeks in the group of patients treated with enalapril for all hormones except adrenaline. There were no correlations between these changes in hormone levels. Summarily, there was a pronounced but variable neurohormonal activation in CHF even in patients with similar clinical findings. This activation was reduced by enalapril therapy. The results suggest that the effect of enalapril on mortality is related to hormonal activation in general and the renin-angiotensin system in particular.

Nifedipine vs isosorbide dinitrate

Elkayam and colleagues[31] in Los Angeles, California, performed a prospective, randomized, double-blind, crossover study to compare the efficacy and safety of vasodilation with nifedipine with that of isosorbine dinitrate and their combination as treatment for CHF. Twenty-eight patients with New York Heart Association Functional class II or III chronic CHF due to LV systolic dysfunction were studied. All patients were maintained on a constant dose of digitalis and diuretics throughout the study. Eight weeks of therapy with nifedipine alone or in combination with isosorbide dinitrate resulted in a significantly higher incidence of CHF deterioration necessitating hospitalizations and/or additional diuretics. Twenty-four percent of patients required hospitalization during nifedipine therapy and 26% required hospitalization during nifedipine/isosorbide dinitrate combination therapy in comparison to 0% requiring hospitalization during isosorbide dinitrate therapy alone. The total number of CHF worsening episodes was 9 among patients on nifedipine, 3 among patients on isosorbide dinitrate, and 21 among patients on nifedipine/isosorbide dinitrate combination. A comparison of 8 patients who had clinical deterioration on nifedipine with the remainder of the patients demonstrated no significant difference in LVEF, or maximal oxygen uptake during exercise. Treadmill exercise time demonstrated a comparable improvement on all three drug requirements 2 and 4 hours after drug administration. The investigators concluded that the administration of nifedipine alone or in combination with isosorbide dinitrate in patients with CHF due to LV systolic dysfunction who demonstrate relative stability during isosorbide dinitrate therapy results in frequent clinical deterioration necessitating treatment. Worsening CHF can not be predicted by resting LVEF or functional capacity as measured by maximal oxygen uptake. These findings demonstrate the potential hazard associated with the use of nifedipine for vasodilation in patients with mild to moderate CHF due to LV systolic dysfunction.

Nitroglycerin

To determine whether a 72-hour infusion of nitroglycerin produces hemodynamic improvement in patients with severe CHF and to assess

the contributing role of various possible causes of hemodynamic tolerance to nitroglycerin, 19 patients received an infusion of nitroglycerin 1.5
μg/kg/min for 72 hours in a study reported by Dupuis and associates[32]
from Montreal, Canada. In a subgroup of patients (n = 10), there was an
increase in stroke work index and a decrease in ventricular filling pressures throughout the infusion and even after it was discontinued. Tolerance to the hemodynamic effects of nitroglycerin was partially reversed
8 hours after the infusion was stopped. Neurohumoral changes occurred
but appeared to play only a minor role in the development of nitroglycerin
tolerance. The hematocrit fell 9 ± 5%, which suggests that an increased
intravascular volume contributed to tolerance. In summary: 1) a 72-hour
infusion of nitroglycerin improves ventricular function in some patients
with severe CHF; 2) volume shifts from the extravascular to the intravascular compartments may, at least in part, be responsible for nitroglycerin
tolerance; and 3) reflex neurohumoral activation may also play a small
role in nitrate tolerance.

Bucindolol

The hemodynamic effects of β-adrenergic blockade with bucindolol,
a nonselective β-antagonist with mild vasodilatory properties, were studied by Eichhorn and colleagues[33] in Dallas, Texas, in patients with CHF.
Fifteen patients underwent cardiac catheterization before and after 3
months of oral therapy with bucindolol. The LVEF increased from 0.23
to 0.29, and end-systolic elastance, a relatively load-independent determinant of contractility, also increased. Both LV stroke work index and
minute work increased despite reductions in LV end-diastolic pressure.
These data demonstrate improvements in myocardial contractility after
beta-adrenergic blockade with bucindolol. At a matched heart rate of 98
beats per minute, the time constant of LV isovolumic relaxation was
significantly reduced by bucindolol therapy, and the relation of the time
constant to end-systolic pressure was shifted downward with therapy.
These data suggest that chronic beta-adrenergic blockade with bucindolol improves diastolic relaxation but does not alter myocardial chamber
stiffness. Myocardial oxygen extraction, consumption, and efficiency were
unchanged despite improvements in contractile function and mechanical work. Thus, in patients with CHF, chronic beta-adrenergic blockade
with bucindolol significantly improves myocardial contractility and minute work, yet it does not do so at the expense of myocardial oxygen
consumption. Additionally, bucindolol improves myocardial relaxation
but does not affect chamber stiffness.

The sympathetic hyperactivity of CHF may worsen cardiovascular
function by down-regulation of myocardial β-receptors. For this reason,
β blockade is proposed to be useful in CHF. Bucindolol is a new β-blocker
that has intrinsic nonadrenergically-mediated vasodilation and may be
valuable in the treatment of CHF. To test this hypothesis, Pollock and
associates[34] from Charlottesville, Virginia, randomized 19 patients with
CHF in a double-blind protocol to 3 months of treatment with bucindolol
(n = 12) or placebo (n = 7). Significant improvement was seen in the
bucindolol group using invasive and noninvasive tests; treadmill time
increased from 445 to 530 seconds, Minnesota Living With Heart Failure
Questionnaire score improved from 61 to 40, cardiac output increased
from 4.0 to 4.7, and systemic vascular resistance decreased from 1,888 to
1,481. Also, peak exercise heart rate and pulmonary capillary wedge pressure decreased significantly with treatment. There were no changes in

the placebo group. The authors concluded that bucindolol may be an effective treatment for CHF when administered chronically and that its non-adrenergic vasodilation may be an important feature.

Xamoterol

The Xamoterol in Severe Heart Failure Study Group[35] from Stockholm, Sweden, randomized 516 patients with New York Heart Association Class III or IV CHF despite treatment with diuretics and angiotensin converting enzyme inhibitors in a double-blind between-group comparison to xamoterol 200 mg (352 patients) or placebo (164 patients) twice daily for 13 weeks. There was no difference between the treatments in loss of clinical signs. Visual analogue scale and Likert scores indicated that breathlessness was less severe with xamoterol, but there was no difference in exercise duration or total work done. Xamoterol reduced maximum exercise heart rate and systolic BP, did not affect the number of VPCs after exercise, showed no arrhythmogenic activity, and had variable (agonist and antagonist) effects on 24 hour heart rate. On intention-to-treat analysis 32 (9.1%) patients in the xamoterol group and 6 (3.7%) patients in the placebo group died within 100 days of randomization.

Enoximone

Uretsky and co-investigators[36] in Pittsburgh, Pennsylvania, in the enoximone multicenter trial group conducted a double-blind, randomized, placebo-controlled trial of oral enoximone, a phosphodiesterase inhibitor, in 102 out-patients (50 receiving enoximone and 52 receiving placebo) with moderate to moderately severe congestive heart failure. All were on a long-term regimen of digoxin and diuretics with vasodilators and converting enzyme inhibitors. Symptom score was obtained, and exercise testing was performed monthly for 4 months. There were no differences between groups in symptoms or exercise duration at the end of 4 months. A subgroup undergoing analysis of oxygen consumption with measurement of anaerobic threshold during exercise showed an increase in anaerobic threshold at 1 month with enoximone compared with placebo. This improvement was not sustained at 4 months. The dropout rate was significantly higher with enoximone than with placebo. Adverse effects other than death were slightly, but not significantly, higher with enoximone than with placebo. During therapy, 5 deaths occurred in the enoximone group, and none occurred in the placebo group. Two deaths were sudden, 2 were from progressive CHF, and one was from AMI. With intention-to-treat analysis and inclusion of patients who were removed from therapy because of lack of drug study effect, 10 deaths occurred in the enoximone group, and three occurred in the placebo group. All five enoximone and three placebo-treated patients who died after therapy was discontinued died from terminal CHF. This study does not demonstrate improvement in exercise capacity or symptoms with 16 weeks of enoximone therapy compared with placebo in patients with CHF receiving digoxin and diuretics without vasodilators and does not provide evidence that enoximone is beneficial in the long-term therapy of chronic CHF. The unexpectedly worse survival rate with enoximone therapy raises concerns about a possible detrimental effect of enoximone in the dose range given in this study.

Procainamide vs tocainide vs encainide

Many newer antiarrhythmic agents are said to cause minimal myocardial depression, but their hemodynamic effects have not been invasively evaluated and compared in patients with severe chronic heart failure. In a randomized crossover study, Gottlieb and co-workers[37] in New York, New York compared the hemodynamic responses to single oral doses of procainamide (750 mg), tocainide (600 mg), and encainide (50 mg) given to 21 patients with severe chronic CHF. Cardiac performance decreased with all three drugs, but the magnitude of deterioration differed among the three agents. Stroke volume index decreased with procainamide, tocainide and encainide, but the decline was significantly greater with encainide than with procainamide. Similarly, LV filling pressure increased with tocainide and encainide, but not with procainamide; the increase was significantly greater with tocainide and encainide than with procainamide. These deleterious hemodynamic effects were accompanied by worsening symptoms of CHF in 6 patients with encainide and 7 patients with tocainide but in only 2 patients with procainamide. Serum levels for all drugs were in the therapeutic range. In conclusion, although the 3 type I antiarrhythmic agents tested may all adversely affect LV function in patients with CHF, encainide and tocainide are more likely than procainamide to cause hypodynamic and clinical deterioration.

Moricizine

Patients with VPCs and CHF have an increased risk of sudden death, yet suppression of arrhythmia in this population is frequently complicated by proarrhythmia and by the negative inotropic effects of antiarrhythmic drugs. Pratt and associates[38] from Houston, Texas, and Boston, Massachusetts, evaluated the safety and efficacy of moricizine in patients with clinical CHF. The New Drug Application data base submitted to the Food and Drug Administration was analyzed. A total of 908 patients were treated with moricizine for ventricular arrhythmias; CHF developed in 49 of them (5.4%). Of the 908 patients, 374 had a history of CHF, 326 of whom tolerated moricizine for a mean of 97 ± 217 days. New-onset CHF occurred only once ($\frac{1}{546} = 0.2\%$). Recurrence or exacerbation of clinical CHF during treatment with moricizine occurred in 48 of 374 patients (13%), 28 of whom continued treatment with alteration in CHF therapy. The mean LVEF of those patients in whom CHF developed was 26%. It is important to note that patients with a history of CHF were as likely to have suppression of VPCs (defined as ≥75% reduction) as those without a history of CHF. In fact, suppression of arrhythmia was achieved as often in patients with LVEF <30% as in those with more preserved LVEF. Of the 374 patients with a history of CHF, 15 (4%) had a proarrhythmic event within 14 days of therapy. The incidence of sudden cardiac death in this group was 0.8%. These proarrhythmia rates compare favorably with those of other antiarrhythmic drugs. In conclusion, morcizine has a good safety profile and appears to be well tolerated in patients with mild CHF, in whom suppression of VPCs is often achieved.

References

1. Massie BM, Packer M: Congestive heart failure: Current controversies and future prospects. Am J Cardiol 1990 (Aug 15);66:429–430.

2. Ferrick KJ, Fein SA, Ferrick AM, Doyle JT: Effect of milrinone on ventricular arrhythmias in congestive heart failure. Am J Cardiol 1990 (Aug 15);66:431–434.

3. Kulick DL, Rahimtoola SH: Vasodilators have not been shown to be of value in all patients with chronic congestive heart failure due to left ventricular systolic dysfunction. Am J Cardiol 1990 (Aug 15);66:435–438.

4. Massie BM: All patients with left ventricular systolic dysfunction should be treated with an angiotensin-converting enzyme inhibitor: A protagonist's viewpoint. Am J Cardiol 1990 (Aug. 15);66:439–443.

5. Cohn JN: Nitrates are effective in the treatment of chronic congestive heart failure: The protagonist's view. Am J Cardiol 1990 (Aug 15);66:444–446.

6. Anderson JL: Should complex ventricular arrhythmias in patients with congestive heart failure be treated? A protagonist's viewpoint. Am J Cardiol 1990 (Aug 15);66:447–450.

7. Podrid PJ, Wilson JS: Should asymptomatic ventricular arrhythmia in patients with congestive heart failure be treated? An antagonist's viewpoint. Am J Cardiol 1990 (Aug 15);66:451–457.

8. Packer M: Are nitrates effective in the treatment of chronic heart failure? Antagonist's viewpoint. Am J Cardiol 1990 (Aug 15);66:458–461.

9. Poole-Wilson PA: Future perspectives in the management of congestive heart failure. Am J Cardiol 1990 (Aug 15);66:462–467.

10. Katz Am: Future perspectives in basic science understanding of congestive heart failure. Am J Cardiol 1990 (Aug 15);66:468–471.

11. Ghali JK, Cooper R, Ford E: Trends in hospitalization rates for heart failure in the United States, 1973–1986. Arch Intern Med 1990 (April);150:769–773.

12. Francis GS, Johnson TH, Ziesche S, Berg M, Boosalis P, Cohn JN: Marked spontaneous improvement in ejection fraction in patients with congestive heart failure. Am J Med 1990 (Sept);89:303–307.

13. Roubin GS, Anderson SD, Shen WF, Cloog CYP, Alwyn M, HIllery S, Harris PJ, Kelly DT: Hemodynamic and metabolic basis of impaired exercise tolerance in patients with severe left ventricular dysfunction. J Am Coll Cardiol 1990 (April);15:986–94.

14. Keogh AM, Baron DW, Hickie JB: Prognostic guides in patients with idiopathic or is-chemic dilated cardiomyopathy assessed for cardiac transplantation. Am J Cardiol 1990 (Apr 1);65:903–908.

15. Kelly TL, Cremo R, Nielsen C, Shabetai R: Prediction of outcome in late-stage cardio-myopathy. Am Heart J 1990 (May);119:1111–1121.

16. Pye M, Rae AP, Cobbe SM: Study of serum C-reactive protein concentration in cardiac failure. Br Heart J 1990 (Apr);63:228–230.

17. Gottlieb SS, Baruch L, Kukin ML, Bernstein JL, Fisher ML, Packer M: Prognostic impor-tance of the serum magnesium concentration in patients with congestive heart failure. J Am Coll Cardiol 1990 (October);16:827–31.

18. Middlekauff HR, Stevenson WG, Woo MA, Moser DK, Stevenson LW: Comparison of frequency of late potentials in idiopathic dilated cardiomyopathy and ischemic car-diomyopathy with advanced congestive heart failure and their usefulness in pre-dicting sudden death. Am J Cardiol 1990 (Nov 1);66:1113–1117.

19. Vasiljevic JD, Kanjuh V, Seferovic P, Sesto M, Stojsic D, Olsen EGJ: The incidence of myocarditis in endomyocardial biopsy samples from patients with congestive heart failure. Am Heart J 1990 (December);120:1370–1377.

20. Port JD, Gilbert EM, Larrabee P, Mealey P, Volkman K, Ginsburg R, Hershberger RE, Murray J, Bristow MR: Neurotransmitter depletion compromises the ability of in-direct-acting amines to provide inotropic support in the failing human heart. Cir-culation 1990 (March);81:929–938.

21. Francis GS, Benedict C, Johnstone DE, Kirlin PC, Nicklas J, Liang C, Kubo SH, Toretsky Yusuf S, for the SOLVD Investigators: Comparison of Neuroendocrine Activation in Patients with Left Ventricular Dysfunction With and Without Congestive Heart Fail-ure. Circulation 1990 (November);82:1724–1729.

22. Sullivan MJ, Green HJ, Cobb FR: Skeletal muscle biochemistry and histology in ambu-latory patients with long-term heart failure. Circulation 1990 (February);81:518–527.

23. Levine B, Kalman J, Mayer L, Fillit HM, Packer M: Elevated circulating levels of tumor necrosis factor in severe chronic heart failure. N Engl J Med 1990 (July 26);323:236–241.

24. Anand IS, Malhotra RM, Chandrashekhar Y, Bali HK, Chauhan SS, Jindal SK, Bhandari RK, Wahi PL: Adult subacute mountainsickness—a syndrome of congestive heart failure in man at very high altitude. Lancet 1990 (Mar 10);335:561–565.

25. Coats AJS, Adamopoulos S, Meyer TE, Conway J, Sleight P: Effects of physical training in chronic heart failure. Lancet 1990 (Jan 13);335:63–66.

26. Jaeschke R, Oxman AD, Guyatt GH: To what extent do congestive heart failure patients in sinus rhythm benefit from digoxin therapy? A systematic overview and meta-analysis. Am J Med 1990 (Mar);88:279–286.

27. Kiyingi A, Field MJ, Pawsey CC, Yiannikas J, Lawrence JR, Arter WJ: Metolazone in treatment of severe refractory congestive cardiac failure. Lancet 1990 (Jan 6);335:29–31.

28. Deedwania PC: Angiotensin-converting enzyme inhibitors in congestive heart failure. Arch Intern Med 1990 (Sept);150:1798–1805.

29. Osterziel KJ, Dietz R, Schmid W, Mikulaschek K, Manthey J, Kubler W: ACE inhibition improves vagal reactivity in patients with heart failure. Am Heart J 1990 (November);120:1120–1129.

30. Swedberg K, Eneroth, Kjekshus, Wilhelmsen, for the CONSENSUS Trial Study Group: Hormones Regulating Cardiovascular Function in Patients with Severe Congestive Heart Failure and Their Relation to Mortality. Circulation 1990 (November);82:1730–1736.

31. Elkayam U, Amin J, Mehra A, Vasquez J, Weber L, Rahimtoola SH: A Prospective, Randomized, Double-Blind, Crossover Study to Compare the Efficacy and Safety of Chronic Nifedipine Therapy With That of Isosorbide Dinitrate and Their Combination in the Treatment of Chronic Congestive Heart Failure. Circulation 1990 (December);82:1954–1961.

32. Dupuis J, Lalonde G, Lebeau R, Bichet D, Rouleau JL: Sustained beneficial effect of a seventy-two hour intravenous infusion of nitroglycerin in patients with severe chronic congestive heart failure. Am Heart J 1990 (September);120:625–637.

33. Eichhorn EJ, Bedotto JB, Malloy CR, Hatfield BA, Deitchman D, Brown Marilyn, Willard JE, Grayburn PA: Effect of B-Adrenergic Blockade on Myocardial Function and Energetics in Congestive Heart Failure Improvements in Hemodynamic, Contractile, and Diastolic Performance with Bucindolol. Circulation 1990 (August);82:473–483.

34. Pollock SG, Lystash J, Tedesco C, Craddock G, Smicker ML: Usefulness of bucindolol in congestive heart failure. Am J Cardiol 1990 (Sept 1);66:603–607.

35. Xamoterol in Severe Heart Failure Study Group: Xamoterol in severe heart failure. Lancet, 1990 (July 7);336:1–6.

36. Uretsky BF, Jessup M, Konstam MA, Dec GW, Leier CV, Benotti J, Murali S, Herrmann HC, Sandberg JA, for the Enoximone Multicenter Trial Group: Multicenter Trual of Oral Enoximone in Patients With Moderate to Moderately Severe Congestive Heart Failure Lack of Benefit Compared With Placebo. Circulation 1990 (September);82:774–780.

37. Gottlieb SS, Kukin ML, Medina N, Yushak M, Packer M: Comparative hemodynamic effects of procainamide, tocainide, and encainide in severe chronic heart failure. Circulation 1990 (March);81:860–864.

38. Pratt CM, Podrid P, Greatrix B, Borland RM, Mahler S: Efficacy and safety of moricizine in patients with congestive heart failure: A summary of the experience in the United States. Am Heart J 1990 (January);119:1–7.

Miscellaneous Topics

In hypothyroidism

Pericardial effusion is reported to occur in 30% to 80% of individuals with hypothyroidism. These earlier studies were conducted when the diagnosis of hypothyroidism was only suspected and was confirmed only in the presence of classic clinical features. In contrast, the diagnosis has recently been established in the early mild stage or more often in an asymptomatic stage because of more frequent or routine determinations of thyroid function tests, especially in the elderly. Thus the individuals in the older studies were severely hypothyroid at the time of diagnosis and may not be representative of the present hypothyroid population. For this reason, 30 individuals with hypothyroidism were evaluated with echocardiography to reassess the evidence of pericardial effusion in this disorder in this report by Kabadi and Kumar[1] from Phoenix and Tucson, Arizona, and Des Moines and Iowa City, Iowa. Only 2 individuals had pericardial effusion, and in only 1 of them with severe disease could the pericardial effusion be attributed to hypothyroidism, since it resolved on the patient's attaining the euthyroid state. Thus the incidence of pericardial effusion was only 3% to 6%, depending on the inclusion of 1 or both individuals, an extremely infrequent occurrence when compared with that of previous studies. Moreover, the occurrence of pericardial effusion in hypothyroidism appears to be dependent on the severity of the disease. Thus pericardial effusion may be a frequent manifestation in myxedema, an advanced severe stage, as previously found, but a rare association of hypothyroidism, an early mild stage, because of the timeliness with which the latter condition is nowadays detected.

In rheumatoid arthritis

Hara and associates[2] from Rochester, Minnesota, described clinical characteristics and actuarial survival of a consecutive cohort of 41 patients with rheumatoid arthritis and clinical pericarditis seen at their clinic from 1970 to 1987 and followed until death or through 1987. The survivors were followed up for a median of 5.1 years. Approximately three-fourths of the patients had acute pericarditis, the remainder having recurrent acute pericarditis, chronic pericarditis with effusion, or chronic constrictive pericarditis. Most patients had symmetrical joint swelling, morning stiffness, subcutaneous nodules, rheumatoid factor, and classic radiographic changes of rheumatoid arthritis. Common extra-articular features included fatigue, loss of weight, and fever. Dyspnea or orthopnea, typical pericardial pain, peripheral edema, tachycardia, tachypnea, a diminished mean BP, a pericardial friction rub, jugular venous distention, rales, radiographic evidence of cardiomegaly and pleural effusions, and abnormal echocardiograms were the most common cardiac manifestations. An elevated erythrocyte sedimentation rate and anemia were other common laboratory findings. The cohort demonstrated decreased survival in comparison with an age- and sex-matched North Central white population (from the upper midwestern USA), especially during the first year after diagnosis. Increasing age, the presence of other heart disease, an increasing total number of other extra-articular manifestations of rheumatoid arthritis, jugular venous distention, and a lower mean BP were associated with decreased survival.

Postpericardiotomy syndrome

Although the postpericardiotomy syndrome is a common complication of cardiac operations, the most effective drug regimen for the treatment of this condition has not been established. Horneffer and associates[3] from Baltimore, Maryland, designed a study to evaluate the effectiveness of nonsteroidal antiinflammatory drugs (NSAIDs) in the treatment of postpericardiotomy syndrome, in a double-blind, placebo-controlled randomized trial with a 10-day course of ibuprofen or indomethacin. Of 1019 adult patients undergoing cardiac operations during a 14-month period, a diagnosis of postpericardiotomy syndrome was made in 187, and 149 were enrolled in the study. Diagnosis was based on the presence of at least 2 of the following: fever, anterior chest pain, and friction rub. Drug efficacy was defined as the resolution of at least two of these criteria within 48 hours of drug initiation. Ibuprofen and indomethacin were 90% and 89% effective, respectively, and both were significantly more effective than placebo (62.5%). The occurrence of side effects, including nausea, vomiting, renal failure, and fluid retention, was low in all groups (13% for ibuprofen, 16% for indomethacin, and 17% for placebo). Length of hospital stay, incidence of ischemic events, and accumulation of significant pericardial effusions were similar in all groups. The results of this study demonstrate that both ibuprofen and indomethacin provide safe and effective symptomatic treatment for postpericardiotomy syndrome.

Colchicine therapy

Recurrence is one of the major complications of pericarditis. Treatment of recurrence is often difficult, and immunosuppressive drugs or surgery may be necessary. Guindo and co-workers[4] in Barcelona, Spain, conducted an open-label prospective study of nine patients treated with colchicine (1 mg/day) to prevent recurrences. All patients had suffered at least 3 relapses despite treatment with acetylsalicylic acid, indomethacin, prednisone, or a combination. Pericarditis was classified as idiopathic in 5 patients, postpericardiotomy in 2, post-myocardian infarction in 1, and associated with systemic lupus erythematosus in 1. For statistical analysis, investigators conducted a paired comparison design. All patients treated with colchicine responded favorably to therapy. Prednisone was discontinued in all patients after 2–6 weeks and colchicine alone was continued. After a mean follow-up of 24 months, no recurrences were observed in any patient; there was a significant difference between the symptom-free periods before and after treatment with colchicine. This study suggests that colchicine may be useful in avoiding recurrence of pericarditis, although these results need to be confirmed in a larger, double-blind study.

Tamponade after endomyocardial biopsy

Craven and associates[5] from Salt Lake City, Utah, described 3 patients who had perforation of the RV wall and fatal cardiac tamponade following endocardial biopsy to evaluate CHF. The number of endocardial biopsies at this institution at the time of the third death was 2,372, resulting in an overall mortality rate of 0.13%. Of the 2,372 biopsies, 2,136 (90%) were performed to evaluate cardiac graft rejection and 236 (10%) were performed for other reasons. All the patients who died belonged to the latter group. None of the cardiac transplant patients have had fatal ventricular perforation—a significant difference. At our institution, the frequency of mortality following endocardial biopsy in the noncardiac transplant patients is 1.3%. Patients who have ventricular endocardial biopsy of native hearts rather than transplanted hearts may be at increased risk for fatal perforation.

KAWASAKI DISEASE

Pahl and associates[6] from Pittsburgh, Pennsylvania, performed cardiac catheterization and coronary arteriography in 29 patients with Kawasaki disease suspected of having coronary artery abnormalities because of echocardiographic abnormalities, CHF, prolonged fever, or cardiac arrest. Angiographically documented coronary artery abnormalities were present in 22 of 26, with 19 having right and 20 left coronary artery involvement. The majority had diffuse involvement of both vessels. Clearance of contrast media from the coronary arteries was significantly prolonged in patients with coronary aneurysms as compared with the control group. In 15 patients who underwent follow-up catheterization 6 months to 7 years after initial study, complete resolution was observed in only 37% of affected coronary artery resegment. In 4 patients, 3 of whom were asymptomatic, severe stenotic or occluded coronary segments were found on elective catheterization and coronary artery bypass surgery was performed in 2 of these patients. Echocardiography did not detect any of these stenoses. Echocardiography is the most important modality for initial diagnosis and serial evaluation. These authors make a strong case for angiographic assessment in patients with suspected coronary artery abnormality. In this study only 33% of patients with coronary aneurysms had complete resolution in comparison to the previous data suggesting 50% of patients will resolve aneurysms. Angiography is an essential tool and should be used in conjunction with noninvasive methods to determine the presence or progression of coronary artery obstructive lesions after the diagnosis of Kawasaki disease has been made.

Niwa and associates[7] from Chiba, Japan, performed magnetic resonance imaging in patients with Kawasaki disease following AMI to assess the usefulness of the technique in detecting myocardial infarction and coronary artery lesions. In 6 patients (group A), the interval after AMI was from 7 days to 7 months, and in 5 patients (group B) it was from 1 to 4 years. Imaging was performed with a superconducting magnet with spin-echo sequence and electrocardiographic-gated multiple slices of 5 mm thickness. Myocardial signals were increased in group A, and the region of high signal intensity corresponded to the site of AMI. The signal intensity within the myocardium was homogenous in 5 patients in group B. Coronary arteries were visualized in 20 of 22 instances. Signals within the coronary artery were observed in all 14 instances with poor contrast runoff from the coronary aneurysm, and 11 of these vessels showed high signal intensity. In all 6 instances in which large aneurysms with severe stenosis were present, signals in the coronary artery were increased. In contrast, high signal intensity in the coronary artery was not observed in 5 of 6 instances with good contrast runoff. Signals in the coronary arterial cavity and high signal intensity in the coronary artery persisted in 5 of 6 instances with turbulent coronary flow. The findings of increased coronary arterial signals suggested stagnant blood flow in the coronary aneurysm. In conclusion, magnetic resonance imaging was a useful modality for assessment of myocardial infarcts and coronary artery lesions in Kawasaki disease.

To elucidate the incidence and natural history of valvular heart disease in Kawasaki syndrome, Akagi and associates[8] from Kurume and Omura, Japan, analyzed patients who were found to have a new heart murmur after the onset of the disease. Among 1215 patients they found 13 (1.1%) with valvular disease (12 with MR and 1 with AR). These patients were compared to 30 who did not have valvular lesions. The duration of fever was longer and the incidence of coronary artery lesions significantly higher than in those without valvular disease. Heart murmurs disappeared within 2 months after the onset of valvular heart disease in 5 patients, whereas in another 6, all involving valve prolapse, they persisted for ≥2 years. It was postulated that 2 different mechanisms may be responsible for the variation in the duration of valvular heart disease: one, which disappeared spontaneously, was attributed to pancarditis; the other, which persisted, was due to dysfunction in valve and papillary muscles as a result of ischemia.

TRANSESOPHAGEAL ECHOCARDIOGRAPHY

Seward and associates[9] from Rochester, Minnesota, described their initial investigation of wide-field ultrasonic cardio-thoracic tomography utilizing a transesophageal transducer. Examination included manual rotation of an esophageal transducer 180 to 360 degrees to visualize contiguous related structures. The photographs they produced in their manuscript are absolutely magnificent and assuming that they are representative indicate that wide-field transesophageal cardiothoracic ultrasound tomography holds promise for excellent demonstration of cardiothoracic and mediastinal anatomy.

Transesophageal echocardiography is a rapidly expanding diagnostic procedure. Conventional transesophageal endoscopes allow imaging from a single array mounted in the horizontal plane. Seward and associates[10] from Rochester, Minnesota, introduced the clinical application of biplanar imaging, which incorporates a second orthogonal longitudinal plane. Their clinical experience with 291 patients who underwent biplanar transesophageal echocardiography was described, and the examination, technique, and result of anatomic correlations unique to this new examination were discussed and illustrated (Figures 10-1–10-5). They concluded that biplanar imaging adds substantially to the comprehensive anatomic delineation of certain cardiac structures.

Stumper and associates[11] from Rotterdam, The Netherlands, performed transesophageal echocardiographic imaging in the longitudinal axis and found that the technique provided unique images of intracardiac anatomy, although their interpretation remains difficult. A heart specimen was cut according to the echocardiographic imaging planes to elucidate the morphologic details (Figure 10-6). These results suggested that longitudinal transesophageal imaging complements the transverse axis approach. It gave new imaging information on the RV outflow tract and the pulmonary trunk, the AV valves, the ventricular septum, the cardiac apex, and the thoracic aorta. In particular, it showed the entire length of the RV outflow tract. When longitudinal imaging was used in combination with transverse imaging almost all the thoracic aorta could be examined. Imaging in the longitudinal axis may also allow better assessment of the mechanisms of atrioventricular valve regurgitation.

Pearson and associates[12] from St. Louis, Missouri, studied the safety and utility of transesophageal echocardiography in the evaluation of critically ill patients in the intensive care unit setting. Sixty-two studies were performed in 4 different intensive care units on 61 patients with a mean age of 58 ± 14 years (range 25 to 78 years). Indications for the study included suspected aortic pathologic conditions (18 patients), cardiac source of embolus (16 patients), postmyocardial infarction complications

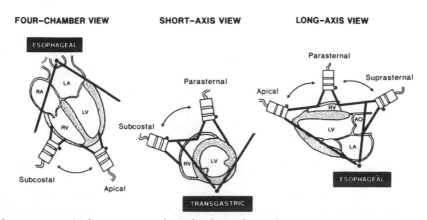

Fig. 10-1. For biplanar transesophageal echocardiography, image orientation conforms to conventions used in precordial two-dimensional echocardiographic presentations. Frontal or four-chamber views are displayed with cardiac apex or anterior structures at bottom of image, posterior or basal structures at top, right heart structures to the left, and left heart chambers to the right. Short-axis views are displayed with posterior structures at bottom, anterior structures at top, and left heart structures to viewer's right. Long-axis views (sagittal or longitudinal images) are displayed with basal structures to the right, apical structures to the left, anterior structures at top, and posterior structures at bottom of image. AO = aorta; LA = left atrium; LV = left ventricle; RA = right atrium; RV = right ventricle. (Modified from Henry and colleagues. By permission of The American Heart Association, Inc.) Reproduced with permission from Seward, et al.[10]

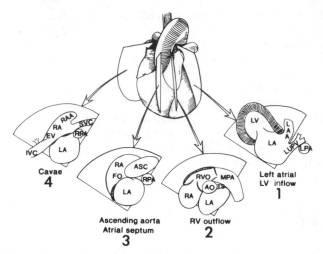

Fig. 10-2. Primary longitudinal views in biplanar transesophageal echocardiography. With top of endoscope in neutral long-axis orientation within esophagus, four views are obtained by rotation of scope from left side toward right side of heart. Sequentially imaged structures in sagittal plane (from right to left in illustration) are left ventricular-left atrial two-chamber view (section 1), right ventricular outflow long-axis view (section 2), ascending aorta-atrial septal view (section 3), and caval, right atrial, and atrial septal view (section 4). AO = aorta; ASC = ascending aorta; EV = eustachian valve; FO = fossa ovalis; IVC = inferior vena cava; LA = left atrium; LAA = left atrial appendage; LPA = left pulmonary artery; LUPV = left upper pulmonary vein; LV = left ventricle; MPA = main pulmonary artery; RA = right atrium; RAA = right atrial appendage; RPA = right pulmonary artery; RV = right ventricle; RVO = right ventricular outflow; SVC = superior vena cava; TS = transverse sinus. Reproduced with permission from Seward, et al.[10]

(6 patients), and suspected infective endocarditis (5 patients). Studies were performed at bedside with the use of small amounts of intravenous sedatives. The probe was passed successfully in 61 of 62 attempts. Diagnoses that were missed by surface echocardiography, including aortic dissection, LA thrombus, ruptured papillary muscle, and prosthetic valve vegetation were clearly identified by transesophageal echocardiography, which facilitated appropriate management in these cases. In cases in which no pathologic condition was identified, transesophageal echocardiography was useful in ruling out intracardiac shunt, in assessing LV function, and in excluding significant valvular pathologic conditions. No serious complications were recorded, and the procedure was, in general, very well tolerated.

The capability of transesophageal versus transthoracic echocardiography as a diagnostic tool in clinical practice was prospectively examined in 86 consecutive cases in a report by Pavlides and associates[13] from Royal Oak, Michigan. A conclusive diagnosis was possible in 95% with transesophageal, whereas the same result was achieved in 48% by transthoracic echocardiography. Specifically, transesophageal echocardiography provided a conclusive diagnosis in 14 of 16 cases of infective endocarditis, while transthoracic gave this result in 4 of the 16 cases. Similarly, transesophageal echocardiography allowed a conclusive diagnosis in 11 of 11 instances of aortic dissection, while transthoracic gave this indication in 2 cases. Transesophageal echocardiography was similarly effective in 8 of 8 cases of atrial thrombi, whereas transthoracic echocardiography gave the diagnosis in 3 of 8 cases. In 5 subjects with intracardiac masses, transesophageal echocardiography gave a conclu-

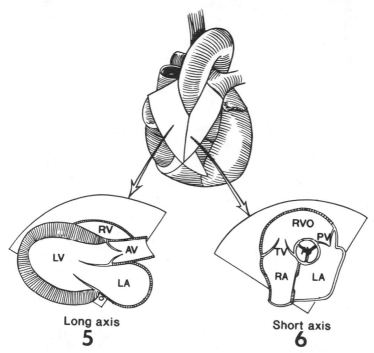

Fig. 10-3. Biplanar transesophageal echocardiographic secondary (off-axis) long- and short-axis views in longitudinal plane. Leftward (lateral) flexion of tip of endoscope reorients longitudinal plane into long-axis view of left ventricle (section 5). Rightward (medial) flexion reorients longitudinal array into short-axis plane relative to aortic valve (section 6). AV = aortic valve; PV = pulmonary valve; TV = tricuspid valve; other abbreviations as in Figure 10-2. Reproduced with permission from Seward, et al.[10]

sive diagnosis in all 5, whereas transthoracic echocardiography was able to diagnose conclusively in only 1 individual. In 7 patients with MR, transesophageal echocardiography gave the conclusive diagnosis in all 7 and transthoracic echocardiography was able to provide this information in 4. Transesophageal echocardiography was able to provide a conclusive diagnosis in 4 patients with AR, and transthoracic echocardiography gave the same information in 2 of the 4. In 14 patients with prosthetic valve dysfunction, transesophageal echocardiography gave the diagnosis in 12 and transthoracic gave it in 8 patients. Both methods gave a conclusive diagnosis in 13 out of 13 cases of MS. Also, transesophageal echocardiography provided a conclusive diagnosis in 8 of 8 patients with adult congenital heart disease and transthoracic gave this information in 4. Transesophageal echocardiography obviated 5 planned cardiac catheterizations, 8 computed tomography scans, and 1 magnetic resonance imaging session; whereas transthoracic echocardiography was only able to obviate 2 cardiac catheterizations. Treatment was altered in 24% of cases by transesophageal echocardiography versus the same result in 10% of cases with transthoracic echocardiography. When it is clinically indicated, transesophageal echocardiography is a powerful diagnostic tool, with a significant impact on patient course and treatment. Nevertheless, transthoracic echocardiography remained efficacious in 48% of this selective group of patients, and the 2 techniques are complementary.

Transesophageal echocardiography provides a unique view of the interatrial septum. Schwinger and associates[14] from New York, New York,

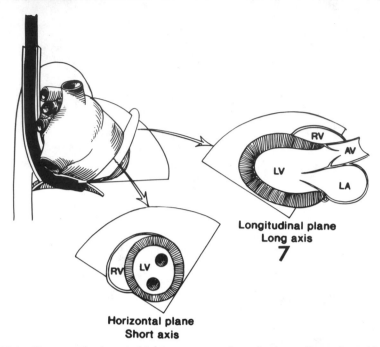

Fig. 10-4. Transgastric views in biplanar transesophageal echocardiography. With tip of endoscope in fundus of stomach, short- and long-axis views of left ventricle can be obtained. Longitudinal plane is oriented to correspond to conventional image orientation with inferoposterior wall at bottom of image, basal structures to the right, apex to the left, and anterior wall at top of image (section 7). Abbreviations as in Figures 10-2 and 10-3. Reproduced with permission from Seward, et al.[10]

reviewed results of 119 transesophageal studies to: 1) study the detailed anatomy of the interatrial septum, 2) to determine the thickness of the interatrial septum at different times during the cardiac cycle, 3) determine the effect of age, and 4) evaluate the thickness of the interatrial septum in relation to various disease states. From the transesophageal view the interatrial septum extends from the right posteriorly toward the left and anteriorly. The more inferior aspect of the septum courses in a more direct posteroanterior direction and is more difficult to accurately visualize. The atrial septum is thickest peripherally and gradually narrows toward the more centrally located fossa ovalis. A region of constant thickness is frequently present between the most peripheral aspect of the interatrial septum and the fossa ovalis. Schwinger and colleagues standardized the measurement of the thickness of the septum by measuring it only at this region of constant thickness in the plane that visualized the fossa ovalis. The mean thickness at this point was 6 ± 2 mm. The thickness correlated weakly with the age of the patient. These results agree with previously published autopsy findings. Thickness was not affected by the presence of significant disease of the AV valves, AF, or an ASD. The thickness increased to 7 ± 2 mm with atrial contraction during sinus rhythm. The mean thickness of the septum primum covering the fossa ovalis was 1.8 ± 0.7 mm. The septum primum was significantly thicker in patients with disease of the AV valves (2.0 ± 0.6 mm) compared to those without significant disease of the AV valves (1.6 ± 0.7 mm). Transesophageal echocardiography allows detailed anatomic study of the interatrial septum. Thickening during atrial systole and alterations

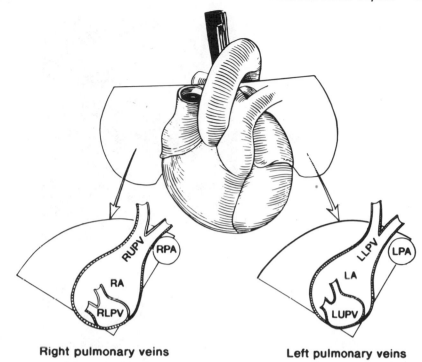

Right pulmonary veins   **Left pulmonary veins**

Fig. 10-5. Diagram illustrating technique of imaging pulmonary veins. By rotating long-axis scan plane leftward, left upper and lower pulmonary veins (LUPV and LLPV) are imaged, whereas far rightward rotation images right upper and lower pulmonary veins (RUPV and RLPV) in longitudinal plane. LA = left atrium; LPA = left pulmonary artery; RA = right atrium; RPA = right pulmonary artery. Reproduced with permission from Seward.[10]

in patients with valvular heart disease can be appreciated. A standardized approach should be used to measure the thickness of the interatrial septum.

Patients with unexplained stroke or other embolic phenomena are often referred for echocardiography. The aortic arch is not usually visualized in detail during routine echocardiography; however, with the introduction of transesophageal echocardiography, this area may be seen with great resolution. Tunick and Kronzon[15] from New York, New York, recently studied 3 patients who had embolic events, and transesophageal echocardiography showed a new and unexpected finding; large, protrusive plaques in the aortic arch and descending aorta, which had mobile projections that moved freely with the blood flow. These lesions could be responsible for embolic syndromes, especially after catheter manipulation in the aorta.

Hofmann and associates[16] from Freiburg and Hamburg, Germany, examined prospectively by transthoracic and transesophageal echocardiography 153 patients aged 16 to 60 years (mean 42) who had arterial embolic events. Patients older than 60 years and those with evidence of extracranial carotid artery occlusive disease were excluded. Eighty-four patients had a cerebral ischemic event, 50 patients had embolic events in an abdominal organ or limb, and 19 patients had acute retinal ischemia. The transthoracic echocardiographic examination was normal in 92 patients (60%), whereas only 65 patients (42%) had normal findings after both transthoracic and transesophageal examination. Intracardiac masses, including valvular vegetations, were found in 39 patients (25%), including

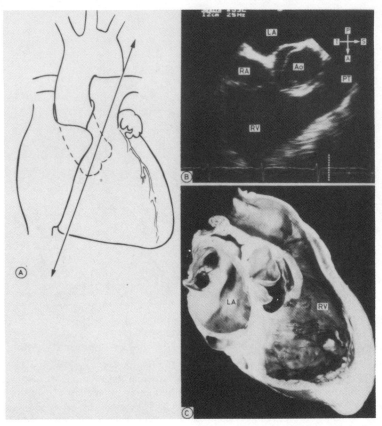

Fig. 10-6. (A) Diagram showing the scan plane that displays the right ventricular outflow tract. This is obtained by tilting the transducer laterally from position 3 in Fig. 1. (B) Longitudinal axis scan through the right ventricular cavity (RV), the right ventricular outflow tract, and the proximal pulmonary trunk (PT). Centrally the aortic root (Ao) is cut obliquely. Posteroinferiorly, a segment of the right atrium (RA) is seen together with a portion of the atrioventricular junction and the anterosuperior leaflet of the tricuspid valve. (C) a corresponding anatomical section, LA, left atrium. See Fig. 2 legend for other abbreviations. Reproduced with permission from Stumper, et al.[11]

27% of patients with cerebral embolism and 32% of these with peripheral embolism, but in none of the patients with retinal ischemia. Forty-seven patients (31%) had valvular disease, 10 (7%) had wall motion abnormalities, 23 (15%) had abnormalities of the interatrial septum, and 9 patients (6%) had diseases of the thoracic aorta. Cardiovascular abnormalities were frequently found by echocardiography in patients with arterial emboli. The transesophageal technique significantly increased the chance of detecting such abnormalities, especially intracardiac masses.

CARDIAC TRANSPLANTATION

Key references

Griffith[17] from Pittsburgh, Pennsylvania, provided a list of key references (59 articles) on cardiac transplantation.

Widening donor criteria

To combat the continuing shortage of ideal donor hearts, Sweeney and associates[18] from Houston, Texas, have used cardiac allografts from high-risk donors for critically ill recipients. The authors defined high-risk donor variables as age greater than 40 years, systemic (noncardiac) infection, cardiopulmonary resuscitation greater than 3 minutes, ischemic time >5 hours, weight >20% less than that of the recipient, and requirements for high doses of inotropes. Of the 305 donors the authors used, 73 (24%) have been high-risk, with 59/73 (81%) exhibiting one variable, 12/73 (16%) exhibiting 2 variables, and 2/73 (3%) exhibiting 3 variables. No correlation was found between the number of donor variables and a poor postoperative result. No infectious complications occurred in 17 patients receiving hearts from potentially infected donors. Hospital mortality rates (30 day) for recipients of high-risk donor versus non-high-risk donor hearts were 8.2% and 6.9%, respectively (not significant). The 1-, 6-, and 12-month actuarial survival rates were 92%, 81%, and 76% for the high-risk donor group and 94%, 80%, and 78% for the non-high-risk donor group (not significant). Among survivors with high-risk donor hearts, mean LVEFs were 0.54 ± 0.08 at 3 months, 0.55 ± 0.08 at 1 year, and 0.54 ± 0.09 at 2 years after transplantation. These results suggest that accepting less than ideal donor hearts can be safe and might be considered when better options are not available.

In infants and children

Boucek and associates[19] from Loma Linda, California, reviewed the results from their first 25 patients who underwent orthotopic cardiac transplantation in infancy for lethal cardiac disease. Diagnosis of recipients was hypoplastic left heart syndrome in 80%. The ages ranged from birth to 7 months and 21 of 25 patients are alive with follow-up from 4 to 40 months (84% survival rate). No late deaths have occurred with long-term immunosuppression using cyclosporine and azathioprine. Rejection surveillance was performed noninvasively with only 1 child requiring biopsy. Donors died from a variety of traumatic and metabolic causes, including sudden infant death syndrome. Most donors had a history of cardiac arrest requiring cardiopulmonary resuscitation. One-third were receiving inotropic support at the time of cardiac evaluation. These authors present outstanding results for short term follow-up with infant transplantation. The overall survival is significantly better than older patients at this point. In addition, they have been able to avoid biopsy in these infants in whom this procedure would be difficult and potentially hazardous.

Pahl and associates[20] from Pittsburgh, Pennsylvania, reviewed coronary angiograms and autopsy data from 21 of 30 children who underwent orthotopic heart transplantation and survived the perioperative period. The age ranged was 5 months to 16 years with a mean of 11 years. Six patients had coronary artery disease and 5 of these patients died 6 months to 3 years after transplant. Deaths were sudden and unexpected. Coronary angiography demonstrated several types of lesions, including concentric narrowing, tubular segmental lesions, and abrupt obliteration of major vessels. Risk factors assessed included hypertension, hyperlipidemia, cytomegalovirus infection, type of immunosuppressive regimen, number of rejection episodes, and major histocompatibility antigen mismatches. Only the frequency and duration of rejection episodes seemed to be more prevalent in patients with CAD. These authors show a disturbing number of patients with CAD. Continued surveillance with yearly coronary angiograms is needed in a larger patient group with different regimens including patients who are not on long-term steroids.

For neoplastic disease

Cardiac transplantation traditionally has been reserved for individuals with in-stage CHF in whom there is no history of other life-threatening systemic disorders. In most transplant centers, patients with a history of malignancy and severe CHF have not been considered acceptable candidates for cardiac transplantation. Edwards and associates[21] from Stanford, California, and Rochester, Minnesota, performed 8 cardiac transplants in 7 patients with a history of neoplastic disease. Six patients had already received treatment for lymphoproliferative disorders and in 1 case, a patient underwent a transplant after treatment for adenocarcinoma of the colon. Six of the 7 patients were discharged from the hospital and in that group, the 1-year post-transplant survival rate was 71%. This was comparable to an overall 1-year survival rate of 80% for patients undergoing a cardiac transplant at the authors' center during the same period of time. At follow-up averaging over 2 years, there has been 1 case of recurrent neoplasia. One patient with evidence of radiation-induced pulmonary damage died of respiratory failure 2 days after transplantation. One patient required retransplantation because of intractable rejection and subsequently died from infectious complications. Immunosuppressive therapy in these patients has not been associated with an increased risk for neoplastic recurrence or for the development of post-transplant lymphoproliferative disorders. The current study demonstrates that in a carefully selected group, previously treated neoplastic disease should not represent a contraindication to cardiac transplantation.

Hyperlipidemia

To determine the prevalence, time course and factors responsible for hyperlipidemia after cardiac transplantation, Rudas and associates[22] from London, Canada, studied 83 consecutive 1-year survivors. By 1 year, 83% of patients had serum total cholesterol levels >5.2 mmol/L (200 mg/dl) and 28% of the patients had serum total cholesterol higher than the age- and sex-matched 95th percentile. At the end of 1-year follow-up, serum total cholesterol correlated with the recipient age, the preoperative cholesterol level, the actual dose of maintenance prednisone at 1 year and the cumulative 1-year steroid dose (Figure 10-7). Similarly, the serum triglyceride level at 1 year correlated with the pretransplant level of serum triglycerides, recipient age and cumulative 1-year steroid dose (Figure 10-8). Patients with a pretransplant diagnosis of CAD had a significantly higher level of serum total cholesterol and triglyceride levels at 1 year. Heart transplant recipients with body mass index $\geq$25 kg/m^2 also presented with significantly elevated serum total cholesterol and triglyceride levels at 1 year compared with nonobese patients. Hyperlipidemia occurs frequently and is detected within the first month after heart transplantation. Optimal management of this problem requires further study.

Atherosclerosis is the leading obstacle to long-term survival in cardiac transplant patients. Increases in plasma triglycerides and lipoprotein cholesterol levels occur after transplantation and they may contribute to transplant atherosclerosis. The etiology of this increase in unclear. Su-

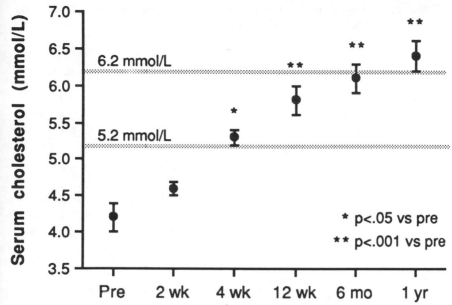

Fig. 10-7. Time course of serum total cholesterol levels over the first year after cardiac transplantation (mean ± standard error of the mean). Reproduced with permission from Rudas, et al.[22]

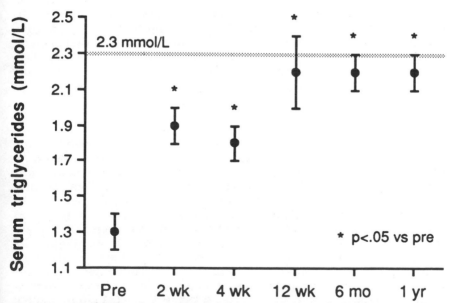

Fig. 10-8. Time course of serum triglyceride levels over the first year after cardiac transplantation (mean ± standard error of the mean). Reproduced with permission of Rudas, et al.[22]

perko and associates[23] from Stanford and Berkeley, California, investigated the inaction of immunosuppressive medications with plasma triglycerides, LDL cholesterol, HDL cholesterol, the HDL subclasses HDL_2 and HDL_3 cholesterol, and hepatic and lipoprotein lipase activity in 72 consecutive cardiac transplant patients compared to 51 healthy control subjects (Table 10-1).

TABLE 10-1. *Triglyceride and lipoprotein cholesterol values. Reproduced with permission from Superko, et al.*[23]

	Transplant Patients	Control Subjects
Triglyceride (mg/dl)	178 ± 137	99 ± 41*
Total cholesterol (mg/dl)	243 ± 64	210 ± 34*
HDL cholesterol (mg/dl)	47.0 ± 17	49.6 ± 13
HDL$_2$ cholesterol (mg/dl)‡	8.0 ± 10	9.7 ± 11
HDL$_3$ cholesterol (mg/dl)‡	38.8 ± 11	39.9 ± 5
HDL$_2$ cholesterol (mg/dl) (%)‡	14 ± 16	17 ± 12
LDL cholesterol (mg/dl)	163 ± 55	141 ± 28†
Hepatic lipase (μmol/FAA/ml/hr)	11.8 ± 3.5	5.9 ± 1.9*
Lipoprotein lipase (μmol/FAA/ml/hr)	−0.4 ± 2.0	1.7 ± 1.1*

* $p < 0.001$; † $p < 0.005$; ‡ HDL$_2$ cholesterol was obtained for 51 of the 72 transplant patients.
Values are mean ± standard deviation.
FAA = fatty free acid; HDL = high-density lipoprotein; LDL = low-density lipoprotein.

Without corticosteroid therapy

Although the etiology of allograft CAD, a major limiting factor in long-term survival after cardiac transplantation, is poorly understood, it is undoubtedly in part immune mediated and not detected by routine endomyocardial biopsy. Therefore, it is possible that withdrawal of maintenance corticosteroids, although providing other short- and long-term benefits, could increase the prevalence of allograft CAD by permitting undetected immune-mediated vascular injury to occur. To assess whether corticosteroid-free maintenance immunosuppression increased the prevalence of allograft CAD, Ratkovec and associates[24] from Salt Lake City, Utah, reviewed serial angiograms of 102 patients (49% not receiving corticosteroid maintenance therapy) who underwent heart transplantation after March 7, 1985. Multiple variables including serum cholesterol, recipient and donor age, sex, BP, rejection frequency and severity, early rejection prophylaxis protocol (polyclonal vs monoclonal T-cell agents), and corticosteroid use were examined in relation to allograft CAD by univariate and multivariate analyses. Allograft CAD was identified in 21 patients (7 severe, 4 moderate, and 10 mild). The prevalence by Kaplan-Meier life-table analysis was 17% at 1 year and 25% at 2 years (Figure 10-9). No further allograft CAD was detected among patients undergoing angiography at 3 years. Increased allograft CAD was not noted in patients withdrawn from maintenance corticosteroids when compared with their corticosteroid-requiring counterparts. In fact, with each 1 gm increment in cumulative corticosteroid use, a slightly increased risk (1.04) of allograft CAD was noted (Cox regression model). None of the other variables correlated with the prevalence of allograft CAD. Thus, withdrawal of maintenance corticosteroids is not associated with an increased risk of early allograft CAD and minimization of corticosteroids may lead to a decreased long-term incidence of CAD in cardiac transplant recipients.

Cyclosporine-treated results

To elucidate the long-term effects of cyclosporine, Grattan and associates[25] from Stanford, California, retrospectively studied 310 con-

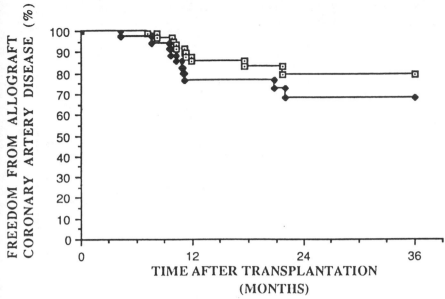

Fig. 10-9. Freedom from allograft coronary artery disease after cardiac transplantation in patients receiving less than 10,000 prednisone equivalents (—⊡—, n = 67) and in patients receiving more than 10,000 prednisone equivalents (—♦—, n = 35). When cumulative corticosteroids are analyzed as a continuous variable, an increased risk (1.04) of allograft coronary artery disease is observed with each 1000 mg increment in cumulative corticosteroids (p<0.05, Cox regression model). Cumulative corticosteroids were calculated as prednisone equivalents assuming prednisone 1 mg = methylprednisone 0.8 mg = hydrocortisone 4 mg and includes all corticosteroids administered from the time of operation. Reproduced with permission from Ratkovec, et al.[24]

secutive patients who had undergone cardiac transplantation since December, 1980 and in whom immunosuppression had been maintained with cyclosporine. The ages of recipients ranged from 1 month to 64 years and of donors from 1 month to 48 years. The actuarial survival rates for cyclosporine-treated patients were 81% at 1 year and 60% at 5 years and were significantly greater than those for previous patients not treated with cyclosporine (Figure 10-10). Their actuarial prevalence of rejection was 60% at 1 month and 87% at 1 year; 206 patients are living. The actuarial prevalence of lymphoma development was 4.6% at 5 years but has been significantly lower with the current immunosuppression protocol of lower doses of cyclosporine, and OKT3 in place of rabbit antithymocyte globulin. Infection remains the most common cause of death (Figure 10-11). Recipients less than 50 years of age had a significantly higher actuarial survival than older recipients (Figure 10-12). Male and female recipients had similar overall prevalence of survival and rejection, but men died of graft atherosclerosis significantly more frequently. Rehabilitation has been successful in 85% of patients surviving 1 year after transplantation. Of those surviving 1 year, 96.5% were in New York Heart Association class I. Thus, the results of orthotopic cardiac transplantation have improved since the introduction of cyclosporine and have allowed measured liberalization of the criteria for recipient selection.

Hypertension is a frequent complication of cyclosporine-induced immunosuppression, but the underlying mechanism is unknown. In anesthetized animals, the administration of cyclosporine increases sympathetic-nerve discharge, which may contribute to hypertension. To

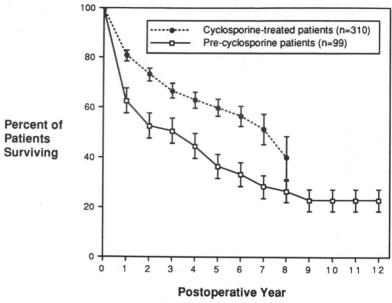

Fig. 10-10. Patients treated with cyclosporine had a significantly higher survival rate than had patients not treated with cyclosporine (p < 0.005). Reproduced with permission from Grattan, et al.[25]

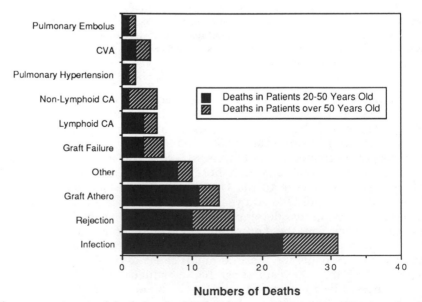

Fig. 10-11. Causes of death for all adult patients are shown; with subdivisions in each category for deaths in patients 20 to 49 years old and in patients 50 years or older. Reproduced with permission from Grattan, et al.[25]

determine whether cyclosporine-induced hypertension is accompanied by sustained sympathetic neural activation in patients, Scherrer and associates[26] from 3 medical centers (Dallas, Texas, Madison, Wisconsin, and Richmond, Virginia) recorded sympathetic action potentials using intraneural microelectrodes in the peroneal nerve in heart-transplant recipients receiving azathioprine and prednisone alone (n = 5) or in

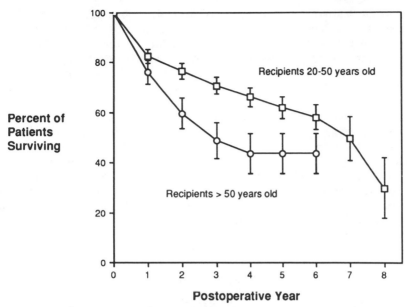

Fig. 10-12. Cyclosporine-treated patients 50 years of age or older (n = 82) had a significantly lower survival rate than had cyclosporine-treated patients 20 to 49 years of age (n = 177, p < 0.01). Reproduced with permission from Grattan, et al.[25]

combination with cyclosporine (n = 14). The authors performed the same studies in 8 patients with myasthenia gravis who were receiving cyclosporine and 8 who were not, in 5 patients with essential hypertension, and in 9 normal controls. Heart-transplant recipients receiving cyclosporine had higher mean arterial BP (± SE) than those not receiving cyclosporine (112 ± 3 vs 96 ± 4 mm Hg) and a 2.7-fold higher rate of sympathetic-nerve firing (80 ± 3 vs 30 ± 4 bursts per minute). For patients with myasthenia gravis, similar doses of cyclosporine were associated with smaller elevations in mean arterial BP (100 ± 2 mm Hg, as compared with 91 ± 4 mm Hg in those not receiving cyclosporine) and in the rate of sympathetic-nerve firing (46 ± 3 bursts per minute, as compared with 25 ± 4 bursts per minute). Sympathetic activity in patients with heart transplants or myasthenia gravis who were not being treated with cyclosporine was no different from that in patients with essential hypertension or in normal controls. Cyclosporine-induced hypertension is associated with sympathetic neural activation, which may be accentuated by the cardiac denervation that results from heart transplantation.

This article was followed by an editorial entitled, "Cyclosporine, Sympathetic Activity, and Hypertension" by Allyn L. Mark.[27] Mark concludes with the following sentence: "By demonstrating striking increases in sympathetic activity in patients receiving cyclosporine, Scherrer et al., have advanced our knowledge of the pathogenesis of cyclosporine-induced hypertension and, in a broader context, have again focused attention on the role of the sympathetic nervous system in the pathogenesis of human hypertension."

Cardiac arrhythmias

Jacquet and colleagues[28] in Pittsburgh, Pennsylvania, studied type and consequences of cardiac arrhythmias early after heart transplantation in

25 cardiac transplant patients monitored for 728 days from the day of surgery to discharge or death. A subset of 15 patients had sinus node function studies with overdrive suppression performed weekly at the time of endomyocardial biopsy. Results revealed sinus bradycardia in 10 patients (40%) and junctional bradycardia in 6 (24%). Supraventricular tachycardia in the form of atrial tachycardia, atrial fibrillation and atrial flutter occurred in 11 patients (44%). VT developed in 15 patients (60%) and was nonsustained in all. Cardiac pacing for 1,403 hours was used in 9 patients with a pulse rate less than 50 beats/minute; 7 patients recovered and permanent pacing was necessary in 2. In the patients with sinus node function studies, 7 had clinical bradyarrhythmia and each had an abnormal sinus node recovery time greater than 1,400 ms and abnormal corrected sinus node recovery time in at least one study. These 7 patients also had a significantly prolonged ischemic time (236 ± 26 minutes versus 159 ± 68 minutes). Thus, cardiac arrhythmias, especially VT and brady-arrhythmia, occur more commonly after orthotopic heart transplantation than has been reported previously. Sinus node dysfunction due to prolonged organ ischemic time, antiarrhythmic drug use or surgical trauma may contribute to these arrhythmias.

Ultrasonic backscatter in acute rejection

Cyclic variation of integrated ultrasonic backscatter was noninvasively measured by Masuyama and co-workers[29] in Stanford, California in the septum and LV posterior wall using a quantitative imaging system to assess the alterations in the acoustic properties of myocardium associated with acute cardiac allograft rejection. The study population consisted of 23 cardiac allograft recipients and 18 normal subjects. In each cardiac allograft recipient, 1–8 studies were performed, each with 24 hours of RV endomyocardial biopsy performed for rejection surveillance. The magnitude of the cyclic variation of ultrasonic backscatter in the posterior walls was 5.9 dB in normal subjects and 6.2 dB in the cardiac allograft recipients without previous or current histological evidence of acute rejection. A significant decrease in the septal ultrasonic backscatter was observed in cardiac allograft recipients with LV hypertrophy. Ultrasonic backscatter studies were done before and during moderate acute rejection in 11 recipients. During moderate acute cardiac rejection, the magnitude of the cyclic variation in ultrasonic backscatter decreased from 6.7 to 5.1 dB in the posterior wall and from 4.2 to 2.9 dB in the septum. These data suggest 1) the magnitude of the cyclic variation in ultrasonic backscatter of the septum is different in cardiac allografts with cardiac hypertrophy and normal subjects, possibly reflecting regionally depressed myocardial contractile performance and 2) acute cardiac rejection in humans is accompanied by an alteration in the acoustic properties of the myocardium. This change is detectable by serial measurement of the magnitude of the cyclic variation in ultrasonic backscatter, both in the septum and in the posterior wall.

PERIPHERAL VASCULAR DISEASE

Prevalence in the USA

Peripheral arterial occlusive disease of the extremities is an important cause of morbidity and health care expenditures among the elderly. Data from the National Hospital Discharge Survey and National Vital Statistics System were used to assess its impact in the USA in this report by Gillum[30] from Hyattsville, Maryland. In 1985 to 1987, an estimated 229,000 men and 184,000 women per year were discharged with any diagnosis of chronic peripheral arterial occlusive disease. Discharge rates were much higher in men and increased sharply with age. Lower extremity arteriography was performed during 88,000 hospitalizations and aorta-iliac-femoral bypass procedures were done during 31,000 hospitalizations per year. Numbers of procedures increased markedly since 1979. An estimated 60,000 men and 50,000 women per year were discharged with any diagnosis of acute peripheral arterial occlusive disease. Embolectomy or thrombectomy of lower limb arteries was listed for 28,000 discharges per year. Few deaths were attributed to peripheral arterial occlusive disease. Although these data are limited by likely incomplete reporting and by the nonspecificity of diagnostic codes, they provide an indication of the magnitude of the problem. An aging population and advances in surgical techniques suggest continued monitoring using multiple data sources. Vigorous primary prevention programs are needed to lessen the impact of all atherosclerotic diseases.

Frequency of coronary and cerebrovascular disease

Smith and colleagues[31] in London, UK, analyzed the Whitehall study in which 18,388 subjects aged 40–64 years completed a questionnaire on intermittent claudication. Of these subjects, 147 and 175 were deemed to have probable intermittent claudication and possible intermittent claudication, respectively. Within the 17 year follow-up, 38% and 40% of the probable and possible cases, respectively, died. Compared with subjects without claudication, the probable cases suffered increased mortality rates due to CAD and cerebrovascular disease, but the mortality rate due to noncardiovascular diseases was not increased. Possible cases demonstrated increased mortality rates due to cardiovascular and noncardiovascular causes. This difference in mortality pattern may be due to chance. Possible and probable cases still showed increased cardiovascular and all-cause mortality rates after adjusting for coronary risk factors (cardiac ischemia at baseline, systolic blood pressure, plasma cholesterol concentration, smoking behavior, employment grade, and degree of glucose intolerance). Intermittent claudication is independently related to increased mortality rates. It is not a rare condition, and simple questionnaires exist for its detection. The latter can be usefully incorporated in cardiovascular risk assessment and screening programs.

Dipyridamole thallium scintigraphy

The prognostic value of long-term risk stratification of patients with peripheral vascular disease who undergo intravenous dipyridamole thallium scintigraphy has not been well studied. Younis and colleagues[32] from St. Louis, Missouri, screened 131 patients with peripheral vascular disease who underwent intravenous dipyridamole thallium testing to determine cardiac event rates over an average follow-up of 18 ± 10 months. Of the 131 patients, 111 subsequently had peripheral vascular surgery. The patients with abnormal thallium scans after dipyridamole had a significantly higher risk of death or AMI both in the perioperative phase (7% vs 0%) and at late follow-up (17% vs 6%). The risk of a cardiac event was 2-fold greater when a reversible as compared to a fixed thallium defect was present. Multivariate analysis selected the number of thallium segments with perfusion defects, prior history of angina pectoris, and chest pain during dipyridamole testing as perioperative predictors of a cardiac event. A reversible thallium defect was the only predictor of death or nonfatal AMI during late follow-up. Thus intravenous dipyridamole thallium scintigraphy is a useful noninvasive test for risk stratification of patients before peripheral vascular surgery and provides prognostic information as to the risk of a cardiac event in the 2-year period after the test. A reversible thallium defect is associated with a significant increased risk and would indicate that coronary angiography should be considered and preoperative CABG.

Cholesterol embolization

Rosman and associates[33] in Detroit, Michigan have described the clinical characteristics of 13 patients with cholesterol embolization. Embolization occurred spontaneously in 2 patients and after a vascular procedure in 11. Acute but vague symptoms were reported by 11 of 13 patients, including skin findings of purple toes or livedo reticularis (Figure 10-13) and renal dysfunction were present in 12 patients, 5 of whom required dialysis. Blood pressure elevation occurred in all 13 patients, eosinophilia in 9 of 10, and elevated sedimentation rate in 5 of 6. Death occurred within 6 months in 3 of these patients. Two distinct patterns of cholesterol embolization were observed: mild (5 patients) and severe (8 patients). Compared with the severe pattern, patients with mild cholesterol embolization had early symptoms less frequently, less severe renal insufficiency, including a serum creatinine of 1.7 vs 7.4 mg/100 ml, respectively, less of an increase in BP, and later development of skin lesions (14 vs 6 weeks, respectively). The presence of cholesterol embolization is often subtle and may go unrecognized, especially in its mild form. As vascular interventions increase in elderly atherosclerotic and hypertensive patients, the incidence of this disorder will probably increase as well.

Transluminal atherectomy

Johnson and associates[34] in Richmond, Virginia, and Redwood City, California used an atherectomy device to obtain tissue for gross and light microscopic analysis in 218 peripheral arterial stenoses resected from 100 patients. One hundred seventy of these lesions were primary stenoses and 48 were restenoses subsequent to prior PTCA or atherectomy. Microscopically, primary stenoses were composed of atherosclerotic plaque (150 lesions), fibrous intimal thickening (15 lesions) or thrombus alone (5 lesions). Atherosclerotic plaques had a variable morphology and in one-third of cases were accompanied by abundant surface thrombus that probably contributed to the severity of the stenosis. Most patients with fibrous intimal thickening or thrombus alone had typical atherosclerotic plaque removed elsewhere from within the same artery. Intimal hyperplasia with or without underlying residual plaque was found at 36 sites of restenosis, the remaining 12 consisting of plaque only. Intimal hyperplasia had a distinctive histologic appearance and one associated with smooth muscle cell proliferation within a loosely fibrous stroma. Superimposed thrombus may have contributed to arterial narrowing in 25% of hyperplastic and 8% of atherosclerotic restenoses.

von Pölnitz and associates[35] in Munich, Federal Republic of Germany, used the Simpson atherectomy catheter to treat 60 patients with a total

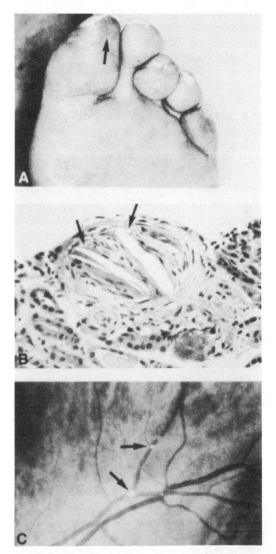

Fig. 10-13. A, Left foot of a patient with the severe pattern of cholesterol embolization. The great toe shows a demarcated area (arrow) of cyanosis resulting from ischemia. B, Renal biopsy showing multiple cholesterol clefts (arrows) in a glomerulus. C, Cholesterol crystals lodged inside a retinal arteriole (arrow). Reproduced with permission from Rosman, et al.[33]

of 94 lesions comprising 63 stenoses and 31 occlusions of the superficial femoral (n = 77), popliteal (n = 8), iliac (n = 8) and anterior tibial (n = 1) arteries. The immediate angiographic success was 90% for both occlusions and stenoses and clinical success was obtained in 82% of patients. The stenoses were reduced from 83 ± 13% to 17 ± 18% acutely and to 31 ± 26% at 6 months. The occlusions were reduced from 100% to 9 ± 9% initially and to 60 ± 34% at 6 months. Angiographic restenosis occurred in 24%, including 23% in concentric, 11% in eccentric, and 47% in total occlusions. At 1 year, 72% of patients had clinically patent arteries with maintained Doppler index and walking distance. Three of 4 patients having repeat atherectomy had a second restenosis. Thus, atherectomy using the Simpson atherectomy device is relatively safe and effective in the treatment of peripheral vascular disease, and it appears to be par-ticularly useful in the treatment of eccentric stenoses.

Graor and Whitlow[36] in Cleveland, Ohio, treated 112 patients with superficial femoral artery stenosis or occlusion with percutaneous atherectomy. Patients were considered to have a simple lesion if the occluded or stenotic arterial segment was <5 cm and a complex lesion if the length of the occluded segment was >5 cm. All atherectomies were performed in the superficial femoral and popliteal arteries. Urokinase-induced thrombolysis was used in conjunction with atherectomy in 16 patients. Atherectomy was successful if there was less than 20% residual stenosis determined by arteriography. Initial atherectomy results and 30 day patency were 100% successful in the group with simple lesions and 93% in the group with the complex lesions. At a mean follow-up of 12 months and a range of 5 to 24 months, there was a continued patency rate of 93% and 86%, respectively in the two groups. In the patients who had restenosis, all pathologic specimens obtained during the second procedure demonstrated myointimal hypoplasia and organized thrombus. Eight complications of the procedure occurred, including one fatal AMI. The complication rate was 3.5% with the simple lesion and 8.3% with the complex ones. With the exception of AMI, the complications were associated with catheter entry site hematomas. Thus, femoropopliteal atherectomy has a relatively high rate of success and low morbidity and mortality for both simple and complex arterial lesions and represents a viable alternative therapy, at least in the short term, for patients with peripheral vascular disease.

Laser assisted balloon angioplasty

In 12 patients (aged 64 years) with femoropopliteal occlusions (1–27 cm length) that could not be recanalized by standard guidewire balloon angioplasty techniques, Leon and co-workers[37] in Bethesda, Maryland, performed percutaneous laser assisted balloon angioplasty by use of a new fluorescence guided dual laser system. Plaque detection by 325-nm laser excited fluorescence spectroscopy provided real time feedback control to a 480-nm pulsed dye laser for atheroma ablation. By means of a common 200-μm optical fiber, after diagnostic fluorescence sensing, computer algorithms directed a fire or no fire signal to the treatment laser for selective plaque removal. Laser recanalization was successful in 10 of 12 patients; this procedure was followed by definitive balloon angioplasty in 7 of 12 patients with increased ankle/arm indexes. In laser and balloon angioplasty failures, all femoropopliteal occlusions were heavily calcified, and there were two mechanical guidewire perforations without clinical sequelae. Ablation of calcified lesions required higher pulse energies and greater total energy per centimeter of recanalized tissue. Fluorescence spectroscopy was helpful in flush occlusions and correctly identified plaque, underlying media, and thrombus by changes in fluorescence intensity, shape, and peak position. Thus, when fluorescence guided laser angioplasty was used in a subgroup of patients refractory to standard angioplasty techniques, primary recanalization and subsequent balloon angioplasty of femoropopliteal occlusions was successful in 83% and 58 of the patients, respectively. Importantly, treatment of heavily calcified lesions accounted for all of the failures and will require modified delivery systems to create larger primary channels and to increase catheter tip control, which should improve clinical results in the future.

Aortic dissection

Chirillo and associates[38] from Padova, Italy, retrospectively analyzed 290 patients with spontaneous aortic dissection occurring between January 1976 and June 1987. Their article appeared in April 1990. Dissection was always documented by retrograde aortography and data were collected from 11 catheterization laboratories operating in northeastern Italy. The results show that over a 12-year period there was an increase in cases, an increase in the number of operations and a decline in operative mortality (Figures 10-14 and 10-15). Multivariate discriminant analysis demonstrated that AMI, persistent shock and persistent central neurologic deficit were significant independent predictors of operative mortality in type A patients. Only persistent shock was significantly related to higher operative mortality in type B patients. Late deaths occurred in 14/118 operated patients, and were mostly secondary (directly or indirectly) to aortic dissection. Discharged patients underwent frequent medical checks and chronically received drugs to control hypertension and reduce inotropism. Most of them (74%) were asymptomatic: Careful post-operative medical assistance is necessary to guarantee the long-term success of surgical treatment. Aortic dissection was classified according to the Stanford Type A/B nomenclature based on the presence or absence of involvement of the ascending aorta irrespective of the site of the primary intimal tear and regardless of the extent of distal propagation.

Roberts and Roberts[39] from Bethesda, Maryland, described clinical and necropsy findings in 12 patients who had fatal aortic dissection with the entrance tear in the transverse aorta. The 12 patients represent 7% of 182 autopsies of spontaneous aortic dissection studied by them. The ages of the 12 patients at death ranged from 37 to 87 years (mean, 67

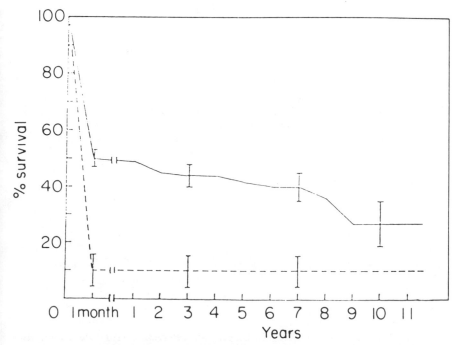

Fig. 10-14. Actuarial survival curves for type A patients (——— = operated patients; ---- = non-operated patients). Reproduced with permission from Chirillo, et al.[38]

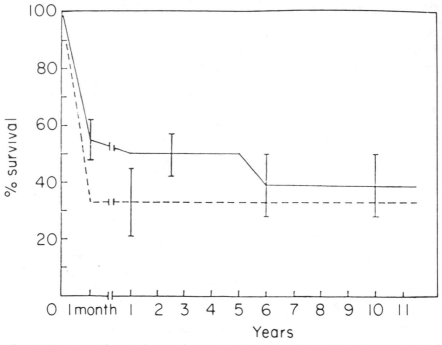

Fig. 10-15. Actuarial survival curves for type B patients. Mortality is higher for non-operated patients than for surgical patients, even if the difference is not as evident as for type A patients. (——— = operated patients: ---- = non-operated patients). Reproduced with permission from Chirillo, et al.[38]

years). Eight were men; 8 had a history of systemic hypertension, and 10 had hearts of increased weight. Diagnosis of aortic dissection was made during life in only 4 of the 12 patients. All 12 patients died of rupture of the false channel within 2 weeks of onset of signs or symptoms compatible with dissection. The direction of aortic dissection from the entrance tear was entirely retrograde in 4 patients, entirely anterograde in 4 patients, and in both directions in 4 patients. Hemopericardium occurred in the first group, left hemothorax in the second group, and either in the last group. Of the 8 patients in whom the ascending aorta was involved, the retrograde dissection in each extended to the aortic root, 6 had pulmonary adventitial hemorrhage, and 4 had involvement of the arch arteries by dissection. In the 4 patients with strictly anterograde dissection, none had dissection in the arch arteries. Thus, tear in the transverse aorta causes a dissection that is usually fatal, that often dissects retrogradely, and that may mimic dissection from a tear in ascending aorta. Aortic dissection from a tear in transverse aorta requires early operative intervention.

PULMONARY DISEASE

Pulmonary embolism

To determine the sensitivities and specificities of ventilation/perfusion lung scans for acute pulmonary embolism, the Prospective Investigation of Pulmonary Embolism Diagnosis (PIOPED) investigators[40] prospectively studied a random sample of 933 of 1,493 patients. Nine hundred and thirty-one underwent scintigraphy and 755 underwent pulmonary angiography; 251 (33%) of 755 demonstrated pulmonary embolism. Almost all patients with pulmonary embolism had abnormal scans of high, intermediate, or low probability, but so did most without pulmonary embolism (sensitivity, 98%; specificity, 10%). Of 116 patients with high-probability scans and definitive angiograms, 102 (88%) had pulmonary embolism, but only a minority with pulmonary embolism had high-probability scans (sensitivity, 41%; specificity, 97%). Of 322 with intermediate-probability scans (sensitivity, 41%; specificity, 97%). Of 322 with intermediate-probability scans and definitive angiograms, 105 (33%) had pulmonary embolism. Follow-up and angiography together suggested that pulmonary embolism occurred among 12% of patients with low-probability scans. Clinical assessment combined with the ventilation/perfusion scan established the diagnosis or exclusion of pulmonary embolism only for a minority of patients—those with clear and concordant clinical and ventilation/perfusion scan findings.

To better characterize the morbidity from pulmonary embolism, Lilienfeld and associates[41] from New York, New York, and Minneapolis, Minnesota, examined hospital discharge data for all acute care facilities (except for the Veterans Administration Medical Center) in the Minneapolis-St. Paul metropolitan area in each year from 1979 to 1984 for persons aged 30 to 74 years. For each person in whom the discharge diagnosis included pulmonary embolism, the age, sex, year of admission, and vital status at discharge were recorded. Annual age-sex-specific and age-adjusted sex-specific hospitalization rates were calculated. Similar analyses were undertaken for case fatality. With the exception of men <55 years of age, all groups experienced significant decline in the pulmonary embolism discharge rate. No significant temporal changes were observed in any of the case fatality rates. These data suggest that changes in pulmonary embolism mortality in the United States from 1979 to 1984 may reflect declining occurrence of the disease and are likely not the result of changes in case fatality.

Primary pulmonary hypertension

Although the mechanisms involved in the pathophysiology of primary pulmonary hypertension have not yet been delineated, thrombosis has been implicated. Eisenberg and co-workers[42] in St. Louis, Missouri, designed a study to determine whether thrombin activity as reflected by plasma concentrations of fibrinopeptide A, a marker of the action of thrombin on fibrinogen, is increased in patients with primary pulmonary hypertension. To evaluate fibrinolytic activity, the investigators measured plasma concentrations of tissue-type plasminogen activator, plasminogen activator inhibitor-1, and cross-linked fibrin degradation productions. The investigators studied 31 patients with primary pulmonary hypertension. Plasma fibrinopeptide A concentrations measured by radioimmunoassay were elevated. Fifteen minutes after administration of 5,000 units of heparin, fibrinopeptide A concentrations decreased. In 21 of 30 patients, fibrinopeptide A concentrations after heparin administration were less than half the preheparin levels, a response consistent with inhibition of thrombin by heparin and the short half-life of fibrinopeptide A. Despite evidence for marked thrombin activity, plasma concentrations of cross-linked fibrin degradation products were normal in all but 4 patients. Plasminogen activator inhibitor-1 activity was elevated in 19 of the 27 patients in whom it was measured, potentially limiting the fibrinolytic response. The elevations of fibrinopeptide A indicate that thrombin activity is increased in vivo in patients with primary pulmonary hypertension. Thus, sequential assays of plasma markers of thrombosis and fibrinolysis in vivo may help identify those patients who may benefit from treatment with anticoagulants.

Epoprostenol sodium (prostacyclin) administered intravenously is considered the standard for assessing the ability of the pulmonary circulation to vasodilate. At present, epoprostenol sodium is an investigational drug that has limited availability. In contrast, acetylcholine, also a pulmonary vasodilator, is readily available. Therefore, Palvesky and coworkers[43] in Philadelphia, Pennsylvania assessed the feasibility of using acetylcholine as an alternative to prostacyclin in testing for the capacity of the pulmonary vasculature to vasodilate. Twenty-three patients with primary pulmonary hypertension received incremental infusions of prostacyclin and acetylcholine to predetermined maximal infusion rates as part of a battery of vasodilator agents administered according to standard protocols; the administration of the different agents was timed to avoid synergistic effects. Of all the agents tested, prostacyclin and acetylcholine were most consistently effective in evoking acute pulmonary vasodilation, and both seemed to distinguish patients capable of manifesting acute pulmonary vasodilation from those who were not. However, at maximal doses set by protocol, prostacyclin generally elicited a greater vasodilator response than acetylcholine. The difference in magnitude of response may have been due to use of prescribed dosages of acetylcholine that were submaximal. In other respects, the two agents were similar; both were equally well tolerated, and side effects were mild and resolved rapidly when the vasodilator infusions were stopped. The investigators concluded that in the majority of patients with primary pulmonary hypertension, acetylcholine appears to be an effective and available substitute for prostacyclin in screening for pulmonary vasodilator responsiveness.

MISCELLANEOUS TOPICS

Management guidelines in intensive care units for chest pain, pulmonary edema, and syncope

Eagle and associates[44] from Boston and West Roxbury, Massachusetts, developed consensus management guidelines for patients admitted with chest pain, pulmonary edema, and syncope (Table 10-2).

Preoperative risk assessment for cardiac surgery

The Veterans Administration Preoperative Risk Assessment Study for Cardiac Surgery was authorized by the Department of Veterans Affairs to improve the quality assurance of cardiac surgery by assessing pre-operative risk factors and relating them to operative mortality.[45] Data were received on 10,480 patients over a 2-year period. Preoperative risk variables were subjected to univariate and multivariate logistic regression analyses. Significant variables for CABG after logistic regression analysis in order of importance are previous cardiac operation, priority of operation, New York Heart Association functional class, peripheral vascular disease, age,

TABLE 10-2. Reproduced with permission from Eagle, et al.[44]

APPENDIX

A: Guidelines for Admission to the Coronary Care Unit (CCU)/Intensive Care Unit (ICU)

I. Chest Pain and Suspected Myocardial Infarction

1. New chest pain with electrocardiogram (ECG) evidence of ischemia or infarction not known to be old.
2. New chest pain suggestive of ischemia, without ECG evidence of ischemia, of >30 minutes' duration, especially in setting of diaphoresis.
3. Characteristic angina of increasing frequency, severity, duration, and/or requiring less provocation (including new rest pain).
4. Chest pain known to be, or suggestive of, ischemia associated with any of the following:
   a. Hypotension
   b. Congestive heart failure
   c. More than five unifocal premature ventricular beats per minute not known to be chronic
   d. Complex ventricular ectopy activity (VEA); multifocal, consecutive, R on T
   e. Second- or third-degree atrioventricular (AV) bundle-branch block (BBB)
   f. New hypoxia
5. Chest pain suggestive of myocardial ischemia in the setting of other major life-threatening or acute organ system failure: eg, sepsis, pneumonia, gastrointestinal (GI) bleeding, diabetic ketoacidosis.

II. Pulmonary Edema

1. Pulmonary edema with associated chest pain or other symptoms suggestive of myocardial infarction.
2. Pulmonary edema with ECG evidence of one or more of the following:
   a. Myocardial ischemia
   b. Myocardial infarction
   c. Ventricular tachycardia or complex VEA
   d. Bradycardia <40 beats per minute
   e. New Mobitz type II AV block or "complete" heart block
   f. Sinus arrest or pauses >2 seconds
   g. Pacemaker failure to capture or sense
3. Pulmonary edema related to suspected or proven pulmonary embolism.
4. Pulmonary edema in patients with known or suspected severe valvular disease affecting aortic or mitral valves.
5. Pulmonary edema in patients requiring:
   a. Continued care for respiratory distress after initial treatment
   b. Ventilatory support
   c. Blood pressure support
   d. Invasive venous or arterial monitoring

III. Syncope

1. Syncope with associated chest pain or other symptom suggestive of myocardial infarction.
2. Syncope with ECG evidence of one or more of the following:
   a. Myocardial ischemia
   b. Myocardial infarction
   c. Supraventricular tachycardia with rate >120 beats per minute
   d. Ventricular tachycardia or complex VEA
   e. New Mobitz type II AV block or "complete" heart block
   f. Sinus arrest or pauses of >2 seconds
   g. Pacemaker failure—failure to capture or sense appropriately
3. Syncope related to suspected or proven pulmonary embolism, GI bleeding, or aortic dissection.
4. Syncope of uncertain cause in "high-risk" patients with one or more of the following:
   a. Known ischemic heart disease, congestive heart failure, or renal failure
   b. Known prior tachyarrhythmias: ventricular tachycardia or accelerated supraventricular tachycardia
   c. Known or suspected prior bradyarrhythmias: second- or third-degree AV

block or sinus pause/arrest
   d. Unexplained orthostatic hypotension
   e. Known or suspected cardiac outflow obstruction: aortic stenosis, hypertrophic cardiomyopathy, idiopathic hypertrophic subaortic stenosis, pulmonic stenosis, pulmonary hypertension, or atrial myxoma
   f. In association with new or suspected new neurological event: transient ischemic attack, cerebral infarction, or cerebral hemorrhage
   g. Unexplained syncope in the elderly (>65 years) in whom associated *comorbid conditions* raise the suspicion of cardiac or neurological cause for syncope
   h. Recurrent unexplained syncope: two or more episodes in past 6 months

B: Guidelines for Continued ICU/CCU Stay

I. Chest Pain and Suspected Myocardial Infarction

1. Suspicion of myocardial infarction justifies up to 24 hours.
2. Confirmed acute myocardial infarction within 48 hours.
3. Any of the following complications occurring within 48 hours:
   a. Ventricular tachycardia or fibrillation
   b. Sustained hypotension
   c. New second- or third-degree AV block
   d. Infarct extension by ECG or enzyme analysis
   e. Decompensated congestive heart failure
4. Any of the following complications occurring within 24 hours:
   a. Recurrent ischemic chest pain or ongoing infarction pain
   b. Complex VEA
   c. New first-degree heart block, sustained bradyarrhythmia, or new BBB
   d. New supraventricular tachycardia
   e. Temporary pacer
   f. Mechanical ventilator

II. Pulmonary Edema

1. Confirmed myocardial infarction within 72 hours.
2. Repeated episode of pulmonary edema within 72 hours.
3. Any of the following complications within 48 hours:
   a. Ventricular tachycardia or fibrillation
   b. Sustained hypotension or hypoxia (PO$_2$ <60 mm Hg)
   c. High-risk bradyarrhythmias: sinus pause > 2 seconds, new Mobitz type II AV block, new third-degree AV block
   d. Rapid supraventricular tachycardia with hemodynamic compromise:ischemia, shock, or pulmonary congestion from congestive heart failure
   e. Status epilepticus
   f. Uncontrolled hypertension
   g. Active GI bleeding (>1 U/24 h)
4. Any of the following complications within 24 hours:
   a. Altered mental status with threat of aspiration
   b. Temporary pacemaker
   c. Ischemic chest pain
   d. Complex VEA
   e. New Mobitz type 1 AV block or sinus bradycardia at rate <40 beats per minute

III. Syncope

1. Confirmed myocardial infarction or aortic dissection justified up to 48 and 72 hours of ICU stay, respectively.
2. Any of the following complications justifies up to 48 hours of ICU stay:
   a. Ventricular tachycardia or fibrillation
   b. New sustained hypotension or hypoxia (PO$_2$ <60 mm Hg)
   c. High-risk bradyarrhythmias: sinus pause >2.5 seconds, new Mobitz type II

AV block, new third-degree AV block
   d. Rapid supraventricular tachycardia with hemodynamic compromise: coronary ischemia, shock, or pulmonary congestion

C: Guidelines for Continued Post-ICU/CCU Stay

I. Chest Pain and Suspected Myocardial Infarction

1. Transfer from ICU/CCU following acute myocardial infarction within 9 days.
2. Transfer from ICU/CCU following coronary insufficiency within 5 days.
3. Transfer from ICU/CCU following chest pain of uncertain etiology within 2 days.
4. Pulmonary or systemic embolus occurring within 7 days.
5. Any of the following complications occurring within 5 days:
   a. Recurrent ischemic pain (>10 minutes duration)
   b. VEA or arrhythmia requiring antiarrhythmic therapy
   c. New or worsening congestive heart failure
6. Invasive diagnostic study (eg, angiography) within 24 hours.
7. Cardiac or other major surgery within 14 days.
8. Comorbid conditions requiring parenteral therapy (eg, transfusions or intravenous antibiotics) up to 24 hours.

II. Pulmonary Edema

1. Transfer from ICU following acute myocardial infarction or pulmonary embolism within 9 days.
2. ransfer from ICU following coronary insufficiency or major GI bleeding within 5 days.
3. Any one of the following complications within 5 days:
   a. VEA requiring treatment or monitoring
   b. Bradyarrhythmia requiring placement of temporary or permanent pacemaker or change in drug therapy
   c. Recurrent pulmonary edema or persistent, symptomatic congestive heart failure
4. Invasive study within 24 hours.
5. Major surgery within 14 days.
6. Comorbid condition requiring parenteral therapy within 24 hours.

III. Syncope

1. Transfer from ICU following acute myocardial infarction, pulmonary embolism, or aortic dissection within 9 days.
2. Transfer from ICU following coronary insufficiency or major GI bleeding within 5 days.
3. Transfer from ICU following syncope of uncertain cause within 3 days.
4. Any one or more of the following complications justifies up to 5 days:
   a. VEA requiring antiarrhythmic therapy or monitoring
   b. Bradyarrhythmia requiring placement of temporary or permanent pacemaker or alteration of drug therapy
   c. New or worsening congestive heart failure
5. Invasive diagnostic study justifies up to 24 hours.
6. Major surgery justifies up to 14 days of additional hospitalization.
7. Comorbid condition requiring parenteral therapy justifies up to 48 hours after discontinuation of intravenous therapy.

The guidelines put forth in this article are not presented as rigid tools for monitoring or providing health care. In this study, they were used to measure variation in health care delivery and to explore reasons for this variation. While the guidelines may serve physicians in providing general strategies for care, they cannot replace clinical judgment and continuing monitoring of care by expert clinicians.

---

pulmonary rales, current diuretic use, and chronic obstructive pulmonary disease (Figures 10-16–10-18). For patients undergoing valve or other cardiac operations with or without CABG, those variables found to be significant after multivariate logistic regression analysis are priority of operation; age; peripheral vascular disease; great vessel repair; all other except AVR, MVR; and cardiomegaly (Tables 10-3 and 10-4). By identifying these current risk factors and the coefficients from the multivariate stepwise logistic regression analysis, expected mortality can be calculated. The authors propose that the ratio of observed to expected mortality is a better measure of quality of care than unadjusted mortality.

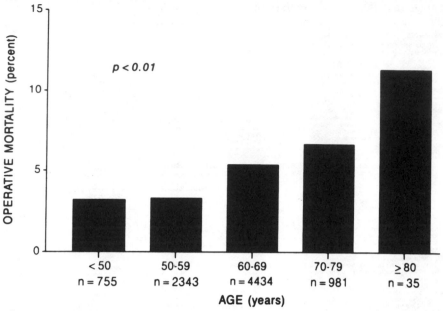

Fig. 10-16. Effect of age on operative mortality for patients undergoing coronary bypass grafting. There is a marked increase in mortality for patients 80 years old or older (11.4%) versus younger patients (4.8%). Reproduced with permission from Grover, et al.[45]

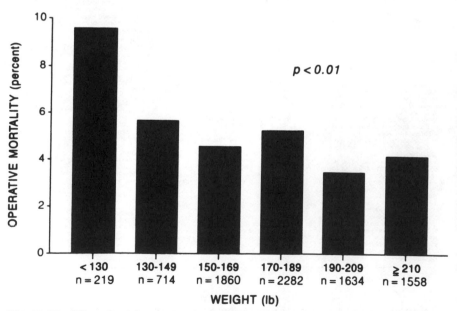

Fig. 10-17. Effect of weight on operative mortality for patients undergoing coronary artery bypass grafting. Of interest is the fact that low weight, less than 58.5 kg (130 lb), is associated with a greater operative mortality than higher weight and obesity. Reproduced with permission from Grover, et al.[45]

Septic shock

Septic shock in humans is usually characterized by a high cardiac output, a low systemic vascular resistance, reversible depression of LVEF,

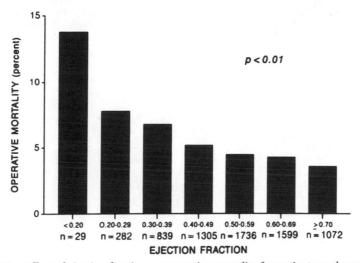

Fig. 10-18. Effect of ejection fraction on operative mortality for patients undergoing coronary artery bypass grafting. There is a progressive increase in operative mortality as ejection fractions decrease with a 13.8% operative mortality for patients with ejection fractions less than 0.20. Reproduced with permission from Grover, et al.[45]

TABLE 10-3. *Relationships of preoperative continuous variables to operative mortality for patients having coronary artery bypass grafting*[a]. *Reproduced with permission from Grover, et al.*[45]

| Variable | Survivors | | | Nonsurvivors | | | |
	No.	Mean	± SD	No.	Mean	± SD	p Value
Age	8,136	61.0	8.0	412	63.2	7.8	0.002
Weight (kg)	7,877	82.67	14.04	390	80.64	15.17	0.009
BSA (m²)	7,856	1.96	0.2	389	1.94	0.18	0.007
Creatinine	6,925	112.27	70.72	339	123.76	44.2	0.023
(μmol/L [mg/dL])		(1.27)	(0.8)		(1.4)	(0.5)	
PaO$_2$ (mm Hg)	2,943	79.2	11.9	154	77.2	13.0	0.042
FEV$_1$	2,481	2.7	0.7	104	2.4	0.7	0.001
Height (cm)	7,859	172.5	7.75	389	171.75	7.25	0.084
PaCO$_2$	2,994	37.1	6.0	158	36.6	5.0	0.252
LV systolic pressure (mm Hg)	5,247	131.1	23.4	245	135.8	25.9	0.003
Aortic systolic pressure (mm Hg)	5,317	130.6	23.6	256	135.6	26.1	0.001
PA systolic pressure (mm Hg)	1,789	30.1	11.0	101	32.4	11.4	0.047
PA wedge pressure (mm Hg)	1,804	13.1	6.5	107	14.9	7.6	0.005
Cardiac index (L/min/m²)	1,787	2.9	1.0	100	2.6	0.7	0.001
LV ejection fraction	6,525	0.54	0.14	337	0.50	0.15	0.001
Left main stenosis (%)	5,626	23.1	32.1	289	36.4	37.9	0.001
LAD stenosis (%)	7,424	82.7	21.0	362	86.0	19.9	0.008
Right (with PDA) stenosis (%)	7,241	82.3	27.2	361	86.9	22.8	0.006
Circumflex (with marginals) stenosis (%)	7,063	75.5	29.0	352	79.3	26.2	0.017
MD's estimate of operative mortality (%)	6,315	4.9	4.8	322	10.0	11.6	0.001
Distal disease score	4,615	1.8	1.8	231	2.3	1.9	0.001
LV contraction score	6,322	8.3	3.6	290	9.5	4.1	0.002
LVEDP (mm Hg)	5,152	15.9	7.8	240	17.0	8.6	0.051
Right atrial pressure (mm Hg)	1,629	6.5	4.1	93	6.6	4.2	0.722
LVEDV (mL)	1,633	144.3	58.5	69	148.1	64.1	0.596

[a] During the 2-year period of this study, 8,569 patients underwent coronary artery bypass grafting; 414 (4.8%) died.

BSA = body surface area; FEV$_1$, = forced expiratory volume in 1 second; LAD = left anterior descending coronary artery; LV = left ventricular; LVEDP = left ventricular end-diastolic pressure; LVEDV = left ventricular end-diastolic volume; MD = surgeon or cardiologist; PA = pulmonary artery; PaCO$_2$ = arterial carbon dioxide tension; PaO$_2$ = arterial oxygen tension; PDA = posterior descending coronary artery; SD = standard deviation.

TABLE 10-4. *Discrete variables predictive of operative mortality for patients having coronary artery bypass grafting. Reproduced with permission from Grover, et al.*[45]

Variable	Variable Absent			Variable Present			p Value
	No. of Patients	Operative Deaths	%	No. of Patients	Operative Deaths	%	
COPD	6,048	262	4.3	2,092	134	6.4	0.001
IV nitroglycerin preoperatively	6,546	247	3.8	1,477	139	9.4	0.001
Prior cardiac operation	7,645	299	3.9	888	111	12.5	0.001
History of CHF	7,092	304	4.3	1,176	97	8.2	0.001
Current diuretic use	5,958	234	3.9	2,063	146	7.1	0.001
Peripheral vascular disease	6,128	240	3.9	1,889	144	7.6	0.001
Cerebrovascular disease	6,850	293	4.3	1,165	91	7.8	0.001
Pulmonary rales	7,465	323	4.3	523	63	12.0	0.001
Resting ST depression	6,496	271	4.2	1,394	109	7.8	0.001
Preop IABP	8,028	363	4.5	279	44	15.8	0.001
Cardiomegaly (roentgenogram)	6,850	290	4.2	1,163	97	8.3	0.001
Old MI (> 30 days)	3,606	135	3.7	4,482	249	5.6	0.001
Recent MI (< 30 days)	6,657	284	4.3	1,499	111	7.4	0.001
Rest angina	3,500	120	3.4	4,404	267	6.1	0.001
Exertional angina	622	18	2.9	7,425	364	4.9	0.024
NYHA functional class							
I	...	...	...	251	2	0.8	0.001[a]
II	...	...	...	1,555	36	2.3	
III	...	...	...	3,417	132	3.9	
IV	...	...	...	2,523	201	8.0	
Priority of operation							
Elective	...	...	...	5,229	183	3.5	0.001[b]
Urgent	...	...	...	2,149	127	5.9	
Emergent	...	...	...	634	80	12.6	
No. of stenotic vessels							
0	...	...	...	26	0	0	0.001
1	...	...	...	448	10	2.2	
2	...	...	...	1,862	64	3.4	
3	...	...	...	4,443	255	5.7	
Left main stenosis ≥ 50%	4,210	163	3.9	1,705	126	7.4	0.001
Pleural effusion	2,892	150	5.2	42	7	16.7	0.006
General medical condition							
Good	...	...	...	1,488	38	2.6	0.001[c]
Fair	...	...	...	1,826	87	4.8	
Poor	...	...	...	319	60	18.8	

[a] Significance: $p < 0.001$ for class IV versus classes I, II, and III.   [b] Significance: $p < 0.001$ for emergent priority versus urgent and elective priorities.   [c] Significance: $p < 0.001$ for poor general condition versus good and fair general condition.

CHF = congestive heart failure;   COPD = chronic obstructive pulmonary disease;   IABP = intraaortic balloon pump;   IV = intravenous;   MI = myocardial infarction;   NYHA = New York Heart Association.

and transient LV dilatation. The relation of LV to RV function in septic shock is poorly understood. To evaluate RV vs LV performance and to evaluate the relation of biventricular performance to survival, Parker and associates[46] from Bethesda, Maryland, performed serial hemodynamic and radionuclide angiographic studies in 39 patients with septic shock. RVEF was calculated using the 2 regions of interest method. There were 22 survivors and 17 nonsurvivors. Comparing initial with final (after recovery for survivors; within 24 hours of death for nonsurvivors) studies, each survivor's cardiovascular performance returned toward normal, with significant increases in mean arterial pressure, LV and RVEF, and RV stroke work index. Their profiles also demonstrated significant decreases in central venous pressure, pulmonary artery wedge pressure, pulmonary artery mean pressure, and LV and RV end-diastolic volume indices. From initial to final study in the nonsurvivors, there was a statistically significant increase in heart rate but no change in any other cardiovascular parameter, indicating a persistence of the initial cardiovascular dysfunction until death. Comparing serial studies, the pattern of change in RV vs LV function was very similar (same direction in 82% of patients). Thus, myocardial depression in human septic shock affects both ventricles simultaneously with a similar pattern of dysfunction.

Parrillo and associates[47] from Bethesda, Maryland, provided a splendid review of observations in septic shock, which in their view is the most common cause of death in intensive care units. Although sepsis usually produces a low systemic vascular resistance and elevated cardiac output, strong evidence (decreased EF and reduced response to fluid administration) suggests that the ventricular myocardium is depressed and the ventricle dilated. In survivors, these abnormalities are reversible. Failure to develop ventricular dilatation in nonsurvivors suggests that dilatation is a compensatory mechanism needed to maintain adequate cardiac output. With a canine model of septic shock that is very similar to human sepsis, myocardial depression was confirmed using load-independent measures of ventricular performance. Endotoxin administration to humans simulates the qualitative, cardiovascular abnormalities of sepsis. The pathogenesis of septic shock is extraordinarily complex. Diverse microorganisms can generate toxins, stimulating release of potent mediators that act on vasculature and myocardium. A circulating myocardial depressant substance has been closely associated with the myocardial depression of human septic shock. Therapy has emphasized early use of antibiotics, critical care monitoring, aggressive volume resuscitation, and, if shock continues, use of inotropic agents and vasopressors. Pharmacologic or immunologic antagonism of endotoxin or other mediators may prove to enhance survival in this highly-lethal syndrome.

Hospital deaths on a cardiac surgical service

McGrath and associates[48] from Browns Mills and New Brunswick, New Jersey, reported results of cardiac operations from January 1982 through December 1985 in 3,772 patients having operations for coronary or other acquired heart diseases. Operative mortality increased from 4% in 1982 to 7% in 1985 by X^2 analysis. There was an increase over time of patients older than 70 years. Female patients increased from 31% in 1982 to 35% in 1985. The percentage of patients having isolated CABG decreased from 69% in 1983 to 60% in 1985, and hospital mortality after this procedure increased. Patients requiring more complex procedures including multiple-valve operations or combined valve replacement or repair plus by-pass grafting increased from 1982 through 1985. Reoperations for multiple-valve procedures or combined valve repair or replacement plus CABG also increased, particularly for patients more than 70 years of age. Changing practice patterns have had a negative impact on surgical results. This evolution in cardiac surgical practice has important implications related to peer review and quality-assurance screening, diagnosis-related group reimbursement, and reporting of surgical outcomes to governmental agencies.

Outpatient cardiac catheterization

Lee and associates[49] in Durham, North Carolina, determined the feasibility and cost-saving potential of substituting outpatient for inpatient cardiac catheterization in 986 consecutive procedures. Patients were classified prospectively as to their eligibility for outpatient cardiac catheterization. Resource consumption was recorded and cost savings calculated by analyzing the specific supply and personnel costs that could be changed as a result of inpatient versus outpatient status. Among 986 patients who underwent diagnostic catheterization, 240 (24%) were outpatients, 279 (28%) were inpatients that had no exclusion criteria for outpatient catheterization and 467 (47%) were inpatients who had one or more exclusions for outpatient catheterization. The most common reasons for exclusion from outpatient catheterization were CHF (22%), unstable angina (15%), noncoronary heart disease (14%), recurrent AMI (11%) and severe noncardiac disease (9%). Inpatients with no exclusions for the outpatient procedure were often older, they had lower EFs, and they had more triple vessel CAD. The cost of the catheterization procedure itself was not different between inpatients and outpatients, but laboratory testing was more frequent among inpatients and "room and board" costs were higher. Although the difference in hospital charges for inpatients and outpatients was $580, a rigorous analysis indicated that the potential cost savings was only 38% of this amount, or $218 per eligible patient. Thus, approximately half the patients undergoing cardiac catheterization at a large referral center are eligible for an outpatient study with substantial cost savings.

Left ventricular morphometrics in normal children

Franklin and associates[50] from London, UK, used 2-dimensional and m-mode echocardiography and arterial blood pressure to study LV morphometrics and contractility in 44 normal children, aged 2 to 12 years. LV end-systolic and end-diastolic length, diameter, wall thickness, volume and mass all showed linear increases with body surface area. Shortening and ejection fractions, velocities of circumferential fiber shortening, morphometric ratios and endocardial meridional and circumferential stress all remained constant. A load-independent measure of normal resting LV contractile state was determined by relating the rate corrected velocity of circumferential fiber shortening to end-systolic endocardial meridional and circumferential stress. These data provide a quantitative basis for assessment of myocardial hypertrophy afterload and contractile state in children.

Coronary dimensions in aortic stenosis and in hypertrophic cardiomyopathy

To examine the "adequacy" of basal coronary flow in ventricular hypertrophy, Kimball and associates[51] from Toronto, Canada, evaluated the relation between proximal coronary artery dimensions and regional ventricular mass in patients with AS and in those with HC. Coronary artery size was determined by quantitative coronary arteriography while global/ regional ventricular mass was calculated using computer-processed biplane 2-dimensional echocardiography. In comparison to 18 "normal" subjects, left anterior descending coronary dimensions were significantly larger in those with hypertrophy (normal 3.32 ± 0.54, AS 3.82 ± 0.71, HC 4.72 ± 0.81 mm), with progressive increases in left anterior descending/ circumflex coronary diameter ratios (normal 1.04 ± 0.14, AS 1.18 ± 0.19, HC 1.25 ± 0.31). Compared to the AS group, indexed anteroseptal mass was greater in the HC subjects (AS 40.9 ± 8.9 vs HC 72.1 ± 21 g/m²). Both septal width/left anterior descending coronary diameter ratios (AS 3.61 ± 1.06 vs HC 4.85 ± 1.17 mm/mm) and indexed anteroseptal mass/left anterior descending coronary diameter ratios (AS 11.2 ± 3.0 vs HC 15.6 ± 3.4 g/m²/mm) were greater in HC subjects. Increased coronary dimensions were observed in both AS and HC, with the greatest changes noted within the left anterior descending distribution in HC, but when analyzed with respect to regional ventricular mass, these subjects demonstrated relative "inadequate" enlargement in coronary artery diameters. Underdeveloped epicardial coronary arteries may contribute to anteroseptal myocardial ischemia, with resultant angina pectoris, increased ventricular ectopic activity and sudden death in HC.

Electrocardiographic criteria of left ventricular hypertrophy

Numerous electrocardiographic criteria, which are largely dependent on fixed voltage threshholds, have been proposed for the diagnosis of LV hypertrophy. Levy and colleagues[52] in Farmington, Massachusetts, examined the electrocardiographic criteria for LV hypertrophy in 4,684 subjects of the Framingham Heart Study who underwent echocardiographic study for LV hypertrophy. Echocardiographic LV hypertrophy was detected in 290 men and 465 women. Electrocardiographic features of LV hypertrophy were present in 3% of men and 1.5% of women. The overall sensitivity of the electrocardiographic diagnosis of LV hypertrophy was 7%, whereas specificity was 99%. Sensitivity of the electrocardiogram for LV hypertrophy was marginally lower in women than in men. Obesity and smoking were inversely related to sensitivity in both sexes combined. In contrast, sensitivity of the electrocardiogram increased with age. These findings suggest that electrocardiographic detection of LV hypertrophy can be improved by incorporating information about noncardiac factors that impact on electrocardiographic sensitivity for LV hypertrophy, presumably by attenuating QRS voltage. New strategies that take into consideration sex, age, smoking status, and obesity might improve the sensitivity of the electrocardiogram without diminishing specificity.

Thrombosis of central venous catheters

To determine whether a very low dose (1 mg) of warfarin is useful in thrombosis prophylaxis in patients with central venous catheters, Bern and associates[53] from Boston, Massachusetts, randomly assigned 121 patients to receive or not to receive 1 mg of warfarin beginning 3 days before insertion of a central venous catheter and continuing for 90 days. Subclavian, innominate, and superior vena cava venograms were done at onset of thrombosis symptoms or at 90 days into the study. Eighty-two patients completed the study. Of 42 patients completing the study while receiving warfarin, 4 had venogram proven thrombosis. All 4 had symptoms from venous thrombosis. Of 40 patients completing the study while not receiving warfarin, 15 had venogram-proven thrombosis and 10 had symptoms from thrombosis. There were no measurable changes in the coagulation values assessed due to this warfarin dose except in occasional patients who had become anorectic because of their disease or chemotherapy. Thus, very low dose warfarin can protect against thrombosis formation without inducing a hemorrhagic state. This approach may be applicable, of course, to other groups of patients.

Digoxin intoxication

Antman, and collaborators[54] from Boston, Massachusetts, treated 150 patients with potentially life-threatening digitalis toxicity with digoxin-specific antibody fragments purified from immunoglobulin G produced in sheep. The dose of antibody fragments was equal to the amount of digoxin or digitoxin in the patient's body as estimated from medical histories or determinations of serum digoxin or digitoxin concentrations. Seventy-five patients were receiving long-term digitalis therapy, 15 had taken a large overdose of digitalis accidentally, and 59 had ingested an overdose of digitalis with suicidal intent. The clinical response to anti-body fragments was unspecified in 2 cases, leaving 148 patients who could be evaluated. One hundred nineteen patients had resolution of all signs and symptoms of digitalis toxicity, 14 improved, and 15 showed no response. There were 14 patients with adverse events considered to possibly or probably have been caused by antibody fragments; the most common events were rapid development of hypokalemia and exacerbation of congestive heart failure. No allergic reactions were identified in response to antibody fragments. Of patients who experienced cardiac arrest as a manifestation of digitalis toxicity, 54% survived hospitalization. Reasons for partial responses and nonresponses, in descending order of frequency, were underlying heart disease that was the true cause of some of the presumed manifestations of digitalis toxicity, too low a dose of antibody fragments, and treatment of patients who were already moribund. Thus, a treatment response can be expected in at least 90% of patients with solid evidence of advanced or potentially life-threatening digitalis toxicity.

Digoxin intoxication has been reported to be a common adverse drug reaction with an in-hospital frequency of 6% to 23% and an associated mortality rate as high as 41%. In this report by Mahdyoon and associates[55] from Detroit, Michigan, a retrospective analysis was conducted to assess the accuracy of diagnosis, the morbidity and mortality of digoxin intoxication, and its frequency in hospitalized patients with CHF. The medical records of 219 patients discharged with the diagnosis of digoxin intoxication between 1980 and 1988 were reviewed. Patients were classified as follows: 1) definite intoxication—patients with symptoms and/or arrhythmias suggestive of digoxin intoxication that resolved after discontinuation of digoxin; 2) possible intoxication—patients with symptoms and/or arrhythmias suggestive of digoxin intoxication in the absence of documented resolution after discontinuation of digoxin, or the presence of other clinical illnesses that could possibly account for those findings; 3) no intoxication—patients whose symptoms or electrocardiographic abnormalities were clearly explained by other associated clinical illnesses and persisted after withdrawal of digoxin. Only 43 patients (20%) with definite intoxication were identified. The majority of patients discharged with the diagnosis of digoxin intoxication (133 or 60%) were classified as possibly digoxin intoxicated, and 43 patients (20%) had no clinical evidence to support this diagnosis. To estimate the frequency of digoxin intoxication, also reviewed were the medical records of 994 patients admitted in 1987 with CHF. Of these, 563 were receiving digoxin and in 27 the diagnosis of digoxin intoxication was made by their clinicians. The review showed that only 4 were definitely intoxicated (0.8%), and the diagnosis could not be excluded in another 16 (4%). It was concluded that the diagnosis of digoxin intoxication remains difficult, and its frequency and mortality in hospitalized patients is currently much lower than was previously reported.

New transpulmonary ultrasound contrast agent

Feinstein and associates[56] in Chicago and Maywood, Illinois; Houston, Texas; Rotterdam, The Netherlands; Indianapolis, Indiana, and Loma Linda, California, used myocardial contrast echocardiography consisting of sonicated albumin microspheres ("Albunex") given by intravenous injections in 71 patients at three independent medical institutions to evaluate the utility of contrast angiography when coupled with 2-dimensional echocardiographic examination. The quality of cardiac chamber opacification was qualitatively assessed by two independent blinded observers using a grading system of 0 to +3 with 0 indicating an absence of contrast effect and +3 indicating full opacification of the cardiac chambers. All injections were well tolerated and no serious side effects were noted in any of the patients. Cavity opacification ≥ +2 was seen in the RV in 212 (88%) of 240 intravenous injections and in the LV in 151 (63%) of 240 injections (Figure 10-19). The degree of ventricular cavity opacification appeared to be dose and concentration related. This multicenter clinical study demonstrates that this contrast agent appears to be safe when administered intravenously and achieves significant transpulmonary passage in a majority of patients.

A new myocardial perfusion agent

Hendel and colleagues[57] in Worcester, Massachusetts, utilized technetium-99m-labeled teboroxime, a new boronic acid adduct of techne-

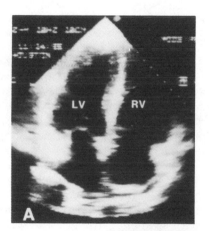
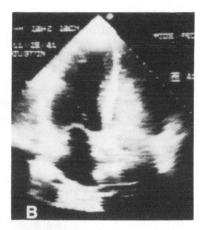
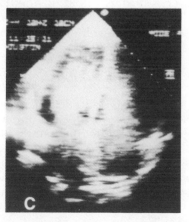

Fig. 10-19. Serial frames from a single intravenous injection in a patient whose heart was imaged from an apical four chamber view. A, Baseline image without contrast; B, early image showing contrast in the right ventricle; C, contrast opacification of both left and right ventricles. In these images, the left atrium and left ventricle (LV) are on the left and the right atrium and right ventricle (RV) are on the right. Reproduced with permission from Feinstein, et al.[56]

tium dioxime that demonstrates favorable characteristics in preliminary studies in which its ability to assess myocardial perfusion has been evaluated to study 30 patients undergoing planar study with teboroxime at rest and after maximal treadmill exercise. Post-exercise scans were completed in an average of 4 ± 1.6 minutes with 5 ± 1.5 minutes required for the views at rest. The results were compared with coronary arteriography, thallium-201 scintigraphy after treadmill exercise testing, or both. Diagnostic agreement as regards abnormal vs normal results occurred in 28 of the 30 patients. Findings of AMI and ischemia were concordant in 89% and 86% of patients, respectively between teboroxime and thallium-201. Delayed post-exercise images obtained 5 to 10 minutes after exercise demonstrated rapid disappearance of exercise-induced defects found on the initial post-exercise views. Thus, this new imaging agent appears promising as another technetium-labeled myocardial perfusion agent allowing the relatively noninvasive evaluation of myocardial perfusion.

New nongeometric echocardiographic technique

Zoghbi and associates[58] in Dallas and Houston, Texas, used a new nongeometric echocardiographic technique for measurement of RV and LV volumes. With this method, all images are taken from one point on the chest wall as the transducer is tilted through the ventricle. No geometric assumptions about ventricular shape are made and all images are acquired from the best echocardiographic window. The digitized points may be used to make a 3-dimensional reconstruction of the ventricle. Twenty-four patients underwent echocardiographic studies within 2 hours before angiography. At catheterization, volumes determined by the bi-plane area-length method ranged between 95 and 368 ml at end-diastole and between 15 and 303 ml at end-systole. A good correlation was observed between ventricular volumes by angiography and echocardiography at end-diastole and end-systole. Correlation between volumes by the two techniques was also good. Ventricular EF ranged between 18 and 84% at angiography and correlated well with echocardiographic measurements. Thus, the echocardiographic tilt method provides accurate determination of LV volume and EF. This nongeometric method offers the potential for detection of RV volume and 3-dimensional display of the heart.

Some good cardiologic books published in 1990

1. O'Rourke RA, Pohost GM, editors. *Principles and Practice of Cardiovascular Imaging.* Boston: Little, Brown and Company, 1991:880, $175.00.

O'Rourke and Pohost, as J. Willis Hurst states, know low technology, and as this book indicates, they also know high technology. The 2 editors call this ". . . . a unique book providing comprehensive information on the sometimes confusing array of diagnostic methods for evaluation of the cardiovascular system." They may be right too.

2. Gersh BJ, Rahimtoola SH, editors. *Acute Myocardial Infarction.* New York: Elsevier, 1991:524, $84.00.

This multiauthored (49) book, the first of a new series entitled *Current Topics in Cardiology* and edited by Shahbudin H. Rahimtoola, is a comprehensive monograph on acute myocardial infarction. It is well done.

3. Gould KL. *Coronary Artery Stenosis.* New York: Elsevier, 1991:323, $99.00.

The title of this book provides little indication as to its contents. It describes pressure flow characteristics, physiologic behavior, and quantitative geometry of coronary stenosis experimentally in vivo and clinically using the most advanced invasive arteriographic analysis and noninvasive perfusion-metabolic imaging available. The first part of the book concerns anatomic and functional characteristics of coronary artery stenoses, and the second part, positron emission tomography of the heart. Although a scholarly book, it may be too "heavy" for most cardiologists.

4.   Grossman W, Baim DS, editors. *Cardiac Catheterization, Angiography, and Intervention.* Fourth edition. Philadelphia: Lea & Febiger, 1991:698, $59.50.

5.   Bashore TM, editor. *Invasive Cardiology: Principles and Techniques.* Toronto: B.C. Decker Inc., 1990:318, $65.00.

6.   Serruys PW, Simon R, Beatt KJ, editors. *PTCA. An Investigational Tool and a Non-operative Treatment of Acute Ischemia.* Dordrecht: Kluwer Academic Publishers, 1990:404, $125.00.

7.   Abela GS, editor. *Lasers in Cardiovascular Medicine and Surgery: Fundamentals and Techniques.* Boston: Kluwer Academic Publishers, 1990:480, $150.00.

The Grossman and Baim book has been the classic in this arena, but it is now getting some competition. It provides, as the editors state, "clear and concise descriptions of the major techniques currently used in cardiac catheterization . . . and the growing field of interventional cardiology."

The Bashore book is more expensive and contains far less information than the Grossman and Baim book.

The multiauthored Serruys et al book describes the effects of balloon-induced myocardial ischemia on the electrocardiogram, coronary blood flow dynamics, cardiac muscle metabolism, left ventricular function, and measures to counter these effects, including reperfusion, in unstable angina pectoris and acute myocardial infarction. The subject matter is of interest but the preparation of the product is not ideal. The word "Ischemia" is spelled on the title page as "Ischema."

The multiauthored Abela book describes the most up-to-date technology and procedural approaches of laser angioplasty using the various laser systems.

8.   Messerli GH, editor. *Cardiovascular Drug Therapy.* Philadelphia: W.B. Saunders Company, 1990:1709, $84.00.

9.   Antonaccio MJ, editor. *Cardiovascular Pharmacology.* Third edition. New York: Raven Press, 1990:556, $75.00.

The Messerli book discusses >100 cardiovascular agents and various therapeutic strategies by 184 authors. The Antonaccio book by 22 authors is a more basic pharmacologic book with less information and it costs nearly as much as the Messerli book. The Messerli book will be popular.

10.   Kaplan NM. *Clinical Hypertension.* Fourth edition. Baltimore: Williams & Wilkins, 1990:466, $63.00.

11.   McMahon FG. *Management of Essential Hypertension: The Once-A-Day Era.* Third edition. Mount Kisco, New York: Futura Publishing Company, Inc., 1990:684, $59.50.

The new edition of both the Kaplan and McMahon books are good. Both are single authored (which I like). The Kaplan one is my favorite despite the 220 more pages in the McMahon book for essentially the same price.

12.   Grundy SM with illustrations by DuPrey LP. *Cholesterol and Atherosclerosis: Diagnosis and Treatment.* Philadelphia: J.B. Lippincott Company, and New York: Gower Medical Publishing, 1990:176, $55.00.

This book is outstanding. Its magnificent illustrations and beautiful layout make it unique and a most desirable addition to any personal or institutional cardiovascular library.

13.   Davidson DM. *Preventive Cardiology.* Baltimore: Williams & Wilkins, 1991:300, $48.00.

14.   Frohlich ED, editor. *Preventive Aspects of Coronary Heart Disease.* Philadelphia: F.A. Davis Company, 1990:239, $70.00. (Cardiovascular Clinics 20/3).

The Davidson book is single authored and easily readable. The Frohlich-editored book is a stronger one.

15.   Gillette PC, Garson A Jr, editors. *Pediatric Arrhythmias: Electrophysiology and Pacing.* Philadelphia: W.B. Saunders Company, 1990:703, $195.00.

This textbook, by 31 authors, is probably the best thus far for diagnosis and treatment of arrhythmias in children and young adults.

16.   Rosen MR, Janse MJ, Wit AL, editors. *Cardiac Electrophysiology: A Textbook Prepared in Honor of Brian F. Hoffman.* Mount Kisco, New York: Future Publishing, Inc., 1990:1195, $160.00.

This book has contributions from 101 authors, including virtually all prominent investigators in this arena. Any book dedicated to Brian Hoffman must be a good one.

17.   El-Sherif N, Samet P, editors. *Cardiac Pacing and Electrophysiology.* Third edition. Philadelphia: W.B. Saunders Company, 1991:784, $145.00.

The last edition of this book was 1980, and that book dealt only with cardiac pacing. This third edition has been much expanded by the 109 authors and is quite comprehensive.

18.   Horowitz LN, editor. *Current Management of Arrhythmias.* Philadelphia: B.C. Decker, Inc., 1991:436, $75.00.

This multiauthored book summarizes recent developments in diagnosis and management of cardiac arrhythmias. Each chapter presents the views of the authors of that chapter rather than a compilation of many views.

19. Saksena S, Goldschlager N, editors. *Electrical Therapy for Cardiac Arrhythmias, Pacing, Antitachycardia Devices, Catheter Ablation.* Philadelphia: W.B. Saunders Company, 1990:731, $95.00.

This is mainly pacing but there is more. The 83 contributors represent viewpoints from 30 medical centers. A fine book.

20.   Touboul P, Waldo AL, editors. *Atrial Arrhythmias. Current Concepts and Management.* St. Louis: Mosby Year Book, 1990:521, $75.00.

This book describes current concepts of the mechanisms responsible for atrial arrhythmias and their therapy by 108 contributors.

21.   Hurst JW. *Ventricular Electrocardiography.* Philadelphia: J.B. Lippincott Company and New York: Gower Medical Publishing, 1991:312, $55.00.

A beautiful book stressing the vector method of interpretation of the 12-lead electrocardiogram by a masterful teacher.

22.   Goldberger AL, Goldberger E. *Clinical Electrocardiography, A Simplified Approach.* Fourth edition. St. Louis: Mosby Year Book, 1990:348, $31.95.

One of the fine books from which to learn basic electrocardiography.

23.   Jawad IA. *A Practical Guide to Echocardiography and Cardiac Doppler Ultrasound.* Boston: Little, Brown and Company, 1990:379, $40.00.

Another echo-Doppler book that physicians should buy, read, and then give to their echocardiography technicians.

24. Garson A Jr, Bricker JT, McNamara DG, editors. *The Science and Practice of Pediatric Cardiology.* Philadelphia: Lea & Febiger, 1990:1–668 (Volume I), 669–1616 (Volume II), and 1617–2557 (Volume III), $395.00.

These 3 volumes have it all. They require time and money. A big year for Tim Garson—2 major books in 1990.

25. Snider AR, Serwer GA. *Echocardiography in Pediatric Heart Disease.* Year Book Medical Publishers, Inc., 1990:379, $125.00.

A superb book.

26. Higgins CB, Silverman NH, Kersting-Sommerhoff BA, Schmidt K. *Congenital Heart Disease. Echocardiography and Magnetic Resonance Imaging.* New York: Raven Press, 1990:395, $135.00.

Two major diagnostic techniques from investigators in the forefront of their fields applied to a single type of cardiovascular disease—the result is an excellent product.

27. Soto B, Pacifico AD. *Angiography in Congenital Heart Malformations.* Mount Kisco, New York: Futura Publishing Company, Inc., 1990:669, $175.00.

This beautifully prepared book contains 37 chapters and 745 illustrations, most of which are angiograms, mainly axial views. This book may be the best thus far on this subject.

28. Clark EB, Takao A, editors. *Developmental Cardiology. Morphogenesis and Function.* Mount Kisco, New York: Futura Publishing Company, Inc., 1990:732, $135.00.

This monograph represents the Proceedings of the 3rd International Symposium on the Etiology and Morphogenesis of Congenital Heart Disease held in Tokyo in November 1989. The first symposium was held in 1978 and the second in 1983 and each also resulted in a book. The present book brings in "the disciplines of cellular and molecular biology, extracellular matrix, cell migration and interaction. . . ." into the morphogenesis of congenital heart disease.

29. Baumgartner WA, Reitz BA, and Achuff SE, editors, and illustrated by Schlossberg L. *Heart and Heart-Lung Transplantation.* Philadelphia: W.B. Saunders Company, 1990:406, $138.00.

30. Cooper DKC, Novitzky D, editors. *The Transplantation and Replacement of Thoracic Organs. The Present Status of Biological and Mechanical Replacement of the Heart and Lungs.* Dordrecht: Kluwer Academic Publishers, 1990:543, $225.00.

31. Thompson ME, editor. *Transplantation.* Philadelphia: F.A. Davis Company, 1990:271, $75.00.

Although the Baumgartner et al book is by 28 authors, most are from the same institution (The Johns Hopkins Medical Institutions). It is comprehensive and beautifully prepared. Some of Leon Schlossberg's drawings are in color. When a book cannot be written by a single author, a book from a single institution is advantageous. I like this book best of the cardiac transplant books thus far available. The Cooper et al and Thompson books also are good, but I prefer the book by the Baltimore group.

32. Gay WA Jr with illustrations by Roselius E. *Atlas of Adult Cardiac Surgery.* New York: Churchill Livingstone, 1990:189, $125.00.

This book contains 86 full-page drawings of various operative approaches to many *acquired* heart diseases for which surgical repair has been effective. The commentaries in the text accompanying the illustrations are brief and usually fill only a small portion of the page. The consequence is much wasted space.

33. Waldhausen JA, Orringer MB, editors. *Complications in Cardiothoracic Surgery.* St. Louis: Mosby Year Book, 1991:460, $110.00.

As Frank Spencer states in the foreword, this book is "a unique and valuable contribution in that no single book previously has concentrated in one source the available information about the numerous complications that can occur." The 86 contributors provide a valuable reference source.

34. Goldberger E. *Treatment of Cardiac Emergencies.* Fifth edition. St. Louis: The C.V. Mosby Company, 1990:429, $44.95.

The topics include syncope, cardiac arrest, cardiogenic shock, arrhythmias, conduction disturbances, acute myocardial infarction, cardiopulmonary emergencies, hypertensive emergencies, aortic dissection, and cardiac tamponade, and apparatuses used for their treatment.

35. Soler-Soler J, Permanyer-Miralda G, Sagrista-Sauleda J, editors. *Pericardial Disease. New Insights and Old Dilemmas.* Dordrecht: Kluwer Academic Publishers, 1990:244, $102.50.

This book is not a comprehensive one on pericardial disease. Rather, it reviews several controversial aspects based on experiences primarily of the editors from Barcelona.

36. Bharati S, Lev M. *The Cardiac Conduction System in Unexplained Sudden Death.* Mount Kisco, New York: Futura Publishing Company, Inc., 1990:399, $115.00.

37. Rossi L, Matturri L. *Clinico-pathological Approach to Cardiac Arrhythmias—A Color Atlas.* Torino: Centro Scientifico Torinese Editore, 1990:325, $120.00.

Bharati and Lev discuss the findings in the conduction system in approximately 100 patients dying "suddenly and unexpectedly, instantaneously or within 24 hours after the onset of symptoms without any evidence of trauma" and they illustrate findings in 75 cases. These illustrations, which number 229, are almost entirely photomicrographs. The authors concluded that "the conduction system was abnormal in *all* (their italics) cases studied." The epicardial coronary arteries in their cases were "usually normal. The maximal changes were found in the bundle of His. . . ."

Rossi and Matturri also are recognized authorities on the morphologic aspects of arrhythmias and conduction disturbances. This book contains 248 color figures, also mainly photomicrographs of the conduction system. Neither book contains electrocardiograms or graphics from electrophysiologic studies. Although both are detailed anatomic descriptions of conduction tissue abnormalities, there is little in either book useful to clinical cardiologists.

38. Conti CR. *Introduction to Clinical Cardiology.* New York: Raven Press, 1991:288, $36.00.

39. Goldberger E. *Essentials of Clinical Cardiology.* Philadelphia: J.B. Lippincott Company, 1990:433, $49.95.

40. Sokolow M, McIlroy MB, Chetlin MD. *Clinical Cardiology.* Fifth Edition. Norwalk, Connecticut: Appleton & Lange, 1990:659, $37.50.

41. Kloner RA, editor. *The Guide to Cardiology.* Second edition. New York: Le Jacq Communications, 1990:546, $44.00.

The Conti book is new and different. It is not intended to be as extensive as the other 3. It is quite personable, easy to read, and focuses on the appropriate approach by cardiologists to the 50 subjects under discussion. Although it is intended primarily for house officers and cardiology fellows, there are gems here for the clinical cardiologist. Chapter 2—"Communicating with Patients and Physicians"—is terrific. The usefulness or lack thereof of clinical trials is stressed. My only criticism of the Conti book would be the selection of references appearing at the end of each chapter under "Suggested Reading." More effort could have gone into selecting the most outstanding sources, including the classics, for each of the subjects under discussion.

The Goldberger book is a revision of the book, *Textbook of Clinical Cardiology*, which appeared in 1982 by the same author. The present book is half the size of the 1982 product. The Sokolow et al book is a revision of the one appearing in 1986. The Kloner-edited book is a revision of his 1984 first edition. For interns, residents, and cardiology fellows, the price of the Kloner book is $30.00. All 3 are intended primarily for non-cardiologists seeking cardiologic information.

42.   Roberts WC, editor, Mason DT, Rackley CE, Willerson JT, Graham TP Jr, and Karp RB. *Cardiology 1990*. Boston: Butterworth-Heinemann 1990:494, $75.00.

For some reason I continue to mention this annual book in this column every year. The book is not widely known because the publisher has few cardiology titles, the book is not presented on publishers' row at the 2 major cardiologic meetings in the USA, and maybe the authors have a few deficiencies. Nevertheless, take a peek and you will find 802 articles, each appearing in 1989, summarized, and those on the same subject are lumped together. To assist in the reading are 126 figures and 66 tables. Despite some biased views, I highly recommend this red book.

43.   McDougall JA with recipes by McDougall M. *The McDougall Program. Twelve Days to Dynamic Health*. New York: NAL Books, 1990:436, $19.95.

44.   Ornish D. *Dr. Dean Ornish's Program for Reversing Heart Disease*. New York: Random House, 1990:631, $24.95.

Dr. George Burch once said that "every doctor should read a diet book before he[she] retires." During the last few years I have sought out diet books and now have about 50 of them. The 2 titles above are among the better ones appearing in 1990. McDougall is the author of the 1985 book entitled *McDougall's Medicine. A Challenging Second Opinion* in which he provides the evidence for the role of dietary fat in certain cancers, osteoporosis, systemic hypertension, diabetes mellitus, certain types of arthritis, and some urinary disorders. His present book describes his 12-day plan for reversing some serious illnesses. This approach is not popular with some physicians but Dr. Nathan Pritikin was ahead of his time and persons like McDougall are similar advocates.

Ornish's 1-year study using a pure vegetarian diet plus other endeavors appeared in *Lancet* in 1990, and this book provides a step-by-step guide into his program for preventing and reversing heart disease. He is the author also of the 1982 book called *Stress, Diet & Your Heart*. McDougall and Ornish are on the right road and we need to get on it also.

References

1. Kabadi UM, Kumar SP: Pericardial effusion in primary hypothyroidism. Am Heart J 1990 (December);120:1393–1395.
2. Hara KS, Ballard DJ, Ilstrup DM, Connolly DC, Vollertsen RS: Rheumatoid pericarditis: Clinical features and survival. Medicine 1990;69:81–91.
3. Horneffer PJ, Miller RH, Pearson TA, Rykiel MF, Reitz BA, Gardner TJ: The effective treatment of postpericardiotomy syndrome after cardiac operations: A randomized placebo-controlled trial. J. Thorac Cardiovasc Surg 1990 (Aug);100:292–296.

4. Guindo J, de la Serna AR, Ramio J, de Miguel Diaz MA, Subirana MT, Ayuso MJP, Cosin J, deLuna AB: Recurrent Pericarditis Relief with Colchicine. Circulation 1990 (October);82:117–1120.

5. Craven CM, Allred T, Garry SL, Pickrell J, Buys SS: Three cases of fatal cardiac tamponade following ventricular endocardial biopsy. Arch Pathol Lab Med 1990 (Aug);114:836–839.

6. Pahl E, Ettedgui J, Neches WH, Park SC: The Value of Angiography in the Follow-up of Coronary Involvement in Mucocutaneous Lymph Node Syndrome (Kawasaki Disease). J Am Coll Cardiol (November) 1989;14:1318–1325.

7. Niwa K, Tashima K, Kawasoe Y, Okajima Y, Nakajima H, Terai M, Nakajima H: Magnetic resonance imaging of myocardial infarction in Kawasaki disease. Am Heart J 1990 (June);119:1293–1302.

8. Akagi T, Kato H, Inoue O, Sato N, Imamura K: Valvular heart disease in Kawasaki syndrome: Incidence and natural history. Am Heart J 1990 (August);120:366–372.

9. Seward JB, Khandheria BK, Tajik AJ: Wide-field transesophageal echocardiographic tomography: Feasibility study. Mayo Clin Proc 1990 (Jan 1);65:31–37.

10. Seward JB, Khandheria BK, Edwards WD, Oh JK, Freeman WK, Tajik AJ: Biplanar transesophageal echocardiography: Anatomic correlations, image orientation, and clinical applications. Mayo Clin Proc 1990 (Sept);65:1193–1213.

11. Stumper O, Fraser AG, Ho SY, Anderson RH, Chow L, Davies MJ, Roelandt JRTC, Sutherland GR: Transoesophageal echocardiography in the longitudinal axis: Correlation between anatomy and images and its clinical implications. Br Heart J 1990 (Oct);64:282–288.

12. Pearson AC, Castello R, Labovitz AJ: Safety and utility of transesophageal echocardiography in the critically ill patient. Am Heart J 1990 (May);119:1083–1089.

13. Pavlides GS, Hauser AM, Stewart JR, O'Neill WW, Timmis GC: Contribution of transesophageal echocardiography to patient diagnosis and treatment: A prospective analysis. Am Heart J 1990 (October);120:910–914.

14. Schwinger ME, Gindea AJ, Freedberg, Kronzon I: The anatomy of the interatrial septum: A transesophageal echocardiographic study. Am Heart J 1990 (June);119:1401–1405.

15. Tunick PA, Kronzon I: Protruding atherosclerotic plaque in the aortic arch of patients with systemic embolization: A new finding seen by transesophageal echocardiography. Am Heart J 1990 (September);120:658–660.

16. Hofmann T, Kasper W, Meinertz T, Geibel A, Just H: Echocardiographic evaluation of patients with clinically suspected arterial emboli. Lancet 1990 (Dec 8);336:1421–1424.

17. Griffith BP: Cardiac transplantation. Ann Thorac Surg 1990 (July);50:161–162.

18. Sweeney MS, Lammermeier DE, Frazier OH, Burnett CM, Haupt HM, Duncan JM: Extension of donor criteria in cardiac transplantation: Surgical risk versus supply-side economics. Ann Thorac Surg 1990 (July);50:7–11.

19. Boucek MM, Kanakriyeh MS, Mathis CM, Trimm III RF, Bailey LL: Cardiac Transplantation in Infancy: Donors and Recipients. J Pediatr (February) 1990;116:171–176.

20. Pahl E, Fricker RJ, Armitage J, Griffith BP, Taylor S, Uretsky BF, Beerman LB, Zuberbuhler JR: Coronary Arteriosclerosis in Pediatric Heart Transplant Survivors: Limitation of Long-Term Survival. J Pediatr (February) 1990;116:177–183.

21. Edwards BS, Hunt SA, Fowler MB, Valantine HA, Stinson EB, Schroeder JS: Cardiac transplantation in patients with preexisting neoplastic diseases. Am J Cardiol 1990 (Feb 15);65:501–504.

22. Rudas L, Pflugfelder PW, McKenzie FN, Menkis AH, Novick RJ, Kostuk WJ: Serial evaluation of lipid profiles and risk factors for development of hyperlipidemia after cardiac transplantation. Am J Cardiol 1990 (Nov 1);66:1135–1138.

23. Superko HR, Haskell WL, DiRicco CD: Lipoprotein and hepatic lipase activity and high-density lipoprotein subclasses after cardiac transplantation. Am J Cardiol 1990 (Nov 1);66:1131–1134.

24. Ratkovec RM, Wray RB, Renlund DG, O'Connell JB, Bristow MR, Gay WA Jr, Karwande SV, Doty DB, Millar RC, Menlove RL, Burke JL, Lappe DL, Tsagaris TJ, Sutton RB, Jones KW: Influence of corticosteroid-free maintenance immunosuppression on allograft coronary artery disease after cardiac transplantation. J Thorac Cardiovasc Surg 1990 (July);100:6–12.

25. Grattan MT, Moreno-Cabral CE, Starnes VA, Oyer PE, Stinson EB, Shumway NE: Eight-year results of cyclosporine-treated patients with cardiac transplants. J Thorac Cardiovasc Surg 1990 (Mar);99:500–509.
26. Scherrep U, Vissing SF, Morgan BJ, Rollins JA, Tindall RSA, Ring S, Hanson P, Mohanty PK, Victor RG: Cyclosporine-induced sympathetic activation and hypertension after heart transplantation. N Engl J Med 1990 (Sept 13);323:693–699.
27. Mark AL: Cyclosporine, sympathetic activity, and hypertension. N Engl J Med 1990 (Sept 13);323:748–750.
28. Jacquet L, Ziady G, Stein K, Griffith B, Armitage J, Hardesty R, Kormos R. Cardiac rhythm disturbances early after orthotopic heart transplantation: Prevalence and clinical importance of the observed abnormalities. J Am Coll Cardiol 1990 (October);16:832–7.
29. Masuyama T, Valantine HA, Gibbons R, Schnittger I, Popp R: Serial measurement of integrated ultrasonic backscatter in human cardiac allografts for the recognition of acute rejection. Circulation 1990 (March);81:829–839.
30. Gillum RF: Peripheral arterial occlusive disease of the extremities in the United States: Hospitalization and mortality. Am Heart J 1990 (December);120:1414–1418.
31. Smith GD, Shipley MJ, Rose G: Intermittent Claudication, Heart Disease Risk Factors, and Mortality. Circulation 1990 (December) 82:1925–1931.
32. Younis LT, Aguirre F, Byers SH, Dowell S, Barth G, Walker H, Carrachi B, Peterson G, Chaitman BR: Perioperative and long-term prognostic value of intravenous dipyridamole thallium scintigraphy in patients with peripheral vascular disease. Am Heart J 1990 (June);119:1287–1292.
33. Rosman HS, Davis TP, Reddy D, Goldstein S. Cholesterol embolization: Clinical findings and implications. J Am Coll Cardiol 1990 (May);15:1296–9.
34. Johnson DE, Hinohara T, Selmon MR, Braden LJ, Simpson JB. Primary peripheral arterial stenoses and restenoses excised by transluminal atherectomy: A histopathologic study. J Am Coll Cardiol 1990 (February);15:419–25.
35. von Pölnitz A, Nerlich A, Berger H, Höfling B. Percutaneous peripheral atherectomy: Angiographic and clinical follow-up of 60 patients. J Am Coll Cardiol 1990 (March);15:682–8.
36. Graor RA, Whitlow PL. Transluminal atherectomy for occlusive peripheral vascular disease. J Am Coll Cardiol 1990 (June);15:1551–8.
37. Leon MB, Almoger Y, Bartorelli AL, Prevosti LG, Teirstein PS, Chang R, Miller DL, Smith PD, Bonner RF: Fluorescence guided laser assisted balloon angioplasty in patients with femoropopliteal occlusions. Circulation 1990 (Jan);81:101–106.
38. Chirillo F, Marchiori MC, Andriolo L, Razzolini R, Mazzucco A, Gallucci V, Chioin R: Outcome of 290 patients with aortic dissection: A 12-year multicenter experience. Eur Heart J 1990 (Apr);11:311–319.
39. Roberts CS, Roberts WC: Aortic dissection with the entrance tear in transverse aorta: Analysis of 12 autopsy patients. Ann Thorac Surg 1990 (Nov);50:762–766.
40. Prospective Investigation of Pulmonary Embolism Diagnosis Investigators: Value of the ventilation/perfusion scan in acute pulmonary embolism: Results of the prospective investigation of pulmonary embolism diagnosis (PIOPED). JAMA 1990 (May 23);263:2753–2759.
41. Lilienfeld DE, Godbold JH, Burke GL, Sprafka JM, Pham DL, Baxter J: Hospitalization and case fatality for pulmonary embolism in the twin cities: 1979–1984. Am Heart J 1990 (August);120:392–395.
42. Eisenberg PR, Lucore C, Kaufman L, Sobel BE, Jaffe AS, Rich S: Fibronopeptide A Levels Indicative of Pulmonary Vascular Thrombosis in Patients with Primary Pulmonary Hypertension. Circulation 1990 (September);82:841–847.
43. Palevsky, HI, Long W, Crow J, Fishman AP: Prostacyclin and Acetylcholine as Screening Agents for Acute Pulmonary Vasodilator Responsiveness in Primary Pulmonary Hypertension. Circulation 1990 (December) 82:2018–2026.
44. Eagle KA, Mulley AG, Skates SJ, Reder VA, Nicholson BW, Sexton JO, Barnett GO, Thibault GE: Length of stay in the intensive care unit: Effects of practice guidelines and feedback. JAMA 1990 (Aug 22/29);264:992–997.
45. Grover FL, Hammermeister KE, Burchfiel C, Cardiac Surgeons of the Department of Veterans Affairs: Initial report of the veterans administration preoperative risk assessment study for cardiac surgery. Ann Thorac Surg 1990 (July);50:12–28.

46. Parker MM, McCarthy KE, Ognibene FP, Parrillo JE: Right ventricular dysfunction and dilatation, similar to left ventricular changes, characterize the cardiac depression of septic shock in humans. Chest 1990 (Jan);97:126–131.

47. Parrillo JE, Parker MM, Natanson C, Suffredini AF, Danner RL, Cunnion RE, Ognibene FP: Septic shock in humans: Advances in the understanding of pathogenesis, cardiovascular dysfunction, and therapy. An Intern Med 1990 (Aug 1);113:227–242.

48. McGrath LB, Laub GW, Graf D, Gonzalez-Lavin L. Hospital death on a cardiac surgical service: Negative influence of changing practice patterns. Ann Thorac Surg 1990 (Mar);49:410–412.

49. Lee JC, Bengtson JR, Lipscomb J, Bashore TM, Mark DB, Califf RM, Pryor DB, Hlatky MA. Feasibility and cost-saving potential of outpatient cardiac catheterization. J Am Coll Cardiol 1990 (February);15:378–84.

50. Franklin RCG, Wyse RKH, Graham TP, Gooch VM, Deanfield JE: Normal Values for Noninvasive Estimation of Left Ventricular Contractile State and Afterload in Children. Am J Cardiol (February) 1990;65:505–510.

51. Kimball BP, Lipreti V, Bui S, Wigle ED: Comparison of proximal left anterior descending and circumflex coronary artery dimensions in aortic valve stenosis and hypertrophic cardiomyopathy. Am J Cardiol 1990, (Mar 15);65:767–771.

52. Levy D, Labib SB, Anderson KM, Christiansen JC, Kannel WB, Castelli W: Determinants of sensitivity and specificity of electrocardiographic criteria for left ventricular hypertrophy. Circulation 1990 (March);81:815–820.

53. Bern MM, Lokich JJ, Wallach SR, Bothe A Jr, Benotti PN, Arkin CF, Greco FA, Huberman M, Moore C: Very low doses of warfarin can prevent thrombosis in central venous catheters: A randomized prospective trial. An Intern Med 1990 (Mar 15);112:423–428.

54. Antman Elliott, Wenger T, Butler V, Haber E, Smith T: Treatment of 150 Cases of Life-Threatening Digitalis Intoxication With Digoxin-Specific Fab Antibody Fragments Final Report of a Multicenter Study. Circulation 1990 (June);81:1744–1752.

55. Mahdyoon H, Battilana G, Rosman H, Goldstein S, Gheorghiade M: The evolving pattern of digoxin intoxication: Observations at a large urban hospital from 1980 to 1988. Am Heart J 1990 (November);120:1189–1194.

56. Feinstein SB, Cheirif J, Ten Cate FJ, Silverman PR, Heidenreich PA, Dick C, Desir RM, Armstrong WF, Quinones MA, Shah PM. Safety and efficacy of a new transpulmonary ultrasound contrast agent: Initial multicenter clinical results. J Am Coll Cardiol 1990 (August);16:316–24.

57. Hendel RC, McSherry B, Karimeddini M, Leppo JA. Diagnostic value of a new myocardial perfusion agent, teboroxime (SQ 30,217), utilizing a rapid planar imaging protocol: Preliminary results. J Am Coll Cardiol 1990 (October);16:855–61.

58. Zoghbi WA, Buckey JC, Massey MA, Blomqvist CG. Determination of left ventricular volumes with use of a new nongeometric echocardiographic method: Clinical validation and potential application. J Am Coll Cardiol 1990 (March);15:610–7.

Author Index

Subject Index

Numbers in italic indicate figures. Page numbers followed by a t indicate tables.